An Introduction to Children with Language Disorders

An Introduction to Children with Language Disorders

Fifth Edition

Vicki A. Reed
James Madison University

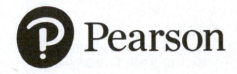

330 Hudson Street, NY NY 10013

Editorial Director: Kevin Davis
Executive Portfolio Manager: Julie Peters
Managing Content Producer: Megan Moffo
Portfolio Management Assistant: Maria Feliberty
Executive Product Marketing Manager: Christopher Barry
Executive Field Marketing Manager: Krista Clark
Manufacturing Buyer: Carol Melville
Cover Design: Carie Keller, Cenveo® Publisher Services
Cover Art: Fanatic Studio/Getty Images
Editorial Production and Composition Services: Cenveo® Publisher Services
Full-Service Project Manager: Susan McNally, Revathi Viswanathan
Text Font: Stone Serif ITC Pro

Credits and acknowledgments for materials borrowed from other sources and reproduced, with permission, in this textbook appear on appropriate page within text, or below.

Library of Congress Cataloging-in-Publication Data
Names: Reed, Vicki, author.
Title: An introduction to children with language disorders / Vicki A. Reed, James Madison University.
Description: Fifth edition. | Boston : Pearson, [2017] | Includes bibliographical references and indexes.
Identifiers: LCCN 2017003341 | ISBN 9780133827095 | ISBN 0133827097
Subjects: LCSH: Language disorders in children.
Classification: LCC RJ496.L35 R44 2017 | DDC 618.92/855—dc23 LC record available at https://lccn.loc.gov/2017003341

NC 09.02.2022 1013

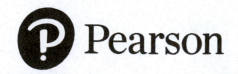

Print Edition
ISBN-10: 0-13-382709-7
ISBN-13: 978-0-13-382709-5

31 2022

I have been blessed to have so many wonderful friends and mentors.
This book is dedicated to you for letting me stand on your shoulders.
Thank you from the bottom of my heart.

Contents

PART TWO Children with Language Disorders

Preface

OVERVIEW OF THE BOOK

The focus of this book continues to be about children who do not acquire language normally. It is intended both for students who are learning about children's language disorders in order to help the children and for professionals wanting to update their knowledge in order to serve the children better. Language is the most powerful and important human ability. It affects educational achievement, relationships, and entire lives. Children with language disorders do not have easy access to this ability and are at a severe disadvantage. They struggle with learning and with human interactions; a language disorder alters a child's relationships with caregivers, undermines academic success, disturbs interpersonal relationships, limits vocational potential, and isolates the child from mainstream society.

This edition continues the organizational structure of the previous edition. There are three parts. The first provides an overview/review of normal language in two chapters—the bases of language and communication and normal language development in children and adolescents. Nine chapters that focus on the language difficulties of different populations comprise the second part of the book. Several of these chapters address language problems associated with children with intellectual disabilities, specific learning disabilities, autism spectrum disorder, auditory impairments, cultural and linguistic differences, and acquired language impairment, plus a chapter that looks at language issues associated with other special populations of children, such as gifted children and those with cleft palate. Two other chapters discuss the language of preschoolers with specific language impairment and adolescents with language impairment. These two chapters bookend the chapter on children with specific learning disabilities. The ordering of the three chapters is purposeful, attempting to convey the progression of specific language impairment in preschool children through the early school years and into and through adolescence. A main message is that the language impairment does not disappear and it is not "cured." Across the nine chapters in this section of the book, a number of the topics covered in the chapters are those often overlooked in other texts on language disorders in children. Each chapter includes considerations for intervention associated specifically with the population of children discussed in the chapter. The third part of the book consists of three chapters that focus on intervention for children with language disorders—a chapter on assessment, one on intervention, and a third, unique chapter on augmentative and alternative communication as an intervention approach with children with language difficulties.

NEW TO THIS EDITION

Although the overall organization of the previous edition has been retained, this new edition contains considerable changes. An aim in revision was to include new content related to topics. Another aim was to reflect changes in the field of child language disorders. As a result, some topics have been expanded while others have been reduced. Some reordering of topics has also occurred to reflect current thinking and practices. Examples of "what's new" are the following:

- The authors for some of the contributed chapters have changed. This edition welcomes Geraldine P. Wallach, Marsha Longerbeam, Jeff Sigafoos, Stacey Pavelko, Sarah E. Hegyi, and Kate L. Anderson as either new sole authors or coauthors.
- Across chapters, new tables have been included and a number of tables and figures from the previous edition have been significantly revised where new data are available; other tables and figures from the previous edition have been omitted.
- New content reflecting current information is evident throughout the book.

- Although all chapters have been updated, three chapters have undergone major revisions and expansions—Chapter 4, "Language and Children with Learning Disabilities," Chapter 6, "Language and Children with Intellectual Disabilities," and, in particular, Chapter 7, "Language and Children with Autism Spectrum Disorder"—in order to reflect new diagnostic criteria.
- Where specific published language tests are referred to in several of the chapters, newer versions of the tests are cited when appropriate.
- Since the previous editions, increasing recognition of discourse issues beyond narratives has emerged in our thinking about children with language impairment. Therefore, discussions of expository discourse have been expanded and are more frequent in several chapters.

We hope readers will find that these and other new features offer current information and perspectives and reflect the shifts in thinking and knowledge over the last several years. Children with language disorders depend on professionals providing services based on current knowledge.

ACKNOWLEDGMENTS AND THANK-YOUS

A book, whether a new or revised edition, involves the efforts of many people. I am deeply grateful to the authors who offered their expertise and knowledge in their contributed chapters. I am also very thankful for the hard work of many responsible, conscientious, and bright undergraduate and graduate students who assisted with the revisions. I anticipate that their exceptional personal commitment to the project foreshadows their success as professionals and their ability to help and advocate for children with language disorders. And, the reviewers—Amy Ann Cocanour, University of Nevada, Reno; Ruth Crutchfield, SLP.D., CCC-SLP, University of Texas Pan American; Shana Goldwyn, Fitchburg State University; Johanna Price, Western Carolina University—offered suggestions and comments that helped improve this edition. Importantly, however, are the people in our personal lives. These individuals assist us to keep our balance, as well as our focus. They were truly significant factors in helping this edition see the light of day. We hope you know that you have our thanks, but more importantly, you have our hearts.

Vicki A. Reed

PART 1

Aspects of Normal Language and Communication

1

Language and Human Communication

AN OVERVIEW

LEARNING OBJECTIVES

After reading this chapter, you should be able to

- Explain what comprises communication
- Describe the components of language
- Describe comprehension and production and the relationship between these various communication modes
- Explain the various communication modes
- Explain the biological, cognitive, and social bases of human communication

When two people talk with each other, one person usually speaks while the other person listens. The speaker encodes thoughts into mental representations of words and sentences and changes these into a continuous stream of speech sounds or acoustic energy. The speech sounds travel through the air in the form of sound waves (acoustic energy) and reach the listener's ear. The listener then decodes the sound waves into a stream of speech sounds, the speech sounds into the intended string of words, and the string of words miraculously into what the speaker originally thought. A breakdown in any step along the way may result in miscommunication or even a failure to communicate. Importantly, both the speaker and the listener must share the same code or symbolic system of what sounds and words represent what thoughts. Put simply, they must share the same language.

This book is concerned with the symbolic process of communication called language and the ways in which children do or do not use it. Before we can examine children's language disorders, however, we, like the speaker and the listener, must share the same language. Therefore, the purpose of this chapter is to overview for the reader the foundations of human communication and other topics that provide a platform for discussing children's language disorders. We discuss the terms *communication, language, speech,* and *extralinguistic elements of communication,* and we look at the different components of language and the relationship between understanding and using language. We also consider different communication modes. Finally, we review some of the biological, cognitive, and social bases of human communication. The content of the chapter is built primarily on two pillars—information that is now recognized as relatively "common" knowledge for respective topics and knowledge provided by foundation researchers in their areas. Inclusion of many of the citations in the chapter thus attempts to recognize their early, still relevant, and important contributions to the study of child language disorders.

COMMUNICATION

Communication refers to the sending and receiving of messages, information, ideas, or feelings. It is a broad term that encompasses not only the physical production of speech and the symbolic nature of language but also any behavior or action that conveys a message. For example, a throat clear may convey a message that a person has a sore throat. A baby's cry conveys needs or discomforts that require attention. In these instances, the spoken word is not essential.

Communication is not limited to humans. Other animals communicate. Unlike other animals, however, humans have the ability to communicate highly complex thoughts, feelings, and ideas through the use of language. Humans also have the capacity for speech. Extralinguistic behaviors, which are discussed below, additionally contribute to the communicative process.

Language

Language is a code in which we make specific symbols stand for something else. Bloom (1988) defines language as "a code whereby ideas about the world are represented through a conventional system of arbitrary signals for communication" (p. 2). According to this definition, coded symbols refer to real things, concepts, or ideas, and the things that the symbols represent are the *referents.* In the English code, there is no reason why an animal with four legs that is noted for tail wagging and barking is labeled a *dog.* Such an animal could as easily be coded as a *sloot*—and perhaps it is, in a code system other than English. Although the symbols are arbitrary, the symbols and their appropriate referents must be mutually agreed on by members of a community using the code if the code is to be meaningful. In this sense, language is a *convention* (Bloom, 1988).

Language is also a system in which *rules* or regularities guide which coded symbols may be combined with other symbols and in what order and what symbols can be used in what situations. These rules or regularities are predictable and can be used to identify what are and are not acceptable uses of language. For example, in the English language, the word order in the sentence "The ball is not red" is acceptable and considered correct, whereas the word order in the sentence "The ball not is red" violates accepted rules even though the words in the two sentences are identical.

The number of rules that delimit a language is finite. Once these finite rules are learned, however, a person can generate an infinite variety of meaningful messages by combining and recombining the symbols according to the agreed-on rules. The system of rules that results in the ability to produce an infinite number of expressions gives language its creative feature. By applying systematic rules, a language user can generate expressions never used or heard before, and another user of the same language can understand those expressions by employing the same rules. Every day, humans create sentences never spoken or written before, and they hear or read sentences and paragraphs they have never before encountered.

Because a language consists of regularities or sets of rules, members of a language community (including children) must learn the rules and induce the regularities in order to use the language. Among the rules that must be learned are those that determine who can say what to whom when and how. Language is, therefore, a *learned* or acquired behavior.

The ability to learn language is considered an innate human ability. Most infants are born with the capacity to acquire language, but this does not mean that infants inevitably use language. Even with the capacity to acquire language, infants still need to *learn* the language or code of the linguistic community in which they are reared.

Speech

Speech is the oral expression of language. It involves the sensorimotor processes by which language users reproduce the coded symbols that are stored in their central nervous systems so that others can hear the symbols. Consequently, speech production requires the neurological control of physical movements to create sound patterns. These sound patterns are produced as a result of respiration, phonation, resonation, and articulation. *Respiration* refers to the coordinated, rapid muscular activities of the chest (which controls the lung action). Respiration provides the air in which a speech sound wave travels. Without air, there would be no way of phonating. *Phonation* refers to the production of sound through vibration of the vocal cords (vocal folds) in the larynx. Once a sound has been created, it resonates in the vocal tract (pharynx, oral cavity, and nasal cavity). Finally, the *articulators* (including the tongue, jaw, lips, and palate) are used to modify the sound into a vowel or a consonant. A consonant is produced by constricting the airstream, whereas a vowel is produced without significant constriction of the airstream through the mouth. An important point is that language is the code, whereas speech is the sensorimotor production of that code.

Extralinguistic Aspects of Communication

As we saw previously, communication can be any behavior or action that conveys a message. If a speaker said, "The baby's sleeping," in a quiet whisper accompanied by a frown and an upright open-hand gesture in front of the listener, the speaker's original thought and, therefore, communicative intention may have been not to comment on the fact that the baby is asleep but to stop the listener from waking the baby by speaking loudly. A term often used to refer to behaviors such as loudness, frowning, or using gesture is *extralinguistic communication.* These may enhance or even change the linguistic code. Extralinguistic elements include paralinguistics, nonlinguistics (nonverbal communication), and metalinguistics.

Paralinguistics. Paralinguistics refers to the melodic components of speech that modify the meaning of the spoken message. Melodic components include stress, pitch, and intonation. *Stress* is the relative loudness with which certain syllables in words are produced. For example, in the word *blackbird,* if the first syllable is said more loudly than the second syllable, the meaning is a specific type of bird. If there is no difference in stress between the syllables, the meaning is any bird that is black. If we take the word *pervert,* it is difficult to know whether the written word refers to a *pervert* (noun) or the act *to pervert* (verb). In spoken English, stress can communicate meaning. Stress can also be used for contrastive emphasis within utterances. One speaker might say, "I like the *red* jacket," whereas a second speaker might say, "I like the *blue* jacket." In doing so, the second speaker contrasts the color *red* with the color *blue* through the use of stress.

Pitch and intonation can also modify the meaning of a spoken message. Ladefoged (2006) describes *pitch* as the "auditory property of a sound that enables a listener to place it on a scale going from low to high" (p. 295). *Intonation,* on the other hand, refers to the patterns of rises and falls in pitch within and across utterances. Pitch and intonation both enhance a spoken message. For example, pitch can convey personal characteristics of speakers, such as their gender, age (to some extent), and emotional state. Changes in pitch can also alter the meaning of a word, as is seen in tone languages such as Mandarin Chinese, Thai, and Vietnamese. Intonation can be used to convey syntactic information. For example, the sentence "He went skydiving" could be said as a statement of fact, with falling intonation at the end of the utterance, but the same sentence could be expressed as a question or surprise, with rising intonation at the end of the utterance. In both examples, the sequence of speech sounds remains the same, but a difference in meaning is signaled by the intonation pattern.

The combination of these melodic components of speech creates prosody. Because prosody is superimposed on the segments of an utterance (e.g., the speech sounds, words, or phrases), the melodic components are often referred to as *suprasegmental* devices. These act above the level of a segment to enhance the overall meaning of an utterance to convey an emotion or an attitude. Without paralinguistics our speech would sound robotic or dull, that is, like computer speech.

Nonlinguistics (Nonverbal Communication). The nonlinguistic aspect of communication is sometimes referred to as nonverbal communication. *Proxemics,* one aspect of nonverbal communication, refers to the ways that use of space and physical distance between speakers communicate. Another way speakers communicate nonverbally is with body language, or *kinesics.* Kinesics refers to the way in which body movements are used for communication, such as with gestures to point to objects or head shakes to signal "no."

In many respects, nonverbal communication can be considered a system itself. In his now classic, insightful, and sometimes humorous book on nonverbal communication, Hall (1990) described ways in which unspoken communication is so very important and can vary by cultures. To emphasize the importance of nonverbal communication in human interaction, he entitled his book *The Silent Language.* Consciously or unconsciously, we engage in nonverbal communication, sometimes to emphasize concurrent oral messages, sometimes to contradict simultaneous oral messages, and sometimes to substitute for oral messages. For example, the utterance "That chocolate caramel fudge looks nice" could mean that the speaker thinks chocolate caramel fudge is appealing. But when spoken by a customer in a candy store, accompanied by pointing and leaning toward a piece of chocolate caramel fudge displayed in the store window, it could mean that the customer would like to purchase some fudge. Our understanding and use of nonverbal cues can largely determine the quality and effectiveness of our interpersonal relationships. In fact, some suggest that nonverbal communication carries more than half of the social meaning in interpersonal communication situations. When we are in a foreign country and unable to communicate through the use of speech and language, we often resort to using nonlinguistic cues to communicate and hope that those cues are appropriate symbols for that country. It is important to know that nonlinguistic behaviors, like specific words, are not always universal in what they communicate and that cultures differ in uses of and meanings associated with specific elements of nonverbal communication. A nod of the head in the United States or Australia indicates agreement ("yes"), while the same gesture in Bengal indicates "no" (Axtell, 1991).

Because inaccurate or ineffective interpretation and use of nonverbal communication can lead to problems in establishing and maintaining social relationships with others, an awareness of nonverbal communication, the nonlinguistic elements that make up particular nonverbal systems, and the ways in which these influence relationships are important. Some children who struggle with language experience deficits in the ability to understand and express nonverbal cues correctly. Such difficulties can result in the development of poor self-images and self-concepts, potentially leading to even more impaired interpersonal relationships.

Metalinguistics. The third extralinguistic element of communication is metalinguistics. The prefix *meta-* as it is used in *metalinguistics* means something like "beyond" or "higher" or "transcending," not unlike how it is used in the word *metaphysics.* As such, *metalinguistics* refers to the ability to use language to communicate or talk about and to analyze language. It involves thinking about language, seeing it as an entity separate from its function as a way of communicating, and using language to judge the correctness of language and to correct it; it is an awareness of the components of language, and it is seeing language as a tool and controlling how we use language. For example, identifying and generating rhyming words involves metalinguistic ability.

Frequently, monitoring whether our messages are understood and consciously deciding how to clarify them involve metalinguistic skills. If we return to our example of the customer requesting a piece of chocolate caramel fudge using the utterance "That chocolate caramel fudge looks nice," the response of the sales assistant would provide the customer with information about the success of his or her utterance. If the sales assistant nods agreeably but fails to begin to pick up the piece of fudge, then the customer would recognize a need to rephrase the request, perhaps in a way that makes it an explicit request. Alternatively, the sales assistant might say, "Pardon, what did you say?" from which the customer would become aware of a need to correct or clarify the utterance in order to be understood.

A Bit More about the Relationships among Speech, Language, and Communication

Communication involves the sending and receiving of messages. Although it can be as simple as a sneeze, it can also be a complex symbolic code expressed through the action of respiration, phonation, resonation, and articulation accompanied by paralinguistic and nonlinguistic cues. Figure 1.1 shows how the various terms we have discussed (speech, language, paralinguistics, nonlinguistics, metalinguistics, and communication) relate to one another. Sometimes, we may communicate just using nonlinguistic behaviors, such as raising our eyebrows or frowning. We may also communicate using language without speech, as is the case with writing.

It is also important that we differentiate further between the two key terms *speech* and *language*. As our definitions so far have indicated, language and speech are closely related but are not the same. The two sentences "The dog is black and white," and "Is the dog black and white?" consist of the same sounds. However, the order of the sounds and therefore the order of the words in the two sentences are different, as is the resultant meaning of the two sentences. As another example, to produce the sentences "I want it to *fit*," and "I want it to *sit*," a child must only alter speech movements slightly to produce the difference between "f" and "s." Yet the meaning of the two sentences is quite different based on the one speech sound variation.

It is possible for a child's code system (language) to be intact but for the same child to have difficulty with the articulation of speech sounds. For example, a child who has an interdental lisp and says "th" for "s" might say the words *thing* and *sing* the same way, but from the context we can tell that the child knows the words mean different things:

I can "thing" Old McDonald has a Farm.

I don't like that thing.

It is also possible for a child's speech production to be intact but for the child's language system to be deficient. As examples, a child who says, "I want it no to go," "The gooses are flying," or "I don't

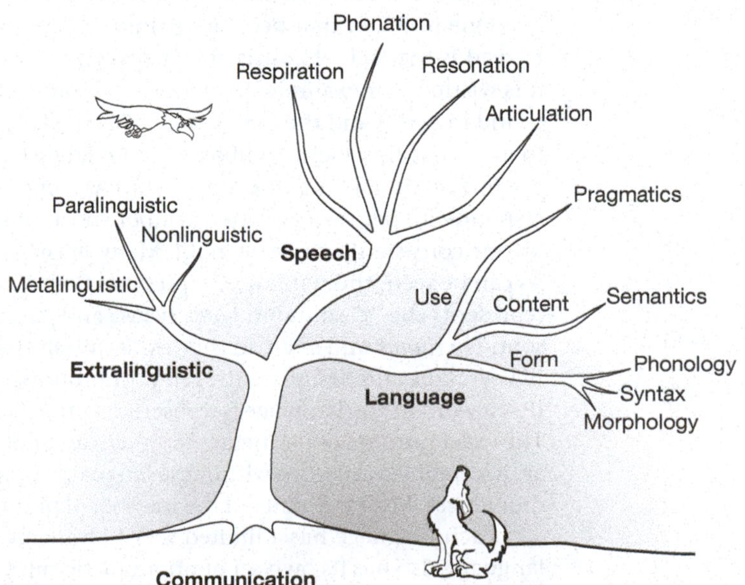

FIGURE 1.1 | Components of Communication

want for you to sick," with well-pronounced sounds in a highly fluent manner, is demonstrating problems with language, not speech.

COMPONENTS OF LANGUAGE

Spoken languages are made up of components. Some authors call these *elements,* some call them *parameters,* and others call them *aspects.* Whatever they are labeled, the intent is to break language into parts in order to discuss and describe it. Often, we consider there to be five basic components of language: (1) phonology, (2) semantics, (3) syntax, (4) morphology, and (5) pragmatics. Each is part of a system and is therefore governed by regularities and sets of rules that all speakers of a specific language must learn if they are to communicate effectively. Although we can discuss each of these components separately, they are all interrelated in language functioning, as we will see in later chapters.

Phonology

When we utter a word such as *fish,* we produce a string of speech sounds that represent the word *fish,* beginning by lightly biting the bottom lip with the top front teeth, then producing the vowel sound, then using the tongue to produce the sound "sh." If people who understand English were to hear the production of this string of speech sounds, they would know that the word was *fish.* A listener who understands and speaks a language other than English would not know what was being said. This idea of using a specific set of speech sounds in a particular sequence within a language to communicate meaning is the essence of phonology. *Phonology* is, therefore, language based and relates to the phoneme patterns that are governed by the rules of a specific language which lead to meaning within the language. To appreciate this definition, we need to examine the concept of speech sounds, or *phonemes,* more closely.

Phonemes are sounds that distinguish one meaningful word from another. When we look at a string of speech sounds in words, we see that by changing just one speech sound within a word, we can differentiate one word from another. For example, in the word pair *cat/rat,* sound differences occur in the initial positions of the words. The sounds that create these meaning differences (in this case, "c" and "r") are phonemes. By replacing the "c" in "cat" with other sounds to create *rat, mat, hat, fat, pat, that,* we discover that "r," "m," "h," "f," "p," "th" are also phonemes of English because they result in words with different meanings. Phonemes can be classified as either vowels (*mat, met*) or consonants (*hat, pat*).

One problem that becomes painfully clear as we watch children attempting to learn to read is the lack of consistency between the way an English sound is said and the way it is written. For example, the letter "c" is pronounced as a "k" sound in *cat* and as an "s" sound in *center,* and the long vowel "a" is spelled *ay* in *bay, a* in *fade,* and *ea* in *break.* Trying to use usual alphabetic symbols to write English as it is said is very difficult. This is where the International Phonetic Alphabet (IPA) comes to the rescue. It is a system that has a correspondence between a written symbol and a sound. That is, a spoken sound is represented by one consistent printed symbol. Many of the symbols of the IPA are shown in Table 1.1. As can be seen, the symbol /s/ represents the "s" sound in *sun* and *cement;* the symbol /dʒ/ represents the "j" sound in *jump, badge,* and *fudge;* and the symbol /θ/ represents the "th" sound in *thumb* and *tooth.* In this text, symbols that occur between / / indicate that they are IPA symbols and designate the relevant pronunciation as shown in Table 1.1. In using the IPA, a word in the language is transcribed on paper to match the way a speaker produces it. The exact number of phonemes in American English is difficult to determine because there are acceptable variations within the language. Some of these variations result from dialectal differences. Most estimates of the number of phonemes suggest that there are 40 to 46.

Each language has a limited set of phonemes that makes up the sound system; each language also has its own set of phonotactic rules or rules governing which phonemes can be combined with other phonemes and in what order. In English, *ksont* is not a word and never could be, even though all the individual sounds that make up the word are acceptable

TABLE 1.1 | The International Phonetic Alphabet

Consonants				Vowels and Diphthongs			
Voiceless		*Voiced*					
Symbols	*Key Words*	*Symbols*	*Key Words*	*Symbols*	*Key Words*	*Symbols*	*Key Words*
p	pig	b	big	i	feet	u	food
t	to	d	do	ɪ	hit	ʊ	foot
k	coat, key	g	goat	e	cake	o	toll
f	fine	v	vine	ɛ	head	ɔ	fog
θ	thumb	ð	the	æ	pack	ɑ	father
s	cider, sun	z	zipper	ʌ	dug	ɒ*	law
ʃ	she	ʒ	vision, azure	ə	sofa	aɪ	time
tʃ	chair	dʒ	gem, huge	ɝ	fur	aʊ	house
h	hello	m	me	ɚ	mother	ɔɪ	toil
ʍ	when	n	new	ɜ*	bird	ju	fuse
		ŋ	ring	a*	mad		
		l	letter				
		r	run				
		w	we				
		j	yes				

**These vowels occur in some eastern and/or southern American speech patterns.*

English phonemes. On the other hand, *skont,* which is also not an English word, potentially could be a word in the language because the sequence of phonemes is possible. We see the application of English phonotactic rules in Lewis Carroll's opening passage to his literary classic "Jabberwocky": "Twas brillig, and the slithy toves did gyre and gimble in the wabe: All mimsy were the borogoves, and the mome raths outgrabe." English speakers are able to read the passage aloud and sound like they are producing acceptable English because the nonsense words abide by the phonotactic rules. If Lewis Carroll's opening passage began with something like "Ksee ngot, and the lsiyth ptosv did yger and rgilbe in the wabeh," we would struggle to pronounce many of the words because they fail to conform to the phonotactic rules of English. Children learning the phonological system of their language must learn to use not only the acceptable set of phonemes but also the phonotactic rules for combining these phonemes sequentially into words.

Semantics

Semantics deals with the referents for words and the meanings of utterances. At a basic level, semantics involves the vocabulary of a language, or the lexicon. Sequences of phonemes combine to form words. The words are then used to represent items, attributes, concepts, or experiences. As we know, many words can have multiple meanings depending on the situations in which they are used. *Peel* can refer to the rind of a piece of fruit or the act of stripping or tearing off. In identifying the meanings of words, we typically think of the dictionary meanings. These dictionary meanings are the *referential meanings* or denotative meanings of words. However, words may have *connotative* or *emotionally associated meanings.* These meanings can, in fact, be so strong as to actually produce physical responses to the word. To many, the word *snake* can create chills even though the denotative meaning of the word refers to one of several kinds of limbless reptiles.

A word and its referents can trigger associations with another word and its referents. In some instances, the associated words belong to the same category as the original word. For example, the word *cow* may trigger one to think of *pig, horse,* and *sheep.* In other instances, the associated word or words may be the category for the original word—*animal* or *farm animal.*

Words can be categorized and recategorized through the process of abstraction. In the process of categorizing words, we identify or abstract the similarities among the referents for the words and use the similar characteristics to form another category that is also labeled. In his classic explanation of the hierarchical organization of meaning and word relationships, Hayakawa (1964) used the example of Bessie the cow to demonstrate the categorization and abstraction of referents. One of the lowest levels of categorization of Bessie is that of "cow," some of the abstracted characteristics of which include animal, four legs, tail, milk giver, and *moo*. This category of abstracted qualities ignores the individual differences among all the other cows that make up the group and focuses only on the similar characteristics. The similar characteristics or attributes form the category "cow." However, cows have characteristics similar to chickens, pigs, and horses. Those abstracted similar characteristics can be categorized and labeled as "livestock." The term *livestock* becomes a superordinate category for cows, chickens, and pigs. In turn, livestock is similar to all other salable farm items, and based on these attributes, a new category of "assets" is abstracted. "Livestock" is now subordinate to the superordinate category of assets. The abstracted similar attributes of all possible assets allow the formation of a new category—"wealth." Each time a new category was created, we increased our level of abstraction, and with each level of abstraction, we moved farther and farther away from the concrete, or that which can be perceived by the senses. "Wealth" is an abstract concept. Its attributes cannot be perceived by the senses; therefore, its referents are said to be relatively abstract.

The use of superordinate and subordinate categories in the lexicon helps to bring order to our experiences. By categorizing and labeling our experiences, it is not necessary for us to treat each experience as a totally new one. Because we have finite memories, this skill is efficient and allows us to store cognitively more information than if it were not used. Children learning the semantic system of their language must acquire a categorization system somewhat consistent with that of others in the language community. Much of the educational system does, in fact, center on teaching children the categorization of attributes and how to move from superordinate categories to subordinate categories and vice versa—for example, units of instruction on colors, animals, and transportation.

Not only does the semantic component of language deal with the lexicon, but it also involves the meanings conveyed by the relations among words. This aspect of semantics is termed *relational meaning*. In fact, some words, such as *an* or *if*, really take on meaning only as they are used with other words. Furthermore, when the individual meanings of words interrelate in a multiword statement, the statement takes on a meaning that goes beyond the separate words. This meaning is the statement's *propositional meaning* and is partly derived from the logical relationships inherent in the sequence of words. In the sentences "The boy climbs the tree," and "The tree climbs the boy," the words are identical. The first sentence is plausible, while the second is not, even though the individual words within the sentences retain their usual referents. The order in which the words are arranged imposes certain restrictions on the logical relationships among the words, and these restrictions are violated in the second sentence.

Earlier, in discussing semantics, reference was made to the multiple meanings of individual words. In situations where a word may have several different referents, we typically determine its meaning from the contexts in which it is used and its relationship to other words uttered. We can use the word *table* to illustrate the derivation of meaning by employing cues regarding the word's logical relationship to other words in a sentence. Although *table* has several meanings, we can surmise from the sentence "The table was too small to use six chairs" that the referent for the word is a piece of furniture; from the sentence "As the rains continued, the table continued to rise" that the referent is probably a water level rather than a floating part of a dining set, although this could be plausible; and from the sentence "The table contained numbers she had never seen before" that the referent for the word is an organized grouping of numerals such as those of a statistician. However, using the word in some sentences may not aid in deriving the word's meaning. For example, the sentence "Read about the table" gives us no clue as to the meaning of *table*. This is referred to as an *ambiguous statement,* and in these instances we must depend on previous utterances or the situation in which the sentence is expressed to determine the referent of *table*. Verbal humor is frequently based on multiple meanings of words.

Two other aspects of semantics involve figurative meaning and inferential meaning. *Figurative meaning* goes beyond meaning that can be derived from literal interpretations of phrases. For example, "It's raining cats and dogs" is implausible if interpreted at its literal level. Metaphors, similes, proverbs, and idioms all involve figurative meanings. Inferential meaning refers to meaning that is derived not from what is stated explicitly but from the logical relationships of statements. As an example, consider the following sequential statements:

> Sally went to the restaurant and ordered from the standard menu. She loved her wantons and fried rice.

The kind of restaurant is not stated explicitly. Yet we are able to derive sufficient information through inferential meanings to increase the odds of making a correct, educated guess of a Chinese restaurant. Learning in school requires students to make an enormous amount of inferences to succeed, and increasing skill in inferring meaning is required with advancing grades.

Syntax

All languages have systems of syntax, or sets of rules that govern how words are to be sequenced in utterances and how the words in an utterance are related. Phonemes combine to form words, and words combine to form phrases, clauses, and sentences. In the same way that phonological rules govern what phonemes can be combined in what order, syntactic rules determine what words can be combined in what order to convey meaning.

A basic English syntactic rule is the subject + verb + object sequence, which places the actor first followed by the receiver of the action. Although the words in the sentences "The boy hits the girl" and "The girl hits the boy" are identical, reversal of the word order signals a different meaning. Word combinations typically convey more specific information than any of the individual words alone do. For example, a child who utters the word *milk* may be indicating that the item is present, may simply be labeling it, may wish to have more of the item, or may not want it at all. If the child uses the utterance "more milk," additional specificity is obtained, although the child may be indicating that a larger quantity is present or that an increase in the amount is requested. But when the child says, "I want more milk," the child's meaning is specific. If the child says, "More milk I want," the listener may be able to understand the child's wish, but the utterance violates the syntactic rules for the intended meaning. In most instances, however, precise sequencing of words using correct syntactic rules is essential if the exact intended meaning of an utterance is to be conveyed. The words in the sentences "When she was 10 years old, she reported that a dog had bitten her" and "She reported that a dog had bitten her when she was 10 years old" are identical, but the meanings of the two sentences are different, depending on the location of the clause "when she was 10 years old."

The explanation for how children are able to learn what seem to be implicit syntactic rules is a continuing matter of considerable debate. We will not wade into the debate here. What most agree about, however, is that there is a generative element, so that once syntactic rules are learned, numerous sentences or phrases can be generated, and thus numerous ideas can be expressed. Table 1.2 shows a number of the multiple phrases and ideas that are possible with knowledge of a single syntactic rule—article + attributive + noun sequence.

TABLE 1.2 | Use of a Syntactic Rule to Generate Multiple Phrases

Article	+	Attributive	+	Noun
The		Pretty		Dress
A		Big		Doll
An		Old		Apple
The		Tremendous		Crowd
An		Exhaustive		Experience

TABLE 1.3 | Various Transformations and Examples

Transformation Types		
Negation	*Question*	*Negation & Question*
The ball is not red.	Is the ball red?	Isn't the ball red?
The girl does not run.	Does the girl run?	Doesn't the girl run?
The flower is not blooming.	Is the flower blooming?	Isn't the flower blooming?
	What color is the ball?	When isn't the girl running?
	When is the girl running?	Why isn't the flower blooming?
	Why is the flower blooming?	
	What is this?	

Another aspect of syntax is that a *transformational element* is involved. That is, with a set of operational rules, sentences can be changed by adding, deleting, and/or rearranging the words to derive sentences of various types. To illustrate, the sentence "The girl is riding a horse" can, by rearranging the words, be transformed into the question "Is the girl riding a horse?" or, by adding the word *not* in the correct place, transformed into the negative, "The girl is not riding a horse." In both transformations, the meaning conveyed by the first sentence is altered. However, both transformed sentences are based on the structure of the original sentence, "The girl is riding a horse."

Chomsky's (1965, 1981) concepts of syntax and language learning have had a major influence on our thinking about how children acquire language and the syntactic components of the language in particular (e.g., generative transformational grammar). A discussion of his theories and others that have evolved from the theories is not appropriate for this text. However, we can see in Table 1.3 further examples of how we can transform sentences and creatively alter meaning once we know "the rules."

Morphology

Morphology deals with the rules for deriving various word forms and the rules for using grammatical markers or inflections. These derived word forms include plurals, verb tenses, adverbs, superlatives, and many words associated with school curricula, for example, *photosynthesis, polynomial, pseudonym*. Table 1.4 shows how we can use morphology to change meaning.

TABLE 1.4 | Examples of Morphological Derivations of Words

Root Word: *drive*		Root Word: *gentle*	
drives	Third-person singular, present tense or plural noun for motor paths	*gently*	Adverb
drove	Irregular past tense	*gentleness*	Noun
driven	Past participle, functioning as part of a verb form or as an adjective	*gentleman*	Noun
driving	Present participle, functioning as part of a verb form or as an adjective, as in ***driving rain***	*gentlemanly*	Adverb
		ungentlemanly	Adverb

Because morphology is concerned with sequences of phonemes, it is sometimes discussed as part of the phonological system. Sometimes it is considered part of the semantic system because of the meaning derived from the phoneme sequences, and sometimes it is classified as part of the syntactic system because of the interrelationships among varying word forms, their functions within sentences, and word order. Furthermore, morphology is sometimes considered a separate component of language because of the unique rules affecting differing word forms.

Morphology is concerned with meaning, and the smallest meaning units of a language are called *morphemes*. In some instances, the smallest unit or form that conveys meaning is a word, such as *drive* (Table 1.4). Even though the word is composed of phonemes, none of them is meaningful by itself. Therefore, *drive* cannot be broken into smaller units and retain its meaning. *Drive* is a morpheme. In other instances, however, the smallest unit that conveys meaning is not a word. For example, *ing,* when added to a verb, denotes the progressive tense and its associated meaning. Therefore, when *ing* is added to the verb, it signals a meaning that is somewhat different from the meaning *drive* alone. While *ing* is not a word, it is still a morpheme.

There are basically two classes of morphemes: roots and affixes. *Roots* are words that cannot be divided into any smaller units, while *affixes* are morphemes that are attached to roots in order to alter meaning. In the word *driving,* the root is *drive,* and the affix, in this case a suffix, is *ing.* In the word *redo,* the root is *do,* and the affix, in this case a prefix, is *re.* Sometimes the affix involves deriving a grammatical form and conveying grammatical information, such as *ing* on *drive.* Other terms used for such affixes are inflections, inflectional morphemes, grammatical markers, and grammatical inflections. In other instances, the affix involves deriving an altered word meaning that conveys semantic information, such as the *re* on *do.* A term used for these affixes is *derivational morphemes.*

Another classification of morphemes uses the terms *free morphemes* and *bound morphemes* to identify the two different kinds. A free morpheme is able to occur alone in the language. In the previous example, *drive* is a free morpheme because it can occur meaningfully by itself. However, *ing* is a bound morpheme because it cannot occur by itself and be meaningful; it derives its meaning only when attached to another morpheme. Therefore, its function is bound to that of another morpheme. There is obviously a parallel between free morphemes and roots and bound morphemes and affixes. Words must be viewed in terms of the smallest units of meaning they possess to determine the number and types of morphemes they contain. The word *ungentlemanly* in Table 1.4 contains two free morphemes (*gentle* and *man*) and two bound morphemes (*un* and *ly*).

Examples of common rules for attaching bound morphemes to free morphemes include the formation of plural nouns by adding "s" (pronounced as the /s/ sound) to the root noun (*cat* to *cats*), past-tense verbs by adding "ed" (pronounced as a syllable *uhd*) to the root verb (*bait* to *baited*), superlative adjectives by adding "est" to the root adjective (*short* to *shortest*), and reflexive pronouns by adding "self" to the objective pronoun (*him* to *himself*). However, such rules do not explain the formation of plural nouns for which the "z" sound is used (*home* to *homes*), for which a syllable with "z" (pronounced as *uhz*) is used (*house* to *houses*), or for which the entire word changes (*man* to *men*). The examples do not explain past-tense verbs pronounced with a "t" or "d" at the end (*kick* to *kicked* or *comb* to *combed*), superlative adjectives that use a different word (*good* to *best*), or reflexive pronouns that use "selves" (*them* to *themselves*). The concept of allomorphs is needed to explain such variations. An *allomorph* is a variation of a morpheme that does not alter the meaning of the original morpheme. Table 1.5 lists several examples of allomorphs that are used to indicate noun plurals, verb tenses, and verb person and number.

In some cases, the use of allomorphs is determined by specific rules; for example, to form a noun plural when the root ends with a voiceless consonant, such as "p," add "s" to the root, except when the voiceless consonant is a fricative or an affricative, such as "sh" or "ch," in which case *uhz* is added to the root. However, in English many of the allomorphs to be used are irregular. That is, there are no specific rules governing their application. Why do we pluralize *child* by using *children,* and why do we use *was* as a past tense of *be?* Because no rules can be used for the irregularities, they must simply be memorized. Children, in the

TABLE 1.5 | Examples of Allomorphs for Noun Plurals, Verb Tenses, and Verb Person and Number

Noun Plurals				
book			books	/s/
robe			robes	/z/
twitch			twitches	/əz/
leaf			leaves	
Verb Tenses				
kick	kicked	/t/	kicked	/t/
comb	combed	/d/	combed	/d/
eat	ate		eaten	
ring	rang		rung	
do	did		done	
bait	baited	/əd/	baited	/əd/
tear	tore		torn	
Verb Person/Number				
kick			kicks	/s/
comb			combs	/z/
eat			eats	/s/
ring			rings	/z/
do			does	
have			has	

process of learning the morphology of their language, often overgeneralize the morphological rules and use the rules in place of the irregular allomorphs (*comed* instead of *came, deers* instead of *deer,* and *gooder* instead of *better*). Even adults may have difficulty with some of the irregular allomorphs. Context and/or syntax are often the only ways to determine the meaning of some irregular allomorphs or to know whether an allomorph has been used correctly. For example, *deer* does not change its form from singular to plural. If *deer* is the subject of a sentence, a verb may indicate whether the noun is singular or plural ("The deer is jumping" or "The deer jumping").

Pragmatics

Language is used for specific reasons, and without these there would be no purpose for language. Language helps us achieve communicative or social functions. This aspect of language is referred to as pragmatics. Because the area of pragmatics is concerned with the whys, and therefore, the hows of language use, some prefer to see pragmatics not as a component of language that is equal in status to the other components, such as syntax or semantics, but rather as the "super" component that drives, organizes, and encompasses the other components. This perspective is often referred to as a functionalist model of language.

When we think of people talking with each other, we can visualize each taking turns during which they produce sequences of connected speech; these people are engaging in discourse. Some confusion exists in the literature about two terms often used in discussion of pragmatics—discourse and narrative. For our purposes, *discourse* will be used to refer to the connected flow of language. This frequently relates to conversations and communicative interactions between people, but different kinds of discourse may also occur in, for example, speeches, soliloquies, reports, or explanations of procedures or theories. *Narrative* is one form of discourse, that of telling a story. A narrative is a frequently used logical description of a sequence of events. We employ narratives in discourse when describing a movie we have seen or giving an account of what happened when we went shopping. Stories, as in children's fairy tales or in novels, are another type of narrative. *Expository discourse* is another category of discourse. It is generally a more formal form of discourse and is used to inform. Ukrainetz (2006, p. 250) explains that there "are many expository genres and many different ways of dividing up the expository pie." We see expository discourse in reports, procedures, explanations, analyses, and persuasion, for example. It is a primary form of discourse in school as students advance in grades.

The process of reading is largely a language-based function. This means that when individuals read paragraphs or pages of text, they are engaging in interpretation of print discourse. Consequently, discourse is both a spoken and print form of language use. The same varieties of spoken discourse are seen in print discourse.

Effective language use requires that sequential utterances be related to each other. This aspect of pragmatics, termed *cohesion,* refers to the organization and order of utterances in a whole message so that the individual ideas of each utterance build logically on the previous ones. It is related to discourse. As with the other components of language, the different genres of discourse follow different rules for how they are organized, the order of utterances for logical formulation of a message, and methods of gluing these utterances and the organization together for good cohesion. The following is part of a classic example, provided by Wiig and Semel (1984), in which cohesion problems are illustrated in the sequential utterances of a boy engaging in narrative discourse, in this case a narrative retell as he attempts to relate the plot of a television show:

> So he was scared to tell John-boy that he stoled his poem, but he didn't really. He just got an idea from John-boy's poem. And then John-boy was trying to figure out what who shot this man he knows. And then the man stole the chickens and then that night he bring 'em back. (p. 288)

The adequate inclusion of temporal words and grammatical inflections indicating time references to help listeners orient themselves to the interrelationships of ideas and events and the use of appropriate referent identification for pronouns are parts of delivering coherent messages. Another important aspect of delivering coherent messages involves using not only coordinating conjunctions (e.g., *and, so*) but also subordinating conjunctions (e.g., *because, if, when*) to produce complex sentences that contain more than one proposition and convey relations among the propositions. Adverbial conjuncts (e.g., *nevertheless, however*) are other devices that contribute to cohesion.

Being able to provide coherent messages also depends, in part, on determining what listeners already know about the topics under discussion. Shared knowledge between listener and speaker is not given emphasis or, in some cases, even reported. However, knowledge that only the speaker has must be stated in order for a listener to comprehend a message. This aspect of pragmatics is termed *presupposition* and refers to the provision of sufficient but not too much information for adequate listener comprehension. Appropriate use of presuppositions requires that a speaker gauge listeners' needs for specificity and frames of reference. We have all experienced irritation with speakers who waste valued communication time reporting what is obviously known without proceeding to the key parts of a message. In contrast, we have attempted to engage in conversations in which we were unable to follow the speaker's sequence of ideas because adequate background information was not supplied.

The concept of presupposition is related to theory of mind (TOM). TOM refers to an individual's ability to understand and interpret another person's knowledge and beliefs, particularly when they are different from one's own perspectives (Baron-Cohen, 1989, 2000). It is important to understand what another person might believe or know in order to formulate our messages in a way that meets the needs of our listeners. Ability with TOM is a skill that children learn as they mature and an ability that has been found to be problematic for many children with language disorders. We will, therefore, see TOM discussed again later in this text.

When individuals fail to make appropriate presuppositions and then cast their messages inappropriately, a communication breakdown is likely to occur. When this happens in written language, the writer often does not have an opportunity to repair the breakdown. However, when the communication breakdown occurs in spoken language, the opportunity to repair may be possible and we are generally required to attempt to repair it. In conversation, the process of repair is twofold. First, speakers are obligated to identify when listeners have not understood their messages and supply additional information or modifications of the ways in which previously given information was delivered. Second, listeners must signal their lack of understanding. These signals may be verbal, such as the statements "I don't understand," "What did you say?" or "Would you repeat that please?" Or listeners may use nonverbal cues, such as puzzled facial expressions, to indicate that they have not understood.

During a conversation, both the speaker and the listener take turns responding to each other's utterances. One part of this rule-governed behavior is that one does not interrupt or talk over the other. However, turn taking also involves acknowledging the previous utterances but without repeating unnecessary content and expanding the content of the conversation with appropriate additional information. Such behavior facilitates topic maintenance. Topic maintenance requires that a person about to speak abide by the constraints of the topic created by a previous speaker and reply with responses appropriate to the topic. For example, an appropriate response and one that would continue the topic to the statement "I bought a new car" would be "What kind is it?" In contrast, the response "It's cold outside" would be startling and disconcerting to the previous speaker and would probably discontinue the first topic, if not the interaction. However, there are times when we wish to change a topic that has already been introduced. These are referred to as *topic shifts*. Topic shifting is acceptable if it is not done so frequently that our conversational partners begin to think we are uninterested in them and if it is done smoothly rather than abruptly.

One reason written communication is often thought of as being a more advanced and complex form of language use than spoken language is that the writer does not have the advantage of "real time" communication repair. The reader is not there when the writer writes. Consequently, the writer has a greater load, for example, to presuppose what the reader will know at the time of reading, to organize ideas in cohesive ways that build the writer's propositions in ways that conform to the reader's likely knowledge level, to select the appropriate language structures (syntax, morphology) and words for both the reader's needs and the meaning of the message, and to choose the appropriate genre for the propositions to be put forth in the written message. Managing the load requires a high level of language competency in the spoken form to transfer to the written form and knowledge of the rules of written discourse. This in part explains why students who struggle with their spoken language generally struggle to achieve competency in reading and writing.

In certain situations with certain people, specific rules dictate the way we are supposed to communicate. For example, it would be very inappropriate during an interdisciplinary educational staffing on a child to relate the results of testing as "Sally sure did ace the hearing test but bombed the IQ test." In contrast, it might be acceptable to say to a friend and colleague that "Tom aced the continuing ed. course he took." Several researchers have described different styles or registers of communication, some of which are intimate, casual, consultative, formal, and frozen (Joos, 1976). Effective use of language involves determining in communicative situations which styles are appropriate and wording messages accordingly.

Language also functions as a means of engaging in human relationships. Adolescents, for example, are known for their use of language as a way of establishing and maintaining peer friendships (Thurlow, 2005). Language is also an avenue for initiating relationships. As an example, if we wish to meet a person sitting next to us in an audience, we might ask what time the performance is expected to start even though we already know. The function of the utterance in this instance is not to acquire information but rather to make contact. The same query, of course, could be made for the purpose of receiving information, and another important function of language is to acquire information. For most adults, messages often serve more than one function at the same time, and adults usually vary their messages appropriately between direct and indirect speech acts. That is, they use alternative forms of language to accomplish similar purposes, depending on the context and the person to whom they are addressing the messages. While an imperative (a direct speech act, such as "Close the door") might be acceptable in some instances, a question (an indirect speech act, such as "Can you close the door?") is more appropriate in others. As we can see, the form (syntax, phonology, semantics, and morphology) of a message does not always correspond to the intents or functions of the message. And certain ways of using language vary from context to context. What is socially and culturally acceptable in one situation violates the appropriate rules in another. Competency with pragmatics might well be considered social competency (Prutting, 1982).

Another aspect of communication that contributes to the tapestry of skills that make up communicative competency that deserves additional attention is fluency. *Fluency* in the delivery of messages refers to the number of false starts, hesitations, fillers, and revisions that take place as speakers say their utterances. These fluency interrupters are often referred to as speech disruptions or mazes and should not be confused with stuttering, which is a speech disorder. While mazes or speech disruptions occur in most people's speech, they interfere with communication if they are too frequent or long. They can sometimes indicate language impairment when they represent difficulties in formulating syntactic or morphologic structures or rapid retrieval of words from our mental lexicons. However, we sometimes use particular fluency disruptors deliberately to help convey part of our message. For example, if we wish to appear thoughtful about what we are saying, we might introduce more hesitations and false starts into our utterances than if we said the same thing with total assurance. As discussed previously in the chapter, extralinguistic aspects of communication such as paralinguistic and nonlinguistic devices can also be used to enhance or even change the linguistic meaning of an utterance. The ability to use such devices falls within the pragmatic component of language.

Children, in the process of learning the form and content of language, must also learn how to handle the many aspects of pragmatics to communicate effectively in a variety of situations. As we have seen, among the many aspects are the following:

1. The various functions and acts that utterances serve and the shift among different discourse genres for different functions
2. The coherence of sequential statements
3. The fluency with which messages are delivered
4. The ability to take turns during dialogues and at the same time maintain topics of conversation
5. The provision of adequate information for listeners to comprehend spoken and written messages without supplying redundant information
6. The responsibility to repair communication breakdowns and request additional information when messages are not understood
7. The appropriate use of nonverbal communicative cues
8. The codes or styles of communicative behavior employed in different situations, that is, our ability to code switch

Skill in employing these elements, combined with the ability to use the phonological, semantic, syntactic, and morphological systems accurately, embodies what we refer to as *communicative competency* or *proficiency.*

COMPREHENSION AND PRODUCTION

In our discussion on the pragmatic aspects of language, we saw that language use often involves at least two people interacting in a communicative situation—the sender of a message (speaker or writer) and the receiver of a message (listener or reader). In spoken language interactions, the people typically take turns in the roles of sender and receiver. This communicative process is referred to as *dyadic communication.* However, the notion of turn taking breaks down when we consider printed language; although the sender writes, the message to the receiver is delayed so turn taking is limited. Mobile communication alternatives are modifying the sender-receiver relationships in terms of turn taking. Although the speed of message sending and receiving is less in mobile than in usual print modes, it does not equate to turn taking speed or the quantity of communicative cues available in real-time dyadic communication.

Regardless of communication mode, a basic assumption is that for the communicative act to be complete, both the sender and the receiver must use the same code and know the same rules of the language. The sender takes an idea and applies the appropriate language rules to put the idea into code. In spoken language, the sender then transmits the code through speech production. Also in spoken language, the listener hears the sound transmission, applies the same language rules to match the code with the one already neurologically stored, and then, one hopes, comprehends the message. In other words, the sender *encodes* the message, and the receiver *decodes* the message. Terms often used interchangeably with *encoding* are *expression* and *production,* while *reception, understanding, interpretation,* and *comprehension* are terms often considered synonymous with *decoding.*

It is generally agreed that for adults in most situations, comprehension skills are greater than production abilities. For example, for most of us, our understanding vocabularies are superior to our expressive vocabularies (the words we use to convey our thoughts to others). There has also been a general belief that this superiority of comprehension over production applies to children in their acquisition of language. This belief appears reasonable when one considers the superiority of receptive to expressive skills in adults and when one observes that very young children often appear to understand much more language than they produce.

The research on the acquisition of comprehension and production skills in children has, however, yielded some conflicting results. It appears that in some situations children's comprehension of language does precede their production. This certainly is true in the early stages of language learning. However, in other situations, production abilities appear superior. Factors such as the definition of comprehension being used, the degree of comprehension being measured (e.g., depth and/or breath of comprehension of the word *snake*), and the amount of contextual support attached to the comprehension tasks likely affect how we interpret the relationship between production and comprehension. It may be that the relationship between comprehension and production changes with age. It may also be that comprehension and production are related but distinct skills. As Miller and Paul (1995) write, "One thing we have learned is that language comprehension and production, while following predictable patterns of acquisition in most children, do not always correspond perfectly to each other, even in an individual child" (p. 1).

COMMUNICATION MODES

In our discussion of comprehension and production, the primary focus was placed on hearing as the input modality for comprehension, and speaking as the output modality for production. These are the input–output modalities that make up the auditory–oral system for language. The auditory–oral system is the most common way of using language and the one that most children acquire first. However, other combinations of input–output modalities that people may use include the visual–graphic (reading and writing) and the visual–gestural systems, as shown in Figure 1.2.

Auditory–Oral System: Hearing and Speech

The functional components of the auditory–oral system are hearing and speaking. Phylogenetically, humans heard and comprehended before they read, and they spoke before they acquired the ability to write. In the history of the human species, we have been hearing and talking for a very long time, and our bodies have had lots of time to evolve to

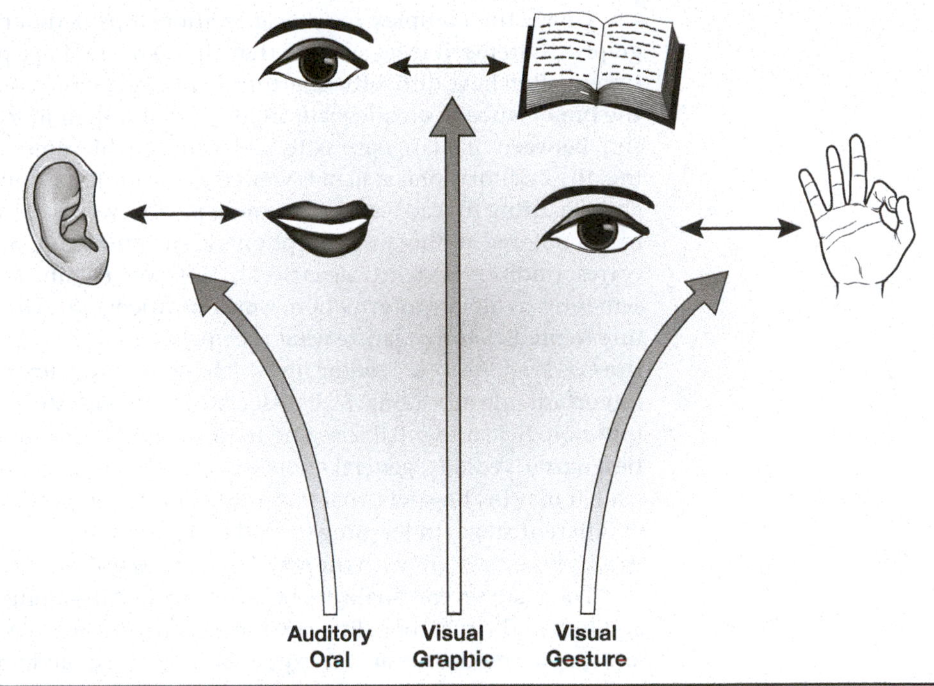

FIGURE 1.2 | Modes of Communication

support these functions well. By comparison, we have been reading and writing for only a short time, and our bodies have not had quite the same amount of time to evolve to support these functions as well. In many ways, the auditory-oral mode for language is also more flexible than the visual-graphic mode. Vision is a unidirectional sense, whereas hearing is multidirectional. We can see in only one direction at a time, but we can hear sounds originating from many directions despite the positions of our heads. Furthermore, we can talk when our hands are busy, but we cannot write. Speaking needs no special instruments, whereas writing requires the use of a pencil, pen, or a keyboard.

Children typically learn to use the auditory-oral system before they learn to use the visual-graphic system. That is, they can listen and speak before they know how to read and write. Developmentally, maturation of the physiological bases for audition and speech occurs before those used for reading and writing. Yet developmental maturation is not the only reason for children's earlier proficiencies with the auditory-oral system. For most Western languages, writing evolved as a system of visual symbols used to represent auditory symbols. The auditory-oral system is generally the basis of the visual-graphic system.

Visual–Graphic System: Reading and Writing

In the visual-graphic system, reading is employed as the input mode, and writing is used as the output mode. As indicated above, reading and writing are relatively newly acquired human skills, so the neurophysiological bases of these functions have not had as much time to establish themselves in humans as the neurophysiological bases of listening and speaking. Nevertheless, the functions of reading and writing are closely related to the auditory-oral system. In many respects, the visual-graphic system is a code for another code—the auditory-oral system. As a code, language symbolizes experiences and thoughts. This code can then be represented by a system of sounds combined to form words and sentences. However, these sounds (which are themselves a code) can be recoded and rerepresented as visual rather than auditory symbols. That is, reading and writing are codes for hearing and speaking, which themselves are codes for the actual experiences or ideas. In the process of learning the visual-graphic language system, children learn a new coding system based on a previously learned code system.

Given the complex reciprocal relationships between the auditory–oral and visual–graphic systems, it is no surprise that children who have problems with the auditory–oral system often have difficulties learning to read and write. Most professionals emphasize both the importance of an adequate auditory–oral system in learning to read and the relationship between oral language skills and reading achievement. In a bottom up theory of reading, the auditory–oral system is viewed as the underpinning of learning to read such that a child learning to read learns to segment printed words, decode letters in them, match them to some stored auditory model (phonetic and phonemic segmentation), and then retrieve a corresponding word (lexical retrieval). However, reading also involves using already known semantic–syntactic information, world knowledge, and information about discourse structure to predict and organize what is being seen on the printed page. This is consistent with the *top-down theory* of reading, in which higher-order linguistic and cognitive skills play an important role in reading. Skills associated with both the bottom-up and top-down theories (phonological and syllabic segmentation, rapid lexical retrieval, semantic–syntactic abilities, narrative skills, general knowledge level) have been found to be factors in learning to read. It may be, however, that these different skills play more prominent roles in the process at different stages in learning to read and in different children at different times. This perspective is consistent with the *parallel,* or *interactive, theory* of learning to read.

There are several analogies between the visual–graphic and auditory–oral systems. The auditory and visual modalities are the receptive aspects of the two systems, whereas the oral and graphic modalities are the expressive aspects. The auditory component is based on a set of sounds that combine to form spoken words; the visual component is based on a set of letters that combine to form written words. Just as oral production for speech is a sensorimotor process, the same is true for graphic production for writing. Reception for the auditory–oral system involves transduction (conversion of waves into neural impulses) and auditory perception and processing of sound waves. Similarly, reception for the visual–graphic system involves transduction and visual perception and processing of light waves. Rules govern the use of both systems.

Although there are several analogies between the auditory–oral and visual–graphic systems, there are also differences. One difference is the sequence in which the two systems are usually acquired. Furthermore, although rules govern both systems and although some rules are similar, there are also different rules. One obvious difference deals with punctuation. Another relates to spelling. These are not factors in the auditory–oral system. Another difference deals with the level of grammatical complexity. The semantic–syntactic level used in the auditory–oral system is generally less complex than that found in the visual–graphic system once one progresses beyond the early learning stages. Still another difference relates to the amount of context that is available to aid understanding, a factor that we encountered previously in this chapter. Reading and writing are more decontextualized modes of communication than listening and speaking. That is, fewer cues to decipher and impart meaning are available in reading and writing compared to listening and speaking. We cannot point or use facial expressions to communicate in reading and writing, although graphs, illustrations, and pictures are attempts to supplement written material. Another difference is that speech consists of sounds that occur over time, and these are generally temporary and fleeting. Writing consists of marks in space that are relatively permanent and can be referred to repeatedly. However, it is faster to speak than to write, and most children acquire the auditory–oral system without formalized instruction, whereas carefully planned instructional processes are typically offered in schools in order to teach children to read and write. Finally, while use of the auditory–oral system can develop independently of the visual–graphic system, proficiency with the visual–graphic system is exceedingly difficult to achieve without first acquiring some proficiency with the auditory–oral system. This point will be reiterated in later parts of this text.

Visual–Gestural Systems

Consistent with our earlier discussions, the visual modality combined with gestures, body postures and movements, and/or facial grimaces can be used as communication modes. A form of a visual–gestural communication system, nonverbal communication with its nonlinguistic elements, was discussed previously, and that discussion will not be repeated here.

Here we introduce readers to two other forms of visual–gestural communication systems: manual communication and other forms of augmentative/alternative communication. We include brief discussions of these two systems because they are used with some children who have language and/or speech disorders.

Manual Communication. Manual communication, or sign language, is sometimes used by people who are deaf or severely hearing impaired. Children with other speech and/or language problems also sometimes use manual communication. There are many forms of manual communication. Some use manual signs that correspond closely to or match exactly the sequence of morphemes in English syntax. Other forms are actually languages different from English. One is American Sign Language (ASL), which, as the name implies, is a language communicated through the visual–gestural modalities used in the United States. However, other English-speaking countries, for example, England and Australia, have different signed languages, such as Auslan in Australia. Just as speakers of one language, such as Greek, will not understand speakers of another language, such as Cantonese Chinese, users of ASL cannot be expected to understand users of Auslan and vice versa.

Understanding that ASL is a language and not English expressed through gestures raises several questions about the education of children who are hearing impaired. For example, are we, in teaching reading and writing to children who already know ASL, attempting to teach them to use a visual–graphic system of a language (English) for which they have little background? Is this a second-language visual–graphic system for them? For those children who acquire some oral communicative skills, are these oral skills based on a different language than the one they may already know (ASL)?

Augmentative/Alternative Communication. In addition to manual communication, a number of augmentative/alternative communication (AAC) systems rely primarily on visual–gestural modes for communication. With professionals' increased understanding of and emphasis on communication, greater use of AAC for individuals with speech and/or language problems has evolved. Advances in technology in general have also facilitated the development of a wide variety of more sophisticated, efficient, and flexible AAC systems. Later in this text, we will discuss AAC in more depth as an intervention for some children with language disorders.

BIOLOGICAL, COGNITIVE, AND SOCIAL BASES OF HUMAN COMMUNICATION

Communication is a complex linguistic, biological, cognitive, and social phenomenon. All these factors are involved in language functioning, but the ways in which they interact are not fully understood. Earlier in this chapter, we discussed some of the linguistic and social bases of language. Here, we introduce some of the biological and cognitive bases of language and include some additional discussion of social bases of language. Volumes have been written on each of these topics. We cannot hope to cover them in depth in one chapter. Rather, this chapter provides an overview or, for some readers, a refresher.

Biological Bases of Communication

In the previous section on communication modes, we read that hearing and speaking were identified as the primary modalities used in spoken languages. Although other modalities, such as vision and gesture, may contribute to the total communicative process, our discussion here provides an overview of the major physical bases of auditory–oral language: the ear, the speech mechanism, and the nervous system.

Hearing and Listening

Basic Anatomy and Physiology of the Ear. The ear is the sensory mechanism that receives sound waves and converts them into mechanical, hydraulic, and finally electrical/electrochemical energy (neural impulses). If the ear is not adequately sensitive to a variety of sound

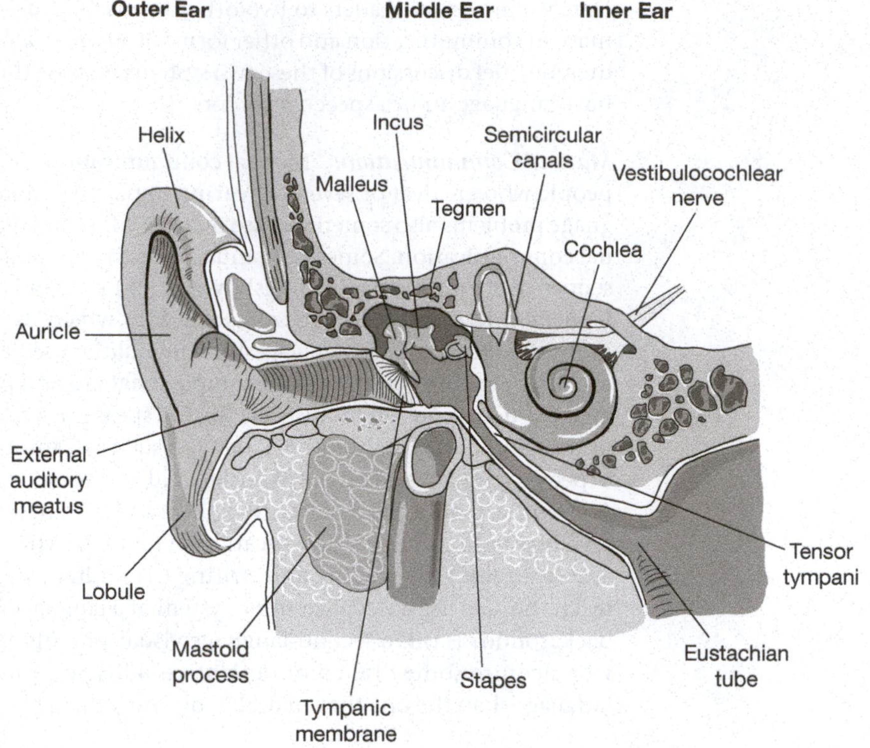

FIGURE 1.3 | The Ear

frequencies (the psychological parallel is pitch) and intensities (the psychological parallel is loudness), auditory information needed to receive and understand the spoken code of others is prevented from being converted to neural impulses and reaching the brain.

The ear consists of three main parts: the outer ear, the middle ear, and the inner ear. Together these are the peripheral hearing mechanism (Figure 1.3). In the *outer ear,* the auricle and ear canal (external auditory meatus) collect sound waves and funnel them toward the middle ear, where the waves hit the eardrum (tympanic membrane) and make it vibrate. The movement of the eardrum, now mechanical energy, is transferred to three small bones of the *middle ear*—the malleus, incus, and stapes—which pass the movement to the inner ear. The major structure for hearing in the *inner ear* is the cochlea. The *cochlea* contains a membranous structure suspended in fluid. As the mechanical energy in the middle ear reaches the inner ear, the fluid is set in motion. Mechanical energy now becomes hydraulic energy. As the fluid moves, it impinges on the membranous structure in the cochlea that also contains fluid and the end organ of hearing, the *organ of Corti.* Rows of cells that contain protruding hairs (*inner hair cells, outer hair cells*) extend from the organ of Corti to the membrane so that as the fluid moves, it causes the membrane to move, and the result is a rubbing or shearing action on these parts of the organ of Corti. This rubbing converts the hydraulic energy to neural energy, which travels to the brain via cranial nerve VIII (the vestibulocochlear, or auditory, nerve). The brain interprets the neural energy it receives.

Biological Basis for Listening to Speech. The middle and inner ears reach their adult size at 20 weeks' gestation. The auditory nerve is developed by the 24th week of gestation. Newborn infants thus enter the world having listened to their internal environment (e.g., mother's blood flow and heartbeat) and external environment (e.g., mother's speech, music, and environmental noises) for some months. They enter the world with some idea of what it sounds like. Infants can in fact discriminate between a variety of speech sounds and linguistic boundaries within weeks and months following their birth. Infants as young as 4 weeks old have also been found to attend longer to facial (lip) movements that match the vowels being heard than those that do not match the vowels being heard (Kuhl, 1990; Kuhl & Meltzoff, 1988).

Apparently, infants' attending skills are intermodal in that they associate lip movements with the appropriate speech sounds. How infants and toddlers actually learn to process incoming auditory stimuli, however, and understand the speech they listen to is a more complex phenomenon.

Speech and Talking

Basic Anatomy and Physiology of the Speech Mechanism. The anatomical structures used to produce speech are actually parts of the respiratory and digestive systems (Figure 1.4). The exhaled air from the lungs provides the basic source of energy for speech. It is this air that is modified by the vocal folds in the larynx ("voice box") and/or the vocal tract—pharyngeal (throat), oral (mouth), and nasal (nose) cavities above the vocal folds—that results in speech. The physical production of speech requires the processes of respiration, phonation, resonation, and articulation.

The *larynx,* located in the front of the neck, houses the *vocal folds.* The function of the larynx is not solely or primarily the production of sound. Rather, the larynx and vocal folds serve to stop foreign objects (such as food) from entering the airway and as such keep us alive. If we want the larynx to produce voice, then respiration and phonation are needed in addition to the functioning of the larynx. *Respiration* involves the inhalation and exhalation of air from the lungs. *Phonation* involves the use of the exhaled air from the lungs in conjunction with changes in subglottic air pressure to create vibrations of the vocal folds.

During the production of approximately one-half of the English consonants, the vocal folds do not move to phonate, or produce voice. Hence, these sounds are termed *voiceless consonants.* The production of voiceless consonants merely requires the air from the lungs to pass unobstructed through the vocal folds into the vocal tract. If a hand is placed lightly against the front of the neck (where the larynx is located) and the consonant /s/ is produced with no accompanying vowel, no vibration is felt. However, during production of all vowels and the remaining consonants, the vocal folds vibrate to create a voiced sound. Thus, phonemes that require vocal-fold vibration are termed *voiced sounds.* Vocal-fold vibration, or phonation, can be felt when a hand is held lightly on the front of the neck as a sound, such as /z/, is produced. The size of the vocal folds and the rate at which they vibrate are primary factors in determining the pitch of a person's voice. Generally, the faster something vibrates, the higher is the pitch.

After the exhaled air passes through the larynx, it travels through the vocal tract (including the pharyngeal, oral, and or nasal cavities), as shown in Figure 1.4. When the vocal folds have vibrated and therefore vibrated the air, a sound wave is produced, and the vocal tract acts like a resonator, much like the main body of a cello. *Resonation* involves modifying the

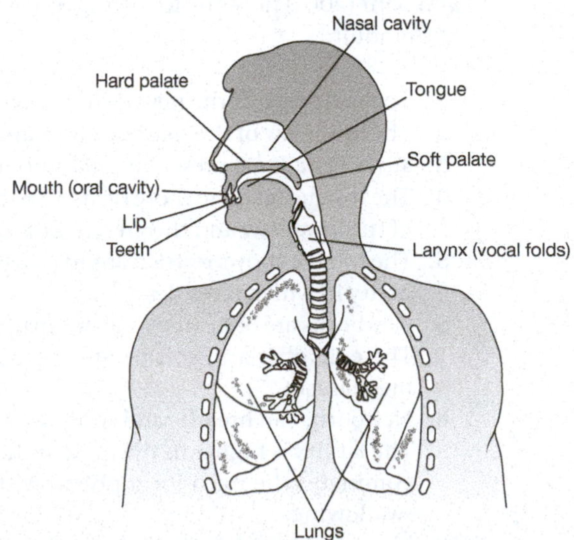

FIGURE 1.4 | The Speech Mechanism

sound generated by the vocal folds by changing the shape and size of the spaces in the vocal tract, which results in some parts of sound waves being emphasized and others being dampened. The outgoing air (whether or not the vocal folds are vibrating) also hits barriers in the form of the palate (the roof of the mouth), the tongue, lips, and teeth. These barriers, some of which are movable, such as the tongue, are the articulators, and the different positions they take give the outgoing air (vibrating or not) different characteristics, that is, *articulation*.

The *impedance* (obstruction, barrier) of the air is greater for consonants than vowels. Some obstructions for consonants are complete and are then released (e.g., /p/, /t/, /k/), while other obstructions allow for an obstructed but continuous flow of air (e.g., /s/, "sh"). The type of obstruction is called the *manner of formation*. The place in the mouth where obstruction occurs for consonants (e.g., lips–teeth for /f/ or back of the tongue for /k/) is termed the *place of articulation*. The different positions of the articulators cause sound energy to be concentrated in different frequencies. For example, /s/ and /z/ have sound energy concentrated in higher frequencies, whereas /f/ and /v/ have sound energy concentrated in lower frequencies. If a consonant is voiced, such as /z/, the mouth noises created by the articulators are superimposed on the vibrating air created by the vibrating vocal folds. Therefore, voiced sounds have a fundamental frequency from the vocal-fold vibrations, which is comparatively low, and concentrations of sound energy in certain other higher frequencies (mouth noises) because of the obstructions of the articulators. For most English vowels and consonants, the exhaled air is directed into the oral cavity, or mouth. However, production of three English phonemes ("m," "n," and "ng") requires that the air be directed into the nasal cavity to create a nasal resonance (*nasalization*). The effect of the air in the nasal cavity can be felt if an index finger is placed lightly along the boney side of the nose while saying a prolonged /n/. As all three nasal sounds are voiced, the nasal resonance is superimposed on vocal-fold vibration.

For vowels, all of which are voiced, as we have noted, the articulators place few obstructions in the way of the exhaled air. Instead, movement of the articulators changes the internal shape of the mouth cavity in order to give each vowel its unique sound. These changes concentrate sound energy in different frequencies. For each vowel, energy concentration occurs in identifiable bands at different frequencies, including the low-frequency one associated with the vocal-fold vibrations. The frequency location of the higher-frequency bands of energy gives each vowel its unique acoustic features. The bands of energy are called *formants,* which are particularly important for receiving and perceiving speech and play important roles in what children with hearing impairments might be able to detect and perceive.

Biological Basis for Speech Production. Infants' vocal tracts become adultlike over the first 3 years of their life. Unlike the ear, which is born ready to listen to speech, the infant vocal tract differs from the adult and so is not in such a ready state for producing speech. Hillis and Bahr (2001) note the following differences between the newborn's vocal tract and that of the adult:

1. The oral space of the newborn is small.
2. The lower jaw of the newborn is small and somewhat retracted.
3. Sucking pads are present in infants but not in adults.
4. The tongue takes up more relative space in the newborn, because of the diminished size of the lower jaw and the presence of sucking pads in the cheeks.
5. The tongue shows restrictions in movement, partially because of the restricted intraoral cavity in which it resides.
6. Newborns are obligated mouth-breathers. They do not breathe through their noses.
7. The epiglottis and soft palate are in approximation in the newborn as a protective mechanism.
8. Newborns can breathe and swallow at the same time.
9. The larynx is higher in the neck of the newborn than in the older infant or adult. This eliminates the need for sophisticated laryngeal closure to protect the airway during swallowing.
10. The Eustachian tube in the infant lies in a horizontal position. It assumes a more vertical angle in the adult. (pp. 17–18)

Over the first 3 years of life, the vocal tract anatomy and function of a child change. For instance, tongue muscle tone increases, tongue movements become dissociated from jaw movements, lip closure improves, the larynx moves farther down the vocal tract, and more sophisticated movements (including elevation) of the larynx occur during swallowing (Hillis & Bahr, 2001). Together, these changes coincide with an improvement in the child's ability to articulate. Thus, although the speech production mechanism is devoted primarily to breathing and swallowing, it develops into a marvelous platform for speech production.

The Controller and Interpreter: The Nervous System

Basic Anatomy and Physiology of the Nervous System. Two major divisions of the nervous system are integrally involved in communication: the central nervous system (CNS) (brain and spinal cord) and the peripheral nervous system (PNS) (cranial and spinal nerves). A third division, the autonomic nervous system, regulates the presumably involuntary bodily functions, such as stomach and bowel contractions and heartbeat. Since this last system affects speech and language only indirectly, it will not be discussed here.

The Central Nervous System. At its superior end, the spinal cord forms a structure known as the *brain stem* (Figure 1.5). The cerebrum (often referred to as the *brain*) sits on top of the brain stem and surrounds it, much as a mushroom top surrounds the upper stem of the mushroom. The wrinkled outer surface of the cerebrum is the *cortex.* The cerebellum is located below the cerebrum and behind the brain stem. Like the cerebrum, the cerebellum also has a wrinkled outer surface called a cortex. The wrinkles of both structures are the result of folds in the surfaces. Each ridge created by these folds is known as a *gyrus,* or *convolution,* and each indentation caused by the folds is called a *sulcus,* or *fissure.* These convolutions and fissures provide us with landmarks in order to describe the brain. These also result in greater brain surface area than would a smooth surface.

Both the cerebellum and the cerebrum are divided into left and right hemispheres. Each cerebral hemisphere is further divided into four lobes. The most anterior lobe is known as the *frontal lobe.* The *parietal lobe* lies behind the frontal lobe and is separated from it by the *central fissure.* Behind the parietal lobe is the *occipital lobe.* The *temporal lobe* is on the side and separated

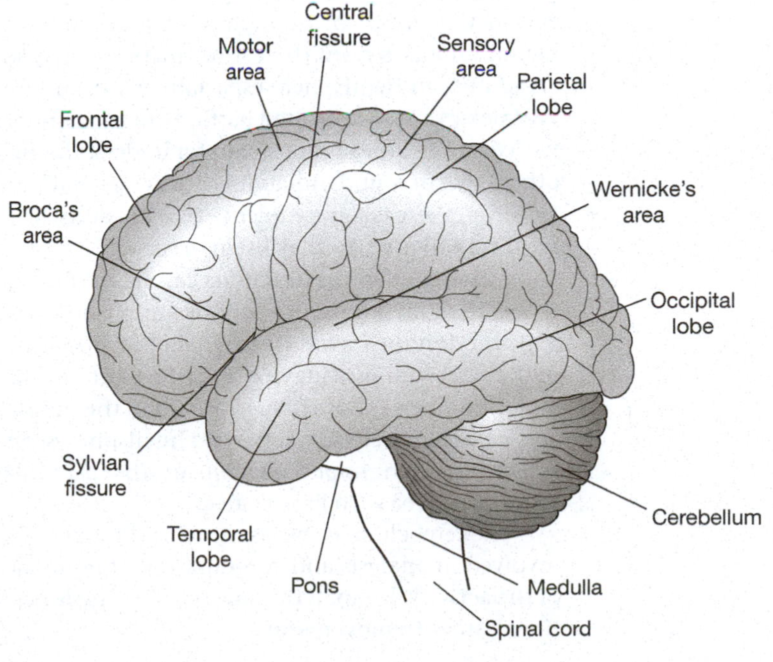

FIGURE 1.5 | The Brain

from the frontal lobe by the *Sylvian fissure*. The area around the Sylvian fissure is known as the *perisylvian area*, which contains the *planum temporale* in the upper portion of the temporal lobe in the perisylvian area. The planum temporale is well implicated in language function.

The cells that make up the nervous system are referred to as *neurons*. Most neurons contain a nucleus (contained within a cell body), an array of dendrites extending from one side of the nucleus—which conduct impulses toward the nucleus—and an axon extending from the other side of the nucleus—which conducts impulses away from the nucleus. When a neural impulse is generated by the nucleus of a neuron, the impulse travels along the axon until it reaches another cell. The point at which one neuron meets another is referred to as a *synapse*. The neural impulse then crosses the synapse and continues its journey onto adjacent cells via chemicals known as neurotransmitters. Curiously, the power and complexity of the human brain are due not to the number of neurons but rather to the rich array of interconnections (particularly dendritic connections) between neurons.

As the result of studies investigating the effects of damage to parts of the brain on neurological functions and, more recently, studies using newer neuroimaging techniques, we know that certain functions in adults are generally related to different parts of the cerebral cortex. The *motor area* is located in the frontal lobe in front of the central fissure. Neural impulses are sent from the motor area to various muscles of the body, including those involved in speech production, in order to produce movement. For most adults, regardless of which hand is dominant, the left cerebral hemisphere is the primary controller of speech and language. For the majority of the population, the left frontal lobe in front of the motor area and above the Sylvian fissure is a region known as *Broca's area*. This area programs speech production. It coordinates neural signals that then travel to the motor area (also located in the frontal lobe but in front of the central fissure) and subsequently to the articulators. Congruent with the left hemisphere's dominance for speech and language, Broca's area in the left frontal lobe is typically described as more convoluted than the corresponding area in the right hemisphere. Furthermore, for adults, damage to Broca's area in the left hemisphere impairs speech production, whereas damage to the same area in the opposite hemisphere typically results in no discernible disturbance of speech production. The sensory area of the cerebrum is located in the parietal lobe just behind the central fissure. This area receives neural impulses from various parts of the body and uses this information to help control functions in those parts of the body.

Many of the functions of the temporal lobe are involved in receiving and processing auditory stimuli. For example, the auditory (vestibulocochlear) nerve, which transmits neural impulses from the ear to the brain, courses toward the temporal lobe. An area in an adult's left hemisphere especially important for the comprehension of oral language—Wernicke's area—is located partially in the temporal and partially in the parietal lobe. The left Wernicke's area is dominant for understanding spoken words. In contrast, processing of other types of sounds, including music, generally takes place largely in the right hemisphere. However, there is some evidence that in adults, both the right and the left temporal-parietal areas are active when they listen to speech.

Although certain functions can be attributed to specific parts of the cerebral cortex, there are tremendous interactions among areas of the brain, interactions requisite for normal functioning, including language learning and function. One way in which the structure of the cerebrum provides for functional interrelationships among cortical areas is via its association fibers. These fibers, located in the interior of the cerebrum, interconnect various cortical areas, including lobes and hemispheres. The largest and most important interhemisphere fiber is the *corpus callosum*. Another particularly important association fiber connects Wernicke's area with Broca's area.

The cerebellum is the last structure of the CNS to be discussed. This structure is integrally involved in analysis and coordination of motor activity, although it does not initiate any of the activity. Its analytic and coordinating functions result in the ability to produce well-timed, smooth movements.

The Peripheral Nervous System. The PNS is made up of 12 pairs of cranial nerves and 31 pairs of spinal nerves. The cranial nerves extend from the brain stem primarily to the neck and head areas, and the spinal nerves extend from the spinal cord to the remaining lower parts

TABLE 1.6 | Seven Cranial Nerves Involved in Language and Speech

Number of the Nerve	Name	Functions
V	Trigeminal	*Sensory*—face; jaw; mouth *Motor*—jaw; soft palate
VII	Facial	*Sensory*—taste; mucous membrane of soft palate and pharynx *Motor*—face; lips
VIII	Vestibulocochlear (auditory)	*Sensory*—hearing; balance
IX	Glossopharyngeal	*Sensory*—taste; mucous membrane of pharynx, middle ear, and mouth *Motor*—pharynx
X	Vagus	*Sensory*—mucous membrane of pharynx, larynx, soft palate, tongue, and lungs *Motor*—larynx; pharynx
XI	Accessory	*Motor*—soft palate; larynx; pharynx; neck
XII	Hypoglossal	*Sensory*—tongue *Motor*—tongue

of the body. Many of the nerves contain both sensory fibers (which travel to the CNS and provide it with information) and motor fibers (which transmit commands from the CNS to various parts of the body). Cranial nerves are identified by both roman numerals and names. Seven of these 12 pairs of cranial nerves are especially important for speech and language functions (*see* Table 1.6). These nerves carry the command signals originating in the CNS to the specific muscles of speech production that they innervate. Their sensory fibers then feed back to the CNS information about the performances of muscles. This allows the CNS to monitor the activities and send corrective signals if necessary. Furthermore, information about the acoustic characteristics of a speech signal, sent to the CNS via the auditory nerve, augments other sensory data about an organism's speech and language performance.

Neurological Basis for Human Communication. Much of our discussion thus far has centered on the adult nervous system. Care must be taken when attempting to draw parallels between adult and child neurological functioning. The nervous systems of children are immature. Like the speech production mechanism, the newborn's nervous system, particularly the CNS, has further anatomical and physiological advances to come. This can be seen by the sheer difference in weight of the human brain. At birth, the infant's brain weighs only 25 percent of the adult brain weight. However, 5-month-old fetuses may have complete sets of neurons. Rather than more neurons, an increase in the interconnections between the neurons results in the increasing brain weight in a child's postnatal brain development. If we focus on the areas of the brain involved primarily in communication development, according to Hillis and Bahr (2001), by about 3 months of age dendritic branching becomes "more advanced in the oral area of the cortical motor strip than in Broca's area and in the right hemisphere than in the left hemisphere" (p. 3). By around 2 years of age, dendritic branching is thought to become more complex in Broca's area and throughout the rest of the left hemisphere, and by 6 years of age, dendritic branching in Broca's area is more advanced than the oral region of the motor cortex (Hillis & Bahr, 2001). Thus, children are born with the neurological *potential* for speech and language acquisition. With exposure and experience, children's brains change and learn to understand and produce speech and language.

Having noted that certain parts of the adult brain are dedicated to linguistic functions and that children's brains gradually develop the rich array of interconnections seen in the adult brain, children's brains differ from those of adults in one particularly important aspect. Children's brains are described as having more *plasticity* and less cerebral *localization* and specialization than those of adults. Consequently, the effects on language seen from focal CNS damage in adults may not be seen in children. Damage limited to left-hemispheric areas in children appears not to account fully for the presence of developmental language disorders as opposed to language disorders seen in children who have acquired language problems as a result of childhood trauma or disease. Although we have come a long way in our knowledge, we do not currently have a thorough understanding of how the brain works, including its functioning with regard to learning language and speech initially and subsequently performing activities related to learned language and speech. This explains, in part, why we still do not have all the answers regarding language disorders in children.

Cognitive Bases of Language

What Is Cognition? For months before birth, an infant was curled up in a protective and nurturing environment. The day of birth brings with it a new environment to get to know and understand if he or she is to survive. Thus, cognition is the process of getting to know the environment and to make sense of it, a process that starts at birth or earlier and continues throughout life as stimuli, events, and environment continuously change.

According to Piaget (1954), infants have psychological structures (schemas or schemata) that allow them to process and organize incoming stimuli. Over time, these schemas adapt or change in response to incoming stimuli. In Piaget's pursuit to understand the development of cognition, he proposed a series of stages through which children progress as they learn to "get to know" the world in which they live. Specifically, Piaget proposed four stages of cognitive development: (1) the sensorimotor stage from birth to about 2 years, (2) the preoperational stage from about 2 to 7 years, (3) the concrete operations stage from about 7 to 11/12 years, and (4) the formal operations stage from about 11 years to 14/15 years. These are described in more detail in Table 1.7.

Within the first year of infancy, specifically during the sensorimotor stage of cognitive development, children develop a particularly important cognitive ability that enables them

TABLE 1.7 | Characteristics of Piaget's Stages of Cognitive Development

Sensorimotor (0–2 years)
Substage 1: 0–2 months
Reflexive sensorimotor behavior Reflexive vocal/prelinguistic behavior
Substage 2: 2–4 months
Coordinated hand–mouth movements Coordinated eye–hand and auditory orienting movements Anticipatory gestures
Substage 3: 4–8 months
Begins to act motorically on objects Searches for objects Babbles and imitates sounds
Substage 4: 8–12 months
Begins to recognize own ability to cause objects to move Early stages of walking Searches for objects based on memory of last location Uses first word

TABLE 1.7 | *Continued*

Sensorimotor (0–2 years)
Substage 5: 12–18 months
Experimentation with objects' functions and properties Imitates models' behaviors when models present Walks Evidence of object permanency
Substage 6: 18–24 months
Represents objects internally Problem solving with thought Acquires basic cause–effect relations Uses memory for deferred imitations Uses words when referents not present
Preoperational (2–7 years)
Preconceptual: 2–4 years
Experiences difficulty with sub- and supraclassifications Uses transductive reasoning (inferences from one specific to another specific) Over- and underextends word meanings
Intuitive: 4–7 years
Thought guided by perceptions Deals with only one variable at a time Lacks conservation and reversibility Employs improved but still inadequate classification skills Egocentric Concreteness of thought
Concrete Operations (7–11/12 years)
Uses effective classification skills Acquires conservation and seriation skills Uses coordinated descriptions Employs logical causality Reasoning limited to concrete operations Less egocentric
Formal Operations (11/12–14/15 years)
Uses hypothetical and prepositional reasoning Demonstrates lack of egocentricity Employs adequate verbal reasoning and logical "if . . . then" statements Can deal with the abstract Uses deductive and inductive thought processes

to learn more about the world in which they live—they learn to create symbolic mental representations. That is, they learn to represent their environment in their brains, not just as it occurs in the here and now. This is important for language acquisition. Recall that earlier in this chapter we defined language as a code in which we make specific symbols stand for something else. Thus, it would seem that cognition and language are related. However, there is no universal agreement concerning the nature of the relationship. Does cognitive development for specific mental processes occur *before* the acquisition of language structures? Does language influence cognition? Are the developments of language and cognition separate entities that become entwined at some point? If so, when? Finally, how do language and cognition influence each other? We have no definitive answers to these questions yet, although a number of theoretical positions regarding the relationship of language and cognition have been advanced.

The Relationship between Cognition and Language. The relationship between cognition and language is not completely understood but many theories about this relationship have been proposed. The theories have been known to cause scholarly debates among their proponents, some more heated than others. An in-depth discussion of the theories is not appropriate for this text, so the following sections present a few of the more prominent perspectives of the earlier theorists whose work has provided foundations for our thinking about language and cognition today and whose work has, therefore, influenced many of the intervention approaches that are used with children with language disorders.

Dependency of Language on Cognition. According to one view of the relationship between language and cognition, language use is a function of cognition, and its acquisition is dependent on underlying cognitive processes. Proponents of this position strongly support the notion of cognitive precursors to language, that is, prerequisite cognitive abilities that children need to develop before learning various language skills. This viewpoint is sometimes referred to as the *strong cognition hypothesis*.

Piaget is one of the best-known advocates of this position. According to Piaget, children progress through each of the cognitive developmental stages he proposed (*see* Table 1.7) in order, without skipping any of them, and each stage of development is the foundation for each succeeding stage. As children progress through the stages, they acquire the necessary cognitive operations that lead to the development of successively higher levels of language. Piaget, therefore, believes that thought precedes language. Language use is a reflection of underlying cognitive skills.

A related view of language functioning as dependent on cognition is the *weak cognition hypothesis.* This position proposes that cognition accounts for many of a child's language abilities but not all of them. There remain some aspects of language that do not derive directly from cognition. Rice (1983) referred to this as a partial "mismatch" between language and cognition and presented, as examples of the mismatch, "language acquisition not rooted in parallel change in meanings, linguistic competence exceeding the supposed cognitive base, and language-specific difficulties with the expression of meanings" (p. 353).

Language and Cognition as Separate (but Sometimes Related) Entities. A differing point of view concerning language and cognition is that although language and cognition are related, cognitive activity without language and language without underlying cognitive bases are both possible. For example, a composer or a sculptor at work is not necessarily directed by language processes (Langacker, 1968). From this perspective, cognition without language is possible. In contrast, Vygotsky (1962) proposed that language without appropriate underlying cognitive bases also occurs. He cited examples in which children correctly use conjunctions, such as *because, but,* and *if,* before they understand the logical relationships expressed by the terms.

Vygotsky (1962) also suggested that the developments of language and thought stem from different roots. A child progresses independently through a "preintellectual language" period and a "prelinguistic thought" phase. Although these lines of development are separate for some time, the two developmental processes do eventually merge. The child's thought then becomes verbal and language rational. According to Vygotsky (1962), once the union of language and thought has occurred, language becomes the foundation of further cognitive development:

> The . . . [language] structures mastered by the child become the basic structures of his thinking. . . . The child's intellectual growth is contingent on his mastering the social means of thought, that is, language. (p. 51)

The *local homology model* offers a different point of view (Bates, 1979; Bates, Benigni, Bretherton, Camaioni, & Volterra, 1977). Some have observed that certain cognitive and linguistic skills develop at the same time but not necessarily in a predetermined order. That is, a specific language ability sometimes emerges first, and in other instances a cognitive ability appears. This perspective suggests a correlative relationship between language and cognition for some skills at certain points in time, but the particular correlation between cognitive and language skills may not be maintained over time. Both language and cognition are seen as distinct functions that derive from a common but separate source. This model has found considerable favor with a number of professionals and researchers in the child language area.

Language Mediation of Cognition. Although there may not be agreement on the exact nature of the early relationship between language and cognition, many suggest that, once acquired, language does mediate many of our cognitive processes. Although Piaget believed that in the earlier stages of a child's development thought precedes language use, he stressed the importance of language in the acquisition of conceptual thinking in the later stages of a child's development.

Both Vygotsky (1962) and Luria (1961) have proposed that language mediates cognitive activity. They used their concepts of *inner speech* and language as a *second signal system* to explain. Vygotsky (1962) and Luria (1961) viewed inner speech as thought processes that take place in the form of words. Once language and thought have merged (as previously discussed), thinking occurs in terms of language or word meanings.

Vygotsky's concepts of inner speech led him to disagree with Piaget on the role of children's *egocentric* speech. Piaget described the egocentric speech of young children as speech that occurs with no intent to communicate with others, whether or not others are present, or with no attempt to consider the informational needs of others in communication. It is speech emanating from children who see themselves as the centers of the universe, without communicative concern for others. According to Piaget, egocentric speech disappears as children develop, and socialized speech—speech aimed specifically at interpersonal communication—emerges. Vygotsky, however, proposed that the egocentric speech of children is a forerunner of inner speech. He viewed the function of egocentric speech as an overt act of thought, or putting thought into expressed words. According to Vygotsky, the acts of expressing cognitive processes in words are children's ways of guiding and regulating their actions and thoughts. He suggested that as children develop, they are able to turn the overt expressions of thought inward into language, which is used for the same purposes of regulating and guiding thoughts and actions but is not heard by others, that is, inner speech. In contrast to Piaget, Vygotsky described egocentric speech as evolving into inner speech rather than disappearing and being replaced by socialized speech.

The discussion of egocentric speech functioning to regulate and guide thought and action and then evolving into inner speech for the same guiding and regulating purposes leads us to Luria's view of language functioning as a second signal system. As children interact with the environment and the verbalizations of adults, complex connections between perceived phenomena and words are formed (Luria & Yudovich, 1971). Initially, adult verbalizations in the presence of stimuli serve to guide children's behaviors, either to focus the children's attention on specific, essential features of stimuli or to modify and direct their actions in certain directions. That is, in the early developmental stages, the regulation (or direction) of children's cognitive activities and behaviors is externally controlled by the verbalizations of adults that occur simultaneously with perceived phenomena. Because of the connections between these perceptions and others' verbalizations, children eventually begin to use the verbalizations internally to regulate their own behaviors. Through this process, children learn to use language to direct their own thoughts and actions. Language becomes a mediator of cognition and purposeful behavior. For Luria, language is the basis of the development of higher mental processes because of the second signal function it plays in mediating experiences.

We have seen here several different views on the relationship between language and cognition. What we generally agree on, however, is that there is a relationship and that the relationship is different at different stages of development.

Information Processing. Information processing refers to the ways in which we deal with incoming stimuli and what we do in our heads to figure them out. There is considerable discussion in the literature about the role of various aspects of information processing in children's language learning and language disorders (e.g., Coady & Evans, 2008; Graf Estes, Evans, & Else-Quest, 2007; Leonard et al., 2007; Montgomery, Evans, & Gillam, 2009; Windsor,

Milbrath, Carney, & Rakowski, 2001). Several information processing models have been proposed, and in comparing models it is not unusual to find that they include different component processes, label the processes differently, and use different definitions for what appear to be similar processes. Furthermore, no one information processing model has been universally adopted. Ellis Weismer and Evans (2002) suggest that information processing accounts related to children's language disorders fall mostly into two broad groups—those emphasizing generalized processing and those focusing more on specific aspects of processing. Among the specific processing accounts, two aspects of processing are frequently discussed—phonological processing, which deals with the processes involved in the ability to mentally manipulate phonological aspects of language such as word rhyming or breaking words into their components, and temporal auditory processing, which deals more specifically with the ability to perceive brief acoustic events that comprise speech sounds and track changes in these as they occur quickly in others' speech. Among the generalized processing accounts, speed of processing (e.g., Miller, Kail, Leonard, & Tomblin, 2001), attentional capacity (e.g., Finneran, Francis, & Leonard, 2009), and overall processing capacity (Ellis Weismer, Evans, & Hesketh, 1999; Montgomery, 2000) are among those prominent in discussions.

Processing linguistically based (verbal) information involves such functions as the following:

- Selecting the elements of a verbal message to attend to
- Temporarily storing the representations of those elements in memory
- Keeping those representations active in our short-term memory so that they do not fade, disappear, or decay before we are finished working with them
- Organizing our cognitive functions and directing them to undertake particular tasks with the representations, that is, our analysis of the representations
- Choosing where and how to store the analyses of the representations in longer-term memory for future use—or in some cases not sending the analyzed information to long-term memory store

It can also involve how and when we access the stored information at a later date, the form in which it is available to us, and the degree to which the original elements are or are not distorted as a result of all the processing. On a small scale, it is not unlike what we do when someone tells us a new telephone number and we need to walk into another part of the house to dial it. Most of us attend carefully to presentation of the number and then make a conscious (cognitive) effort to keep the number rumbling around in our heads so that we can actually "hear" the number silently in our heads as we move to the other room. We do not want any part of the auditory representation of the complete number to disappear on us. If the number is one we believe we need only once, many of us promptly let the auditory representation of the number in our heads decay after dialing it. That is, we forget the phonological representation, "phonological" because the numbers are words to us and the words are made up of phonemes. If we believe we will need the number again at a later time after we dial it, we undertake different processing strategies to move it into our long-term memory, or we record it somewhere else in a different form. If we do the latter, we need to be able to find it when we need it—another memory process. If we decide to store it in our heads, we still need to be able to find and retrieve it when we need it—a different processing and memory process. Some of the associated terms encountered in information processing literature are *verbal working memory, working memory, short-term memory, auditory short-term memory, auditory processing, phonological processing, phonological memory,* and so on. Different terms are obviously associated with different accounts of information processing.

If we have inefficient or slow processing, smaller temporary storage capacities or resource limitations, poor working memories, problems dealing with fleeting, transitory auditory stimuli, or poor executive override and control of our processing, the elements we need to retain for processing incoming stimuli will decay in our heads before we have a chance to go through all the other processes we need to do with them for them to make sense, be usable, or learn from. Something we also need to keep in mind is that while we are trying to process one thing, other information is coming our way. "System overload" is possible if tasks to be processed are too hard or too fast for us and/or our systems are too fragile to deal with what might be quite easy tasks for another individual with a more robust system. These ideas find their way into concepts about children and their language impairments when we talk about trade-offs between different aspects of language performance, children's repetition of nonsense words as a way of assessing their information processing of phonological aspects of language, rehearsal strategies, central auditory processing disorder, and many other topics related to children's language learning or their problems with language. These are among the concepts associated with information processing ability that readers will encounter in different parts of this text. In fact, our upcoming discussion of metacognition is not devoid of notions related to information processing.

Metacognition. Earlier in this chapter, we introduced the concept of metalinguistics. Like metalinguistics, metacognition relates to the ability to stand back from what we know and the cognitive skills that we have and to consciously analyze, control, plan, and organize them. As adults, we can think about our thinking and can decide what learning and cognitive strategies we might want to use in specific situations. We can even monitor our performance and may decide to employ different learning or cognitive strategies. For example, if we need to memorize a list, we might choose to use any of several types of rehearsal strategies—saying the list over and over, writing the list over and over, or making up sayings (associations). If one strategy does not work, we may choose to abandon it for another or to use several strategies simultaneously. In other instances, we may ask ourselves, "What else do I know with which I can associate this new piece of information?" or "How can I organize this information so it makes sense?" These are all metacognitive activities.

In order to engage in metacognitive activities, we need to *decenter,* that is, be less egocentric. Like metalinguistics, true metacognition in children is a later-developing skill, with some suggesting a shift to metacognitive abilities occurring sometime in the early elementary grades. These grades tend to correspond to about the time children enter Piaget's concrete operations stage (Table 1.7). Another shift to higher-level, more refined metacognitive skills is generally seen at about grade 6, or 11 to 12 years of age, about the time children enter Piaget's formal operations stage.

Not surprisingly, metacognitive skills are important in school success. Expectations for how children are to solve problems and approach learning increase as children progress through school. By high school, students are expected to monitor and plan their own learning and to think and reason with adultlike abilities. We suspect some relationship between metacognitive and metalinguistic skills, but, as with the relationship between cognition and language generally, the exact nature of the relationship is not clear. We do know, however, that many children with language disorders evidence problems with metacognitive tasks as well as problems with metalinguistic tasks.

Social Bases of Human Communication

At birth, babies seem to have an innate tendency to seek social interaction. For example, newborns are particularly attracted to faces despite never having seen one. They will maintain their gaze at the face of an adult who is holding them and even show evidence of imitating facial movements of the adult. We can see how such eye gaze and facial imitations could logically influence an infant's communication development. In fact, as we will see later in this text, infant's problems in engaging in early eye gaze and facial imitations may be early warning signs of the presence of possible autism spectrum disorders.

In this section we will see that the social influences in children's language-learning environments play a major role in their acquisition of language and the rules that govern how the code is used in context. What follows is a short discussion of the social bases of communication. We look at infant–caregiver attachment and the nature of infant–caregiver interactions. We also look at two skills that are integral to social interaction and language learning: imitation and reinforcement.

Infant–Caregiver Attachment. During the first few months of an infant's life, he or she does not appear to mind being held by strangers or being briefly separated from caregivers. However, as infants get older, they begin to show definite signs of attachment. They may cry or become distressed when separated from familiar caregivers. By the time infants learn to crawl, they may display attachment by following their parents and actively seeking to maintain contact with them.

There are several reasons infants become attached to their caregivers. Certainly, one reason for this behavior is that specific adults take care of the infant's basic needs. However, there seems to be more to the behavior; healthy infant–caregiver attachment may be the result of parents and infants sharing a unique system of communication. Caregivers become familiar with the ways their infants communicate needs and wants. The relationship is reciprocal. Infants learn that their caregivers are the ones who "understand" them and meet needs. In other words, there appears to be an interactional, communicative component to the infant–caregiver attachment.

Infant–Caregiver Interaction. Both infants and caregivers have behaviors that are conducive to communication development. As we read previously, infants have a preference for looking at the human face. Caregivers reciprocate by spending time gazing at their infant's face while producing a wide array of facial expressions that in turn sustain the infant's interest. Such early interactions provide a social foundation for speech and language development.

Infant Behaviors during Infant–Caregiver Interactions. Certain infant behaviors appear to stimulate adults to respond in specific ways. One of the main behaviors or attributes of an infant that seems to motivate adults to attend to them and respond to their needs is their helplessness. As we have also seen, infants prefer looking at the face. This is assisted by the fact that an infant's best visual acuity is around the distance from the adult face to the infant being cradled in an adult's arms. Infants also show a preference for their mother's voice. Other infant behaviors that seem to act as positive reinforcers of adults' language stimulation include eye gaze, smiling, and reciprocal touch and vocalization. As children become capable of producing some speech, they provide verbal feedback to adults in terms of what has and has not been comprehended, and they signal understanding by increasing their attention to the adults. Thus, children actually regulate the type of input they receive from caregivers so that the input can match what language models the children need to learn from at different developmental levels.

Caregiver Behaviors and Language during Infant–Caregiver Interactions. When adults interact with infants, they typically demonstrate a communication style different from the way they communicate with peers. Some of these behaviors include the following:

- Vocalizing in response to an infant's smile
- Moving in closer to the infant
- Engaging in eye gaze with the infant
- Holding and cuddling the infant in their arms
- Imitating the infant's behavior
- Waiting for the infant to respond to the adult's behavior, such as a smile or vocalization, and as such engaging the infant in turn taking
- Engaging in rituals and routines such as "peekaboo"

Caregivers have also been shown to tune in to and respond to the different types of cries produced by their infants (hunger, pain, and anger cry). The caregiver's responses may, in fact, teach infants that a cry results in attention, and therefore, if they want attention, they initiate a cry.

In addition to the array of adult behaviors listed previously, the speech and language used by adults when conversing with infants and young children differs. Most investigations of adults' communication with young children have focused on mothers. Consequently, results tend to focus on discussions of *motherese,* or *infant-directed speech,* terms used to describe the unique characteristics of caregiver language patterns to young children. Table 1.8 summarizes a number of the unique characteristics of these patterns.

TABLE 1.8 | Characteristics of *Motherese/Infant-Directed Speech*

Short utterances
Syntactically simple but grammatically well-formed utterances
More concrete nouns and verbs and fewer modifiers in utterances
Proper nouns replacing pronouns
Length and complexity varied as a function of children's ages and language skills
Higher pitched than speech addressed to adults
Rising intonation patterns rather than falling patterns at the ends of the utterances
Duration of spoken words longer
Overall rate of speech slowed
Obvious pauses occur between individual utterances in mothers' speech
More than one stressed word in utterances
Stressed words typically substantive words rather than function words

As infants become young children and begin to use speech and language, not only do adults appear to modify their verbal input, but they also appear to alter the ways they respond to children's utterances. For example, corrections of young children's inaccurate utterances tend to be corrections of content (semantics) rather than morphosyntactic or phonological corrections. As children get older, however, mothers begin to correct these latter aspects of their children's utterances. During parent–child communicative interactions, adults have been found to respond to what the children say by using expansions and recasts of the children's utterances, with semantically contingent responses that may be paraphrases of the children's comments. Furthermore, adult responses tend to consist of frequent repetitions of messages.

Thus, it would seem that infant–caregiver interactions lay the foundation for speech and language acquisition. Infants seem to be prewired for social interaction. They also engage in certain behaviors that elicit responses from the adults around them. They become attached to caregivers who understand and respond to the ways in which they communicate. Primitive as these early communicative attempts may be, they pave the way for more complex symbolic communication. Caregivers also seem to have an ability to respond to infants that not only meets their needs but also provides them with a sociolinguistically rich environment that fosters speech and language acquisition.

Infant–Caregiver Interactions and Language Disorders: A Possible Link? Infants' responses to adult inputs can motivate the adults to continue their language-facilitating behaviors, discontinue them, or modify the behaviors to some that are less beneficial for language learning. Parents of children with language disorders have sometimes been criticized for not providing adequate and appropriate language stimulation for their children. However, this may not be a totally fair judgment. For the most part, parents of children with language disorders have been found to provide language stimulation similar to the stimulation that parents of younger children with normal language acquisition provide. In other instances, parents of children with language disorders may engage in some types of child–adult interactions that are less conducive to children's language learning. We must be careful, however, not to overgeneralize. In light of our previous discussion, it may be that the children, because of their disorders, do not provide the reinforcement for the parents to engage in appropriate language stimulation activities. It appears that children with a disability may not respond to parents' attention in ways that positively reinforce the parents to provide appropriate language stimulation.

Imitation and Reinforcement. The roles of imitation and reinforcement in language acquisition have been debated. Much of this debate has probably resulted from differing definitions of the terms. Imitation, if viewed as children's exact reproductions of adults' utterances, cannot account fully for the language-learning process. If that were the entire basis of language and speech acquisition, children would not produce novel utterances. On the other hand, if we view imitation in light of Bandura's (1971) concept of social, observational learning, in which adults provide numerous models from which children abstract the key elements to form rules for behavior, then imitation that encompasses the rules, not exact duplications of the models, may well be involved in language learning.

This discussion does not imply that imitation in the form of exact duplications has no role in language learning, although its role may change as a function of age and/or language skill. Young children approaching the end of the sensorimotor stage of cognitive development have been found to produce a high percentage of imitative utterances. However, as productive language skills develop, the number of imitative responses decreases as children begin to use a higher proportion of unique, spontaneously generated utterances.

The role of reinforcement in language acquisition is also unclear. Reinforcement, as it is used in conditioning or stimulus–response theories of learning (Skinner, 1957), is not totally sufficient for language learning. Not all of children's early utterances are reinforced, and those that are may not be reinforced in a manner conducive to learning to talk. Yet children do learn to talk. Humans are social beings. If infants find that their early vocalizations and if toddlers discover that their early words establish and maintain adults' interactions with them, then we may consider that reinforcement is operating. Furthermore, adults' expansions and paraphrases of children's utterances, in addition to providing language models, probably serve to reinforce verbal behavior because they also maintain the adults' interactions with the children and support language production.

SUMMARY

In this chapter we have seen that

- Communication refers to the sending and receiving of messages. It can be as simple as a sigh or as complex as a spoken word.
- Extralinguistic aspects of communication include paralinguistics, nonlinguistics, and metalinguistics.
- Language consists of a system of phonological, semantic, morphological, syntactic, and pragmatic rules that are used to put ideas and thoughts into a code in order to communicate them to others and to relate to others. Language is the code; speech is one of several sensorimotor processes that can be used to produce the code.
- Communication involves both comprehension and production, but the relationship between comprehension and production is not fully agreed on.
- Communication can be accomplished through several modes: auditory–oral (hearing and speech), visual–graphic (reading and writing), and visual–gestural modes.
- Communication has biological, social, and cognitive bases.
- Metacognition involves conscious analysis, control, planning, and organization of our thinking.
- Infants have a tendency to seek social interaction, such as a preference for looking at the face, and engage in certain behaviors that make them active partners in their own language learning.
- Caregivers engage in an array of behaviors that facilitate social interaction with infants.

Communication refers to the sending and receiving of messages. For humans, language is the major vehicle for communication. Language comes about as a result of complex interactions among cognitive, physiological, psychological, and sociological factors. Numerous approaches have been taken in attempting to explain these interactions. None alone is sufficient to describe how children learn language. Language is a complicated human behavior that has yet to be explained by any single theory or approach.

2

Normal Language Development

A REVIEW

LEARNING OBJECTIVES

After reading this chapter, you should be able to

- Describe characteristics of infant communication development in the prelinguistic period
- Describe characteristics of language skills of children in the first-word period and aged 1.0 to 2.0 years
- Describe characteristics of language development of children in the two-word period
- Describe major features and characteristics of the language development of preschool and school-aged children
- Describe features and characteristics of language development in adolescence
- Describe features of literacy development and expectations of school and relationships with language

For young children, learning language is a relatively orderly process, although not all children acquire all language abilities in precisely the same order and at identical speed. There is individual variation. Nevertheless, as a general pattern, newly acquired skills are used to modify and augment existing language abilities, and these new abilities are based on earlier learned skills. The process is one of refinement, expansion, and extension. Language learning is synergistic in nature. All components of language—syntax, morphology, semantics, phonology, and pragmatics—interact to evolve gradually into adultlike competence. Although there is variability in individual children's language acquisition, there is also a great deal of consistency. What may be the most amazing aspect of this process is that by about 7 to 8 years of age, most children have learned to use oral language to communicate in basically adultlike fashion. This does not mean, however, that language development stops at these ages. We need to be careful not to fall into the trap of thinking that only uninteresting and minor language development occurs beyond 8 years of age. Many important language skills, especially those essential for higher levels of literacy acquisition and academic success, are not fully acquired until the adolescent years and possibly beyond. For adolescents, however, their continuing language growth is less predictable across individuals than for younger children because what language is acquired varies considerably based on their individual varying life experiences and academic learning. Nevertheless, 7- and 8-year-old children typically produce a wide variety of well-formed sentences containing large numbers of different words with only rare speech production errors. Moreover, they use these sentence types and words effectively and fluently for many different purposes. Language acquisition in adolescence takes advantage of school curriculum, cognitive growth into the formal operations stage, and prior language learning so that language abilities explode in the areas of metalinguistics skills, discourse genres, high-level abstract semantic skills, complex syntax containing multiply embedded relative and other subordinate clauses, and morphologically complex vocabularly.

In this chapter, we will take a quick trip through some of the language achievements of younger children. The discussion is by no means complete, and much more has been written about children's language acquisition. An extensive discussion is well beyond the scope of this book. What this chapter does provide is an overview of some of the major language milestones during early childhood. We will then turn our attention to language development in adolescence. We also take a brief look at language and emergent literacy, the educational sequence of the early grades in which children need to use their language skills to achieve, and reading expectations across primary and secondary grades.

THE PRELINGUISTIC PERIOD: THE FIRST 12 MONTHS

From the moment of birth, newborns communicate. Sucking movements may indicate that a newborn is ready to feed, squinting may indicate digestive upset, and crying may indicate pain. This period during which an infant communicates but does not use language is known as the *prelinguistic period*. To the casual observer, the prelinguistic period may seem quite uneventful. To the trained observer, however, the prelinguistic period is a hive of developmental activity. An incredible amount of learning takes place prior to an infant's first birthday in order for the "first word" to be uttered. The term *infant* is used in this section, in keeping with the Latin form of the word *infans*, which means "one unable to speak."

Prelinguistic Communication Development

To appreciate the communication development of the prelinguistic infant, an understanding of the basic "pragmatic" elements of a speech act is needed. These basic elements include (1) the speaker having an intention to communicate—known as *illocution*, (2) the speaker expressing intention—known as *locution*, and (3) the listener interpreting another's intended utterance—known as *perlocution* (Bates, 1976). During the first 8 months of an infant's life, the focus is on the perlocutionary element of the speech act, and this is therefore known as the perlocutionary period. During this period, caregivers have a vital role to play in facilitating learning because the infant's behaviors are not intentionally communicative but need to be interpreted as communicative. Some of the infant's behaviors that caregivers interpret as communicative include the following:

- Different cries that reflect hunger, pain, or anger
- Facial expressions, including displeasure, fear, sorrow, anger, joy, and disgust
- Eye-gaze patterns, including mutual gaze (prolonged eye contact), gaze coupling (infant and caregiver looking at each other, looking away, and looking back), and deictic gaze (infant looking at an object of interest)
- Moving limbs and making mouth movements, such as opening the mouth, pushing the tongue forward, and smiling, when in a settled state

By about 3 months of age, the infant and caregiver engage in protoconversations. These often consist of the caregiver initiating an interaction, followed by the infant and caregiver engaging in greeting behaviors (mutual smiles and eye gazes). Play dialogue follows the greeting. During play dialogue, the caregiver talks, then pauses to allow the infant time to vocalize during the pause. The dialogue continues until the infant or caregiver looks away.

These are sometimes also referred to as reciprocal interactions between adult and child. Protoconversations are an important experience for the infant, as they teach the infant the basic ingredients of a conversation, including initiating and taking turns. By 6 months of age, many infant–caregiver interactions become triadic because they begin to extend to an object or a toy of interest.

By about 8 months of age, the infant begins to show signs of communicative intent and thus enters the illocutionary period of communication development. This period typically spans the period 8 to 12 months of age. Gestures such as showing objects to adults, requesting items by pointing to them, and giving objects to adults are considered hallmarks of the illocutionary period. During this period, infants are able to follow the eye direction of an adult to locate an object at which the adult looks when the object is present in the infant's visual field. This ability to use joint attention or mutual gaze is important because it provides a basis for pairing words with objects. Another important communication milestone occurs around 8 to 9 months, specifically, the infants' comprehension of spoken words.

By 12 months of age, the infant enters the final stage for the development of the speech act, known as the locutionary period. Between 12 and 18 months of age, children gradually become able to use joint attention to locate objects outside their immediate visual field. Also at about the time of an infant's first birthday, he or she begins to use words to accompany or replace gestures. True language or symbolic representation of thought expressed in words has begun. A major milestone in language development has been achieved. The infant is no longer "unable to speak," has typically begun to walk, and is therefore considered a toddler.

Prelinguistic Vocal Development

The sounds that infants make in the first year of life change from reflexive vocalizations to babbling to the emergence of the first word at approximately 12 months of age. This section reviews the vocal development of the infant over the first 12 months.

Stage 1 (Birth to 2 Months): Reflexive Vocalizations. From birth to approximately 2 months, the infant has a relatively small repertoire of reflexive vocalizations and vegetative sounds. The first reflexive vocalization is the birth cry, which is produced in response to the first breath. Subsequent cries signaling hunger, pain, and anger are considered a reaction to internal stimuli. Other types of reflexive vocalizations include coughing, grunting, and burping. Vegetative sounds include sighs, vowel-like sounds, and grunts associated with an activity, in addition to lip and tongue clicks and other noises associated with feeding.

Stage 2 (2 to 4 Months): Cooing and Laughter. From 2 to 4 months, the infant's range of vocalizations changes with the appearance of cooing, sounds associated with pleasure, and laughter. *Cooing* refers to vowel-like sounds (often "oo") preceded by velar consonant-like sounds such as "g" or "k." Infants are thought to coo when they are in a comfortable state. Infants have also been observed to produce pleasure-like sounds such as "mmmm" during this stage. Laughter emerges around 16 weeks. Crying and primitive vegetative sounds are thought to reduce from about 12 weeks on.

Stage 3 (4 to 6 Months): Vocal Play. From 4 to 6 months, the infant's repertoire of vocalizations expands to include a greater number of vowel-like and consonant-like sounds (including front plosives and nasals) to make way for marginal babbling. In marginal babbling, consonant and consonant-like sounds combine with vowels to create approximated syllables. Some of these productions contain sounds that are consistent with those in the infant's native language but others are not. Productions tend to favor those produced at the front so that we see the emergence of what are called the classic infant "raspberries" as well as lip smack. Intonation variations and other productions such as squeals and yells emerge.

Stage 4 (6 Months and Older): Canonical Babbling. The age 6 months is notable for the beginning of canonical babbling, which consists of reduplicated and nonreduplicated

TABLE 2.1 | Types of Canonical Babbling Seen in Infants from about Age 6 Months and Older

Type of Babbling	Description
Reduplicated	■ Repetitive string of consonant–vowel productions ■ Consonant sound remains constant ■ May exhibit slight vowel changes ■ Example: "mamamama" ■ Tends to predominate in earlier babbling period (i.e., from about 6 months)
Nonreduplicated or variegated	■ Repetitive string of consonant–vowel productions ■ Both consonant and vowel may change ■ Example: "mababena" ■ Tends to emerge somewhat later than reduplicated babbling ■ Becomes frequent at about 12–13 months of age

(or variegated) babbling. Babbling consists of well-formed syllables that contain at least one vowel-like sound and one consonant-like sound that are connected in quick succession. Descriptions of the two types of babbling observed during this stage are found in Table 2.1.

Stage 5 (10 Months and Older): Jargon Stage. The final stage of prelinguistic vocal development coincides with children's production of first words. Jargon refers to series of mostly nonreduplicated (variegated) babbles overlaid with varieties of intonation and stress patterns. Other names for this type of jargon include conversational babble and modulated babble. During this stage, parents are often convinced that their infant is trying to say something, and strangers hearing it might do a double take, believing that the infant has talked to them. First words may in fact be produced among a string of jargon.

The types of consonants produced in jargon include stops, nasals, and glides, and these are also typical of children's first words. Consonant types that do not appear in babbling include fricatives, affricates, and liquids. Predictably, these are not typical sounds of children's first words. These observations provide support for the continuity hypothesis, which, according to Menn and Stoel-Gammon (2008), suggests that "children's phonological patterns in early meaningful speech are linked directly to the patterns that they [children] use in babbling" (p. 72).

THE FIRST-WORD PERIOD

Phonology

Children typically produce their first word around their first birthday. To be considered a true word, it needs to be used consistently in a specific context, and it needs to have a recognizable phonetic form. That is, although the word may not match the adult pronunciation, it needs to closely resemble the adult target. During the beginning stages of phonological acquisition, children show individual variation. For example, although most children use plosive and nasal sounds, one child may favor labial sounds, such as /b/ and /m/, while another child may favor alveolar sounds, such as /d/ and /n/. It is possible that first words are entire phonological units rather than series of individual speech sounds. This would be consistent with an infant's early jargon and babbling patterns. Once children have a single-word vocabulary of about 50 words, they adopt a new, more efficient strategy of treating each word as being made up of individual sounds, and as such they seem to enter a stage in which they pay attention to the phonological rules of the language they are learning.

Semantics

Recall from Chapter 1 that children from birth to about 2 years of age are in Piaget's sensorimotor stage of cognitive development. One of the resulting cognitive achievements is the concept of object permanence, or object constancy, that is, that objects exist in the environment even though they may not be immediately visible. Object permanence is a basis for internal representations of the environment, mental images, or symbols of those objects and events that exist around the children. Many suggest that these internal representations are related to children's ability to use verbal symbols—words.

Lahey's (1988) classic work, still relevant today, identified three broad categories of the types of single words that children use to represent what they learn about the environment: *substantive, relational*, and *social*. Children use *substantive words* to name objects. Many of the words are used to refer to classes or categories of objects. As children learn more about the perceptual or behavioral consistency of objects, they learn that objects with similarly identified characteristics have the same names. Many of these early words are names for objects on which children can act and produce changes, such as *cookie, ball*, and *shoe*. Children at this stage use fewer attributives, such as words referring to color and size, than names for objects. Other types of substantive words refer to objects that children believe exist only as one of a kind. There is only one "Mommy," one favorite blanket, and, to the child, one bottle. In a child's mind, these are unique instances of objects that do not belong to a class of objects.

The second broad category of single-word utterances consists of relational words. *Relational words* describe the relationships or characteristics among objects, including movements of objects, or relationships of an object to itself, such as an object that has suddenly disappeared. Although most children use more substantive words than relational words, the reverse has been noted in some children. Types of relational words include existence, nonexistence/disappearance, recurrence, rejection, denial, attribution, possession, action, and locative action (Lahey, 1988). Table 2.2 lists and explains the types of relational words that children use in the single-word stage. It is important to realize that the same word may actually be used to express several different relations. For example, *no* can be used to indicate

TABLE 2.2 | Relations Expressed in Single-Word Utterances

Relation	Explanation
Existence	An object is present in a child's immediate environment, and the child is attending to it. Examples: *this, that, ball, there*
Nonexistence/ disappearance	An object is expected to be present but is not. An action is expected to occur but does not. An object has been present but disappears. Examples: *all gone, no, bye-bye*
Recurrence	An object reappears. Another object like the one the child is attending to is placed with the first one. An event happens again. Examples: *more, another*
Rejection	The child does not want an object or an event to occur. Example: *no*
Denial	The child rejects the truthfulness of a previous utterance. Example: *no*
Attribution	The child mentions a characteristic of an object or event, usually not shape or color in this stage. Examples: *big, little*
Possession	The child identifies ownership of an object. Examples: *mine, my*
Action	The child identifies or requests an action. Examples: *go, open*
Locative action	The child refers to a change in an object's location. Examples: *here, there, in, up*

Source: Lahey (1988).

rejection, denial, or nonexistence/disappearance. *No* is a very functional, versatile, and important word for children. A noun, such as *ball*, can be used to mean existence or recurrence (hence a relational word) or to label the object (hence a substantive word).

The last broad category of single-word utterances consists of *social words*, such as *hi* and *bye*. These are important words in a child's early repertoire, as they provide a foundation for establishing and maintaining human relationships according to the culture's social code. Although they are important, these words, unlike substantive and relational words, do not lead to later grammatical complexity.

During the single-word-utterance stage, there also seems to be a relationship between a child's phonological and semantic development. Children appear to learn more easily and quickly new words that begin with consonants they have used previously in other words than they do words that begin with consonants they have not yet used, and children exhibit greater phonetic accuracy in saying object words than action words. These observations suggest the notion of synergism among the various components of language in children's development.

Pragmatics

One classification system of the various functions appearing in the communication of very young children that is still used today is that of Halliday (1975). He described seven purposes, or functions, of communicative attempts that occur between approximately 9 to 16 or 18 months of age. Table 2.3 lists and explains these seven functions. Because these functions emerge during part of a period in which children have few words, much of the communication may be accomplished in nonverbal ways. Halliday's (1975) view of communicative functions considered the listeners' responses. On the other hand, Dore (1975), who concentrated on the period during which children are using single words (approximately 12 to 18/24 months), focused on children's intention to use these single-word utterances, with less emphasis on the listeners'

TABLE 2.3 | Children's Functions and Intentions of Their Early Language

Halliday's Functions (9 to 16/18 months of age)		Dore's Intentions (approximately 12 to 18/24 months)	
Function	*Description*	*Intention*	*Description*
		Labeling	To name objects; no response expected
Instrumental	To receive material needs, desired objects, or assistance from others	Answering	To respond to adult's request
Regulatory	To control the behavior of others	Requesting action	To get adult to do something
Interactional	To make interpersonal contact with others in their environment by initiating and/or sustaining contact with other people	Requesting an answer	To get adult to respond to request verbally
Personal	To demonstrate awareness of self and express one's own feelings and individuality	Calling/addressing	To address adult; to get adult's attention
Heuristic	To attempt to have environments or events in the environments explained	Greeting	To acknowledge adult's or object's presence
Imaginative	To pretend or playact	Protesting	To resist or deny adult's action
Informative	To communicate experiences or tell someone something	Repeating/imitating	To model utterance after adult's; no response expected
		Practicing (language)	To rehearse language to self; no response expected

Sources: Dore (1975); Halliday (1975).

reactions to the intents. Dore's (1975) intentions are also shown in Table 2.3. As Prutting (1979) explains, Dore provides a way of identifying children's reasons (intentions) for communication, while Halliday furnishes a way of describing how well the reasons worked or functioned.

During the stage from about 16 or 18 months to 24 months, children use language for different functions. Earlier instrumental and regulatory functions combine with part of the interactional function to form a new function—the pragmatic function (Halliday, 1974). The *pragmatic function* is basically a controlling one that is used to satisfy desires and needs while interacting with people at the same time. Some response from the listener is expected. The newly acquired mathetic function is derived from the more basic personal and heuristic functions in combination, again, with part of the interactional function. The *mathetic function* focuses on language as a tool for learning more about the environment (e.g., asking the names of objects) and for commenting on the environment. In contrast to the pragmatic function, the mathetic function does not always require a response from the listener. Children use a third function during this period: the informative function. In employing the *informative function*, children actually convey information to the listeners. An important achievement occurs by the end of this stage: children learn that language can be multifunctional. That is, one utterance can serve more than one function at a time, a characteristic of most adult communications.

Two aspects of engaging in effective dialogues involve taking one's turn appropriately and helping to maintain the topic of conversation. Children even before the age of 9 months may engage in some rudimentary turn-taking skills in the form of reciprocal interactions. By the time children are 18 to 24 months old, they have learned to participate in dialogues and demonstrate ability in applying rules of turn taking in their dialogues.

THE PERIOD OF TWO-WORD UTTERANCES

Semantic–Syntactic Development

In the second year of life, children gradually expand their single-word vocabularies until they have learned to combine two words in one utterance. This first two-word utterance usually occurs around 18 to 26 months of age. A child's expressive vocabulary at 18 months is about 50 words. Between 18 and 24 months, children experience a lexical growth spurt, and at 24 months of age, they typically have a single-word lexicon of 120 to 300. A vocabulary of at least 50 words is generally considered the minimum prerequisite to beginning to combine two words into one utterance, but most 2-year-old children have expressive single-word vocabularies four to six times greater than 50 words at 2 years of age. Children need a variety of words in order to allow them eventually to use two-word combinations that, in turn, evolve into sentences.

The development that occurs from the single-word to the two-word stage is not haphazard. Children demonstrate an increase in the number of verbs, a reduction in other types of relational words, and an increase in the number of object-class words used in their language as they approach the two-word stage. Some have also suggested that children begin to produce chained single-word productions shortly before they use two-word combinations, although not all agree with this suggestion. *Chained single-word utterances* are two single words that children use in very close succession to each other but, based on stress and intonation patterns, use as individual words. These utterances appear to demonstrate that children are beginning to see more than one aspect of an event. That is, the children seem to identify and talk about relations within one event, such as *ball/roll* or *cookie/gone*. These successive single-word utterances may form a base for the two-word utterances about to occur, such as *ball roll, no cookie*, and *more juice*.

Types of Two-Word Utterances

The two-word utterances that children typically begin to use about their second birthday are often described as reflections of *semantic relations* (Bloom, 1970; Brown, 1973). These two-word productions reflect meaning based on different relationships among the words in the

TABLE 2.4 | Common Semantic Relations

Relation	Example	Structure
Nomination	"That ball"	Demonstrative + N
Nonexistence	"No ball"	No (allgone) + N
Action–object	"Roll ball"	V + N
Agent–action	"Baby cry"	N + V
Recurrence	"More cookie"	More (another) + N
Action + locative	"Jump [on] chair"	V + N
	"Roll here"	V + Loc.
Entity + locative	"Ball [in] chair"	N + N
	"Mommy here"	N + Loc.
Possessor–possession	"Baby ball"	N + N
Agent–object	"Baby [roll] ball"	N + N
Entity–attributive	"Pretty ball"	Att. + N
	"Ball pretty"	N + Att.
Notice	"Hi ball"	Hi + N
Instrumental	"Cut [with] knife"	V + N
Action–indirect object	"Give [to] doggie"	V + N
Conjunction	"Coat [and] hat"	N + N

Source: Brown (1973).

utterances. Children can use the utterance *baby ball* to signify possession ("baby's ball") or to signify the actor and the object of an action ("baby [rolls] ball"). An utterance can indicate two different meanings or two separate relations between the words. Table 2.4 lists a number of the more common semantic relations that Brown (1973) identified in children's two-word productions. As we can see, different semantic relations can be expressed in the same grammatical form, such as noun + noun (N + N) to signify possession, agent–object, and entity–locative. Another significant characteristic of this stage of language use is the absence of morphological endings on the words used. Children do not use the possessive word endings even though their intent is to indicate possession, nor do they use any endings on verbs. Instead, only lexical, or root, forms of words are used.

Brown (1973) has termed this semantic relations period of language development Stage I. During this period, children use about an equal number of one- and two-word utterances. If we average the number of words in many of their utterances, we obtain a mean length of about 1.5. The average lengths of young children's utterances are frequently used as measures of their language growth. Although we can average the number of words that children use in their responses, such an approach does not tell us whether the children are using more complex word endings, such as plural markers. A more common method of arriving at average length is to count the number of morphemes, both free and bound, that occur in the utterances. When children are in Stage I, this averaging procedure also results in a *mean length of utterance* (MLU) of about 1.5 because children are not yet using grammatical inflections, also referred to as grammatical morphemes. In the early periods of language learning, as MLU increases, the complexity of children's utterances generally increases. However, when children begin using more complex sentence forms, this relationship between length and linguistic maturity does not remain as closely associated as in the earlier stages of language acquisition because there are ways other than length to increase syntactic complexity.

THE PRESCHOOL AND EARLY SCHOOL YEARS

From the two-word utterance stage at about 2 years of age, children's language development grows in leaps and bounds. The ability to produce complete and complex sentences is acquired, speech becomes intelligible even to unfamiliar listeners, and vocabulary size explodes.

Phonology

Children learn some sounds before others. This means that the words they say do not always match the adult pronunciation. For example, a child may say *moon* correctly at 2 years because the word contains early-developing sounds; however, words such as *spaghetti* and *spoon* may be pronounced as "detti" and "poon," respectively.

Mastering Production of Speech Sounds. At approximately 2 years of age, children use a repertoire of nine to 10 different consonants in the initial position of words. In the final position of words, these children use five to six different consonants. Between 24 and 39 months of age, children use an average of 2.2 consonant clusters (i.e., two or more consonants together acting like one, such as "sky") in the initial position and 1.7 clusters in the final position of words. With advancing age, children's phonological repertoires increase in terms of both the number of different sounds used and the word positions in which they are used. Most researchers agree that by age 7 or 8, children have fairly well mastered the English phonemes and are producing them correctly in their speech. However, some speech development may continue into fifth grade, or approximately age 10/11.

Several investigations have contributed significantly to our knowledge of when children learn to produce specific sounds (McLeod, van Doorn, & Reed, 2001a, 2001b; Poole, 1934; Smit, Hand, Freilinger, Bernthal, & Bird, 1990; Templin, 1957). Although differences in research designs and criterion levels prevent exact comparisons among results, several similar trends have emerged from the studies. Generally, children learn to master the production of nasal sounds, such as /m/, /n/, and /ŋ/[1]; stop consonants, such as /d/, /k/, /g/, /p/, and /b/; and glides, such as /w/, between 2 and 3 years of age. These phonemes are typically considered early-developing and relatively easy sounds. In contrast, fricative sounds, such as /s/, /z/, /ʃ/, and /ʒ/, and affricates, such as /tʃ/ and /dʒ/, are mastered later, often not until age 7 or 8. However, children do demonstrate variability in the ages at which they acquire individual phonemes (McLeod et al., 2001a, 2001b). There are also trends in terms of when children master the production of the various manners of articulation. For the most part, stop consonants and nasals are typically learned before fricatives and affricates. Furthermore, children often continue to have difficulties with /r/ and /l/ after they begin school.

So far, we have discussed only consonant sound development. Children generally learn to produce the vowels correctly before they acquire the consonant sounds. In fact, vowel production may be mastered by the time a child is 3 years old. It is unusual to see school-aged children making more than occasional errors in their vowel productions.

Producing Words without All the Speech Sounds. Children's simplified pronunciation of words follows patterns known as *phonological processes*. For example, if a child regularly substitutes consonants produced in the front of the mouth (e.g., /t/, /d/) for those that are supposed to be produced in the back of the mouth (e.g., /k/, /g/) and so says *tea* for *key*, the child might be said to be using a fronting process. Or, if a child regularly omits one or more consonants when they occur together as clusters and so says "poon" for *spoon*, the child might be described as using a cluster reduction process.

Several of these processes fall under the three broad classifications of syllable structure, assimilation, and substitution processes. In *syllable structure* processes, young children tend to omit consonants in the final position of words or syllables ("bi" for *bite*), delete unstressed syllables in polysyllabic words ("jama" for *pajamas*), and reduce the number of sounds produced in consonant clusters, such as /bl/ ("bu" for *blue*). *Assimilation* processes are those in

---

1. *See* Table 1.1 for the International Phonetic Alphabet.

TABLE 2.5 | Expressive Vocabulary Growth from the First Year to First Grade

Approximate Age	Approximate Number of Words in Expressive Vocabulary
15 months	10
18 months	50
20 months	150
2 years	120–300
3 years	1,000
4 years	1,600
5 years	2,100–2,200
6 years	2,600–7,000

which one sound in a word affects the production of another sound so that its production is modified. Examples of assimilative processes are "gog" for *dog* or "mam" for *lamb*. When children use both a syllable duplication and an assimilative process simultaneously, an utterance such as "gaga" for *doggie* may be produced. Finally, *substitution* processes are employed when children use one group of sounds, such as stops, in place of another group, such as fricatives. It is not uncommon to hear children say "toap" for *soap*.

As children get older, they discontinue using early phonological processes so that their productions of words approximate those used by adults. Because this learning process takes time, however, any one word may go through several stages in pronunciation. Consequently, just because a child is capable of saying a sound correctly in one word does not mean that the sound will be said correctly in all words that contain it if different phonological processes are operating in the production of the other words.

Semantics

Table 2.5 illustrates what happens to expressive vocabulary size from the first word at about 12 months of age to first grade. In terms of receptive vocabulary, children comprehend their first words at about 8/9 months of age; at about 13 months of age, children comprehend about 50 words. By 6 years of age, their comprehension vocabulary is between 20,000 and 24,000 words, and by 12 years of age, it is about 50,000 words. The size of a child's vocabulary depends, in part, on the experiences and words to which the child is exposed, which means that lexical growth in the early years has rather systematic patterns because infants' and toddlers' early life experiences have largely similar patterns (e.g., bottles, sleep, diapers, caregivers). In contrast, lexical acquisition in later primary and, particularly, in secondary school can take on individualist growth patterns because life experiences for the children and adolescents are more varied and their abilities to take advantage of the semantic richness of school is more varied. With regard to the early years, Rescorla, Alley, and Christine (2001) write that "young children are highly consistent in the words they acquire in their early lexicons" (p. 605). Patterns to what words children acquire and the sequence in which they add words to their lexicons include (Pan & Uccelli, 2008):

- Overextension and underextension of the meanings of words (e.g., overextension such as all four-legged animals being *dogs;* underextension such as *bottle* applying only to the baby's bottle)
- Acquiring words that occur more frequently in their environments
- A general tendency to label first objects and actions, then words that attach attributes to objects or events (*big*), and, finally, words that express temporal, spatial, conditional, and causal relationships

- A shift from classifying words on the basis of perceptual or functional characteristics (concrete classifications) to classifying words according to abstract properties such as temporal–spatial features or animate–inanimate characteristics

There are several ways in which young children are believed to be so good at learning words. One way is with a process known as *fast mapping*. Dollaghan (1987) describes fast mapping as a lexical acquisition strategy in

> which a listener rapidly constructs a representation for an unfamiliar word on the basis of a single exposure to it. This initial representation might contain information on the semantic, phonological, or syntactic characteristics of the new lexical item, as well as nonlinguistic information related to the situation in which it was encountered. (p. 218).

This first meaning may or may not be complete and/or accurate. It does, however, create a basis for further refinement as additional experiences with the word in context occur. Children seem to be able to fast map meaning by having only "incidental" exposures to new words. That is, new words occur in context in a child's ambient environment, and the child is able to discern what the new word means. This is referred to as *quick incidental learning* (QUIL). However, the quick, partial learning of the meaning of new words only starts what is the longer-term, slow mapping process of vocabulary learning. Any new word and its partial meanings need to be remembered, and over time as new contexts are encountered in which a child is exposed to the word, refinements in the meaning need to be made. This longer term refinement of word meaning is sometimes referred to as *slow mapping,* with even more time needed for further refinement and extension of a word's meaning, a process commonly referred to as *extended mapping.*

In addition to fast mapping and QUIL, a number of propositions have been advanced about how children figure out labels for and meanings of words. Some of these are the whole object–versus–object components proposition, the mutual exclusivity proposition, and the novel name–nameless category proposition. The *whole object–versus–object components* proposition (Golinkoff, Mervis, & Hirsh-Pasek, 1994) suggests that children will focus on an entire object as the most likely referent for a new word before thinking about one of the parts of the object or an attribute of the object as the possible referent. According to the *mutual exclusivity* proposition (Markman, 1989; Markman & Wachtel, 1988), a child will assume that a new word applies to an object that does not yet have a name (from the child's perspective) and will not be inclined to give an already-named object a second label, that is, one item, one name, or mutually exclusive labels. Therefore, in a context where a new word occurs and the names for all things are known except one, the new word will be assumed to apply to the unnamed item and will not be another word for one of the other items. The third, the *novel name–nameless category* proposition (Golinkoff et al., 1994; Mervis & Bertrand, 1994), is similar to the mutual exclusivity proposition but adds that children will consider other possibilities, including another name for an object whose label is already known.

The strength of these three propositions as well as others in explaining how children go about figuring out what new names go with what referents is still a matter for discussion. What is certain, however, is that the context in which children encounter words and their referents is central to their word learning. What is also necessary for full knowledge of a word and its referents is multiple exposures to the word in multiple contexts.

Spatial and Temporal Terms. Children's comprehension of spatial (location in space) and temporal (location in time) words develops gradually from about 2 years for *in* as a preposition to about 11 years for terms such as *before* and *after,* with children's understanding of selected spatial and temporal relationships developing throughout Piaget's concrete operational period (about grades 1 to 5 and approximately 7 to 11 years old). In grade 1, children's ability to interpret temporal terms has been found to be greater than their comprehension of spatial relationships. However, after grade 1 children may be able to understand the spatial terms better than the temporal ones, a trend in favor of spatial relationships that continues throughout the primary grades.

Many conjunctions involve temporal concepts (e.g., "She will leave *when* it is convenient" and "We ate breakfast *before* we went to school"), as does the "wh-" question word *when*. And a number of these same terms also occur as prepositions (e.g., "We ate breakfast *before* school). Children generally use these temporal terms as prepositions before using them as conjunctions. Additionally, terms expressing order of events (e.g., *before* and *after*) appear to be learned prior to terms expressing simultaneity (e.g., *while* and *at the same time*).

Spatial relationships are also often expressed by *prepositions*. *In* and *on* are among the first of these word types to be acquired. Some words that function as prepositions also occur as part of a *verb particle*, that is, a multiword construction that functions as a verb, as in "She *put up* a good argument." Like prepositions, these words as verb particles emerge early in children's language and by about 4 to 5 years of age are used with reasonable accuracy. However, Wegner and Rice (1988) suggest that certain words seem to be used more as prepositions (*in*, *on*, and *over*) and others (*up*, *down*, and *off*) more as verb particles.

Other spatial prepositions (e.g., *in front of* and *next to*) are more difficult for children. The referents for these prepositions vary, depending on the children's relationships to objects and the characteristics of the objects. When an object has a front, such as a person, *in front of* relates to the object's front. For an object without a front, such as a ball, *in front of* derives its meaning from the relative positions of the speaker and the object—positions that can vary. Furthermore, *next to* can mean *beside*, *in back of*, or *in front of*, all of which can be very confusing for a child. As might be expected, these types of spatial prepositions develop later.

Deictic Words. Deictic words are terms that have changing referents, depending on who in a communicative dyad is speaking, on the respective locations of objects and people, and on the temporal relationships relative to the speaker and listener (Pan & Uccelli, 2008). The spatial prepositions discussed in the preceding section are deictic in nature. As another example, the referents for *I* and *you* shift as the speaker–listener relationship changes. The terms *here* and *there* and *this* and *that* vary depending on the location of the speaker, listener, and/or objects. Among the deictic verbs are *come*, *go*, *bring*, and *take*. Such words must be confusing for young children, although the literature suggests that children demonstrate some use of deictic shifts for first- and second-person pronouns (*I*, *you*, *me*) sometime between approximately 1 and 2 years of age. Third-person pronouns appear later in children's language, between approximately 2 and 3 years of age, and their development may even continue to 5 years of age and possibly beyond. When children's MLUs approach 4.0, they evidence deictic shifts for the terms *here*, *there*, *this*, and *that*. Other deictic words, such as *come*, *go*, *bring*, and *take*, tend to be learned later, and complete acquisition may extend into children's school years.

Morphology

One way in which young children increase their utterance length is to begin to use grammatical morphemes in their utterances. Recall that in the early two-word combination stage (Brown's Stage I), a child's MLU is 1.5, but no grammatical morphemes are attached to words. When children begin to use grammatical morphemes, their MLUs reach about 2.0. At this point, children progress into Brown's Stage II, acquiring the present progressive *-ing* ending for verbs ("ball rolling") and the prepositions *in* and *on* ("kitty in chair" and "cup on table"). It is important to note, however, that acquisition of a grammatical morpheme, as used in relation to Brown's stages, means that a child uses it correctly in at least 90 percent of the situations in which it is required by adult standards, that is, in 90 percent of the obligatory contexts. Children may use morphemes such as *in* and *on* before this stage but not at the criterion level set by Brown. Table 2.6 summarizes Brown's (1973) findings about the sequence in which children acquire 14 selected grammatical morphemes and indicates the corresponding stages determined by MLU at which the morphemes are acquired. The process of learning these morphemes occurs over several years, and children are developing other language skills during that time. For example, by the time children are 3 years old, they typically demonstrate the use of negative and interrogative sentences as well as basic declarative sentences.

Of the verb forms Brown (1973) investigated, irregular past-tense words such as *ran* and *saw* appear in children's language before regular past-tense verb markers. In learning

TABLE 2.6 | Sequence of Acquisition for Fourteen Grammatical Morphemes

	Morpheme	MLU	Maximum Length in Morphemes	Stage
1.	Present progressive ending (*-ing*)			
2. 3.	*In* and *on*	2.25	7	II
4.	Noun plurals			
5.	Past-tense irregular verbs			
6.	Possessive nouns	2.75	9	III
7.	Uncontractible copula ("Here I am")			
8.	Articles			
9.	Past-tense regular verbs	3.50	11	IV
10.	Regular third-person singular present-tense verbs			
11.	Irregular third-person singular present-tense verbs			
12.	Uncontractible auxiliary ("He was running")	4.00	13	V
13.	Contractible copula ("She's big")			
14.	Contractible auxiliary ("The boy's eating")			

Source: Brown (1973).

morphological rules, children typically acquire a more general rule first and then gradually modify and refine the rule to account for the more specific applications and exceptions, so this initially appears a bit strange. It may be that children simply acquire these irregular verb forms as vocabulary words instead of word form variations derived from lexical verbs. Support for such an interpretation comes from the observation that after children begin to use regular past-tense verb forms correctly, they often incorrectly apply the rules to irregular verbs previously used accurately—so that utterances such as "He runned" and "I seed a dog" are not uncommon (Tager-Flusberg & Zukowski, 2008). This is not inconsistent with research that suggests even some regular past-tense verb endings are first used with specific verb words, that is, as vocabulary items (Pine, 1999).

When regular past-tense forms ("She jumped") appear, not all variations of regular past-tense verbs are acquired at the same time. Learning to use the variety of verb forms that occur in English is especially problematic for many children with language disorders. For this reason, we will take a somewhat closer look at normal verb morphological acquisition. Verbs to which the past-tense allomorph /d/ is added (*climbed*) appear to develop slightly before those to which the allomorph /t/ is attached (*jumped*). Phonological composition influences which allomorphic form is used. In the examples above, the voiceless stop /t/ is used following the final voiceless phoneme in the root, whereas the voiced stop /d/ is used following the final voiced phoneme in the root word. Acquisition of the /əd/ allomorph (*painted*) occurs somewhat later. Use of this allomorpheme is also influenced by the final phoneme in the root. Because it is not possible to produce two stop phonemes sequentially (e.g., /td/) without inserting a vowel, the syllable form of the allomorph /əd/ is used when the root ends in a stop.

There are also different ways in which irregular past-tense verbs are formed. Some use an internal vowel change (*swim*→ *swam*), whereas others use both a vowel and a final consonant change (*catch*→ *caught*). The former types seem to emerge somewhat earlier for children. In one classic study, 7- and 8-year-old children gave fewer than 75 percent correct responses for irregular verbs with internal vowel changes, and only about 40 percent gave correct responses for irregular verbs formed by changing both a vowel and a final consonant (Moran, 1975). Such data indicate that children are continuing to refine some of their morphology in the early school years.

According to Brown (1973), the regular forms of third-person singular present-tense verbs ("She jumps" and "He swims") emerge after past-tense regular forms (*see* Table 2.6). Shortly thereafter, children begin to use irregular forms of third-person singular present-tense verbs (*do* to *does* and *have* to *has*). Of the 14 grammatical morphemes in Brown's investigation, the verb forms involving the contractible copula and auxiliary ("We're big" and "She's running") and the uncontractible auxiliary ("He was running") were the last ones the children acquired.

Table 2.6 indicates that children begin to use regular noun plurals after present progressive verb endings and before irregular past-tense forms (Brown, 1973). Again, there are various forms of regular noun plurals, and there appears to be a developmental sequence for acquisition of these variations. Children's utterances with the plural allomorph /z/ (*pigs*) tend to be more accurate before their utterances containing plural nouns with the /s/ allomorph (*boats*), whereas accurate use of the /əz/ plural allomorph (*houses*) is achieved after the /s/ and /z/ plural forms. The phonological influences on the allomorphemes are the same as those for past tense, as we saw above. Although children begin to use some noun plurals early in their language-learning process, the complete acquisition of plural forms takes several years, with children in the early primary grades potentially still demonstrating problems with plural nouns that require use of the /əz/ ending. The learning of irregular noun plurals (*child* to *children*) seems to lag considerably behind the acquisition of regular forms.

Brown (1973) indicates that children begin to use possessive forms of nouns shortly after the appearances of noun plurals and irregular past-tense verbs (*see* Table 2.6). Possessive forms of nouns are derived in basically the same ways as noun plurals, and their sequence of acquisition appears to be essentially similar. Correct use of the /z/ allomorph (*bug's*) tends to be achieved somewhat before that of the /s/ allomorph (*duck's*), which, in turn, tends to be acquired before the /əz/ ending (*horse's*). We notice that regular forms of noun plurals, possessives, and third-person singular present-tense verbs all use the same word endings, /z/, /s/, /əz/. Therefore, it is not surprising that Brown (1973) found that once the children in his study correctly added the endings to form any one of the three word types (plurals, possessives, or third-person verbs), they used the other two types within 1 year.

Other morphological forms involve derivational morphemes. Unlike grammatical morphemes, derivational morphemes change the part of speech of a word, for example, an action (verb), *to farm,* to a person (noun) who performs the action, *farmer,* or the meaning of a word, for example, *mount* to *dismount.* Among the derivational morphemes are comparatives (*bigger*) and superlatives (*biggest*), noun and adverb derivations (*painter, fireman, violinist, gently, quickly*), and prefixes (*preheat, undone, miscue*). The results of Berko's (1958) classic study indicated that, even by age 7, children had not yet fully acquired the rules for forming comparative and superlative adjectives and for deriving nouns and adverbs. Prefixing also is a difficult skill to acquire because it requires knowledge of the meanings for both the prefix form and the root word. Refinement of morphological rules continues well into the school years, and in the adolescent is a major mechanism by which students advance their vocabulary by acquiring what are known as *morphologically complex words,* that is, words with multiple bound morphemes, e.g., *triangularity*.

Syntax

Syntactic complexity increases both in terms of length and in terms of the types of syntactic structures children learn. Consequently, children extend their previous two-word utterances into multiword utterances and into different sentence forms.

Expanding Two-Word Utterances. Children learn to expand their utterances by combining previously separate semantic relations, such as "baby ball" (possessive) and "ball roll" (agent–action) to form "baby ball roll" (Brown, 1973; Lahey, 1988). Children do not, however, use any new relations in forming these longer utterances. Only previously expressed two-word semantic relations are combined and expanded. The production of the first true sentences is also derived from this combining process. Agent–action ("baby roll") and action–object ("roll ball") combine to form agent–action–object ("baby roll ball"), the subject + verb + object basic English syntactic rule discussed in Chapter 1. With gradually increasing skill in producing the basic sentence form, the child is acquiring the foundation abilities to begin to manipulate that syntactic form to make other types of sentences. As McLean and Snyder-McLean (1999) summarize,

> Between 3 and 4 years of age, typically developing children are able to produce well formed, declarative sentences with generally appropriate grammar. . . . They can ask simple questions using *wh-* words. . . . Future learning will allow children to alter . . . declarative structures to produce interrogative forms. (pp. 170–171)

Acquisition of Negatives. In our discussion of the types of single words that children use, we saw that negative words occur very early in the developmental process. When children begin to combine words, negative utterances are produced by placing the negative marker *no* in front of an element that occurs in the predicate of a sentence, such as a verb or direct object. Utterances like "no milk" and "no go" are typical. Even though children at this stage may produce affirmative sentences with a subject and predicate ("boy roll ball"), the subject is deleted when a negative marker is added. It appears that the use of negation increases the length and complexity of an utterance, which, as a result, can exceed children's linguistic capacities at the time. Perhaps to accommodate these limited capacities, the overall length and complexity of an utterance are reduced to a manageable unit by omitting the subject when a negative is added ("no roll ball"). Furthermore, the subject of a sentence is usually the information shared most between speaker and listener, so its omission tends not to affect communication. Meaning can still be conveyed despite the omission.

Children gradually learn to re-add the subjects to produce negative sentences such as "boy no roll ball." However, before children's negative sentences can evolve into more complex forms, the children need to learn that in English *no* is the negative word used with nouns and that *not* is the negative for verbs. The occurrence of later negative sentences also depends on the use of a copula or auxiliary verb ("The ball is not big" and "The boy is not running"). For sentences in which an auxiliary verb does not occur ("The boy eats"), an auxiliary in the form of *do* must be added ("The boy does not eat" or "The boy doesn't eat"). Although the use of *do* plus a negative is generally considered to be a reasonably complex language skill, the negative words *don't* and *can't* do appear in children's early language productions. These early occurrences of *can't* and *don't*, however, are typically viewed as vocabulary words indicating negation rather than as evidence that children have acquired the operation of adding *do* when an auxiliary is absent. The negatives *won't* and *isn't* also occur in children's early productions although less frequently than *don't* and *can't*.

Negatives can be used to express a number of different concepts (Tager-Flusberg & Zukowski, 2008). For example, with negative utterances, we can reject ("I don't want any"), deny ("That's not a red car"), or signify nonexistence ("It's not here"). Table 2.7 presents six functions of negatives in a suggested developmental sequence and provides examples of each (Bloom & Lahey, 1978). The syntactic representation of these negative functions appears to follow this same sequence. That is, children at a specific developmental level will express nonexistence in a fairly complex way ("It isn't here") while at the same time signifying denial in a less sophisticated manner ("That not a ball").

Acquisition of Questions. Preschoolers' acquisition of interrogative, or question, forms tends to lag somewhat behind their negative utterances. However, before discussing the development of questions, we need to review two types of question forms that can occur in English:

TABLE 2.7 | Suggested Developmental Sequence for Negative Functions

Negative Function	Example and Explanation
Nonexistence/disappearance	"No ball" (The ball is not in the toy box where it belongs.)
	"No milk" (The milk is all gone.)
Nonoccurrence	"No pull" (The toy is stuck and cannot be pulled.)
Cessation	"No turn" (The top has stopped spinning and has fallen over.)
Rejection	"No juice" (I do not want any more juice.)
Prohibition	"No go" (The child is telling Mommy not to leave.)
Denial	"No doggie" (Having been told the Great Dane is a dog, the child does not believe it belongs to the same class as the toy poodle at home.)

Source: Bloom and Lahey (1978).

1. Yes/no interrogatives, characterized as follows:
   - Are labeled as such because the answer to such a query is *yes* or *no*.
   - Involve moving, or transposing, a copula or auxiliary verb to the beginning of the sentence, as in changing the basic sentence "The boy is running" to "Is the boy running?" Transposing reverses the usual sequence of subject and verb; the term *interrogative reversal* is also used to refer to this process.
   - If there is no auxiliary or copula verb in the basic sentence to transpose, as in the sentence "The girl rides the bike," one needs to be added in the form of *do* and then transposed to form the question "Does the girl ride the bike?"
2. "Wh-" questions, characterized as follows:
   - Request information.
   - Require that a "wh-" word, such as *what* or *who*, be added to the beginning of an utterance, which is a process called *preposing*.
   - Need to use "wh-" words that reflect the correct meanings of the utterances, for example:
     What is the boy riding?
     Where is the boy riding?
     When is the boy riding?
     How is the boy riding?
   - Usually involve both a transposing operation and a preposing process ("The boy is riding"→ "What is the boy riding?").

In the early stages of learning to ask questions, children mark their yes/no queries only by using rising inflections, such as "mommy go ↗." These children may also use a limited set of "wh-" questions, although the utterances are not yet in adult form ("What that?" and "Where Mommy going?"). Children learn to prepose with "wh-" words before they learn to transpose verbs. This is a particularly logical pattern, because children are not yet using copula and auxiliary verbs in these early stages; therefore, they have nothing in their utterances to transpose.

Even though children learn to add copula and auxiliary verbs to their basic sentences, their yes/no questions may continue to be marked by rising intonations ("Mommy is gone ↗"), although some children may begin with correct transposing. The children do prepose for their "wh-" questions, but they still do not transpose, so their queries sound something like "What Daddy is doing?" or "Where Mommy is going?" If we examine these forms, we see that the children are using a basic sentence that includes the auxiliary *is* and are simply adding the preposed "wh-" word to the beginning. Gradually, the children begin to transpose for their yes/no questions ("Is the girl eating?"). At this stage, however, they may still fail to transpose copula or auxiliary verbs in their "wh-" questions ("What the girl is eating?"). Children's attempts at negative questions demonstrate the same patterns. Transposing occurs in yes/no questions ("Can't we go?") but not in "wh-" questions ("Why Daddy can't go?"). Finally, children learn to transpose in their "wh-" questions ("What is the girl eating?" and "Why can't Daddy go?").

The choice of which "wh-" word to use in "wh-" question forms requires children to apply semantic concepts (Tager-Flusberg & Zukowski, 2008). *What* and *who* reflect concepts that differentiate between people and things; *where* involves the concept of location. These semantic concepts develop fairly early in children, and, not surprisingly, the "wh-" words reflecting them are among the first to be used in "wh-" questions. Children use *when* and *how* in their questions somewhat later since time and manner concepts are acquired after the three early-developing concepts. Causal relations develop even later. As a result, "wh-" questions with *why* are among the last to be used meaningfully. The word "meaningfully" is used here because children may ask "Why?" as an attention-getting device before they truly understand the concept of causality and use it accurately in "wh-" questions.

Acquisition of Compound and Complex Sentences. The use of a *compound sentence* (a sentence containing more than one independent clause) or a *complex sentence* (a sentence that contains at least one independent clause and at least one dependent clause, also referred to as a subordinate clause) involves the expression of two or more ideas or propositions in the one sentence. (A clause, in contrast to a phrase, contains a subject and verb.) These more advanced sentence forms are created by joining two or more clauses together, often with a linguistic form such as a conjunction or a relative pronoun. This clausal joining process usually begins sometime between 2 and 3 years of age, when a child's MLU reaches about 3.0 morphemes. This approximates Brown's Stage IV (Brown, 1973). The first conjunction that children learn to use is *and*, which usually appears when a child is a little beyond 24 months of age, although it might initially be used for serial naming ("baby and kitty"). For clausal joining, some data suggest that this conjunction is initially employed to conjoin two independent clauses in utterances such as "You do this and I do that" and "The boy runs and the boy jumps" (Tager-Flusberg & Zukowski, 2008). These types of sentences simply require the children to add on to existing utterances in their language. This addition operation is among the earlier transformations that children acquire. However, because many coordinated sentences with *and* contain redundant information, as in "The boy runs and the boy jumps," the redundant elements can be deleted to form sentences like "The boy runs and jumps."

Utterances that contain object complements appear to be the first types of complex sentences that children use. In sentences with object complements, a second basic sentence or clause is used as the object of the verb in the first sentence or clause. For example, in the sentence "I think I have it," the clause "I have it" operates as the object of the verb *think* in the clause "I think." Often included in discussions of object complements are sentences that contain certain types of infinitives. (An *infinitive* is a form of a verb that typically appears with *to*, e.g., "to run," "to go," and the verb itself is unmarked for tense and number, thus appearing in its root form.) In these sentences, an infinitive and its associated words are used as an object of a verb, as in "I want to run fast." Both object complement forms—those with a second basic sentence and those with an infinitive—appear in children's utterances at about the same time. Complex sentences in which a second clause is introduced with a "wh-" adverbial word are acquired shortly after object complement sentences. Examples of these sentence types are "I remember where Mommy is" and "Daddy knows when Mommy comes home." Children tend to use clauses conveying time and location before other "wh-" clauses.

Relative clauses, which are clauses serving as modifiers for nouns (and are therefore a type of adjectival clause), develop somewhat later. A relative clause is often introduced by a relative pronoun, such as *what, who, which, whose*, or *that* ("I see the boys who are running" or "The dog that has the bone is growling"). However, in some instances, the relative pronoun may be omitted ("That's the bed [that] we sleep in"). Children initially use relative clauses to modify predicate nouns ("That is the balloon that I like") and objects ("I see the boy who wears glasses"). They later begin to modify subjects with relative clauses ("The girl who wears glasses sees better"). We see a pattern in which children add to the ends of their sentences before rearranging or adding elements within the sentences (Tager-Flusberg & Zukowski, 2008). The latter process, termed *embedding*, is one of the later-developing transformational operations. Although Limber (1973) indicates that 3-year-old children demonstrate the use of clauses with object complements, "wh-" adverbials, and object relatives, Paul (1981) suggests that the use of all these clause types may not be demonstrated until children are closer to 4 years of age. Embedded relative clauses, having already been identified as later developing, are not used by children at these ages. Embedding usually emerges sometime about kindergarten and is a syntactic operation that continues to develop into adolescence and shows further increasing use into 12th grade (Hass & Wepman, 1974; Loban, 1976). A major shift to the use of clausal constructions occurs at 10 years of age, about the time that students enter secondary school and transition from concrete operations to formal operations cognitively.

Because the construction of compound and complex sentences usually requires the use of connective devices such as conjunctions, accurate use of these sentences involves both the syntactic operations to combine clauses and the selection of appropriate conjunctions to express the correct meanings. In some instances, the semantic task may be more difficult than the syntactic task. We indicated earlier that the conjunction *and* is the first to be acquired by children. Beyond *and*, the exact sequence in which children learn other conjunctions and the ages at which they acquire them are difficult to report. Authors have investigated the use of different conjunctions by children at varying ages and have reported their data in different ways. However, we do know that the frequency with which children use different conjunctions may be related to their knowledge of and facility with the different conjunctions. Thus, the frequency with which conjunctions occur in children's language may provide a clue to their developmental sequence.

In addition to the studies focusing on preschoolers' acquisition of conjunctions, the use of conjunctions by first graders has been examined. In an early but still relevant study, Menyuk (1972) found that, although 95 percent of kindergarten children in her study produced well-formed sentences with the conjunction *and*, only 35 percent of them used adequate sentences with *because*. The conjunctions *if* and *so* were more difficult. Only 20 percent and 19 percent of the first graders produced well-formed sentences with *if* and *so*, respectively. These results certainly suggest that children continue their acquisition of conjunctions past the first grade and into middle and late childhood.

Pragmatics

There are many factors involved in how people use language and what influences their communicative choices in various speaking situations. In this section, we look at children's developing skills in several of these areas—their changing abilities in the functions for which they use language and what they intend to accomplish by its use, their competencies in maintaining a topic and taking turns during a conversation, their uses of presuppositions, their fluency in delivering their messages, and their evolving discourse skills.

Functions of Language. By age 3, children's utterances consistently contain more than one function. This is the third, adultlike stage, and the functions that Halliday (1975) has identified in children's communications in this period are the *interpersonal purpose* (used to relate to other people), the *textual purpose* (used to relate to preceding and following utterances in a dialogue), and the *ideational-experiential purpose* (used to express ideas or events to others).

As we know, the true intentions and functions of some speech acts do not always match the forms of the utterances or their propositional content. As noted in Chapter 1, these are the indirect functions and intentions of speech, and common uses of these indirectives hide the true purposes of utterances in syntactic forms created for the sake of politeness (the interrogative, "Can you open the door?," instead of the imperative, "Open the door") or hint at a purpose by employing content different from the true intent (a child's utterance to a babysitter, "My mommy always lets me stay up late on Fridays," or an adult's remarks, on wishing to have a window closed, "My, it's chilly in here," with no direct reference to the window). In some ways, children's ability to understand and use these indirect speech acts depends partly on their skills in making presuppositions about communicative situations, a topic we discuss in the next section. However, intentions and functions of speech acts are certainly involved.

After about age 3½, children employ these polite devices and hints in their utterances, and they steadily improve with age in their ability to regard requests that contain *please* as more polite than those without it. However, their skill at judging interrogative forms as polite (e.g., "Could I have some candy?") develop later than their skill with *please*. When the children are asked to determine whether a request in the form of an interrogative with *please* ("Could you give me a nut, please?") is more polite than a request in the form of an imperative with *please* ("Give me a nut, please."), even children in the early grades can have difficulty. Use of the polite form—interrogative with *please*—increases steadily between 3 and 7 years, suggesting it takes at least 4 years more after they first start to use indirect polite forms for their use to have many adultlike elements.

Presuppositions. Speakers make presuppositions about what knowledge is shared between speakers and listeners and about what information listeners need to understand messages, and effective speakers modify the form and content of their utterances on the basis of their presuppositions. From this perspective, the use of indirectives, hints, and polite forms can be viewed as part of the presupposition aspect of language use.

For some time, it was believed that children's egocentricity would prevent them from taking a listener's needs into account as they formulated their messages. Surprisingly, however, there is some evidence that, even at the single-word stage, children adapt what limited language they have for their listeners. And, children between ages 3 and 4 change the amount of information they give to listeners relative to their listeners' prior knowledge of communicative topics and ability to share in immediate communicative contexts. The ages of children's communicative partners also influence how preschool children encode their messages. Children at this age use shorter and less complex sentences when talking to younger children than when speaking to their peers or adults.

How children differentially encode new and old information in their utterances is another aspect of presupposition. When this occurs through the use of pronouns, it is referred to as *anaphoric reference* (Tager-Flusberg & Zukowski, 2008). The following example of sequential utterances illustrates what happens as new and old information occur in the content of a message:

> I got new shoes. They're brown and white. But Billy doesn't like them. He liked the black ones.

New information is linguistically emphasized (i.e., named, as in *shoes*), while old information is linguistically deemphasized (i.e., pronominalized). Children in the single-word to approximately the three- or four-word-utterance stages of language learning omit old information in their speech and verbalize information that is new or changing about a situational. As children increase the length of their utterances to approach five words or morphemes, they begin to use pronouns in referring to old information and to name specifically new information.

Use of the definite (*the*) and indefinite (*a* and *an*) articles is also related to the ways in which new and old information is encoded. Although we see children using articles when their MLUs are about 3.5 and they are approximately 2½ to 3 years old (Brown, 1973), accurate use of articles varies, depending on the contexts in which they occur, the amount of shared information between listener and speaker, and whether the information is new or old. In a sequence of utterances, the indefinite article is used to introduce a new referent, and the definite article is employed to encode a previously introduced referent. The following example illustrates this variation:

> I bought a new dress. The dress is red with ruffles.

Because of the shifting use required for articles, we might anticipate that complete acquisition evolves over a number of years. In a classic study, Warden (1976) investigated the developmental changes that occur in the use of articles in children 3, 5, 7, and 9 years old and compared their performances to those of adults. All the children and the adults showed a consistent preference for using the definite article to refer to previously introduced referents. However, the 3-year-old children randomly used either the definite or the indefinite article for introducing initial referents. From 3 years on, there was an increase in appropriate use of the indefinite article for initial referents, but it was not until 9 years of age that the children demonstrated a true preference for using the indefinite article for initial referents. In contrast, adults consistently introduced initial referents with the indefinite article.

Turn Taking, Topic Maintenance, and Revisions. Two aspects of engaging in effective dialogues involve taking one's turn appropriately and helping to maintain the topic of conversation. It appears that children even before the age of 9 months demonstrate rudimentary turn-taking skills in the form of reciprocal interactions. By the time children are 18 to 24 months old, they have learned to participate in dialogues and demonstrate ability in applying rules of turn taking in their dialogues. However, children younger than 5 years have a fair amount of overlap in their conversations with others, but by the time children reach 6 to 8 years they have generally learned how to time their turns so that they occur at appropriate places in dialogues with only a few miscues resulting in overlaps. It is possible classroom experiences in the early grades influence children's learning turn taking skills.

Beyond turn taking, a person's response must relate in some way to a speaker's previous utterance if a topic of conversation is to be maintained. Sometime before age 2, less than half of children's responses to adults' utterances typically maintain the topic of conversation set by the adult. This proportion increases steadily to about 3 years when they can continue a topic in about 50 percent of their responses. However, it is not until approximately age 3½ to 4 that children demonstrate skills in maintaining topics through a number of adjacent comments in a dialogue (Bloom, Rocissano, & Hood, 1976). Brinton and Fujiki (1984) reported that the average number of utterances that even 5-year-old children produced on a single topic during a conversational interchange was five. Additionally, these children covered, on the average, 50 topics in 15 minutes of conversation. The type of activity/context may, however, influence children's ability to maintain topics. Schober-Peterson and Johnson (1989) found that 4-year-old children were able to maintain one topic over as many as 13 to 91 utterances during activities that involved enacting, describing, and problem-solving conversations. Although these children demonstrated considerable topic maintenance skill during activities that promoted these forms of discourse, 75 percent of their topic maintenance utterances were still relatively short.

Not only do children show developmental patterns in their turn-taking skill and topic maintenance ability, they also demonstrate changes with age in the devices they use to maintain topics. As children grow older, they increasingly add new information to a topic to maintain it. Before age 3, children tend to use *focus/imitation* topic maintenance devices (Bloom et al., 1976; Keenan, 1975). That is, they attend to focus on one or more of the words in a previous utterance and repeat or imitate those portions in their succeeding responses. As children approach age 3, their use of focus/imitation devices decreases, while their use of substitution/expansion operations increases (Bloom et al., 1976; Keenan, 1975). In *substitution/expansion*, children add information to the topic of a previous utterance or modify the previous utterance in some way.

Unfortunately, not all utterances in a conversation are understood by listeners. When this occurs, effective speakers revise their messages. Children at about 2 years of age are able to modify their original utterances when their listeners misunderstand, but their modifications typically involve use of phonetic modifications (changing word pronunciations) in attempts to clarify their messages. As children mature, they change their revision strategies and use more word substitutions to modify their communicative attempts. As they approach 5 years of age, they tend to increase the length of subsequent utterances when they know that their listeners have not received the messages adequately. Conversely, they also decrease the length of utterances when they are aware that their message has been understood. The intent of children's messages when there has been a communication failure may affect how successfully the children resolve the communication breakdown. For example, children between 3½ and 5½ years of age may be more successful at resolving their communication failure when the intent of their message was a request than when it was an assertion (Shatz & O'Reilly, 1990).

Fluency. All speakers revise phrases, repeat words, hesitate, use fillers such as "uh," and make false starts in the delivery of messages. These disruptors are often referred to as *mazes*. In fact, preschool children typically go through a period of normal dysfluency. However, most children outgrow this period of normal dysfluency, and once they enter school, the degree to which messages are delivered with a smooth, easily flowing series of words often becomes one of the factors people use, consciously or unconsciously, to evaluate the language proficiency of children (Loban, 1976).

Contrary to what we might expect to see, the overall occurrence of mazes in children's spoken language seems not to decrease with age (Loban, 1976). In fact, as length and complexity of utterances increase with age, so does the number of maze behaviors, although there may be erratic increases and decreases in the number of maze behaviors at different times and during different tasks.

Discourse. As we saw in Chapter 1, there are several forms, or genres, of discourse. Conversation is the earliest occurring form, and our discussion above was focused on children's development of several conversational components. Narratives are a common part of language use but they are not limited to relating information about movies or storybooks. We use narratives when we describe to officials what happened in an automobile accident or when we recount events that occurred during our summer vacation. Narratives are monologues that place heavy demands on logical structure, temporal and causal sequencing, cohesion, and presuppositional abilities. As such, successful narrative ability is a later-developing language skill in children. Narrative discourse emerges in children in the preschool years, but children generally are not successful at producing full narratives until the early school years. In reaching the ability to produce full, cohesive narratives, preschoolers pass through several stages in developing the ability to produce true narratives.

Applebee (1978) proposed six levels of narratives; from least to most complex, these are heaps, sequences, primitive temporal narratives, unfocused temporal chains, focused temporal or causal chains, and proper narratives. Although children between the ages of 2 and 3 years begin to tell fictional narratives and briefly describe what has happened to them (Hughes, McGillivray, & Schmidek, 1997), these narratives are considered to be protonarratives and are characterized by what Applebee (1978) refers to as *heaps*. These are series of unrelated, unsequential statements. Little if any concern for the listener's informational need is present, and beginnings and endings are not obvious. These heaps gradually evolve to sequences (Applebee, 1978). The information in *sequences* is presented in an additive but not temporal fashion.

From about 3 to 5 years of age, children begin to relate narratives that show some concern for temporal sequencing of events. Initially, children's narratives represent what Applebee (1978) terms *primitive temporal narratives*. Although these narratives still do not contain plots or evidence causality, they do present information in a rudimentary temporal sequence and are focused around a central event. These primitive temporal narratives are gradually replaced with narratives characterized by *unfocused temporal chains*. Narratives of this type contain concrete relationships chained in temporal order. Applebee (1978) suggests that the next narrative level is that of *focused temporal or causal chains*. Narratives of this type typically have a main character, and events are presented in a chained manner around the character. Initially, events are chained in a temporal order (Lahey, 1988). Causal chaining generally does not emerge until the early school years, or about 5 to 7 years of age. Focused causal chain narratives are the forerunners of true narratives, which appear at about 7 to 8 years of age (Lahey, 1988).

True narratives not only have central themes and/or characters but also generally include multiple causal chains as well as temporal organization (Lahey, 1988). When children achieve the true narrative level, the narratives have defined episode structure(s) made up of the multiple focused causal and temporal chains referred to above (Stein & Glenn, 1979). Typically, by about 9 years of age, children produce narratives that conform to story grammar structure (Stein & Glenn, 1979). This means that their stories include the following:

- Setting statements
- Initiating event(s)

- Internal responses of characters
- Internal plan(s) to resolve the dilemma(s) in the story
- Attempts at resolution
- Direct consequences
- Reactions

However, children continue to develop in their ability to include more multiply embedded episode structures. We see, then, that children's narratives evolve from those present at about 2 years of age, which are characterized by heaps of unrelated statements, to those produced in the first 2 or 3 years of school, characterized by several embedded episodes containing causal and temporal patterns (Hughes et al., 1997).

When children begin school, they begin to be exposed to a more complex form of discourse, that of exposition. As we know from Chapter 1, expository discourse is designed to inform. It is also a major avenue for children as they acquire increasingly competency in reading and writing. Children read expository discourse to acquire information and children produce written discourse and participate in spoken discourse to demonstrate and share what they have learned. As we will see in subsequent chapters, and particularly in Chapter 4, there is significant reciprocity between spoken discourse, reading discourse, and writing discourse, and as children develop their abilities in one, they develop their skills with the others.

Chapter 1 introduced readers to several of the genres of expository discourse. There is no consensus among authors regarding the number of expository discourse genres or the names for the various genres. And, there is no one requisite organizational format that guides the structure of each genre, unlike narrative discourse which, as we saw above, has a broad organizational framework, for example, a setting, episodes, and temporal orientation. Longacre (1983) used two features, temporal sequence and agent orientation, to explain the overarching frameworks of four types of discourse—procedure, explanation, narrative, and behavioral. Table 2.8 shows the relative prominence of the combinations of the two features for these four genres. For example, narrative discourse has strong emphases on agents (or characters) as well as temporal sequences of events, hence + temporal sequence and + agent orientation. In contrast, explanatory discourse, which consists of texts, such as how dyes work or how keystones function in arches, is less concerned with the who (or agents) and sequences of actions in the provision of the information, hence – agent orientation and – temporal sequence. Campaign speeches, which have a large focus on candidates' promised actions but less focus on the when of the actions, are examples of behavioral exposition and categorized as + agent orientation and – temporal orientation. Lastly, procedural exposition involves considerable attention to sequences of actions in informing about a procedure but generally less concern about the agent of the actions, thus mostly – agent orientation but + temporal orientation.

In contrast to the four genres in the Longacre (1983) example above, Ukrainetz (2006) presented six types of expository discourse: description, enumeration, procedure, explanation, comparison/contrast, and persuasion. We know that conversational and narrative discourse emerges earlier than expository discourse, and that exposition discourse

TABLE 2.8 | Broad Organizational Frameworks for Four Discourse Genres

		Temporal Sequence	
		+ Temporal Sequence	– Temporal Sequence
Agent Orientation	+ Agent Orientation	Narrative	Behavioral*
	– Agent Orientation	Procedure	Explanation

**Connected texts such as campaign speeches, sermons, and some advertisements.*

Source: Based on Longacre (1983).

is generally considered to be a more advanced form of discourse and associated with formal schooling. There does not, however, appear to be a clear developmental sequence in which school children acquire ability to produce the different forms of expository discourse. Beyond broad frameworks, such as that provided by Longacre's (1983) example, each occasion of producing each type of exposition requires students to bring together their knowledge of the topic with many sophisticated language skills, such as complex sentence use with a repertoire of conjunctions to convey precision in organization of content and meaning, and presupposition about the intended audience's prior knowledge of and interest in the topic in order to cast the information appropriately. This means each piece of exposition is relatively uniquely created. These features and requirements of expository discourse support the notion that it is a later developing language skill. Students continue their growth with expository discourse into, throughout, and likely beyond adolescence.

Metalinguistics. Young children who are initially learning language do not understand that what they are saying can be something separate from what they are doing. They do not know that they can talk about language, analyze it, see it as an entity separate from its content, and judge it. They are simply learning language to communicate. When they begin to ask what an object's name is, comment that they have forgotten the word for something, repair their utterances spontaneously, practice words or sounds, rhyme words spontaneously, or say that somebody did not say something correctly, they are showing early metalinguistic awareness.

There is some thought that true metalinguistic skills do not appear until the early school years, suggesting the influence of the educational process in helping children become aware of language as something that can be manipulated and used in learning. Metalinguistic skills develop well into if not throughout high school and possibly even into adulthood.

THE ADOLESCENT YEARS

In contrast to several decades ago when there was a widely accepted belief that the important aspects of spoken language development were complete by about 7 or 8 years of age, we now know that some very interesting aspects continue to develop into and through the adolescent years. We also know that the changes that occur with many of these aspects of adolescent language growth may be gradual, slow, and subtle (Nippold, 2007); become evident only when "the performance of nonadjacent age groups is compared" (Reed, Griffith, & Rasmussen, 1998, p. 166); and/or show up as "spurts and regressions or fluctuations in performance" (Reed et al., 1998, p. 176). In the next sections, several aspects of language that show developmental growth into adolescence are highlighted.

Form

Length of Utterance. Length of utterance is one aspect used to estimate language performance of older children and adolescents. However, unlike measures of utterance length using counts of morphemes that we see used with youngsters, length is typically measured in words when language of adolescents is being investigated. A language sample is also generally segmented into either C-units or T-units.[2] Length of spoken utterance continues to increase up to and during adolescence and even into adulthood (Nippold, Hesketh, Duthie, & Mansfield, 2005; Nippold, Mansfield, & Billow, 2007; Nippold, Mansfield, Billow, & Tomblin, 2008, 2009; Reed, 1990).

2. A C-unit is defined as one independent clause and all dependent/subordinate clauses attached to it. C-unit segmentation of language samples permits inclusion of fragments that occur as the result of conversational interchanges. The definition of T-unit is identical to C-unit, but segmentation of language samples omits fragments for analysis purposes.

Loban's (1976) longitudinal study, which remains, according to Larson and McKinley (2003), "one of the most extensive studies to date" (p. 58), examined a variety of aspects of spoken language development from grades 1 through 12 (about 6 to 7 to 17 to 18 years of age), including utterance length (measured in words).[3] Because of the comprehensive nature of Loban's research, we draw considerably from his work in our discussion of adolescents' syntax.

Loban presented data for three groupings of students. One consisted of students whom teachers identified as having advanced language skills, the second was a group whom teachers identified as having poor language skills, and the third was an artificially contrived grouping created by randomly selecting students from the advanced-language and poor-language groups and pooling the results of their performances. Loban suggested that this last group represented "average" or typical language users. Given what we now know about language impairment in students, knowledge that was not available during the years when Loban collected his data, it is likely that many of the students in Loban's poor-language group might today be identified as having language impairment.

With regard to utterance length, Loban's (1976) results revealed a relatively stable pattern of increasing length throughout the grades for all three groups, a pattern he discounted as resulting from simple verbosity, that is, "an increased use of language without any significant increase in meaningful communication" (p. 25). In his study, utterance length was closely associated with overall syntactic complexity. Additionally, those students whom teachers rated as having advanced language skills consistently used longer statements than their less language-proficient counterparts. By 12th grade, the mean length of utterance (words) for the average-language group was 11.70, compared to the higher mean length of utterance of 12.84 for the advanced-language students and the low mean length of utterance of 10.65 for the poor-language students.

The length-of-utterance data that Loban (1976) reported was collected from language samples of adolescents engaged in conversation and interviews. Nippold et al. (2005, 2007, 2008, 2009) used three different tasks to elicit language samples from the adolescents in their studies—conversation, an expository task involving explanation of a favorite game or sport, and an expository task involving discussion of peer conflicts. Across the different tasks, length of utterance was longer for the older adolescents and/or in the expository tasks, with an advantage for the task involving peer conflicts. Clearly, increasing length of utterance is an indicator of advancing syntax in adolescence, but length can vary as language elicitation tasks vary, an important consideration of assessment of language performance of adolescents.

Dependent/Subordinate Clauses. Complex sentences (which readers will recall contain at least one dependent/subordinate clause in addition to an independent or main clause) are also of interest in adolescent language development, in part because of their importance in acquiring competency with spoken and written expository discourse. Growth in several aspects of complex sentence usage is particularly characteristic of older children and adolescents. Distinguishing features of older students' language include the following:

- Embedding (placing linguistic elements, such as a dependent clause, in the middle of utterances rather than at the end, as in "The man *who came to dinner* ate a lot" versus "The man ate a lot *when he came to dinner"*)
- Using multiple embedding (having more than one dependent/subordinate clause in the middle of utterances, as in "The man *who came to dinner that began quite late* ate a lot")
- Increasing use of clauses located toward the beginning of utterances, such as "*When he came to dinner,* the man ate a lot" compared to clauses toward the ends of utterances, such as "The man ate a lot *when he came to dinner"*

Loban's (1976) work provides us with additional information about other aspects of dependent/subordinate clause usage that continue to develop into the adolescent years:

---

3. Loban used C-units for utterance segmentation and analyses.

- More dependent/subordinate clauses per utterance with advancing age
- Increase in the percentage of words used in the dependent/subordinate clause portions of utterances from 12 to 35 percent between grades 1 and 12

This last finding means that in grade 12, approximately one-third of the words in an adolescent's utterances are part of the dependent/subordinate clauses in their utteracnces. As Loban (1976) stated, "With increasing chronological age all subjects devote an increasing proportion of their spoken language to the dependent clause portion of their communication units" (p. 41). Nippold et al. (2005, 2007, 2008, 2009), in exploring syntactic growth during adolescence, also found increasing use of dependent/subordinate clauses. Findings that adolescents use more conjunctions in their utterances than younger school-age children, including conjunctions that conjoin clauses (Reed et al., 1998), add support for both Loban's and Nippold's findings.

The information above tells us that increasing use and length of dependent/subordinate clauses, especially those embedded in or starting utterances, are characteristics of language development during adolescence. There is, however, another aspect to complex sentence use that is a significant developmental characteristic of adolescent language. This relates to changes in the types of dependent/subordinate clauses used with advancing age. Loban (1976) found that for the "average" language group (i.e., randomly grouped students), the proportion of *noun clauses* (those functioning as nouns in utterances, as in "Ice cream is *what he wants*" or "*What he wants* is a job") increased from grades 1 through 12, while the proportion of *adverbial* clauses (those functioning as adverbs, as in "She will eat *when she comes home*") decreased and the proportion of *adjectival clauses* (which can also be termed *relative clauses*) remained the same from grades 1 through 12. These findings are shown in Table 2.9. By grade 12, about 50 percent of the clauses used were noun clauses, with adjectival and adverbial clauses each accounting for about 25 percent of dependent-clause usage. Recall that object complement clauses are early developing, and object complements function as nouns. Therefore, the fact that the majority of clauses were noun clauses should not be surprising.

Also apparent in Table 2.9 is the different pattern of development for adjectival clauses for the group of students with advanced language skills. These students increased their use of adjectival clauses from grades 1 through 12, in contrast to noun or adverbial dependent clauses. This increase clearly separated language-proficient children and adolescents from those with average and poor language. Loban (1976) concluded that "the evidence seems clear that an exceptional speaker . . . will use a progressively greater percentage of adjectival clauses in oral language, whereas the nonproficient speaker . . . or average speaker . . . will show no such percentage increases in the use of adjectival clauses" (p. 48). He pointed out that the greatest increase in the language-proficient students' uses of adjectival clauses occurred mainly during grades 7, 8, and 9.

TABLE 2.9 | Percentages of Different Clause Types Used by Advanced-, Average-, and Poor-Language Students in Grades 1 through 12

	Noun Clauses		Adjectival Clauses		Adverbial Clauses	
Language Group	*Grade 1 Students*	*Grade 12 Students*	*Grade 1 Students*	*Grade 12 Students*	*Grade 1 Students*	*Grade 12 Students*
Advanced	46%	43%	23%	33%	31%	24%
"Average" (random)	41%	50%	26%	25%	32%	25%
Poor	34%	45%	19%	21%	47%	34%

Source: Loban (1976).

The relationship of adjectival clauses to adverbial clauses also seems particularly revealing about the language development of advanced- versus poor-language students. Although the proportion of adverbial clauses used by the poor-language users decreased from grades 1 through 12, as it did for the advanced-language users, across the grades the poor-language users maintained an overall greater use of adverbial clauses than the advanced-language students. For the poor-language users, their decrease in use of adverbial clauses was paralleled by an increase in the proportion of noun clauses they used. This contrasts with the increase in adjectival clause usage across the grades of the advanced-language users. By grade 12, approximately 33 percent of the dependent/subordinate clauses of the advanced-language users were adjectival clauses compared to about 20 percent for the poor-language users. This is an important difference when use of complex sentences with precise meanings in expository discourse is considered.

Loban's research suggests the importance of increasing use of adjectival (relative) clauses in development of highly proficient language but also shows relatively stable patterns of growth for the "average" language group. However, the combined findings for different types of clause usage, including noun and adverbial clauses as well as adjectival/relative clauses, associated with increasing age during adolescence is less clear from the research of Nippold et al. (2005, 2007, 2008, 2009) on the syntactic development of adolescents. Variations in methodology, particularly the tasks used to sample language, likely contributed to some of the differences. Nevertheless, the importance of knowing the nature of clausal growth in adolescence for assessment and intervention indicates a need to investigate this area further.

Adverbial Connectives. Another characteristic of adolescent language development is the increasing use of linguistic structures that occur relatively infrequently in spoken language (Scott & Stokes, 1995). Adverbial connectives are one category of low-frequency linguistic devices. *Adverbial conjuncts* (forms that indicate a logical relation between utterances, such as "*Nevertheless,* the burned cake was eaten") and *adverbial disjuncts* (forms that indicate an attitude or comment about the utterance, such as "There was, *of course,* some debate about the issue") are two types of these connective devices that link utterances but do so outside of the internal syntactic structure of clauses. The work of several researchers (Crystal & Davy, 1975; Nippold, Schwarz, & Undlin, 1992; Scott, 1984; Scott & Rush, 1985) has contributed to our knowledge of adolescents' uses of these advanced language forms:

- Adolescents use a greater variety of adverbial connectives, use them more frequently, and are more successful at metalinguistic tasks involving them than younger students.
- Teenagers use adverbial conjuncts more frequently than adverbial disjuncts.
- Disjuncts tend to be used by older rather than younger students.
- Adolescents' frequency of use of these forms is less than that of adults.
- Ability in dealing with adverbial conjuncts continues to improve from early adolescence to early adulthood.
- Not all adults achieve full mastery of adverbial conjuncts, especially in written language.

Content

In this section, we will consider the content of language, that is, semantics, or words and meaning. We will take a look at some of the aspects of words, word meanings, and figurative language that continue to develop during the adolescent years.

One obvious measure of semantic development to think about is the number of words in an individual's vocabulary. However, vocabulary size is only part of the picture about adolescents' semantic development. Other parts of the picture involve what types of words they learn and what they do with the words and their meanings. For example, adolescents know more words with abstract meanings than younger children do (e.g., *oppression, simulate, divestiture*) and are able to use words in many more contexts (e.g., *hot* as in "hot food" and "hot topic" or *imperial* as in "imperial persona" and "imperial family"). Recall that morphologically complex words also represent an area for semantic growth during adolescence. A morphologically complex word is one that is derived from attaching prefixes and/or suffixes (bound morphemes) to a root word to form a different word but one that has semantic links with the root. In Chapter 1, an example used was the adjective *gentle,* which was altered into the morphologically complex forms *gently,* an adverb; *gentleness,* a noun; and *ungentlemanly,* an adverb. Derived nouns (*gentleness*) and derived adjectives (*biologic*) are common in texts used in upper elementary and secondary grades (Nippold & Sun, 2008). The comprehension of morphologically complex words of eighth graders, approximately 13/14 years old, has been reported as significantly better than that of fifth graders, approximately 10/11 years old, indicating increasing growth in understanding these types of words with increasing age (Nippold & Sun, 2008). For both age-groups, the derived nouns were more difficult than the derived adjectives. The degree of familiarity, as indicated by their frequency of occurrence in third- through ninth-grade reading materials, was associated with the adolescents' comprehension of the words.

There are several reasons for much of the semantic growth into and during adolescence—educational exposure, life experiences, and cognitive shifts into formal/hypothetical thought levels. As Nippold (2007) points out, these mean that, compared to younger children, adolescents are better able to learn new words and their meanings by doing the following:

- Picking up on cues that morphological markers provide for deciphering meaning of unfamiliar words (*piano, pianist*)
- Using context to decipher meanings of unfamiliar words ("The 80-year-old man enjoyed being referred to as an octogenarian.")
- Taking in the direct instruction to which they are exposed in school and the vocabulary associated with it (e.g., *pyrolytic, trochaic*)

During adolescence, there is a continuing, qualitative refinement in lexical knowledge that is in addition to quantitative growth in the size of the lexicon.

Although vocabulary growth is an important aspect of later language development, there are other, equally important areas of semantic development during adolescence and even into adulthood. These include the characteristics of definitions provided for words, the ability to complete verbal analogies ("feet are to socks as hands are to _____"), and skill in detecting and deciphering statements that are ambiguous ("Pressing the suit led to unpredicted problems"). Adolescence is also a peak period for the use of figurative language, and a number of areas of figurative language feature in the language changes that occur in the teenage years. Among these are verbal humor, idioms, metaphors and similes, and proverbs. Table 2.10 provides a summary of these important areas of semantic growth in adolescence.

Competence in figurative language use is generally not thought of as critical to everyday survival. It is, however, important to adolescents in their academic and social lives. Students across grade levels, including adolescents, frequently encounter figurative language in their classrooms and textbooks, especially in the language arts. According to Lazar, Warr-Leeper, Nicholson, and Johnson (1989), as early as the kindergarten year, about 30 percent of teachers' utterances contained at least one occurrence of a multiple-meaning expression. Five percent of their utterances contained at least one idiom. By eighth grade, 37 percent of teachers' utterances contained at least one occurrence of a multiple-meaning expression, and, of particular interest, the occurrences of utterances containing idioms increased to 20 percent. Success in school has also been found to be associated with students' levels of skill with aspects of figurative language, in particular their ability to comprehend proverbs (Nippold, Uhden, & Schwartz, 1997; Nippold, Hegel, Uhden, & Bustamante, 1998). Additionally, the use of slang and jargon, for which adolescents are renowned, is based primarily on figurative language. In fact, the ability to comprehend and use the slang and jargon of the peer group has been linked to peer acceptance and the ability to establish friendships during adolescence. In discussing later language development of children and adolescents, Nippold (2007) even suggests that "gaining competence with all types of figurative language is an important part of becoming a culturally literate and linguistically facile individual" (p. 17). An adolescent's ability to understand and use figurative expressions *should not be sold short* (to use a figurative expression) as a measure of language development.

TABLE 2.10 | Important Areas of Semantic Growth in Adolescence

Words and Word Meanings	Features
Defining words	Categorical definitions used with increasing frequency ("*Wombat:* an animal"); children's definitions more commonly consist of functions ("*Spoon:* something you eat with") or descriptions ("*Wombat:* A wombat is brown"; "*Wombat*: eats plants") or are idiosyncratic ("*Ball:* the thing Jimmy has") Gradually become more categorical with age ("*Cat:* like a dog") More advanced forms likely to include a superordinate category and include one or more descriptors (i.e., Aristotelian definition) ("*Wombat:* a nocturnal marsupial") May include more than one feature or definition type ("*Ball:* a round, three-dimensional object often used in competitive games") Ability associated with adolescents' reading ability Ability for different word types may develop differently with different patterns (e.g., nouns vs. verbs vs. adjectives)
Verbal analogies *Wing to bird: Fin to _____*	Ability increases from childhood into adolescence but may be a skill not fully acquired until late adolescence or even adulthood Some fifth to eighth graders may approach verbal analogies as free association tasks ("Wing to bird: Fin to swim/water/scales/fish") Ability associated with level of academic performance and word/vocabulary knowledge ("Top to apical: Bottom to _____") Ability associated with world/cultural knowledge ("Democrat to Republican: Labor to _____") (U.S. and Australian political parties) Increase in ability to deal with more complex relationships ("Misfeasance to malfeasance: Misdemeanor to _____") Relationship between cognitive and semantic factors in these tasks not clear
Ambiguities *Playing cards can be expensive.* *The glasses were smeared.*	Statements with more than one meaning that, without context, may be interpreted inaccurately Four types: ■ Phonological ambiguity = homophones ("He saw three pears [pairs]") (Shultz & Pilon, 1973, p. 730) ■ Lexical ambiguity = words with multiple meanings ("She wiped her glasses") (Wiig & Semel, 1984, p. 343) ■ Syntactic or surface structure ambiguity = words in a statement can be grouped in more than one way; interpretation depends on recognition of subtle differences in stress and juncture ("He told her baby//stories"; "He told her//baby stories") (Kessel, 1970, pp. 86–87) ■ Deep structure ambiguity = more than one set of linguistic relationships are possible between words of a statement ("The duck is ready to eat") (Shultz & Pilon, 1973, p. 728) (The duck is going to eat, or the duck has been prepared and someone is about to eat it.) ("I find visiting relatives tiresome") (The act of going to visit relatives is tiresome or relatives who come to visit are tiresome.) Developmental sequence in ability to detect these types in the order listed above ■ Phonological ambiguities: greatest growth rate between 6 and 9 years of age; remains a superior skill compared to other types, at least through grade 10, or about 15 years of age ■ Lexical ambiguities: detected at approximately 10 years of age, although some children in the early elementary grades may respond correctly; remains superior skill to later developing types

TABLE 2.10 | *Continued*

Words and Word Meanings	Features
	■ Syntactic and deep-structure ambiguities: marked development at age 12; little or no skill evidenced earlier ■ Ability to detect syntactic ambiguity may somewhat precede ability to detect deep-structure ambiguities ■ Estimated ages of acquisition: syntactic ambiguities at about 12 years; deep-structure ambiguities at about 12–15 years ■ Some 15-year-olds may continue to have difficulties with both types Often a basis of advertisements (ad for a new car traveling on a highway, "Designed to move you") (Nippold, Cuyler, & Braunbeck-Price, 1988, p. 473)
Figurative language	
Verbal humor	Often based on ambiguities Developmental pattern similar to that for ambiguities
Idioms *Raining cats and dogs* *Slap in the face*	Expressions that have both a figurative and a literal interpretation Comprehension of the figurative meaning of idioms improves with age Gradual growth in understanding into and throughout adolescence In early grades, children may understand literal meaning of idioms; some may also comprehend some of the figurative interpretations Ability associated with reading comprehension level Consistent ability to comprehend figurative meanings not evidenced until adolescence Even older adolescents may not demonstrate complete mastery of idiomatic interpretation Several factors influence idiom comprehension: ■ Frequency of exposure to specific idioms; familiarity; more familiar are more easily understood ■ Manner in which understanding is assessed ■ Degree of supporting contextual information ■ More easily understood when presented in context (e.g., short stories) ■ Harder to understand in isolation (e.g., pointing to pictures depicting the meaning) ■ Providing explanation of idiom is also difficult ■ Transparency; the more transparent, the easier to understand ■ Culture ("Kangaroos in the top paddock," an Australian idiom meaning much the same as "Bats in the belfry") (Reed, 1991, p. 11)
Metaphors and similes *She is a hard person* (metaphor) *The wind was like an arrow looking for its bull's-eye* (simile)	Employing an attribute to describe an entity or to compare entities not literally or typically associated with the attribute or each other Requires acknowledgment of similarities between domains usually seen as dissimilar Common metaphors referred to as *frozen forms;* less common termed *novel forms* Similes: variations of metaphors; inclusion of *like* or the phrase *as (adjective) as;* makes comparison or association explicit Comprehension and use linked to age, cognitive growth, culture, the syntactic forms used to express the metaphor/simile, schooling, semantic growth, and exposure to the forms Similes sometimes thought to be easier than metaphors because of the explicit syntactic form similes employ; research has not fully supported this conclusion Metaphoric comprehension ■ At 7 years of age, children understand some metaphors; appears intuitively based ■ As children enter the concrete operations stage, skill improves considerably ■ Continued improvement into adolescence and the formal thought stage

(*Continued*)

TABLE 2.10 | *Continued*

Words and Word Meanings	Features
	■ In one study (6- to 14-year-olds), only the adolescents understood the metaphors (Winner, Rosenstiel, & Gardner, 1976) ■ Novel forms more difficult than frozen forms Metaphoric use ■ Likely a U-shaped developmental pattern ■ Young children's metaphors generally conventional or frozen forms; any novel forms usually stem from inaccurate perceptions or limited cognitive and linguistic realizations ■ Use of metaphors increases up to the elementary grades ■ In elementary grades, use declines; conforming to educational expectations? ■ Use increases again into adolescent years ■ Adolescence a peak in use of metaphoric productions ■ Frozen forms, not novel forms, predominant even in adolescence
Proverbs *A rolling stone gathers no moss* *Don't put all your eggs in one basket*	Most difficult form of figurative language Later developing than similes, metaphors, and idioms Rudimentary figurative comprehension possibly as young as 7 to 9 years of age if task provides supporting contexts or a receptive task used Proverb explanation a more difficult task Consistent ability in proverb comprehension develops during adolescence and into young adulthood Several factors affect ability: ■ Frequency of exposure; more familiar proverbs easier ("A leopard cannot change its spots" likely easier than "Scalded cats fear even cold water") (Nippold, 2007, p. 218) ■ Word knowledge and word definition ability ■ Culture ("The lion went to the jungle because it ate a deaf ear," a Masai proverb) (Wiig, 1989, p. 7) ■ Amount of formal education, including amount of postsecondary education ■ Degree of concreteness or abstractness of nouns in the proverbs; proverbs with concrete nouns easier Ability associated with level of reading ability

Sources: Achenbach (1970); Armour-Thomas and Allen (1990); Fowles and Glanz (1977); Gardner (1974); Gardner, Kircher, Winner, and Perkins (1975); Johnson and Anglin (1995); Kessel (1970); Nippold (1988, 1991, 1993, 1994b, 1995, 1999, 2000, 2007); Nippold, Allen, and Kirsch (2001); Nippold et al. (1988); Nippold, Hegel, Sohlberg, and Schwarz (1999); Nippold et al. (1998); Nippold, Leonard, and Kail (1984); Nippold and Martin (1989); Nippold, Moran, and Schwarz (2001); Nippold and Rudzinski (1993); Nippold et al. (1992); Nippold and Taylor (1995, 2002); Nippold, Taylor, and Baker (1996); Nippold et al. (1997); Pollio and Pollio (1979); Power, Taylor, and Nippold (2001); Shultz and Horibe (1974); Shultz and Pilon (1973); Spector (1990, 1996); Wiig (1989); Wiig, Gilbert, and Christian (1978); Wiig and Semel (1984); Winner et al. (1976).

Use

Several studies provide indications of developing pragmatic skills in adolescents. Our discussion here focuses on five components of language use: (1) the ability to adapt and modify language, depending on the status of the conversational partner; (2) the various speech acts and functions occurring in communication; (3) ways in which topics are and are not maintained; (4) the paralinguistic features employed; and (5) the nonverbal communicative characteristics of adolescents.

An adolescent who is a competent communicator effectively adapts language to suit the situation (Reed, McLeod, & McAllister, 1999). That is, the adolescent uses code switching and different forms of communication based on the conversational partner's characteristics. Adolescents seem quite aware of the need to place greater importance on certain aspects of communication with particular communication partners than others. In the study by Reed and her colleagues (1999), when grade 10, normally achieving adolescents were asked to rank the order of importance of 14 communication skills in their own communication when they were interacting with their teachers or their peers, communication skills associated with discourse management (e.g., clarification or communication repair for unclear messages) tended to be ranked as more important for interactions with teachers, whereas communication skills associated with empathy and considered to be addressee focused tended to be ranked as more important for communication with adolescent peers. In Larson and McKinley's (1998) longitudinal study, the language development of normally achieving male and female adolescents from grade 7 (12 to 13 years old) through grade 12 (17 to 18 years old) was tracked as they conversed in two situations, one with a same-aged peer and the other with an unfamiliar adult of opposite gender. In adolescent–adolescent conversations, the teenagers used more question types, engaged in more figurative language, introduced more new topics (i.e., evidenced more topic shifts), and used more abrupt topic shifts than in adolescent–adult conversations. These findings support Wiig's (1982) observation that by 13 years of age, adolescents evidence the ability to change from *peer register* to *adult register* and from *formal register* to *informal register.*

Besides being able to adapt their messages according to communicative situations, adolescents should have full use of all communicative functions and speech. The frequency with which adolescents employ different functions and acts appears to vary as a function of both the conversational partner's age and the age of the adolescent speakers themselves. When communicating with peers, adolescents have been described as using more functions designed to entertain and to persuade their peer to feel/believe/do something than when conversing with adults (Larson & McKinley, 1998). Recall from our previous discussion that persuasion has been identified as one type of expository discourse. Although persuading their conversational partner was more evident with peers than adults, when their performance with both conversational partners was pooled, the teenagers showed a pattern of fluctuations in the frequency with which they used persuasion across the grades. Even with the ups and downs in the occurrences of persuasion, the frequency with which this communication function occurred in grades 7 through 12 was actually quite similar. In contrast, the frequency of use of the function of describing an ongoing event increased from grades 7 through 12.

Describing ongoing events can be related to narrative discourse. Nippold (2007) has summarized aspects of narrative ability that improve during the school years and through adolescence. Among these are attempts by older children and adolescents to include more information about the emotions and motivations of the individuals involved in their narratives and to embed episodes or subplots within episodes of the narratives. Johnson (1995) cautions, however, that trying to identify norms for narrative skill is complicated by the fact that there are many different contextually related factors that affect what and how individuals produce narratives.

Other aspects of conversations have been found to change during adolescence. For example, in Larson and McKinley's (1998) longitudinal study, the number of new topics that the adolescents introduced during their conversations decreased from grades 7 through 12, as did their use of abrupt topic shifts. The teenagers did, however, show increases in the number of interruptions during their conversations. For the most part, these findings are consistent with what Nippold (2007) has suggested the literature identifies as characteristics of increasing conversational expertise into adolescence. These include staying on a topic longer, engaging in extended dialogues with conversational partners, and shifting to new topics gracefully.

Although with advancing age adolescents may not increase the frequency with which they use the communication function of persuading the listener to feel/believe/do something (Larson & McKinley, 1998; Nippold, 1994a, 2007), reviews of the literature suggest that there may be refinements in adolescents' execution or application of persuasion. These include greater ability to generate several reasons, rationales, and arguments for a proposition; to control the interactions and discourse; and to use less immature persuasive approaches, such as begging or whining. Other more advanced characteristics of persuasion that Nippold

(2007) identified (i.e., anticipating counterpoints and arguments, adjusting the persuasive strategy to suit listener characteristics, and proposing positive reasons or advantages) relate to the increasing ability of adolescents to adapt their communication to their partners and to see the world from the perspective of their communication partners, which is, in part, related to presupposition. Adolescents' recognition of the importance of being able to take their communication partner's perspective was identified in the Reed et al. (1999) study. These authors found that, although adolescents attached different degrees of importance to specific communication skills depending on whom their communication partners were, the one skill that ranked as relatively important for communication with both teachers and peers was the ability to take the communication partner's perspective. There are several indications in the literature that adolescents' social perspective taking abilities show continuing development during adolescence and that their abilities to consider more fully the perspectives of others in peer relationships become more refined from the period of middle adolescence to later adolescence (Burnett Heyes et al., 2015; Burnett & Blakemore, 2009; Van den Bos, Westenberg, van Dijk, & Crone, 2010).

From Chapter 1, we recall that maze behavior of children—revisions, repetitions, hesitations, and false starts—does not decrease with age. Loban (1976) found that the proportion of maze behavior was the same for children in both grade 12 and grade 1. This was true for all three groups of students—the advanced-, "average-," and poor-language users. Nevertheless, Loban noted erratic increases and decreases in maze behavior in the fourth through ninth grades. Larson and McKinley (1998) found similar fluctuations in grades 7 through 12 and, like Loban, found a similar number of mazes used by adolescents in grade 7 as by those in grade 12. Of particular interest with regard to language impairment was that the poor-language users in Loban's (1976) study exhibited more maze behavior across all grade levels than the "average" language users and much more maze behavior than the advanced-language users.

Findings such as these confirm that there is considerable growth in pragmatic language skills in adolescence. It is during adolescence that teenagers gain adultlike language competency to use in their interactions with others.

LANGUAGE, LITERACY, AND EDUCATION

Language and language-related skills make up the majority of the curricula in school and across all grades. In the early grades, with an emphasis on reading and writing, children's abilities in spoken language, including phonological processing skills, underpin their progress in learning to read and write. With advancing grades in elementary school, children practice their reading and writing, gradually beginning to use these skills for learning content. Learning content exposes the students to more and new language, which as the children progress into adolescence and secondary grades, is used to acquire more content. Along the way students are asked to do increasingly more independent reading and writing with less support from teachers in the process of learning to read and write. Language is, therefore, the primary foundation of literacy and the educational process.

As we have seen, when children enter school, often at the kindergarten level, they typically bring with them a solid base in the spoken (auditory-oral) language system. We know that their spoken language system is wholly developed by age 5, but children beginning kindergarten have usually had 5 years of listening experiences and 4 years of talking experiences. We know that they use fairly well-formed, complex sentences to express their ideas and needs and to ask questions; have a large expressive vocabulary; and understand between 20,000 and 24,000 words. This competence in the spoken language system is a significant factor in learning to read and write. As we will see over and over in this text, children whose listening and speaking skills are well developed most often have better reading and writing skills than those whose spoken language systems were less advanced. Conversely, elementary schoolchildren who struggle in school have regularly been found to have poorer language skills than their academically achieving peers. Oral language development in the preschool years prepares the child for formalized education, and it is integrally related to literacy. As we will see in see later in this text, multiple studies have documented that children's abilities at the end of second, third, or fourth grades in a variety of reading, writing, and reading-related skills, such as decoding printed words, have been predicted by a number of different language skills when the children were toddlers or preschoolers.

Emergent Literacy, Preliteracy, and Reading

Achieving literacy in Western societies is no longer seen as only acquiring the abilities to read and write. Rather, literacy is viewed as engaging in literate behaviors. These include reading spontaneously for pleasure and for learning; writing to convey analyzed and synthesized thoughts and ideas; listening and speaking to argue, persuade, discuss, and plan; and even using computers and the internet to communicate and acquire information. Recent views of literacy have also discarded the notion that literacy begins when children go to school and learn to read and write (Justice & Ezell, 2002). The acquisition of literacy is now seen to begin basically at birth, and toddlers and preschool children are considered to be in the process of becoming literate. *Emergent literacy* and *preliteracy* are terms that have been applied to the development occurring during the preschool years in children's early environments that leads to literacy. These are prereading and prewriting behaviors and skills that develop into conventional reading and writing abilities.

Several factors have been associated with emerging literacy skills in children. One of these is what goes on in preschoolers' homes and their family environment (Justice, Weber, Ezell, & Bakeman, 2002; Skibbe, Justice, Zucker, & McGinty, 2008; Snow, Burns, & Griffin, 1998; van Kleeck, Gillam, Hamilton, & McGrath, 1997). Characteristics of home and family environments that promote literacy include the following:

- A variety of print materials in the environment
- Writing instruments (crayons or pencils) and paper easily available
- Adults who are responsive to the child's attempts to read and write
- Reading and writing as integrated and embedded activities in daily family routine as regular activities of living, such as making lists, writing thank you notes, reading books at bedtime
- Adult–child storybook reading that does the following:
    - Is a social, interactive event
    - Contains routinized dialogue cycles
    - Varies differentially to allow children to take more responsibility for the reading as their language skills grow

Factors such as these are seen as helping to prepare young children for the more formal learning activities they will experience during their elementary and secondary school years. These young children begin school knowing that print represents oral language and, therefore, that it is meaningful and serves a variety of functions. They may even know something about the visual–graphic symbols associated with printed material, including speech sound-to-letter correspondence. Combined with metalinguistic skills, these developmental factors play important roles in children's learning the literacy skills (reading, writing, and spelling) that allow them to engage in literate behaviors, that is, to become literate individuals.

School

The educational system is divided into the elementary and secondary school grades. The primary emphasis of the elementary grades is acquisition of basic learning skills (reading, writing, spelling, and arithmetic abilities), although as children progress into the upper elementary grades, somewhat more importance is placed on using basic skills for content learning. In secondary school, emphasis shifts dramatically to acquiring content-area information, with dramatically increasing expectations for independent learning. At this level, basic skills are assumed to have been acquired.

Stages in Learning to Read The progression that children go through on their route to learning to read has had numerous descriptions. One of those is that of Chall (1996), who described children learning to read as progressing through five stages beginning with formal schooling at entry into kindergarten through high school into adulthood. The following highlights characteristics of these stages.

Stage 1. This stage can be thought of as the "Initial Reading" or "Decoding Stage" in her five-stage framework. This stage corresponds to kindergarten and ages 5 to 7 years. Students learn to associate phonemes in words with the graphemes representing the word in print. Phonics is, therefore, a prominent feature of the stage. Although students likely make word substitution errors, the nature of their errors gives clues as to what they have learned about reading in this initial stage. Initially, as they attempt to read short strings of connected text, they may substitute words that could be semantically possible and fit syntactically, as in reading aloud *The girl is pretty* for the target printed sentence *The girl is throwing.* This type of substitution reflects what linguistic knowledge the student is bringing to the reading task. As students learn more about grapheme-phoneme correspondence as a result of the instructional process, we may see a shift in the emphasis the children put on reading words so that a visually similar word might be substituted for the target but the word substitution might not make sense, such as *The girl is thing.* Gradually a student begins to merge linguistic knowledge with increasing decoding knowledge so word substitutions might be visually similar, semantically plausible, and syntactically acceptable, such as *The girl is three* for the target *The girl is throwing.*

Stage 2. Three accomplishments comprise Stage 2—fluency, confirmation, and ungluing from print. Stage 2 corresponds to grades 2 and 3 and ages 7 through 8 years. Students refine their decoding abilities and practice their reading. As they practice, they encounter redundancies in familiar printed texts, which helps them recognize more quickly and easily words that occur with high frequencies. They experience confirmation in their reading. The practice also increases their reading speed, and because they are better with their decoding skills, they can decipher unrecognized words more quickly. They become more fluent readers as they use greater visual processing. In doing so, they can begin to allocate more of their resources to gleaning meaning from what they are reading and less to the process of deciphering printed words. Thus, they unglue from reading and move toward reading to learn, the next stage.

Stage 3. This stage is the "Reading to Learn" stage. From grades 4 through 8 (possibly 9), corresponding to about 9 to 14 years, students are asked to direct their reading skills to learn information from printed texts and, therefore, learn academic content. The period for Stage 3 covers the upper elementary grades (i.e., grades 4 through 6) and middle school grades (grades 7 through 8/9) and Piaget's concrete operations and formal operations stages of cognition.

Chall considered Stage 3 might more precisely be divided into two substages or periods, with the first corresponding to the upper elementary grades and ages 9 to 11 years. Students are expected to acquire the ability to read relatively long texts typical of adultlike length. However, the reading difficulty level is generally more consistent with grades 4–6. One method of estimating text reading difficulty is a measure known as a "Lexile®" (Stenner, Burdick, Sanford, & Burdick, 2006), which is a metric derived as part of the Lexile® Framework for Reading (Stenner, Burdick, Sanford, & Burdick, 2007). This framework measures students' reading ability as well as measuring the difficulty of text material so that readers can be matched with reading material appropriate for their reading level. The target is for text that the reader can comprehend 75 percent of, which means it is not so difficult that the reader becomes frustrated but is sufficiently challenging that the reader advances in reading ability. In measuring text difficulty, the metric considers both sentence length and the difficulty of the vocabulary in the text.

As students advance into middle school, they enter the second substage of Stage 3. This substage corresponds to approximately ages 12 to 14 years and grades 7 to 8/9. Students improve their reading to learn abilities so that they can typically read text that is adultlike both in length and complexity. At this level, students not only read to learn content but the process also helps them advance their language skills, especially those related to higher level abstract vocabulary, morphologically complex vocabulary, and complex sentences. It is also in these grades and at this reading stage that students start to encounter the challenges of reading expository text associated with different disciplines of the academic areas. The students need to become strategic readers, which means they need to address their reading knowing their purposes for reading the particular material and selecting how they are going to approach their reading. They begin to become "meta-readers." The challenges of dealing with discipline-specific expository texts are discussed in more detail below.

Stage 4. This stage can be thought of as the "Multiple Viewpoints" stage. It corresponds to the high school grades and ages 14 through 18. Students increase in the difficulty of the texts they read and the concepts they encounter. And, as the name implies, students are asked to recognize alternative opinions and contradictions in the material they read. They need to deal more ably with the different ways in which written material is presented in the content areas. That is, they need to become capable "reading code switchers" across the different disciplines.

Stage 5. This stage corresponds to college-level reading, sometimes referred to as the "Construction and Reconstruction—Worldview" stage. Readers read selectively, purposefully, and strategically, choosing what to read, how to read it, and what sections to read. While in Stage 4, they needed to begin to recognize multiple points of view in their reading; in this stage they are expected to analyze and synthesize the viewpoints to construct their own perspectives and viewpoints. Proficient Stage 5 readers deal effectively with their code switching in reading across discipline areas and many are able to even analyze metalinguistically and metacognitively the differences in their reading material across the disciplines. These readers are highly self-controlled readers.

The Elementary Grades: A Brief Overview As readers approach the following information, it would be helpful to keep our immediately preceding information about stages of reading in the fore.

Kindergarten. Kindergarten is often considered as a "readiness" grade to prepare children for the learning experiences to come in first grade. Because of the influence that listening and speaking skills have on reading and writing abilities, kindergarten learning activities frequently focus on further developing the children's spoken language skills. Although kindergarten may emphasize the listening and speaking skills, most children are also introduced formally to reading and writing skills. Kindergartners may learn to recognize the printed words for the days of the week, their classmates' printed names, or the names of printed letters. Learning activities may involve having the children formulate their thoughts and dictate them to the teacher, who writes them for the children. Such an activity emphasizes the relationship between the spoken and printed word and is an initial stage in the development of written composition skills. The children's early experiences with the sensorimotor processes of the visual–graphic language system typically include learning to write the letters of the alphabet and their names and matching sounds to graphemes. The children may also be shown how to improve their drawings of circles and lines, important elements of writing. In some schools, limited formal instruction in reading and writing may be introduced in kindergarten. In other schools, formal instruction in reading and writing is not introduced until first grade.

Another important feature of kindergarten is acculturating children to the scripts and routines of formal group instruction, that is, learning to listen in groups, knowing when to talk and when to be quiet, knowing how to ask and answer questions, and learning how to work quietly alone and to cooperate in groups. Classrooms have a unique discourse style to which students need to acculturate if they are to be able to succeed. This discourse style consists of *IRE* exchanges (i.e., initiate, typically the teacher's role; respond, typically the children's role; and evaluation, typically the teacher's role) (Doell & Reed, 2007; Sturm

& Nelson, 1997). Teachers ask questions to which they obviously already know the answers; students are expected to respond quickly and briefly with answers to these questions if having been given permission to answer; teachers evaluate the quantity and quality of the students' answers. It is within this discourse pattern that orientation and formal instruction in reading typically occurs. Students are challenged, therefore, by the demands of learning not only to read but also to do so in a context that may be quite different from the literacy environment they have experienced at home.

First Grade. Formal reading and writing instruction typically begins in first grade. Children learn to use word recognition skills, acquire information from printed words, distinguish among beginning sounds of spoken words, and read for meaning. In writing, children learn to form both lowercase and uppercase letters and to print short words. Skill levels in writing, however, usually lag behind reading. Although the primary emphasis on language skills in first grade may shift from the auditory–oral system to the visual–graphic system, learning activities continue to involve listening and speaking skills. The children are encouraged to dictate letters and stories; because their writing skills are still limited, the teacher acts as a scribe. Such experiences further demonstrate to children the relationship between the spoken word and the written word and encourage them to learn to write the words they say.

Second Grade. Second-grade curricula emphasize increased skill in listening, speaking, reading, and writing. Children may be asked to rhyme words, follow sequences of orally presented directions, write short stories, increase their spelling vocabularies, and improve printed forms. In reading, the emphasis turns to independence. Students are expected to develop independent word recognition and reading comprehension skills; typically, the curriculum also encourages the children to spend time in independent reading. Learning activities move from concrete, hands-on experiences to abstract, language-related experiences.

Third Grade. Third grade is a transition grade. Increased attention is given to independent reading, with emphasis on reading more complex, longer stories. Instruction in cursive writing typically begins, although printed forms may continue to be used in situations where speed is expected. Children are asked to answer questions by writing sentences and to write increasingly complex paragraphs. Continued emphasis is placed on increasing spelling vocabularies. Children in third grade are also typically expected to proofread and correct their written work. Oral activities include participating effectively in group discussions and making presentations.

Fourth, Fifth, and Sixth Grades. Between third and fourth grade, there is a huge jump in the language demands of school. This transition is one of several points in the course of going to school when students who might have been able to cope with marginal language skills start to experience academic struggles. It is also a time when students who have previously been identified as having language problems may need extra support in order to cope with the language of school. Professionals need to watch children carefully for signs that their language may not be a match for the demands of the curriculum.

The curricular emphases in these upper elementary grades continually shift from learning activities directed to building skills in the auditory–oral and visual–graphic language systems to using these language skills for acquiring content-area information. Students gain information through class discussions and short teacher lectures and demonstrations. Students may even be given independent reading assignments and be asked to write short reports about what they have read. They are expected to use their language skills to seek out information from resources. Without the necessary underlying basic skills in both the auditory–oral and the visual–graphic system, we can see how children can be at risk for failure. We will see a number of times in later chapters how children's early language abilities impact their subsequent success or failure in school.

The Secondary Grades: A Brief Overview. The shift from elementary to secondary education generally occurs somewhere around sixth or seventh grade. The shift from elementary school to middle school is another high-risk transition for students with language problems because the bar for language demands of school is suddenly raised by leaps and bounds. Another risky transition for language demands occurs between middle school and high school. Again, professionals need to be particularly on top of students' performances to make sure they are providing appropriate support and intervention at these points in students' academic progression.

Lectures as the means of instruction become more common, and students are increasingly expected to be able to take written notes on the lecture content. Additionally, students may have different teachers for different subjects. This means that students need to adjust to varying lecture delivery, assignments, and teaching styles. In addition to idiosyncratic language patterns that all language-proficient individuals have, including teachers in their teaching, teachers' language reflects characteristics of the language of their content areas. We see here the influence of discipline-related discourse features in how students need to approach comprehension of content material. Ehren (2010) has delineated several reasons expository text is generally difficult for students, and especially difficult for those who struggle with language:

- Unfamiliarity with the genre of expository text—we have already seen that students typically do not encounter this genre until formal schooling, unlike the experience they might have had prior to school with narrative genre
- Discipline-specific expository genres and even variations in form within a discipline—we have already encountered this issue in how these variations can increase difficulty for students
- Complexity of expository discourse—this includes issues related to, for example:
  - Increased length of material
  - Organizational patterns, often a logical pattern versus the more common temporal order of narratives
  - Impersonal presentation of the text
  - New information presented in the text
  - Technical vocabulary, often in the form of morphologically complex words
- Requirements for considerable inferencing on the reader's part, especially if the author has misjudged readers' prior knowledge of the content; Ehren used the term "considerate texts" (p. 217) to describe expository discourse in which an author has made a concerted effort to presuppose readers' prior knowledge and match text presentation accordingly
- Conceptual density of information crowded into expository texts, an issue escalated in difficulty if students are reading an inconsiderate text with considerable technical and new vocabulary

Independence in all forms of learning is stressed, and teachers expect students to be able to seek out and organize information for themselves. The emphasis is on learning content and on demonstrating what information has been acquired. Acquiring vocabulary associated with specific content areas (e.g., photosynthesis, alliteration, and quadrilateral) is an essential language skill for secondary school success and a major avenue for students being able to increase the sizes of their vocabularies. The larger their vocabularies and the more they can pull apart morphologically complex words into their roots and affixes, the easier it is for them to access additional academic content and increase their vocabularies further. There is also a significant increase in the use of the written mode for demonstrating knowledge, and performance on written tests of content knowledge takes on greater importance.

Children's language skills evolve dramatically from kindergarten on. Although the development is a complex process, with listening, speaking, reading, and writing skills closely related to and interacting with one another, a large part of the early educational achievement in reading and writing depends heavily on the children's abilities with the auditory–oral language system. Later educational achievements depend on both the auditory–oral and the visual–graphic language system and the essential reciprocal interactions between them.

SUMMARY

In this chapter we have seen that

- Babies are born communicating, and before infants use their first words, they engage in many behaviors (e.g., smiling, laughing, and gazing) that convey communication intent and exhibit a range of prelinguistic vocalizations.
- In the one- and two-word stages, children learn the names for objects and relations in their environment; vocabulary growth begins slowly, spurting ahead between 18 and 24 months of age.
- Children's early utterances systematically develop into basic kernel, negative, and question sentences and later into compound and complex sentences.
- Semantic as well as syntactic factors are involved in sentence development.
- Several patterns influence word learning, and there seem to be several principles that apply to children's word learning.
- Children acquire specific grammatical morphemes in a developmental sequence related to increasing mean length of utterance.
- The functions and intentions of language use change as children get older; utterances change from those containing one function to those containing more than one function.
- Young children adapt the form of their language for their listeners; this ability to adapt grows more refined as children become better able to make accurate presuppositions about their listeners. Turn-taking, topic maintenance, and revision skills improve gradually throughout the preschool years and into the school years.
- Children's narratives develop from those produced at about 2 years of age, characterized by heaps of unrelated statements, to those produced in the first 2 or 3 years of school, characterized by multiply embedded episodes with causal and temporal patterns.
- Children learn to deal with expository discourse when they enter school and continue to expand their abilities with this particular form of discourse. Skill with expository discourse is essential for academic success.
- Reading proficiency is acquired throughout the educational experience and progresses through several stages.
- Success throughout the school years depends on a robust language system that continues to develop across the grades.

As this review of normal language development illustrates, there are a great many skills that children must acquire, with the ultimate aim that they will be able to succeed in school, personal relationships, and vocational endeavors. We have seen that the process often follows developmental patterns. These developmental patterns frequently become a basis for planning intervention programs for children who have impaired language skills. These same developmental sequences also provide one way of identifying children who are not progressing appropriately in acquiring their language.

PART 2

Children with Language Disorders

3

Toddlers and Preschoolers with Specific Language Impairment

LEARNING OBJECTIVES

After reading this chapter, you should be able to

- Discuss issues related to identification of young children with language impairment
- Provide an overview of specific language impairment
- Detail the language characteristics of young children with specific language impairment
- Discuss implications for intervention for young children with specific language impairment

This chapter is about toddlers and preschool children who evidence language problems in the apparent absence of other clearly identifiable problems, such as those indicated in the titles of many of the chapters that will follow in this text (e.g., intellectual disability, autism spectrum disorder, hearing impairment, and acquired language impairment). The children we will discuss in this chapter appear on the surface to be essentially typically developing, except for their language acquisition, which does not match that of their peers. Because we cannot attribute their language-learning problems to an identifiable condition, most individuals who work with and study these children have chosen to use the term *specific language impairment* (SLI) to refer to these children, hence the chapter title. Hadley and Short (2005, p. 1344) defined SLI as "a condition characterized by extreme difficulty in language acquisition in the presence of otherwise typical development." Leonard (1998) described these children as those

> who show a significant limitation in language ability, yet the factors usually accompanying language learning problems—such as hearing impairment, low nonverbal intelligence test scores, and neurological damage—are not evident. This is a real curiosity, especially in light of the many language acquisition papers that begin with a statement to the effect that "all normal children" learn language rapidly and effortlessly. The only thing clearly abnormal about these children is that they don't learn language rapidly and effortlessly. (p. 3)

Part of the decision to use the term *specific language impairment* in the chapter title was guided by a desire to distinguish as much as possible the topic of this chapter from other chapters in this text. Using the phrase was not, however, a completely easy choice because of several unresolved issues about these children. Among these are whether the children's language problems are, in fact, specific only to language and whether the language problems of these children reflect language delay or disorder. Another is the possibility that there may be subgroups of these children, in which case SLI might not be one condition but instead several distinct conditions that share some but not all symptoms. How we approach these issues affects what we label the problem. Here is the dilemma about the chapter title. Other issues concern the prevalence data for preschool children with language impairments without obvious concomitant problems, how we identify children who have these language-learning problems, our abilities to predict who will and will not outgrow early language delays, and the intervention implications of these issues. These are topics we address in this chapter. We also discuss some of the language characteristics seen in these young children and introduce assessment and intervention considerations. There is no longer any question that language problems of children in their preschool years signal the real likelihood of later academic, vocational, and social failures, topics taken up further in the two subsequent chapters. ***SLI is an insidious, lifelong disability. And, its prevalence rate makes it the most frequently occurring of all communication disorders, and it is one of the "most commonly occurring neurodevelopmental disorders"*** (Redmond, 2016b, p. 63).

However, before moving too far into discussion of toddlers and preschoolers with SLI, some consideration of the issue of identifying children with language impairment more generally is appropriate. This topic is relevant for many of the children with language disorders whom we will discuss in this text as well as the children with SLI who are the focus of this chapter.

IDENTIFICATION OF CHILDREN WITH LANGUAGE IMPAIRMENT

It may seem strange to think of identifying children with language problems as a major issue. One might think that identifying these children would be straightforward. Certainly, a child whose language performance does not correspond to that of children the same age might be considered to have language problems. However, several questions arise. We know that children who are acquiring language normally can show marked variability in language development. If a child's performance does not correspond to that of other children of the same age, does the difference reflect normal variation or a problem? How do we determine if the difference is normal variation or problematic? If the difference is considered not to be a reflection of normal variability, how much of a difference from expectations constitutes a real problem versus a slowed pattern within normal limits? If a child demonstrates above-average development in areas other than language, such as cognition/intelligence or motor skills, but only average development in language, should we consider the child to have a language impairment? A related issue is how we think about infants who are preverbal, so that oral language performance cannot be observed, or about children who at a particular point in time seem to demonstrate adequate language skills but who have intrinsic factors that may place them at risk for later language performance. Should these children be considered to have language impairments? These are only a few of the questions. The answers to these questions influence which children, as Lahey (1990) writes, "shall be called language disordered" (p. 619) and who may and may not, therefore, receive intervention and what might be the forms of intervention.

Given normal variability in children's language development and in their language performances from one communicative context to another, the standard to which we compare an individual child's performance and the conditions under which we observe that performance are important factors in identification. This latter factor requires that a child's language performance be observed in a variety of contexts, a topic that will be discussed later in this book. Although language developmental milestones provide relevant information about whether a child's performance is similar to or different from these milestones, they provide very little information about the significance of any variations that might be observed. It is the significance attached to the variations that leads to identification of a child as having a language problem. However, deciding on the significance of the variations depends, in part, on the standard to which we compare the performance and how we measure performance.

Mental Age, Chronological Age, and Language Age

The two standards of comparison that have commonly been used are mental age (MA) and chronological age (CA). MA refers to the age level at which a child is functioning on cognitive/intellectual tasks, that is, intellectual level generally measured by intelligence tests. An intelligence quotient (IQ) is often a psychometric indicator that relates a child's MA to CA. In using MA as the standard, children's language performances are compared to those of children with similar MAs. The assumption is that normal children's language performance does not generally differ markedly from their cognitive abilities. When language performance is lower than MA, a language impairment is presumed to be present. That is, there is a gap between MA and language age (LA). Using this standard of comparison raises the controversial issue often referred to as *cognitive referencing,* which is related to the strong cognitive hypothesis discussed in Chapter 1. This means that children's levels of language skills are viewed in terms of their cognitive prowess. There are, however, several problems with this approach, among them:

1. The exact relationship between cognition and language has not been established (*see* Chapter 1). Therefore, it cannot be assumed that cognitive abilities will necessarily always set the limits for or determine language performance.
2. It is generally agreed that there is a reciprocal relationship for most children between cognition and language.
3. Some, but not many, children may have language skills higher than their cognitive skills.
4. There may be different types of intelligence, and a theoretical relationship between these and language has not been demonstrated.
5. From an assessment and intervention perspective, it is possible that many children with intellectual disabilities do not get identified as having a language disorder because there may be little or no gap between their MA and LA. As a result, these children may not receive language intervention services even though they might benefit from intervention.

There is, however, one advantage of this approach. Children who have above-average cognitive skills but language skills significantly below their cognitive levels might be seen as having a language impairment.

A related issue to using MA as a standard of comparison is how a child's cognitive/intellectual abilities are tested in order to determine MA. What we measure as indicators of cognition and language, how we measure them, and when we measure them in children's development impact what we find out about the children's levels in each area of functioning. If intelligence is assessed with a test that includes types of items involving language ability, such as verbal analogies (*Wing to bird; Fin to* _______), the test measures a child's language ability as much as intelligence. An accurate indicator of MA is, therefore, not possible, and it is not possible to separate language ability from intellectual ability. A verbal IQ (VIQ) score is confounded with both language and intelligence. There are some methods of assessing intelligence that minimize the language component, such as tasks requiring recognition and completion of visual patterns as in block designs. A nonverbal IQ (NVIQ) score, or performance IQ (PIQ) score, which is a term also used, is less confounded by language and better reflects intelligence without the language confound. Some intelligence tests are highly verbal in nature, others have tasks that attempt to tap verbal intelligence and nonverbal/performance intelligence separately, and others are primarily nonverbal in nature. In using MA as a standard of comparison when the issue of interest involves language ability, it is essential to know how MA was assessed.

The second standard to which language performance is compared uses CA. Fey (1986) explained it well when he wrote that "with CA referencing, language impairment is defined as a clinically significant departure from what is expected for children of the child's own CA" (p. 36). That is, there is a gap between CA and LA (and MA is not considered). Although this approach resolves the concern about the still unestablished relationship between cognition/MA and language performance, it has certain problems:

1. Children whose cognitive levels exceed their CA but whose language performances correspond to their CA may not be identified as having language problems. These might be very bright or gifted children whose language abilities may prevent achievement at the level that could be expected from their cognitive level.
2. The number of children identified as having language problems may be so large that it strains the professional resources available to serve them. This approach implies, as Fey (1986) explains, that the ultimate goal of intervention for any child identified as language disordered "would be to bring the child's communicative abilities to an age-equivalent level. . . . Unfortunately, this is frequently an unrealistic expectation for many of the children" (p. 36).

Despite the problems associated with the CA–LA gap approach to identifying the children, these may be less serious than those related to the MA–LA comparison. *Of these two standards of comparison, CA is generally the preferred and recommended standard for comparison.* In fact, more recent federal legislation regarding serving children in schools has indicated that the MA–LA comparison (i.e., cognitive referencing) should not be used to qualify children for services in schools and it not considered "best practice" with regard to children with language impairment.

We now return to the issue of what constitutes an important variation from the standard we use. Even in light of our previous discussion, there is justified concern about using age-equivalency measures, such as LA referred to in the preceding discussion. One reason for this concern is that the same delay in terms of age-equivalent performance may not have the same importance for children of different ages. For example, a 1-year delay in language performance for a 10-year-old child may not likely carry the same significance as a 1-year delay for a 3-year-old child. Lahey (1990) argues that a more appropriate approach describes a child's "relative standing with peers" (p. 615) so that normal variability from an average is considered.

Normal Variation, Normal Distribution, and a Statistical Approach

The approach of using normal variability to decide which children's language performances are sufficiently different from their peers' to constitute an impairment is based on concepts surrounding the normal distribution of performance in samples of children of the same age with particular demographic characteristics. It is rooted in statistical approaches to distribution so that the metrics of mean and standard deviations (SD) are considered. Using concepts of normal distribution (i.e., normal curve), we know, for example, that if we measured the receptive vocabulary size of lots of 3-year-old children, about 68 percent of them would have scores falling between –1 standard deviation (SD) below the mean score and +1 SD above, with approximately half on either side of the mean. This range, –1 to +1 SD, is generally considered the "normal" range of performance, and a score below the –1 SD point is often the point at which some unease about a child's performance might occur. Approximately another 13.5 percent of the children would have scores between –1 SD and –2 SD, leaving about another 2.5 to 3 percent of the children having scores below –2 SD. Concern about a child's performance generally escalates the greater the child's score is below the –1 SD point.

Questions are:

- Which cutoff tells us that a child's receptive vocabulary (or any other aspect of language we measure in this way) is sufficiently poor to indicate language impairment?
- What cutoff tells us when the child's performance will cause academic and social difficulties for the child?

In essence, the cutoffs that are frequently used are relatively arbitrary because, as Rice (2000) explains, "there is no intrinsic criterion for where to draw the line between 'normal' and 'affected'" (p. 20). Recall also that if we make the cutoff –2 SD below the mean, there will be only 3 percent of children who will be considered to have impaired language. Bishop (1997) reminds us of the "inherent circularity of statistical definitions" because "if you define a language impairment as a score in the lowest 3%, then 3% of the children will be language-impaired" (p. 23).

Besides standard deviations, other descriptions of language performance based on normal variation, normal distribution, and related statistics include standard scores, percentile ranks, and stanine scores. These are metrics often seen with norm-referenced language tests. To provide some point of reference as to how these metrics correspond to each other, a –1 SD deviation cutoff is commonly about equal to a standard score of 85 (when the SD is 15 and mean is 100), a 17th- to 18th-percentile rank, and a stanine of 3. With regard to identifying children with SLI, a standard of comparison or cutoff at the 10th percentile has been considered as a plausible cutoff for identifying a child's language to be sufficiently problematic to be language impaired. A 10th-percentile rank equates to about –1.25 SD and a standard score of about 80 to 81 (again assuming an SD of 15 and a mean of 100 on the test used to measure the language). This standard of comparison has been shown to have good agreement with speech–language pathologists' judgments of children's language abilities as being impaired (Tomblin, Records, & Zhang, 1996).

However, any test score provides only an estimate of a child's "true" language performance. Assessment and measurement involve errors because humans and their functioning are inconsistent, as are the environments in which we assess and measure, and the instruments that we use are imperfect. Therefore, we need to expect measurement error, which makes any test score an estimate. Better psychometrically developed norm-referenced tests account for measurement error by including a *standard error of measurement (SEM)*. A range (confidence interval) around an obtained standard score can be determined with the SEM by both adding and subtracting the SEM to the obtained score. The larger the range around the obtained standard score, the greater our confidence is that it would include a child's true score. For example, if we want to be 95 percent confident (95 percent confidence level) that a child's true score was within a particular range, the test would provide a metric for the 95 percent confidence level for us to use to determine the confidence interval (e.g., SEM for 95 percent confidence level = ±8; child's obtained standard score on the test = 79; 95 percent confidence interval = 71 to 87). If we are prepared to be less confident, for example, 68 percent confident, about the range within which the child's true score falls, the test might provide a smaller SEM to use in determining the 68 percent confidence interval (e.g., SEM for 68 percent confidence level = ±4; child's obtained standard score on the test = 79; 68 percent confidence interval = 75 to 83). If we have decided that a standard score of 80 to 81 is our cutoff for determining that a child's language is impaired, both confidence intervals in our example here leave open the possibility that the child's language is not impaired because of the upper limit in the two ranges (87 with the 95 percent confidence level and 83 with the 68 percent confidence level) as well as leaving open the possibility that the child does have impaired language. This example illustrates why best practice requires the use of multiple forms of language assessment in making decisions about a child's language status and decisions do not depend solely on norm-referenced tests.

We have another issue to consider when we think about using common metrics to decide when language performance is or is not impaired. In the introduction to this chapter, we noted in Leonard's (1998) description of children with SLI that they would not have low nonverbal intelligence scores. That is, their NVIQs would be at or above the normal level, typically considered to be no lower than –1 SD, or commonly 85 standard score. As we will see in Chapter 6 on language and intellectual disability, the common intelligence test cutoff score for intellectual disability is –2 SD, or 70 standard score. However, some children have NVIQ scores between –1 SD and –2 SD and have language abilities falling below normal (i.e., –1 SD). While these children are unlikely to be considered as having an intellectual disability using the common criteria, they are also unlikely to be seen as having SLI because of their NVIQ level. Because these children have impaired language but do not neatly fall into either the intellectual disability or the SLI classification, some have begun to use the term *nonspecific language impairment* (NLI) to refer to these children to describe these children in assessment and intervention and in research (Catts, Fey, Zhang, & Tomblin, 2002; Leonard, Miller, & Finneran, 2009; Nippold, Mansfield, Billow, & Tomblin, 2009). In providing services to children with language impairment, professionals need to be alert that these children with NLI do not drop through the cracks.

Social Standard

Scores such as percentile ranks and standard scores still do not tell us how much a child's language abilities might interfere with academic and/or social achievements. Using the above cutoff of the 10th-percentile rank, a child whose language performance is at the 10th percentile would be considered language disordered, whereas one whose performance is at the 15th-percentile rank might not. However, it could be that the child at the 15th-percentile rank will experience just as many or more difficulties because of language problems as the one at the 10th percentile. An approach that focuses on variance scores also has the danger of leading professionals to depend too heavily on norm-referenced, standardized tests of language for identifying language-disordered children, a topic discussed in Chapter 13.

There may be a third standard of comparison to consider, that is, a social standard. In using this standard, societal values placed on the degree of language facility and on the degree of success for life functions that are dependent on language facility (e.g., educational success and social success) become important in identifying children (Brinton, Fujiki, & McKee, 1998; Johnson et al., 1999; Leonard, 2014; Rutter, 2008; Silliman & Wilkinson, 2014). Children whose language performances are evaluated as being sufficiently poor to cause potential problems in succeeding within the conditions of societal values could then be seen to have language impairments.

From an educational perspective for school children, this standard has taken root in the requirement that impairments need to have negative academic impact for children to receive services in schools. The odds suggested by research documenting outcomes for children in adolescence and adulthood who were identified with language impairment during preschool years (which readers will encounter in Chapter 5) make it unlikely that the young children will fully escape future negative educational and/or social effects of the impairment. The research now provides professionals with strong predictive abilities about the future for toddlers and preschoolers with SLI. This gives considerable strength to the social standard, especially as a preventative strategy, that is, early identification of (and intervention for) children with SLI to mitigate future negative effects.

Although this standard is harder to measure in numerical terms, it may overcome some of the difficulties inherent in the other standards for identification discussed so far. This may be particularly true if a social standard is used in combination with one of these more traditional standards. It also has the potential to provide a framework for approaching language and language impairments in linguistically-culturally diverse children.

Clinical Markers for SLI

Research attempting to identify clinical markers of SLI in young children may help us in knowing which children have SLI. A *clinical marker* is a behavioral feature or characteristic or a combination of particular features or characteristics that children with SLI have. Because it is either present or absent, a clinical marker is independent of the normal distribution of language ability across the population, and it correctly identifies those children with SLI (i.e., affected children) and does not incorrectly identify other children with normal language as affected. An analogy might be that people with a particular medical condition have a unique combination of hormones in their bodies (i.e., the hormone combination is the clinical marker) that people without the condition do not have. The presence or absence of the hormone combination is not dependent on a normal distribution in the population. When genetic factors are believed to underlie a clinical marker, the term *phenotype* may be used to refer to the clinical marker. Children's abilities with verb tense morphology, nonword repetition (NWR), and sentence recall are three of the directions that the search for an SLI clinical marker has taken. Abilities with one or more of these may have possible genetic bases, so it is possible that they could be phenotypes.

English-speaking children with SLI are renowned for their persisting difficulties with grammatical forms and in particular those related to tense marking on verbs (for example, Leonard, Deevy, Miller, Charest, & Kurtz, 2003; Redmond & Rice, 2001). Rice and her colleagues (Rice, 2000; Rice & Wexler, 1996; Rice, Wexler, & Hershberger, 1998) have reported that tasks examining 5-year-olds' verb form marking abilities correctly identify 97 percent of children with SLI and 98 percent of typically developing children. Findings have also indicated that the longitudinal developmental course of verb tense marking for SLI children is protracted and does not reach adultlike levels of accuracy by 8 years of age. This contrasts with normally developing children, who make almost no errors at that age. At the toddler level, 2-year-olds at risk for SLI have been found to show later onset of tense marking in their language development than even normally developing peers with language development at lower language levels, and toddlers and preschoolers have been shown to be slower to develop tense marking than reported in the literature for normally developing children's language development (Gladfelter & Leonard, 2013; Hadley & Rice, 1996; Hadley & Short, 2005). Verb morphology is a strong candidate as a clinical marker. Given that tense marking should typically emerge in children between 2 and 4 years of age, there is potential that verb morphological skills can be assessed in quite young children, increasing its power as a possible clinical marker useful with toddlers and preschoolers.

The second direction that the search for a clinical marker of SLI has taken is NWR. NWR also appears in the literature with the acronym of *NRT*, which stands for *nonword repetition test/task*. NWR focuses on aspects of children's processing abilities and requires children to repeat nonsense words of varying syllable length and phonological complexity (e.g., Archibald & Joanisse, 2009; Chiat & Roy, 2013; Conti-Ramsden, 2003; Dollaghan & Campbell, 1998; Ellis Weismer et al., 2000; Gathercole, Willis, Baddeley, & Emslie, 1994; Gray, 2003a). Children with SLI generally perform much worse than normally achieving children of the same age and younger children with similar levels of language. And, children's performances on the tasks tend to separate the children with good accuracy into a group without language impairment and those with poor accuracy into a group with language impairments. NWR is a strong candidate as a clinical marker of SLI (Coady & Evans, 2008; Graf Estes, Evans, & Else-Quest, 2007).

As promising as NWR might be for identifying SLI in children, tasks designed to assess this ability in children have been restricted mostly to children 5 years of age and older because of the complexity of performing the tasks (Graf Estes et al., 2007). However, more recently, NWR tasks have been used with children younger than 5 years of age, with some children as young as 2 years old (Chiat & Roy, 2007, 2013; Deevy, Wisman Weil, Leonard, & Goffman, 2010; Gray, 2003a; Roy & Chiat, 2004; Stokes & Klee, 2009; Thal, Miller, Carlson, & Vega, 2005). Because, as we will see later in this chapter, some preschoolers with SLI also have speech sound errors, use of NWR with these children has not been valid and reliable since the tasks generally require accurate production of the sounds making up the syllables in the nonwords. For this reason, Shriberg et al. (2009) developed an NWR test, *The Syllable Repetition Test*, which uses only four consonants, all of which normally developing children acquire early, and only one early developing vowel. Because of the efforts of these and other researchers, there are now nonword repetition tasks that appear to be relatively "toddler and preschooler friendly."

Sentence recall has also emerged as a possible clinical marker of SLI. Sentence recall is sometimes referred to in the literature as *sentence repetition* and *sentence imitation*. Sentence recall has appeared as a task in assessment tools for a long time, including the first American version of the Stanford-Binet intelligence test in about 1916. When the length of a sentence exceeds children's short-term auditory memories but is within the children's comprehension levels and contains morphosyntactic structures also within the children's repertoire, they will generally be able to imitate correctly all elements in an adult's spoken presentation of the sentence. The same children would not, however, be able to repeat a series of random numbers (digits) containing the same number of elements as the sentence because length exceeds the children's short-term memory and presumably because the number series carries no meaning, so there is nothing other than short-term memory to assist the children. The premise with regard to sentence recall tasks is that, in order to perform correctly, children need to rely on their morphosyntactic knowledge in long-term memory (Riches, 2012). If a long sentence contains grammatical elements, for example embedded relative clauses or complex verb forms ("would not be skiing"), that are beyond the children's level of language development, children will typically produce the sentence only with elements that are consistent with those they know. This means they may omit certain grammatical elements or change the elements to fit their language level. Several early tests of syntax for children, for example the Carrow Elicited Language Inventory (CELI) (Carrow, 1974) and the Northwestern Syntax Screening Test (NSST) (Lee, 1971), used a sentence recall format, as do some current child language tests, for example, Clinical Evaluation of Language Fundamentals – 5 (CELF – 5) (Wiig, Semel, & Secord, 2013). Children's performances on sentence recall tasks have suggested that the task is reasonably good at identifying children who have SLI or at predicting those who are at risk for SLI from those who do not or are unlikely to demonstrate later language impairment (e.g., Archibald & Joanisse, 2009; Conti-Ramsden, Botting, & Faragher, 2001; Redmond, Thompson, & Goldstein, 2011; Riches, 2012).

Children's performances in these areas may not serve only as clinical markers of SLI that help identify the presence of SLI. It is also possible that they can serve the role as risk factors for SLI. That is, there may be concern that young children whose performances do not meet the levels of their same-age peers are at risk for SLI, and there may be merit in exploring further the children's language abilities. Thus, tasks incorporating verb tense marking, NWR, and sentence recall might be good at: (1) identifying young children who have SLI; (2) separating young children who have SLI from children who have other conditions, such as ADHD; and (3) predicting which children are at risk for continuing language impairment and which might "outgrow" early language delay.

Challenging and Changing the Child's Language Performance

Among the conundrums facing professionals working with children with possible language impairment is that some toddlers and preschoolers with language impairment that can potentially interfere with academic performance or social interactions might appear at superficial glance to communicate adequately. These children might even attain scores on some norm-referenced language tests that place them within normal limits. However, in such cases their test scores are probably at the lower end of normal limits, and when compared to the scores of their typically developing peers, their scores may be significantly lower, suggesting that their language is not really the same as their peers (Girolametto, Wiigs, Smyth, Weitzman, & Pearce, 2001; Paul, 1996; Stothard, Snowling, Bishop, Chipchase, & Kaplan, 1998). They may also be able to engage in casual, relaxed conversational interchanges (Lahey, 1990), but they may experience difficulties with academic skills closely related to oral language abilities, such as reading, spelling, and writing, and with high-level, demanding discourse language skills, such as narratives (Girolametto et al., 2001; Johnson et al., 1999; Paul, 1996; Stothard et al., 1998; Ukrainetz & Gillam, 2009). These factors have implications for the procedures we use in identifying the children. For this reason, Lahey (1990) suggests that identification should be made under conditions that include stressing or challenging the child's language performance "so that difficulties with performance would most likely be evident" (p. 618).

Children with language impairment should also have more difficulty acquiring particular language skills under conditions of focused instruction than their peers without language problems. Degree of difficulty in learning language targets can be measured in terms of the speed with which new language skills are learned, the amount of teaching effort that is needed, or the accuracy of performance, that is, the quantity of learning. Children with language disorders should therefore require more tries to learn a language target and/or need more and varied stimuli to learn the targets and/or use the targets correctly less often than their typically developing counterparts. These suppositions suggest that another way in which children with language disorders can be identified is by determining how well or poorly they respond to "trial language instruction" or, to be consistent with the terminology currently used in the literature, how well they respond to dynamic assessment. Dynamic assessment is an essential part of the assessment process, and its use is raised in several subsequent chapters and discussed in more detail in Chapter 13.

Risk Factors for Language Problems

Identification also involves predicting which children will ultimately experience problems related to language. There are very young and therefore primarily nonverbal children (e.g., below 1 or 1½ years of age) who may be at risk for language development problems, and there are preschool and school-age children who may not have observable language problems at a specific time but who have a history or other problems that place them at risk for the emergence of later identifiable language difficulties. Tomblin, Hardy, and Hein (1991) suggest that it might be possible to assign neonates to an "at risk for language problems" category based on criteria related to prenatal and perinatal events. The children's development could then be monitored and intervention begun as soon as any problems with language emerged. It might also be possible to institute "preventive intervention" for these children through parent/caregiver training programs even before actual language problems are identified. For older children who have histories or other problems that place them at risk for the emergence of language difficulties, preventive intervention through parental and/or teacher training programs might also be effective.

These approaches depend, of course, on determining what factors place children at risk for language disorders. Some birth factors (e.g., anoxia, hyperbilirubinemia, and kernicterus), chromosomal syndromes (e.g., Down syndrome), and known neurological or physical conditions (e.g., cerebral palsy, hearing loss, and cleft palate) have been linked to potential language problems. Additionally, risk for language problems has been associated with socioeconomic factors and environmental deprivation although these are not always independent of other factors, such as familial or genetic factors. Some have suggested that prematurity may place an infant at risk for later language problems, although this is not always the case. Some of these risk factors are related more to language problems when other conditions exist (e.g., intellectual disability, hearing loss) but are not necessarily known to be risk factors for SLI per se.

There are factors other than these that may more accurately place very young children at risk for later being identified as having SLI. Among those suggested in the literature are (1) a family history of literacy problems and/or communication problems, particularly among members of the immediate family; (2) birth order, with later birth indicating a greater risk; and (3) parents' levels of education, particularly mother's level of education (e.g., Choudhury & Benasich, 2003; Dollaghan et al., 1999; Felsenfeld & Plomin, 1997; Hart & Risley, 1995; Newbury & Monaco, 2010; Plomin, DeFries, McClearn, & McGuffin, 2001; Rice, 2013; Tomblin et al., 1991). Gender of the child, with males appearing to be more at risk than females, is often also cited as a risk factor for SLI. There are, however, conflicting data about whether boys are at greater risk for SLI. Studies using clinical samples of children may tend to show more males as having SLI, whereas studies using population studies may tend to show more equal distribution across genders (Law, Rush, Schoon, & Parsons, 2009). It may be that boys are more frequently referred for assistance with their language than girls. The jury on gender is still out. In a previous section, we also suggested that ability with verb morphological learning, sentence recall, and NWR could be viewed as risk factors for SLI.

Missing from this list of possible risk factors is socioeconomic status (SES). Many children from lower socioeconomic families have language problems, and some of these problems are due to SLI. However, low SES by itself may be an indirect risk factor rather than a core risk factor since SES is often an outcome of some of the risk factors noted above (e.g., lower educational level of mother leading to lower SES and/or family history of literacy/communication problems leading to lower educational level leading to lower SES). Some of the confusion related to the role of SES arises from imprecise differentiation in the literature between language delay and language disorder. Few disagree that low SES is a risk factor for language delay in children, but the question of interest here is about the relationship of SES as a risk factor for impaired language, that is, language disorder.

Caution is important in interpreting these possible risk factors. It is likely that not all factors have been fully determined, that the factors just listed are not invariably associated with language difficulties, and that their interrelationships with other factors have yet to be fully explained. Language learning and language performance are complex human behaviors influenced by multiple factors, so the factors that place children at risk for language impairment are more than likely going to reflect complex interactions. However, in their study of a variety of prenatal and perinatal risk factors for SLI (e.g., parental education, family history of language and/or learning problems, tobacco smoking), Tomblin, Smith, and Zhang (1997) found that, in contrast to risk factors considered to occur during the perinatal period of the children or during their fetal development, SLI in children was more likely to be associated with factors related to their parents that were present before the children were conceived (e.g., parental education, family history of language and/or learning problems). When we think about the implications of these findings, we see the probability of familial transmission of SLI in children.

Despite the limits on the current information, Tomblin et al. (1991) suggest that using an at-risk procedure that places children in a developmental monitoring program in combination with a language screening procedure may aid the identification process. However, if we apply Lahey's (1990) idea, the screening procedure should include tasks that stress the child's language performance. The notion of using high-risk factors with monitoring combined with screening programs is consistent with her suggestion that perhaps two identification categories should be devised. One would be for those children who show problems with language and the other for children at risk for language problems. Using the findings from Tomblin et al. (1997) noted above, it might be possible to begin considering weighting the degree of risk associated with various risk factors.

Table 3.1 summarizes some of the issues we have raised with regard to identifying children with language problems. Although the issues remain, Fey (1986) has offered a practical definition of "who shall be called language disordered" (Lahey, 1990) that is based on one presented in 1983 by Tomblin:

> A child may be viewed as language impaired when the pattern of communicative performance exhibited enables a clinician to predict continued deficits in language development *and* in the social, cognitive, educational or emotional developments which rely heavily on language skills. Furthermore, infants who have biological or behavioral conditions that are commonly associated with future impairments in communicative functioning (e.g., Down's

TABLE 3.1 | Issues in Identification of Children with Language Problems

Issues	Explanations	Considerations
Standards of comparison	Mental age (MA): language performance compared to expectations for child's mental (cognitive) age	Children with language performance higher than MA Relationship between cognition and language not fully established Different forms of intelligence and relationship with language not established Children with intellectual disabilities potentially excluded from being considered language impaired
	Chronological age (CA): language performance compared to expectations for child's CA	Potentially excludes children with above-normal cognitive abilities but with average or below-average language performance from being considered language impaired Too many children identified as having language problems for resources available Implication that goal of intervention is always to achieve age-equivalent language performance

TABLE 3.1 | *Continued*

Issues	Explanations	Considerations
	Social standard: degree of social value attached to verbal ability and aspects of performance linked to verbal ability (e.g., academic achievement and social relationships) and degree to which language problems therefore negatively affect achievement	Hard to measure numerically Not a one-to-one relationship between variance score (e.g., standard score) of language performance and degree of impact on child's current and future life Involves prediction with regard to future problems child might have
Measures of performance	Age equivalency (language age [LA])	Same amount of delay in terms of age equivalence not equally important at different CAs Normal variation in language performance not considered
	Variance measures (e.g., standard scores, percentile ranks, standard deviations, and stanines)	Cutoff point not descriptive of actual problems in real-life language functioning Danger of excessive dependence on norm-referenced, standardized language tests
Clinical markers of SLI	Verb tense marking development, nonword repetition, and/or sentence recall as possible clinical markers of SLI, and maybe phenotypes of SLI	Assessment tools and procedures to use with very young children still being developed Reasons for verb tense marking, nonword repetition, and sentence recall difficulties not fully known but presumed to have underlying neurological bases, likely of genetic origins Other clinical markers may be identified
Identifying underlying language problems	Stress/challenge language performance	Casual language performance and/or norm-referenced language performance may appear normal unless performance stressed to reveal underlying but real language problems Subtle problems can affect language-related academic skills (e.g., reading and spelling)
Predicting future language problems	Identifying children at risk for language difficulties; supplement with screening programs	At-risk factors not completely identified Relationships between factors not fully understood

> syndrome, profound hearing impairment, autistic symptoms) may be viewed as language impaired even before the age at which language forms typically begin to appear. The degree of confidence that a clinician can place in this prediction will determine the severity rating for the child's impairment. (p. 42)

We would add that children with other factors that may place them at risk for language impairment would be identified as, as Lahey (1990) writes, "at-risk for language-related problems" (p. 618) and placed in language developmental monitoring programs.

AN OVERVIEW OF SPECIFIC LANGUAGE IMPAIRMENT

Delay versus Disorder

To say that a child demonstrates a *language delay* implies that language skills are slow to emerge or develop. It also often implies that the order in which the child acquires the skills corresponds to the sequence seen in normal children and that the degree of delay is basically the same for all features or aspects of language so that a child's profile in the different areas of language is relatively flat. There is sometimes the implication that a child with a language delay might overcome the delay and catch up. In contrast, the term *language disorder* denotes a deviance in the usual rate, trajectory, and/or sequence with which specific language skills emerge. This deviance can include differences in the rate of acquisition for skills within one aspect of language (e.g., semantics or syntax), inordinate difficulties with certain features within one aspect of language (e.g., grammatical morphology), differences in the rate of acquisition among various aspects of language (e.g., pragmatic development related to syntactic development), and/or age-appropriate skills in one or more aspects with lags in the acquisition of one or more other aspects of language. Because of asynchrony in the rate of acquisition within and across various language parameters, normal developmental sequence is disrupted. With the term *language disorder*, there may be less of an inference that children might just catch up with their language, with or without intervention.

Despite the differences in these definitions, some have referred to these children with language-learning problems as having a *language delay*, while others have used the term *language disorder* to refer to children with similar language characteristics, frequently without justifying why one phrase has been used over the other. In discussing SES as a risk factor for SLI above, the issue of imprecision in and undifferentiated use of "delay" and "disorder" among professionals has contributed to some of the cloudiness in knowing how SES functions as a risk factor or causal factor for SLI. And the research involving various aspects of language (pragmatics, semantics, syntax, and morphology) has often yielded conflicting interpretations and certainly has not clarified the issue for us (Bishop, 1997; Leonard, 2014). Here and in later chapters, we have tended to use *impairment* and *disorder* interchangeably but have tried to be careful to use *delay* to mean only a lag in development without necessarily implying a disorder.

One reason for these conflicting interpretations of whether language-impaired children show us delay or disorder in their language behaviors is that a problem with any one aspect or component of language will negatively affect other aspects so that the entire language performance appears disturbed. Although we may talk about the components of language separately, in actuality components interact at one time, with one component affecting others (e.g., Hadley et al., 2016; Masterson, 1997; Reed, 1992; Storkel, 2003; Tomblin & Zhang, 2006). What we typically see, however, in children's language is their total performance, and trying to factor out the many aspects of language that can be interacting at any one time is exceedingly challenging (Tomblin & Zhang, 2006). Leonard (2014, p. 41) has recently questioned the "value of continuing the delay-deviance debate."

In light of issues surrounding delay versus disorder, the usefulness of SLI as a construct has been called into question. The language abilities seen in children with SLI might simply represent abilities that are at the lower end of a continuum of normal variation (Leonard, 1987, 1991, 2014; Rutter, 2008). Rather than having a language disorder, the children simply are not as good at learning and using language as other children in the same way that other children might not be as good at learning and using musical skills, for example. Children on the low end of language skill performance would be seen not to have a disorder but rather to reflect the concept of normal variation within and across individuals. Some children are just better at some things than other things, and different children are different in what they are good or weak at learning and doing. From this perspective, it is only because language abilities are so highly regarded in Western societies and because language abilities are so intimately tied to the Western process of formal education and academic success, which are also highly regarded in Western societies, that weaker skills in language could be seen to represent a disorder.

Most researchers and practitioners who work with toddlers and preschoolers who have inordinate language-learning problems in the absence of explicable conditions for language problems reject this position. Leonard (2014, p. 47) has summarized the debate, suggesting that the language patterns the children present make "it apparent that the delay-deviance [referred to in our discussion as 'disorder'] dichotomy is an oversimplification, and can even be misleading." He adds that such a dichotomy "does not adequately describe the various ways children with SLI can differ from typically developing children" (p. 41).

Both the 2013 *Diagnostic and Statistical Manual of Mental Disorders* (5th ed.) (American Psychiatric Association, 2013) and the 2016 *International Statistical Classification of Diseases and Related Health Problems – 10 (ICD – 10)* (World Health Organization, 2016) include conditions (e.g., "expressive language disorder" and "mixed expressive-receptive language disorder" as subcategories of "specific developmental disorders of speech and language") that could be considered generally, but not exactly, descriptive of and similar to SLI. The position that SLI is a condition differentiated from other conditions that include disruptions of language performance suggests that the exceptional problems that some children have in learning and generalizing certain language skills and the continuing difficulties with language that they demonstrate cannot be viewed simply as anything but a disability. The evidence that such children have language and literacy problems that extend into adulthood, as we will see later in this chapter and certainly in Chapter 5, indicates that SLI is not only a childhood disability but rather a lifelong disability. However, one of the problems that confounds the discussion of delay versus disorder is the variety of language problems these children can display, that is, their heterogeneity.

Subgroups of Young Children with Specific Language Impairments

Children with SLI are generally described as a heterogeneous group because of the variation in language performance seen from child to child. It may be that, to understand young children with SLI more fully, we need to consider the possibility that subgroups of these children exist. If this is the case, we need to ask what the relevant subgroups might be.

Some children described as having SLI have difficulties with both language comprehension and expression (Tomblin, Zhang, Buckwalter, & O'Brien, 2003). Other children seem to have problems with language expression but apparently relatively unimpaired comprehension. Two likely subgroups have been implicated, although the relative degrees of difficulties (e.g., lexical retrieval, syntax, and morphology) can vary from child to child:

1. Both comprehension and expression difficulties (i.e., receptive-expressive language disorder)
2. Expression difficulties (i.e., significantly less impaired receptive language with a sizeable gap between it and the more severely impaired expressive language)

Few professionals and little research suggest that children could have comprehension difficulties without exhibiting expression problems, although for some years there was a proposed third group, comprehension-only difficulties. This may still show up as a subgroup in some literature.

This two-group model for subgroups is likely, however, too simplistic, if not inaccurate (Leonard, 2009; Tomblin & Zhang, 2006). The notion that children could have problems with expression in the absence of some comprehension problems has come to be challenged (Leonard, 2009; Tomblin, Mainele-Arnold, & Zhang, 2007; Tomblin & Zhang, 2006). Even though assessment of the children's abilities might not reveal problems with comprehension, as Leonard (2009) writes, "there seems to be no theory of expressive language problems that does not also assume a limitation in language knowledge or a problem in processing language input" (p. 121). The fact that comprehension problems might not be identified in assessment likely speaks more to either our methods of assessing comprehension and language processing (e.g., what we assess and how we assess) or the limited number of available sensitive assessment tasks/tests for assessing quite young children (Leonard, 2009). In addition to issues related to comprehension and expression of language, phonological problems have also been found to co-occur with language problems (Shriberg, Tomblin, & McSweeny, 1999). Additionally, gestures representing symbolic play or used for communicative purposes have been associated with early language difficulties (Thal, Oroz, Evans, Katich, & Leasure, 1995; Watt, Wetherby, & Shumway, 2006), and others have found a relationship between early language deficits and socialization characteristics (e.g., Paul, Looney, & Dahm, 1991).

If we consider only the potential deficit areas mentioned thus far (comprehension, expression, phonology, socialization, and symbolic play gestures), we can see in Table 3.2 some but not all of the combinations that might lead to possible subgroups of children. If we break down expression into the possible specific aspects of language (e.g., semantics,

TABLE 3.2 | Examples of Areas of Deficit Leading to Some Possible Subgroups of Children with Specific Language Impairments

Subgroups	Expression	Comprehension	Phonology	Socialization	Gesture
1	X	X	X	X	X
2	X	X		X	X
3	X	X	X		X
4	X	X	X	X	
5	X	X	X		
6	X	X			X
7	X	X		X	
8	X	X			

pragmatics, syntax, and morphology) that might be problematic, we see even greater complexity in the combinations that could be possible. However, it might not be valid to separate some of these factors because of the overlaps, interrelationships, and associations that are known to operate across linguistic components and among and across other behaviors (e.g., relationships between measures of socialization and use of communicative intentions/functions). Our factors or areas of deficit might not be correct and/or discrete. Other factors and associations have also been implicated with SLI (e.g., behavioral difficulties). Additionally, we would likely need to take account of the relative degree of skill (or deficit) in each of the possible areas. It is possible that the combinations could change in an individual child as CA changes (Conti-Ramsden & Botting, 1999). Our present knowledge has not yet allowed us to overcome the complexity of the task of identifying any valid subgroups, even for what might seem the relatively simplistic expressive-receptive and expressive subgroups. However, developments in the area of the genetics of SLI might yield sufficient information to identify reliable and valid groupings, groupings that might help explain the heterogeneity we see in these children we currently label as SLI. In drawing on the writing of Bishop (2006), Leonard (2009) states that it "is possible that meaningful subtypes might be identified through genetic studies of potential 'endophenotypes' (clusters of related abilities) that arise from theoretical proposals of causal factors in language impairment" (p. 120). The topic of genetic factors as possible causes of SLI will be raised again in the next section. For now, however, we have not been able to identify distinct and stable subgroups.

A Label for It and Reasons for It

In the introduction to this chapter, the dilemma regarding how to title the chapter was raised. Many terms have been used in the literature to label the condition in which language difficulties appear to be the sole problem of these children. Among these terms are SLI, specific language disability, specific language disorder, developmental aphasia, developmental dysphasia, congenital aphasia, language delay, developmental language disorder, expressive and/or receptive language delay, clinical language disorder, language disorder, and slow expressive language development, although this last term tends to be used with toddlers more frequently than with older preschool children. A number of scholars has begun to refer to SLI as a neurodevelopmental disorder. When these children go to school and their language problems begin to cause academic difficulties—a situation that is highly likely to occur—the children may be referred to as learning disabled, language-learning disabled, or specific learning disabled, as we will see in the next chapter.

Without obvious hearing, intellectual, emotional, neurological, or notable environmental deficits, the question of why these children have such a hard time acquiring language is an important one. The search for explanations has sometimes turned to other, less superficial reasons for the existence of the language difficulties.

Neurological Bases. Some authors and researchers have proposed that, in the absence of gross neurological problems, the children's language difficulties must stem from central nervous system dysfunction, and the terms *minimal brain dysfunction* and *minimal brain injury* have been suggested, terms that have also been associated with learning disabilities. In the past, it has been difficult to identify conclusive links between abnormal findings of brain function measurements and the language problems exhibited by children. The general superiority of the left cerebral hemisphere over the right in adults' language functioning has been well established, but we know that early damage to the left hemisphere in children has not been shown to account for the severity or persistence of their language impairments. However, there are many ways in which brain structure and function can vary to disrupt language acquisition.

Most scholars working in the area of SLI agree that there must be neurological correlates and/or substrates for these children's difficulties in language learning and performance. Advances in technology leading to continuing improvements in neuroimaging (e.g., magnetic resonance imaging [MRI], functional magnetic resonance imaging [fMRI]) and event-related neurophysiological procedures (e.g., event-related potentials [ERPs]) have resulted in some of these techniques being used with children with language impairments (e.g., Ellis Weismer, Plante, Jones, & Tomblin, 2005; McArthur, Atkinson, & Ellis, 2009; McArthur & Bishop, 2005; Trauner, Wulfeck, Tallal, & Hesselink, 2000). Using these and other technologies, some differences between individuals with SLI and normally functioning individuals with regard to, for example, neurophysiological measures during auditory and speech processing tasks and semantic and grammatical processing tasks and fMRI/MRI findings for brain morphology and cerebral functioning. These approaches seem to hold promise in unraveling the puzzle, but not all studies have found differences between groups. Cautious optimism seems appropriate; with refinements in technologies and research methodologies together with developments in the area of genetics of SLI, the etiological roots of SLI are likely to be identified. We might not be surprised, however, if multiple neurological (and genetic) roots of SLI are identified. Repeatedly the group of children with SLI is described as heterogeneous with different children showing different language profiles and the same children showing different profiles at different times.

There are two more recent and exciting directions the study of the neurobiology of SLI has taken, although the quantity of research to date is still relatively small. One direction involves using neurophysiological techniques with quite young children to look at the possibility of identifying neurological bases that might eventually be used for early diagnosis of SLI (e.g., Friedrich & Friederici, 2006). The other direction involves examining possible neurological changes occurring as a result of language intervention with children with SLI (Popescu, Fey, Lewine, Finestack, & Popescu, 2009), that is, documenting at a biological level the effects of language intervention.

In thinking about abnormal brain structures and functioning underlying SLI, it is important to realize that these can be related to other findings about possible causes and associations presented in the literature. One of these is genetic bases of SLI, which could lead to altered brain structure and function. We take up discussion of genetic transmission related to SLI later in this chapter. The state of the science is such that we have not yet unraveled the relationships among prenatal neurological development, genetics, postnatal brain morphological development, and even endocrinology. Attempts at unraveling the puzzle continue to be the focus of research.

Language Knowledge and Access to Language Knowledge. Another proposition as to why these children have language problems is that the children have difficulties abstracting from their language-learning environment the requisite implicit language rules, demonstrate incomplete learning of rules, and/or have problems accessing language information that they already know (e.g., Connell & Stone, 1992; Gopnik, 1990; Leonard, Nippold, Kail, & Hale, 1983; Messer & Dockrell, 2006; Rice & Wexler, 1996). That is, the children can take in, process, and acquire at least part of the requisite language information, but they have trouble getting to it and bringing it forward to use it consistently, or they acquire incomplete knowledge of the language rules. The observations that children with SLI are often inconsistent in what they can do with their language lend support to this proposition. For example, children can use appropriate tense-marking morphemes sometimes but not always, or they may sometimes have difficulty retrieving a word to use but at other times are able to use the same word quickly and easily with no latency. But these are observations at a behavioral level about language functioning. The more significant question related to a cause for SLI is what causes these problems in learning their language knowledge in the first place. At best this is a surface account of causation.

Cognitive Deficits. Cognitive abilities of children with SLI have also been the subject of investigation as to the reason for the children's language problems. As we have seen previously, a criterion of SLI is the absence of intellectual disability as the reason for children's language problems. As we saw earlier, a common way in which the intellectual level of these children is established is via tests of nonverbal intelligence, referred to as NVIQ, or performance IQ tests (PIQ). Because the classification of SLI excludes children with intellectual disabilities, children with SLI supposedly demonstrate normal nonverbal intelligence skills.

Nevertheless, deficits in particular aspects of cognitive functioning, such as symbolic play, hypothesis formation and testing, and representational thought, have been associated with SLI in children (e.g., Ellis Weismer, 1991; Johnston, 1994; Rescorla & Goossens, 1992). If the language impairment of these children is, in fact, linked to deficits in their cognitive functioning, the terms *specific* language impairment, *specific* language disability, and *specific* language disorder may be inappropriate. However, deficit cognitive functioning has also not always been substantiated in language-impaired children. The question also arises as to how testing of cognitive ability, particularly NVIQ, can be completely devoid of the influences of language ability (Johnston, 1994). While it might be possible to separate some intelligence measures from language ability in young children, it appears that as children with SLI mature, their language problems have been seen to affect their measured NVIQ. Thus, language impacts nonverbal functioning. And, the measured NVIQ of older children, adolescents, and even adults with SLI has been shown to decline from the previous levels seen in their younger years (Conti-Ramsden, Botting, Simkin, & Knox, 2001; Johnson et al., 1999; Stothard et al., 1998; Tomblin, Freese, & Records, 1992). Of course, if there are cognitive deficits associated with SLI in children, there is the recurring question about the underlying reasons for the deficits.

Information Processing Deficits. Although somewhat related to the notion of cognitive deficits presented above, another direction that the explanation for a causal factor has taken has involved how children process information, that is, an information processing account of SLI (Ellis Weismer & Evans, 2002; Evans, Viele, & Kass, 1997). The basic premise of this explanation suggests that SLI in children stems from problems in how well the children can deal with (process) incoming stimuli and/or use the stimuli in order to learn language and/or acquire information. The general premise is that the children are limited in how much information and/or how quickly they can process the information so that they fail to take in sufficient information in sufficiently complete forms in order to acquire language adequately.

Two broad lines of thought within the information processing account have predominated. One focuses on more generalized information processing limitations. These involve reductions in the speed with which information can be processed and/or constraints on what the children can hold in their working memories in order to process and make sense of incoming stimuli (e.g., Dick, Wulfeck, Krupa-Kwiatkowski, & Bates, 2004; Ellis Weismer, Evans, & Hesketh, 1999; Montgomery, 2005). Working memory is also sometimes known as short-term memory. Some findings have implicated weaknesses in processing nonlinguistic information as well as linguistically based information (e.g., Miller, Kail, Leonard, & Tomblin, 2001). However, not all children show the same weaknesses to the same degree for similar tasks, which certainly confounds conclusions about possible reasons for the language problems and at the same time reinforces the idea that SLI is "multifactorial" (Leonard, 2014, p. 218) in nature.

The second line of thought proposes that the children's information processing problems are more specific to particular processes, such as the temporal processing of rapidly changing auditory stimuli or phonological processing (e.g., Corriveau, Pasquini, & Goswami, 2007; Gathercole, Hitch, Service, & Martin, 1997; Merzenich et al., 1996; Montgomery & Windsor, 2007; Tallal et al., 1996). However, weaknesses in verbal working memory, per our discussion in the preceding paragraph, could relate to observed difficulties with rapid auditory processing or phonological processing. Information processing accounts of SLI have been one of the factors for the emergence of NWR as a possible clinical marker of SLI. The question remains, however, about the possible reasons for the information processing problems; the answers seem to take us back to the possibility of issues related to neurological functioning, per our discussion above.

Behaviorally, many young children with SLI are described as being inattentive, often especially inattentive to spoken language, compared to typically developing, same-age peers. And, logically, children need to attend reasonably well to the stimuli presented to them during NWR tasks in order to perform adequately on the tasks. It is possible that their poor performances on such tasks stem from problems maintaining attention to the auditorily presented nonsense words. Problems with auditory attention have, in fact, been suggested as reasons for the language problems seen in children with SLI.

Using neurophysiological techniques (ERPs) and a narrative discourse task, Stevens and colleagues (Stevens, Fanning, Coch, Sanders, & Neville, 2008; Stevens, Sanders, & Neville, 2006) documented that the children with SLI in their studies, who were instructed to listen to one and not a second narrative presented at the same time, did not differentially attend to the target narrative but instead attended to both. However, the typically developing children did differentially attend to the target auditory stimuli. This suggests that children with SLI may not be able to attend selectively to language-based auditory stimuli. This could make it hard for young children to pick out important elements in the auditory stream of language they hear in order to find the linguistic patterns and abstract these to learn language.

Another way of thinking about the role of attention problems as reasons for young children's difficulties learning language relates to the topic of *(Central) Auditory Processing Disorder [(C)APD]*, which readers will encounter in the next chapter and again in Chapter 8 on auditory impairment and language. As readers will see there, this disorder has been the subject of considerable controversy for decades, including its relationship to language impairment in children. The information processing problem related to deficits possible in temporal processing of rapidly changing auditory stimuli, referred to in the preceding paragraph, is a form of auditory processing. One intervention (i.e., Fast ForWord) that has been reported to be effective in improving the language performances of children with language impairment purportedly rooted in this supposed auditory processing deficit (Tallal et al., 1996) has also met with considerable controversy. In considering the outcomes research on the Fast ForWord intervention, Leonard (2014) has suggested that noted improvements in performances of children with language impairment who took part in the intervention are probably more linked to improving the children's attention than remediating language deficits specifically. In a related theme, results of Moore's (2011) line of research investigating (C)APD has led him to propose that the poor listening performances of most children presumed to have (C)APD are due to reduced working memory or problems with attention.

Attention has been implicated in SLI in still another way—*attention deficit/hyperactivity disorder (ADHD)*. ADHD has been reported to have a sizeable co-occurrence rate with SLI, with wide-ranging estimates of co-occurrence as high as about 75 to 95 percent co-occurrence to under 5 percent (e.g., Gualtieri, Koriath, Van Bourgondien, & Saleeby, 1983; Redmond, 2016a; Snowling, Bishop, Sothard, Chipchase, & Kaplan, 2006; Walsh, Scullion, Burns, MacEvilly, & Brosnan, 2014). However, the majority of studies examining co-occurrence rates of language impairment and ADHD have reported more moderate, centric estimates, such as about 30 to 60 percent (Redmond, 2016a). Concerted research efforts are being directed to trying to tease out the relationship between SLI and ADHD (e.g., Redmond, 2016a, 2016b; Redmond & Timler, 2007), but teasing out those relationships is currently a work in progress.

As with many of the other possible reasons for the inordinate difficulties toddlers and preschoolers with SLI have in learning language, we ask the same question. That is, what has led to the reason? A reason, such as a possible information processing deficit, must logically have a causal underpinning, which again implicates brain functioning, although children's language-learning environments have also been suggested as reasons for the children's language difficulties.

Language-Learning Environment. Children's exposure to language in their environment, or rather the lack of appropriate types of exposure, has been suggested as a reason for the language problems of children with SLI. However, we need to be clear about what we mean about the language-learning environment because we can think of the environment for learning language in terms of quantity or quality of exposure. We know that normally developing children can acquire language without a lot of language stimulation. The point is made fairly clearly with hearing children of deaf parents; most of these children seem not to have difficulties acquiring spoken language if there is a relatively small amount of regular exposure to it. On the other hand, we noted previously that maternal education is sometimes considered a possible risk factor for language disorder. The immediate conclusion might be that this is because of the reportedly greater amount of language stimulation that mothers with more education provide to their children (Hart & Risley, 1995). However, if there are impacts with regard to quantity of maternal input to children's language development, these appear to affect semantic (vocabulary) development rather than other aspects of language ability that are particularly problematic for children with SLI, such as grammatical morphology (Dollaghan et al., 1999; Rice, Spitz, & O'Brien, 1999; Rice et al., 1998). Quantity of language exposure in the environment seems insufficient by itself to be a reason for SLI in children (Bishop, 1997), although it might affect both normally developing and language-impaired children's performances on common measures of language, such as those involving lexical density (size of vocabulary) and length of utterances (Dollaghan et al., 1999). And we need to keep in mind that one of the several criteria that are used to exclude children from being identified as having SLI is severe environmental deprivation such that the deprivation can account for the disruption in language development. Children with SLI generally do not live in environments where insufficient amounts of stimulation for learning language alone can be deemed to be a reason for the children's problems. And there are many studies on preschoolers with SLI that have included children from families with middle and upper-middle socioeconomic status.

In contrast, results of studies looking at the quality of language interactions between mothers and children with SLI give a somewhat mixed picture as a potential reason for the children's problems, at least at first glance. There have been suggestions that mothers of SLI children do not engage in as many of the language interactions with their children that are known to facilitate children's language learning—that is, many of the characteristics of "motherese" and other behaviors such as responses to questions, imitations, or self-repetitions. However, mothers of children with SLI have been found to talk in a similar manner to their younger children whose language is developing normally (e.g., Conti-Ramsden & Dykins, 1991; Warlaumont & Jarmulowicz, 2012), so attributing the reason for children's language learning problems to mothers' communicative interaction styles seems not to stand up consistently to empirical scrutiny. It appears that where differences have been identified, these may be because mothers have adjusted their language levels to those of the children. That is, because the language of children with SLI seems more like that of younger, normally developing children, mothers seem to modify their language and interactions to accommodate their less language-able children. In this way, characteristics of the children seem to drive the language input they receive.

There has been, however, one finding that might point to children with SLI having different language-learning interactions with their mothers than other children. This deals with mothers' use of recasts. *Recasts*, as we will see elsewhere in this book, are responses to a child's utterance that are semantically contingent and include language elements the child used but add or modify the child's utterance in some way that makes it more complex or complete, as in the following:

CHILD: That my teddie.

MOTHER: Yes, that is your big teddie. We'll take it in the car.

Mothers have been found to use recasts with children with SLI differently, including using them less frequently (Conti-Ramsden, 1990; Conti-Ramsden, Hutcheson, & Grove, 1995; Nelson, Welsh, Camarata, Butkovsky, & Camarata, 1995). However, even here it is not clear that the direction of influence is from mother to child as opposed to from child to mother. Mothers of normally developing children reduce their use of recasts as children get older. It could be that, for use of recasts specifically, mothers are responding to the older ages of their children with SLI or their nonverbal cognitive levels rather than the children's lower language levels (Nelson et al., 1995). It is also possible that children with SLI are sufficiently less communicatively interactive with their mothers, so the mothers have fewer interchanges with their children in order to provide recasts. Again, there is the possibility that characteristics of the children affect their language-learning environment as much as if not more than their language-learning environment leading to their language problems. However, this does not rule out a reciprocal interaction in which some of the modifications that mothers make to their children's impaired language inadvertently become less facilitating for the children's language development.

Overall, language-learning environment is not viewed as a probable reason for SLI. Factors in the environment may lead to delays in language learning, particularly vocabulary, but not result in the impairment in language learning that is seen SLI. Nevertheless, language-learning environment can interact with the intrinsic language-learning abilities that a child brings to the task either to moderate the effects of the child's language-learning impairment or to exacerbate them.

Genetic/Familial Bases. Previously we noted that a family history of language, communication, and/or literacy problems is a risk factor for a child having a language impairment. Recall also the findings from the study by Tomblin and his colleagues (Tomblin, Smith, et al., 1997) that suggested that SLI in children was more often associated with risk factors related to their parents' status before the children were even conceived than with various fetal or perinatal risk factors. Among the parental factors were levels of education and family histories of language and/or learning problems, two factors that are not independent of each other.

There is now no question that language impairment has a tendency to run in families and that language-learning environmental influences alone are insufficient to explain the children's language-learning problems (e.g., Bishop, Price, Dale, & Plomin, 2003; Choudhury & Benasich, 2003; Felsenfeld & Plomin, 1997; Flax et al., 2003; Plante, Shenkman, & Clark, 1996; Viding et al., 2003). That is, in many cases there is a likely heritable, genetic basis for the impairment (Conti-Ramsden, Falcaro, Simkin, & Pickles, 2007; Rice, 2013; Rice, Smith, & Gayán, 2009; Vernes et al., 2008). In twin studies, two of the possible clinical markers noted previously (nonword repetition and verb tense marking) have been found to have heritable bases for risk for SLI (Bishop, Adams, & Norbury, 2006).

Twin and adoption studies, along with advances in multivariate genetic analysis, behavioral genetics, and molecular genetics, are moving our knowledge ahead rapidly in this area. For example, longitudinal genetic studies of SLI utilizing growth curve modeling for acquisition of certain language skills have some promise in helping us clarify our perspectives about what leads to SLI (Rice, 2012, 2013). These tie genetic timing mechanisms at a molecular level in brain development to longitudinal acquisition of specific language skills. The timing mechanisms are considered as genetic triggers for starting (onset), speeding up (acceleration), and slowing (deceleration) brain development leading to development of particular behaviors in children. Rice (2013) indicated that the research to date has identified three regulatory genes—*KIAA3019, CNTNAP2,* and *FOXP2*—as candidate genes in the etiology of SLI. Growth curve modeling approaches compare typically developing children's acquisition of a variety of language skills over time to their counterparts with SLI. Rice (2012, 2013) suggests that for a number of language skills, including verb morphology, the modeling shows that children with SLI start their learning of the language skills later than their peers without language impairment (i.e., delayed onset), then appear to acquire the skills at the same rates as their peers (i.e., same rate of development once triggered to start), but then experience a leveling or plateau (i.e., deceleration in learning) before reaching adult-level competency. In other words, the children with SLI start but show a delayed start (for some language skills, 2 years late), then show the same acquisition pace as language-normal children in the acceleration stage but do not catch up because there is no exceptional acceleration, and then they experience deceleration without achieving competency. Rice (2013) writes that studies of these three regulatory genes

> collectively suggest potentially complex interactions among genes along the causal pathway, although definitive evidence is not available to establish regulatory gene effects as part of the aetiology of SLI. The chain of evidence does, however, support the plausibility of such a claim. (p. 230)

We anticipate that the work in the area of genetics in the next several years will add considerably to our understanding. Because SLI overlaps with several other disorders (e.g., speech sound disorders, reading disorders), research directions are exploring if there are particular problematic abilities or clusters of problematic abilities (e.g., verbal short-term memory problems resulting in nonword repetition limitations, attention problems, etc.) that underpin other skills known to be problematic (e.g., verb morphology) that are influenced by a specific gene variation or combination of gene variations.

We have to keep in mind that genetic variations can impact, among other things, development of brain structures and, therefore, brain functions, which might account for some of the differences in brain morphology and functioning seen in the literature, per our previous discussion. Here we see the need to tease out levels of causation and symptomology in our thinking about what leads to SLI and how it manifests. For example, we might hypothesize that something (genetic variation perhaps?) causes (a level 1 cause) affected children's brains to develop differently than unaffected children (a level 2 cause) and therefore function differently (a level 3 cause), possibly in areas of verbal working memory and/or attentional capabilities (a level 4 cause and level 1 symptom), leading to language-learning difficulties (a level 2 symptom), which might then cause (language-learning problems now a level 5 cause) affected children to have social interaction problems and/or reading difficulties (level 3 symptoms). Importantly, this example is hypothetical, but it does illustrate that our thinking about causation of and reasons for SLI needs to eschew simplistic explanations and to aspire to clarity even in the context of still incomplete knowledge. As part of trying to be clear in our thinking about SLI, we are careful to note that not all children with SLI have positive family histories or evidence of genetic transmission, and not all children in families with a history of language problems will themselves have language impairment. Nevertheless, positive family histories of language and/or literacy problems do increase the odds of the children having language problems. Although these situations have several possible sources, which can be consistent with genetic principles, other variables can be implicated. As Bishop (1997) points out, "genes do not act in isolation to cause behaviour" (p. 49), and notions of genetic determinism are, according to Plomin and Dale (2000), "based on misconceptions about genetic research, and on a lack of appreciation of the way complex traits and common disorders are influenced by *multiple genes* [emphasis added] as well as *multiple environmental factors* [emphasis added]" (p. 49).

There are several ways to conceive of environmental factors in combination with genetic transmission of SLI. On the one hand, a child may have one or more predisposing genes for SLI, but the child's environment is one that provides a buffer for the genetic predisposition and limits the emergence of the disabling characteristics of SLI. In another situation, an inherited trait for SLI might be moderated by inserting language intervention into the environment so that it counters the inherited trait and lessens its influence (Bishop, 1997). On the other hand, a child with an inherited SLI predisposition might grow up in a family in which one or both parents also have language impairments, associated literacy problems, difficulties with psychosocial aspects of behavior (which we will see later are often a part of language impairment), and resulting lower socioeconomic conditions. For this child, the environment may exacerbate the inherited trait or, at least, not serve to counter it. Goodyer (2000), in discussing "psychosocial disadvantages" (p. 232) related to the family environment of children with SLI and "environmental adversities" (p. 232) that can therefore impact on the children, writes,

> It may be that there are common genetic components that will be expressed as a familial effect. Also, language and cognitive deficits in a parent may limit the direct help they can give their children. (p. 232)

Figure 3.1 illustrates how genetic and environmental factors might come together to affect a child's language abilities and even continue to have effects in subsequent generations. Plomin and Dale (2000) remind us of the concepts of *assortative mating* and *additive genetic variance*. These concepts refer to the increased likelihood that individuals with similar characteristics or traits tend mate and that the factor of similar cognitive abilities, particularly verbal abilities, has particularly strong influences in selecting mates, more so than behavioral or physical characteristics. This means that, if one adult is particularly strong in verbal ability, that adult will likely mate with another who is also strong in the ability. Over generations, the children of such matings are likely to be high in verbal ability also. This assortative mating, according to Plomin and Dale (2000, p. 48), "increases a particular type of genetic variance called additive genetic variance, which is caused by the independent effects of alleles[1] that 'add up' to affect the trait."

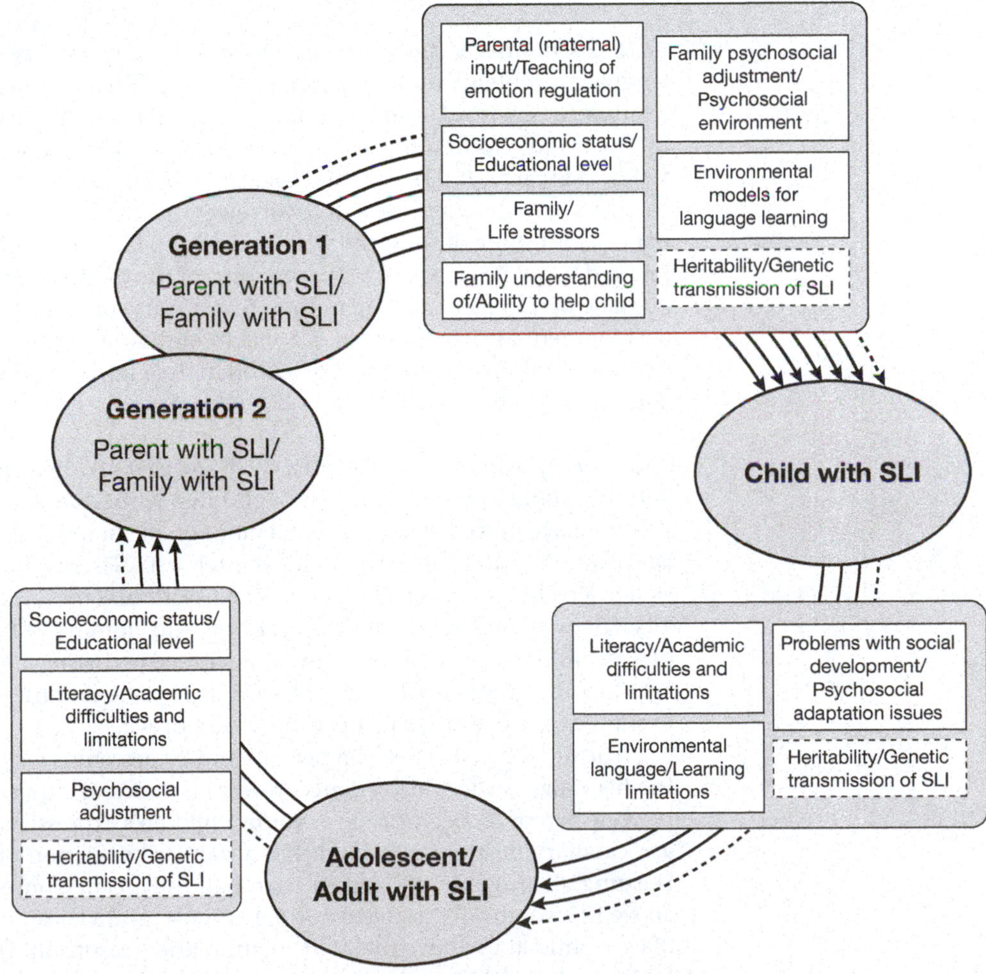

FIGURE 3.1 | Schematic Representation of Some of the Interactions and Effects of Genetic/Familial and Environmental Factors in SLI (© 2002 Vicki A. Reed)

1. Any of alternative forms of a gene (e.g., either the wrinkled-pea gene or the smooth-pea gene) that can occur at a given locus.

Where SLI is concerned, it is probably a mistake to think of the effects of nature (genetics) and nurture (environment) separately and more accurate to consider them as interacting. Language is a complex behavior, so a simplistic explanation about what is wrong in the condition of SLI is unlikely. And the more complex a behavior, as with language, the greater should be our expectations for more interactions among factors. Caution against adopting simplistic explanations of SLI is warranted.

Prevalence

Some young children start off slowly in their language development and then appear to catch up. Other children start off slowly and continue to lag behind and to have problems. Still other children start off slowly, seem to catch up for a while, and then either fall behind again or show problems in different areas related to language, such as literacy and numeracy. Therefore, we may see different prevalence figures at different ages, and these figures are likely affected by what and how we are measuring language.

Vocabulary development is one of the first obvious indices of language growth in very young children. One of the earliest signs that a child may have problems with language is that the first word is used late or that not very many additional words are acquired after the first word.

At 18–24 Months of Age. Between 18 and 24 months of age, signs that a child may have language problems include absence of a vocabulary growth spurt, failing to combine words into two-word utterances, and/or generally talking very little. About 10 to 15 percent of 2-year-old children fit this picture (Klee et al., 1998; Rescorla, 1989; Rescorla, Hadicke-Wiley, & Escarce, 1993). For children at 24 months of age, concern generally focuses on an expressive single-word vocabulary of fewer than 50 single words and no two-word combinations. Yet some of these toddlers do catch up later. The children who catch up are often referred to as *late bloomers*. However, some of the toddlers who demonstrate *slow expressive language development* (SELD)[2] in their first 2 years continue to lag behind in their language development as they grow older. Some longitudinal studies give us hints as to how many of these children continue to lag behind in their language throughout the preschool years and into the school years.

At 3 Years of Age. In reviewing her work and that of others, Paul (1991, 1996) suggests that between about 20 and 75 percent of children who were slow in language development at 2 years of age moved into the normal range on measures of expressive language at 3 years of age (Paul, 1991, 1993; Rescorla, 1993; Whitehurst & Fischel, 1994), the age at which language skill begins to be measured as much by syntactic and morphological abilities as by vocabulary. For twins, however, Dale, Price, Bishop, and Plomin (2003) report that about 45 percent of 2-year-old twins with language delays showed persisting language difficulties at 3 years of age. Together, these results mean that 25 to 80 percent of these SELD 2-year-olds continued to show expressive language delays at 3 years of age.

The difference between 25 percent and 80 percent is very large. One of the reasons for the big range is the wide variance in what is "normal" in very young children. For example, one parent report measure of young children's expressive language at 2 years of age has a vocabulary mean of 300 words but a standard deviation of 175 (Fenson, Dale, Reznick, Hartung, & Burgess, 1990), more than half the mean. Consequently, any vocabulary size above 125 would be considered normal or above, and a vocabulary size of zero or more would place a child at or above the –2 SD point. Other reasons for the big range are the different tools that have been used to assess the children's language, including the varying degrees of specificity and sensitivity of the tools, the aspects of language that were measured, and the

---

2. The current literature on toddlers has so far refrained from using the term *specific language impairment* to refer to these young children. Rather, slow expressive language development (SELD) has been the preferred descriptor. In keeping with this trend, SELD will be used in this section of the chapter.

degree to which language performance has or has not been challenged in the children. Other reasons are the heterogeneity of the groups studied and the children initially being identified at 2 years of age on the basis of their expressive vocabulary size, with some but not all of them having presumably normal comprehension abilities (Ellis Weismer, Murray-Branch, & Miller, 1994; Girolametto et al., 2001; Kelly, 1998; Olswang, Rodriguez, & Timler, 1998; Paul, 1997; van Kleeck, Gillam, & Davis, 1997). Language comprehension of young children is notoriously difficult to assess in toddlers in valid and reliable ways (Leonard, 2009), and the notion that expressive-only language problems actually exist in children with SLI without some degree of receptive problems has been challenged (Leonard, 2009; Tomblin & Zhang, 2006; Tomblin et al., 2007). Prevalence figures might be different if we had accurate information about the children's comprehension.

Of particular note is that vocabulary size of some 2-year-olds with SELD who continue to have language problems in areas other than vocabulary (Paul, 1993; Rescorla, 1993; Whitehurst, Fischel, Arnold, & Lonigan, 1992), even though low vocabulary size was a primary criterion used to identify the children as having delayed language at age 2. What this means is that at 3 years of age, expressive language skills other than vocabulary are below normal expectations. These are often aspects of language related to form, that is, syntax and morphology. As children age, vocabulary size, at least as measured by many norm-referenced tests, is a less reliable indicator of SLI than other language measures.

Others have provided different estimates of continuing language delay in 3-year-olds. Klee et al. (1998) suggest that one-fifth (20 percent) to one-third (33 percent) of 2-year-old children who could be considered as having SELD at 2 years of age continue to be clinically concerning at age 3 years. Paul (1991) reports that 40 to 50 percent of 2-year-olds may continue to have expressive language delays at age 3 years. If we calculate 40 to 50 percent of the 10 to 15 percent figure given for the proportion of 2-year-olds with SELD, we arrive at a 4 to 7.5 percent prevalence figure for expressive language problems in the 3-year-old group. If we use the 20 to 33 percent figure of Klee et al. (1998) to calculate the proportion of the 10 to 15 percent of 2-year-olds with SELD who have problems at 3 years of age, we arrive at a 2 to 5 percent prevalence figure, and if we use the 25 to 80 percent figure, we arrive at a 2.5 to 12 percent prevalence figure for language delay at 3 years of age.

At 4 Years of Age. What is the language of 2-year-old children with SELD like when they are age 4? In compiling the results from her study (Paul, 1991, 1993) and others (Rescorla, 1993; Whitehurst & Fischel, 1994), Paul (1996) has reported that about 45 to 85 percent of 2-year-olds with SELD received scores within normal limits on measures of expressive language at 4 years of age. In another study, at 4 years of age 71 percent of children who had been late talkers had mean lengths of utterance (MLUs) above the 10th-percentile rank (Rescorla, Dahlsgaard, & Roberts, 2000). Reversing the figures from both of these reports, this means that 15 to 55 percent of the 2-year-olds did not move into the normal range at 4 years of age. We need to keep remembering that these figures are proportions of a proportion of the population of 2-year-olds, that is, the 10 to 15 percent of 2-year-olds who have SELD. Therefore, to estimate general prevalence of language impairment at age 4, we need to look at 15 to 55 percent of 10 to 15 percent, or 1.5 to 8.5 percent, which we see is still a considerable range. From a slightly different perspective, in tracking 28 toddlers who had previously been slow to develop their expressive language, Paul and Smith (1993) found that 57 percent of these children had persisting expressive language deficits related to narrative skills at 4 years of age. As Paul (1991) points out, this "finding is particularly significant because narrative skills in preschoolers have been shown to be one of the best predictors of school success" (p. 8). Extrapolated to the general 10 to 15 percent of 2-year-olds with SELD, this estimates that 6 to 9 percent of 4-year-old children might have problems with their narrative skills, a possible portent of coming academic difficulties for these children. Readers might want to keep this 6 to 9 percent estimated prevalence figure in mind.

The language status of preschoolers at 4 years of age and even more so between 4 and 5 years of age likely foreshadows their later language and literacy outcomes. Several authors have noted that children whose language abilities are behind those of their peers at 4 years of age may be in for long-term problems. By "long-term," we mean problems that extend into the elementary and secondary school years and even into adulthood (Rescorla & Lee, 2001; Stothard et al., 1998). It is possible but not confirmed that these children will have demonstrated language comprehension problems in addition to their expressive language weaknesses when they were 4. As we have noted, expressive syntax and morphological abilities are two areas that frequently show particular weaknesses if language problems persist in children to the age of 4, often more so than a vocabulary deficit, which was used to first identify the children as SELD.

At 5 Years of Age. How many of these SELD children will continue to show language problems at 5 years of age? From the results of one study (Whitehurst, Fischel et al., 1991), 5-year-olds who had been slow in their early expressive, but not obviously in their receptive, language development evidenced expressive vocabulary performances and general verbal fluency skills that were not notably different from normally developing 5-year-olds. Given that syntax and morphology are particular problems for most children with SLI and, as we will see later, that many of these children also have problems in interpersonal interactions and psychosocial difficulties, it is unfortunate that this study did not include measures of syntactic or pragmatic abilities. However, the authors reported that, if any problems in the areas of syntax at 5 years of age did exist, they were "subtle and not apparent" (p. 67). These findings might suggest that the children had caught up to their normally developing peers. However, while Bishop and Edmundson (1987) found that many preschool children with language deficits (without nonverbal intelligence deficits) appeared to catch up by 5½ years of age, Conti-Ramsden, Crutchley, and Botting (1997) pointed out that about an equal proportion (40 percent) did not. Paul (1996) reported that, in kindergarten, 75 percent of her 2-year-old toddlers with SELD had moved into the normal range on most measures of language, including achieving syntax scores on samples of their spontaneous language (i.e., their Developmental Sentence Score) that placed them above the 10th-percentile rank. However, 25 percent still exhibited delays in their syntax as well as with other aspects of language. In Rescorla's (1993) study of toddlers with SELD, whom she followed for several years, 15 percent of the children performed poorly on a test of expressive grammatical ability at 5 years of age and were therefore considered to show impaired language, compared to the 85 percent who demonstrated more age-appropriate language performance (Rescorla, 2002). Girolametto et al. (2001) reported that when their 21 children who had expressive vocabulary delays at 2 years of age reached 5 years of age, three of the children (14 percent) scored below the normal range on norm-referenced measures of language. We need to remember that these studies differed on the proportions of the children in the groups who had receptive language problems in combination with their expressive language impairments.

It could seem that most children who have early histories of language delay seem to catch up by the time they are 5 years of age. There may, however, be some real dangers in accepting these findings without more information. Although most of the SELD children in the research of Paul and colleagues (Paul, 1991, 1996; Paul, Murray, Clancy, & Andrews, 1997) scored within normal limits on norm-referenced tests of language at 5 years of age, most of their scores were in the lower range of normal and were significantly lower than their peers who did not have a history of slow language development. Their narrative performance both in kindergarten and in grade 1 continued to be notably poorer than that of the children without histories of language problems (Paul, 2000; Paul, Hernandez, Taylor, & Johnson, 1996; Paul & Smith, 1993). Recall from our previous discussion that Lahey (1990) has suggested that our identification procedures need to examine children's language abilities under conditions that stress the language system. Narrative tasks do just that. The 5-year-old children in the study of Girolametto et al. (2001), most of whom scored within normal limits on norm-referenced measures of language, also performed significantly poorer on these tasks than their peers and had particular problems on higher-level language tasks, such as narratives and perspective-taking language tasks. The SELD children in Rescorla's (2002) research, too, generally performed within normal limits on most language measures at age 5, but their performance was significantly poorer than their peers, and they continued to show poorer performance through to 9 years of age. There was also evidence of emerging reading problems at ages 8 and 9. The children in the Bishop and Edmundson (1987) study who had appeared to "resolve" their early language problems by 5½ years of age had measurable and noticeable academic and language problems at 15 years of age, and their skills with the higher-level language skills of narratives at age 5½ seemed particularly important in terms of what their outcomes were. A picture that emerges suggests that norm-referenced language tests, particularly those that do not tap higher level language abilities or syntax and morphology under conditions that stress children's language abilities, are not the best tools for identifying language impairment. And, when young children with documented language comprehension problems are considered, the chances of continuing language problems at age 5 or beyond increase (Ellis Weismer, 2007). All may not be rosy for these SELD children as they mature, even though some of their test scores might place them in the normal, albeit often lower normal, range.

These outcomes seem to reinforce the concerns expressed by some that early expressive language delay portends the likelihood of future language problems and language-learning-related problems and, therefore, warrants early intervention (Girolametto, Pearce, & Weitzman, 1996; Nippold & Schwarz, 1996; van Kleeck et al., 1997). Those who adopt this position stress the importance of early intervention that tries to take advantage of the neurological plasticity of brains of children younger than 5 years. Rice (2000), in summarizing the work of Dale et al. (1998) on genetic contributions to slow vocabulary development in 2-year-old children and speculating on its implications for later language development, writes that

> the children whose early vocabularies are small, compared to other children, in effect have a qualitatively different status than the children with more robust vocabularies; they are not just at the low end of the normal distribution. In other words, the emergence of first vocabulary items may function much like a clinical marker in affected [i.e., having language impairment] children, although whether or not vocabulary status retains this marker function for older children remains to be seen. It may be that first vocabulary acquisition serves as a valuable indicator of the fact that affected children's language emerges late relative to unaffected children. (p. 28)

The work to develop other markers of SLI in young children with SELD, such as that of Hadley and Short (2005) looking at the onset of verb tense marking in 2- and 3-year-old children and Stokes and Klee (2009) attempting to develop a nonword repetition task able to be used with young children, will likely give us better tools to use with children with SELD, which in turn may help us make more informed decisions about which children with SELD need intervention because their SELD is an indicator of SLI.

Others have suggested that such children should be monitored closely and intervention provided if the children do not appear to be catching up well and early (Paul, 1996, 2000), that is, a "watch-and-see" policy (Paul, 1996, p. 15). From this perspective, SELD should be viewed as a risk factor for SLI but not a disorder (Paul, 1996, 1997; Whitehurst & Fischel, 1994).

Some of the findings about 5-year-olds who as toddlers and preschoolers had slow language development could be interpreted as suggesting a relatively low prevalence rate for children of kindergarten age. However, the experience of professionals who have worked with young children tells us that this may not be true (Johnson et al., 1999). In a large-scale and well-controlled epidemiological study of kindergarteners, Tomblin and his research team (Tomblin, Records et al., 1997) reported that the prevalence of SLI among children in their first year of school, between about 5 and 6 years of age, was 7.4 percent. (This is why readers were earlier asked to keep the estimated prevalence figure derived for 4-year-olds in mind.) As Leonard (1998) comments, "There is no reason to believe that the prevalence of 7.4 percent is artificially high" (p. 20). In fact, Johnson et al. (1999) arrived at an estimate of 6.7 percent. Because children's language abilities at 4 and 5 years of age are quite predictive of what their language, literacy, and numeracy skills will be like as they mature (Catts et al., 2002; Donlan, Cowan, Newton, & Lloyd, 2007; Rescorla & Lee, 2001; Stothard et al., 1998; Tomblin, 2014; Tomblin et al., 2003) and SLI likely does not "get cured" but remains as a lifelong disability with considerable negative consequences (Brownlie et al., 2004; Clegg, Hollis, Mawhood, & Rutter, 2005), it is reasonable to believe that about 6.5 to 7.5 percent of students during their school years, including high school years, will have SLI.

The prevalence rate of about 7 percent is now the commonly accepted rate. This makes the condition the most prevalent of all communication disorders and comparable in prevalence to another, well-recognized neurodevelopmental condition, ADHD. Despite its prevalence, however, preschoolers and kindergarteners with SLI often go unidentified, with any problems they might display attributed to other conditions. Redmond (2016a) comments that SLI has been

> largely unrecognized outside of the research literature and SLI represents a demonstrably under-resourced clinical entity. . . . Longitudinal studies indicate further that the risk of undertreatment rather than overtreatment is more likely for individuals with SLI because the majority of participants did not receive intervention during their academic careers. (p. 134)

A quotation from Rice (2013), describing the children who participated in her longitudinal genetic study of SLI, foreshadows what we will see in the next section and in the next two chapters:

> Most of the . . . [children] were recruited from school clinical caseloads when they were 3–7 years old, in school districts geographically distributed across a wide region. Although they were receiving speech-language therapy at the outset of their participation in the study, ongoing monitoring of the services they were receiving . . . shows that the children were likely to be dropped from speech pathology services by age 7–9 years, although they were likely to receive services for reading or other academic limitations after their speech-language pathology services were discontinued. . . . Thus, there was no common approach to speech-language therapy. (p. 224)

Considerations and Implications. One consideration about trying to determine prevalence is that language deficits may change in their manifestations as children get older, thereby showing effects on language performance differently for certain aspects of language behavior. As we indicated previously, syntax and morphology may be problematic, as might higher-level language skills, such as narrative, even when delays in early vocabulary size might seem to have resolved. We also know that nonword repetition skills, ability to recall sentences, and language comprehension abilities have a high probability of being affected. These factors suggest that tasks, such as complex sentence usage and narrative skill in situations that challenge children's language performance and language processing and language comprehension, need to be utilized with older preschool children to tap their levels of language competency.

Another concern relates to a pattern of normal language development in which 5-year-old children seem to plateau in their language but show a growth spurt again between ages 6 and 7 (Scarborough & Dobrich, 1990). Because normally developing peers may plateau at about 5 years of age, 5-year-old children with histories of SELD may, on the surface, appear to catch up in language use in unchallenging situations. However, when their peers' language skills move ahead again a year or two later, the children with SELD histories may be left behind at a time when acquisition of literacy skills, which are heavily dependent on oral language abilities, becomes critically important in school for future academic success. These children might experience a subsequent growth with particular language skills, but for some children and for some skills, the plateau might mean some of these language behaviors "get stuck" at the plateaued level (Rice, 2013). Certain aspects of language behavior may also plateau at different ages (Rice, 2013; Scarborough & Dobrich, 1990). Therefore, for some children we may see what is an illusion of recovery from early language delay and for different language skills at different times, that is, "illusory recovery." This would create the impression of differing profiles of language adequacy in different children at different ages.

An additional concern relates to what other skills children with SELD might not be learning while they are trying to catch up that their normal language-learning peers have the opportunities to learn because their learning resources are not having to be directed to learning more basic language skills. A "Matthew" effect might operate (Stanovich, 1986), in which case those children who are better at language are better able to take advantage of language-learning opportunities to learn more language, but those who are not good fall further and further behind, and the gap between the language able and language limited children widens with time. It is possible that (1) children with histories of SELD give the illusion of recovery and then relapse; (2) if subgroups of young children with language difficulties exist, children in different subgroups will evidence different patterns of language growth, recovery, and relapse; (3) some language skills may "catch up" but others do not, and findings may depend on which skills have been measured and how these were measured; and (4) SELD children expend learning resources and learning time on trying to catch up, and therefore they "miss out" on other learning—learning that may eventually affect their school performances. Paul (1991) writes that the interpretation of findings suggesting these children "catch up" by 5 years of age needs to consider the following:

- Whether the full range of language skills that are important at this age—and not detectable in measures of expressive vocabulary size, general verbal fluency, or unstructured conversation (such as complex sentence use and narrative skill)—is evaluated
- Whether any recovery that does appear to be completed by age 5 is stable or will again be outpaced by development in normal children over the course of the next year or two, when their rate of language growth accelerates, in conjunction with the acquisition of literacy skills
- Even if oral language skills do appear to remain eventually within the normal range by the end of the preschool period, whether the underlying processes that slowed them down at first continue to operate, now influencing primarily the learning of reading, writing, and spelling, as seems to be the case for so many youngsters with a history of language delay (pp. 9–10)

It is clear that preschoolers with continuing language problems in the apparent absence of other problems run the risk of encountering academic difficulties when they enter school (e.g., Catts et al., 2002; Johnson et al., 1999; Stothard et al., 1998; Zhang & Tomblin, 2000). In fact, in Chapter 5 we shall see that the difficulties created by language problems first evident in the preschool years can continue into and through adolescence and even into adulthood (e.g., Clegg et al., 2005; Snowling et al., 2006). Prevalence data on the occurrence of language problems in school-aged children are, however, conflicting, with some suggesting a fairly dramatic decrease in the prevalence of language impairments in school-aged children (U.S. Department of Education, 2009). Academic difficulties stemming from language deficits frequently lead to school-aged children being referred to as "language-learning disabled" or "learning disabled," a topic taken up in more detail in the next two chapters. As well as an apparent false recovery period for oral language skills in the early school years, this relabeling may account for what Snyder (1984) observed several years ago was the "great disappearing act" (p. 129). That is, once in school, children with SLI may no longer be seen as language impaired in "head counts" of children having disabilities. Rather, they are counted in a different category, most often specific learning disabilities. Recall the quote from Rice (2013) previously in this chapter about children with SLI being dismissed from speech-language services at about 7 or 8 years of age.

Predicting Spontaneous Recovery from Early Language Delay

Which of the children we have been discussing in the previous section are the ones who seem to "outgrow" their early language delays, that is, spontaneously recover from their early delay without intervention, and which do not? This is an important question because, given the insidious and long-lasting effects of language impairment, we want to provide early intervention to those children who need it but do not want to waste professional resources providing intervention to those children who will "outgrow" their delays and do so with no residual negative effects. Intervention with toddlers and preschoolers has positive effects on their language and accelerates their language, but we also know that intervention does not "cure" SLI. The situation may be much like many medical conditions or other disabilities; they do not go away even with the best of practice and intervention, but the effects of the conditions can be moderated with intervention so as to lessen negative impact. As important as it is to be able to predict which toddlers and preschoolers will and will not spontaneously recover from early language delay without negative residual effects, we are not yet very good at doing so with absolute certainty. Dollaghan and Campbell (2009) write, "Findings from a small but growing number of investigations in which predictive accuracy of a variety of early indicators of developmental deficits [language] has been studied directly and found wanting" (pp. 363–364).

Professionals who work with children with SLI become concerned about advice to parents of 2-year-olds who are not talking very much that they should not worry about their child because the child will probably outgrow the early delay. From the previous discussion, we know that such advice might have about a 50/50 chance (splitting the difference on the range of estimates) of being right. For the children for whom the advice was wrong, valuable intervention time has been lost. For 3-year-old children whose language does not match that of their peers, we become even more concerned about such advice, and by 4 years of age, the odds of spontaneous recovery are against the child. However, predicting which children will eventually outgrow their early language delay is not an exact science because we have not yet pinpointed all the factors that affect spontaneous recovery or identified how various factors interact at different ages (Kelly, 1998; Olswang et al., 1998; Paul, 2000). The risk factors for SLI discussed previously in this chapter may provide, perhaps in combination, some direction for professionals in making relatively accurate predictions. However, we have yet to fully investigate the predictive accuracy of these factors in various combinations. Nevertheless, Olswang et al. (1998), in their review of the literature, write that "we know a lot" (p. 23) that can be used to help us make educated predictions so that we lower the odds of being wrong. Table 3.3 lists several of the factors that might provide predictive information about toddlers and preschoolers at risk for continuing language problems.

The possible clinical markers that we have previously referred to also as possible risk factors are listed in Table 3.3 because these might additionally function as factors that can help in predicting which toddlers with SELD might or might not spontaneously recover from their early language delay (Pawlowska, 2014). If 2-year-olds do not seem to be showing the same developmental trajectory for acquisition of early verb morphological markers that is shown by same-age peers without concerns about their early language delay (Hadley & Short, 2005), this could be a signal that the toddlers with SELD may be at risk for experiencing spontaneous recovery. With the development of nonword and even word repetition tasks that may be appropriate for use with toddlers and preschoolers (Chiat & Roy, 2007; Deevy et al., 2010; Gray, 2003a; Shriberg et al., 2009; Stokes & Klee, 2009; Thal et al., 2005), youngsters' performances on such tasks might also add to our ability to predict ongoing language problems for the children. Chiat and Roy (2008) have used a repetition task to predict at 3½ to 4 years of age the language outcomes for toddlers age 2 to 2½ years and have obtained promising results regarding the task's predictive value.

In light of some of the information about comprehension that has been presented so far in this chapter, comprehension skills deserve some special mention. There is increasing evidence that children with delayed expressive language development who also have more notable comprehension deficits are likely to demonstrate poorer outcomes, even into adolescence. For toddlers, Watt et al. (2006) found that comprehension skills of 2-year-old children were significant factors in predicting their receptive and expressive language abilities at 3 years of age. For preschoolers, comprehension deficits may have more impact on peer interactions or parents' reports of their young children's conversational skills than expressive language problems (Gertner, Rice, & Hadley, 1994; Girolametto, 1997). Given the more recent concerns that expressive language deficits may not exist in the absence of some degree of comprehension problems (Leonard, 2009; Tomblin & Zhang, 2006; Tomblin et al., 2007), comprehension abilities of toddlers and preschoolers may need to be seen as having considerable predictive importance. Olswang et al. (1998) have commented that

> the consensus suggests that toddlers with significant expressive and receptive language delays of 6 months or more are more at risk for continued language delay. Further, for those children delayed in both comprehension and production, the larger the comprehension—production gap, the poorer the prognosis. (p. 25)

Language comprehension delays likely play important roles in predicting continuing language deficits in children. Furthermore, toddlers and preschoolers with language comprehension problems are at risk for under-identification, and language comprehension problems in toddlers and preschoolers are at risk for under-identification. Yet, language

TABLE 3.3 | Some Factors Potentially Predicting Continuing Language Problems

Factors	Explanation
Family history	■ Greater risk for children with family member with a history of language, speech, or literacy/learning problems
Mother's education/family SES	■ Lower SES but large proportion of SES level reflected by mother's education ■ Lower educational level of mother implicated for lower vocabulary development but maybe not syntactic complexity and grammatical morphology, except perhaps for implications for assortative mating (Plomin & Dale, 2000)
Communicative intentions, symbolic gestures, and play	■ Production of symbolic gestures in familiar script routines (e.g., bathing a teddy bear) reduced ■ Ability to produce symbolic gestures positively related to comprehension vocabulary level ■ Less frequent use of gesture generally (may be related to reduction in frequency of communicative intentions produced gesturally) ■ Range of communicative intentions used appropriate, but frequency with which they are used is reduced ■ Reduction in frequency with which comment/joint attention communicative intentions used ■ Less use of representational, communicative gesture ■ Greater use of complementary gesture (same meaning as word) and less use of supplementary gesture (add meaning) ■ Grouping and manipulation of play objects but less thematic/combinatorial play
Babbling and phonology	■ Less language growth for children with higher occurrences of vowel babble and greater language growth for children with consonantal babble ■ Greater language growth related to greater babble complexity ■ Less complex syllable structure (e.g., CV versus CVC versus C_1VC_2V) ■ Fewer consonants in phonetic repertoire, with less than four to five at 24 months and limited vowel repertoire ■ Phonological patterns at 36 months that include vowel errors, glottal stops or /h/ substitutions for consonants, many occurrences of initial consonant and final consonant deletion, and back-consonant substitutions for front consonants
Socialization and behavior	■ Possible deficits in social skills (e.g., smiling appropriately, playing social games) ■ More passive communicators who initiate communication and nonverbal interactions less ■ Possibly overactive and difficult to manage; seemingly short attention span ■ Less language growth in children with behavior problems
Comprehension	■ Comprehension language delays accompanying expressive language delays ■ Comprehension delay with large gap between expressive and comprehension abilities
Clinical markers	■ Slower-than-expected acquisition of early verb morphological markers during second year of life ■ Poor performance on nonword and possible word repetition tasks, particularly those that account for early phonological acquisition ■ Difficulties with sentence repetition (sentence recall) tasks
Verb vocabulary size and growth	■ Low proportion of verb words in early vocabulary ■ Slower than expected growth in verb vocabulary ■ Fewer verb words that occur less frequently in the language
Responsiveness to trial intervention/dynamic assessment	■ Evidence of limited learning of a new, targeted language skill under conditions of short-term, intensive learning trials
Narrative production	■ Recounts of experiences shorter than expected for age ■ Difficulties with temporal sequencing of events in stories or experiential recounts ■ Recounts of experiences or story retells more difficult for listener to follow than expected for age
Severity of delay	■ Greater language delay indicating less optimism for spontaneous recovery ■ Very low expressive vocabulary size (zero to eight words) at 2 years of age

comprehension problems may more severely impact children's later academic and social functioning than expressive language deficits.

It is also probably worth a bit more discussion of the early vocabulary of toddlers with early language delay. One aspect of early vocabulary that might inform about the probability of spontaneous recovery is the composition of the vocabulary, particularly for verbs. Olswang et al. (1998) identified several "red flags" (p. 25): (1) a relatively small verb vocabulary compared to other types of words, particularly nouns; (2) reliance on GAP (general all-purpose) verbs, such as *look* or *want*, rather than more specific verbs, such as *walk* or *clap;* and (3) fewer intransitive (not requiring a direct object) and ditransitive (able to either have or not have a direct object) verbs than transitive verbs. Hadley, Rispoli, and Hsu (2016) found that the size of toddlers' verb lexicons was a significant predictor of their syntactic skills about a year later when they were preschoolers, whereas their noun lexicons had much less predictive value for their later syntactic skills. Additionally, the diversity of toddlers' verb vocabulary appears to have some degree of predictive value for later grammatical production (Rispoli & Hadley, 2011). However, Hadley et al. (2016) remind us that the semantics of a particular verb choice often govern the syntactic structure in which it can occur. The authors (Hadley et al., 2016, p. 46) provided the example of the verb *put*, which requires a direct object as well as a locative, i.e., "I put the book on the table." In contrast, the verb *sleep* places no demands on what syntactic structures must follow, i.e., "I sleep" is complete, although there is the option of adding predicate structure, such as "I sleep in the bed." Verb lexical development is not, therefore, divorced from syntactic growth, and syntax is often a particularly deficient component of language for SLI children.

Some verbs occur more frequently than others, for example, *sleep* versus *doze*. We suspect that children who use fewer of the less frequently occurring verbs are more at risk for continuing language problems than those whose verb lexicons include the less frequently occurring verbs. More specific verbs also tend to be less frequently occurring than GAP verbs, as noted above.

There may also be more precise information about size of a child's expressive vocabulary at 2 years of age that might increase our predictive abilities. Although the criterion of using fewer than 50 single words at 24 months of age has been a major guideline for identifying toddlers with SELD, the work of Dale et al. (1998) on the heritability of early vocabulary development suggests that we might need to be more specific about vocabulary size. In this discussion, we need to keep our perspective with regard to the single-word vocabulary size of 2-year-olds, which is somewhere around 130 to 300 (Fenson et al., 1990; Rescorla, Alley, & Christine, 2001). When the vocabulary size of at least one of 2-year-old twin pairs was in the lowest 5 percent of the distribution on a parent report measure, the MacArthur Communicative Development Inventory (Fenson et al., 1990), there was a substantial genetic contribution to the vocabulary size, but the influence of shared environment was found to contribute very little to the vocabulary size (Dale et al., 1998). A vocabulary size of zero to eight words placed the 2-year-old children in the lowest 5 percent. What this suggests is that very low vocabulary size at 2 years of age may have genetic contributions operating that then decrease the probability of spontaneous recovery of the early delay. Professionals might be wise to treat a 2-year-old with very low vocabulary development differently from one with a vocabulary size closer to the 50-word criterion.

This discussion of severity of impairment is also consistent with some evidence that the severity of a child's language delay may also be predictive of recovery (Law, Tomblin, & Zhang, 2008; Olswang & Bain, 1996). That is, the greater the degree of the child's language delay, the less optimistic we might be about spontaneous recovery for the child.

Two other factors might assist us with the task of determining which children will spontaneously recover from early language delay. Previously in this chapter, we noted that children with language impairments would be predicted to be relatively slower to respond to trial language instruction (dynamic assessment) than children without language impairment but with delayed language development. We have also mentioned stressing a child's language ability via narrative production tasks. Narrative skills of children with language impairments have regularly surfaced as one of the areas of considerable and persisting difficulty. Tracking children's developing abilities in narrative production may also help in predicting spontaneous recovery.

Olswang et al. (1998) summarized the current level of knowledge:

> Research has revealed robust trends about language learning in toddlers who are typical and atypical in their language development. These trends have brought to light characteristics that allow us to decide whether we should be seriously concerned about a toddler's actual and potential language growth. The argument being made from this literature is that the magnitude of our concern should directly translate to our recommendations. To our way of thinking, . . . this is not only a reasonable position, but also an ethical and intellectually defensible one. (p. 29)

Using the medical profession's risk factor model may be a way to judge the degree of concern (Thal & Katich, 1996; Whitehurst & Fischel, 1994). This is an additive approach in which the degree of risk for the occurrence of a condition increases with an increase in the number of different known risk factors that are present. The more factors present in or associated with a young child that point to the possibility of future language problems for the child, the greater the concern and, therefore, the more likely that intervention is an appropriate recommendation for the child.

LANGUAGE CHARACTERISTICS OF CHILDREN WITH SPECIFIC LANGUAGE IMPAIRMENT

In this section, we review a number of the language characteristics observed in toddlers and preschool children with SLI. The preceding sections in this chapter have served to foreshadow some of the characteristics we will discuss. And, we need to be aware that not all children will necessarily demonstrate all of these problems and that a problem with one aspect of language can result in problems with other aspects. One example of this was seen in the previous section about the relationship between the semantics of specific verb choices and associated requisite syntactic forms for them. The potentially diverse patterns reemphasize the fact that children with SLI are a heterogeneous group. Additionally, we need to be aware that some of the same types of problems can be observed in school-aged children and adolescents with language disorders, albeit at different levels.

Some Language Precursors

Recognition of and attention to environmental change are important to language acquisition because, without these, a child will not develop the underlying concepts of language. Furthermore, children need to learn that they can be the agents of change. Unless children realize that what they do results in modifications of objects or people's behaviors, they will be unlikely to learn that language is one of the most effective ways of producing change.

Several of the factors listed in Table 3.3 referred to or involved concerns about behaviors and abilities that can be considered precursors to language development, for example, use of symbolic gesture and communicative intentions. As well as participating in reciprocal interactions, establishing joint reference with an adult appears to be important for language acquisition (Delgado et al., 2002; Watt et al., 2006). Early child–adult behaviors of give-and-take play routines and repetitive games such as patty-cake may be prerequisites of conversational turn-taking skills. Some preschoolers with SLI seem to have difficulty participating in these reciprocal routines. These children may also not engage frequently in joint attention or learn to utilize cues provided by joint reference with an adult. With regard to communicative intents, these may be encoded by children with SLI more via gestures and vocalizations than by verbal means, and in particular, as we see from Table 3.3, reduced ability to produce *symbolic* gestures reflecting script routines may predict longer-term language problems.

The relationship between babbling and the production of first words is not fully understood, although the phonetic content of babbled vocalizations likely affects children's early lexicons and may even be a distinguishing feature of some children with language problems. In order to produce a variety of single words, children need to have several different consonants in their repertoires and use these consonants in different distributions and in combinations with different vowels. In this way, the syllable structure of babble might be a precursor to use of first words. When we review Table 3.3, we see that reduced occurrences of certain types of babbling and particular patterns of early phonology might be early indications of language impairment. The impact of limited forms of babbling on language ability beyond 12 months of age was described in a large-scale study by Oller, Eilers, Neal, and Schwartz (1999). In their study of 3,400 infants at 10 months of age, the "infants with delayed canonical babbling had smaller production vocabularies at 18, 24 and 36 months than did infants in the control group" (p. 223).

Phonology

Given the preceding discussion, it is probably not surprising that toddlers and preschoolers with SLI frequently have concomitant phonological problems. The reverse is also true. For example, Shriberg and colleagues (Shriberg & Kwiatkowski, 1994; Shriberg et al., 1999) have reported that most children identified as having phonological problems also have language impairments. Normally developing children are moderately intelligible by about 2 years of age. In contrast, it is not unusual to find 3- and 4-year-old children with SLI who are difficult to understand. However, phonological problems are more likely than language problems to resolve as children mature, and children with speech sound difficulties have been reported as having better long-term academic, social, and vocational outcomes than those with language impairments (e.g., Johnson et al., 1999; Shriberg, Gruber, & Kwiatkowski, 1994; Whitehurst, Fischel et al., 1991).

Some have proposed that problems with phonological acquisition are simply reflections of more general language-learning problems. Others suggest that phonological problems may be characteristics of subgroup membership within the larger, heterogeneous group of specifically language-impaired children. Whatever the relationship between SLI and phonological problems, we know that young children with SLI acquire more quickly single words that begin with consonants they use correctly in other words than words that begin with consonants not yet produced correctly (Leonard, Schwartz et al., 1982). This relationship between phonology and lexical acquisition is consistent with a developmental pattern seen in normally developing toddlers (Schwartz & Leonard, 1982). We also know from one study that about 20 to 30 percent of the preschool children who experienced phonological difficulties apparently not related to concomitant problems in other areas received special education services when they entered school, even though many of the children no longer showed obvious evidence of phonological difficulties at the time of entering school (Shriberg & Kwiatkowski, 1988). This may reflect what we know about phonological problems in the preschool years affecting children's abilities to achieve academically in areas related to linguistic skills, possibly because of phonological processing difficulties.

Semantics

We have indicated that a delay in using the first word (usually emerging at about 12 months of age) and being slow to add lots of words to their vocabularies are frequently the first signs of possible language problems. On the other hand, we have also indicated that vocabulary may be one of the areas in which children who are slow to talk seem to catch up first. However, we must be clear that this does not mean that children with SLI do not have semantic difficulties because many, if not most, have some degree of problems with words and their meanings. These problems are seen most clearly with words and expressions with abstract, nonliteral meanings and those related to the more literate aspects of semantics. Several areas of semantic acquisition that characterize some of the problems young children with SLI exhibit have been identified in the literature and are presented in Table 3.4.

With regard to vocabulary size, we have seen that a delay in using the first word (usually at about 12 months of age) and failing to show a spurt in single-word lexical acquisition

TABLE 3.4 | Several Areas of Semantic Difficulties Experienced by Children with SLI

Areas of Semantic Difficulty	Problems
Size of the lexicon	Smaller vocabularies
Rate of growth of the lexicon	Slower vocabulary acquisition Less lexical diversity
Robustness of word meaning	Less depth of knowledge about word meanings Less known about the meaning of individual words Only partial meanings of a word known
Speed of new word learning	Difficulties learning new lexical items quickly More exposures to a new word in context needed to abstract the meaning of the word
Word finding	Difficulties retrieving words from the cognitive store to use them in quick flow of connected speech The word on the "tip of the tongue"

after emergence of the first word are possible early signs of SLI. Other early delays in semantic development have also been described. Examples of some of the delays that have been reported for young late talkers and children with SLI are the following:

- On average, using their first word at about 23 months of age (Trauner, Wulfeck, Tallal, & Hesselink, 1995), almost a year late in this report compared to normally developing children
- At 24 months of age an expressive vocabulary size of about 17 words compared to 128 to 193 for normally developing children and at 36 months a vocabulary size of 197 words, similar to that of normally developing children at 24 months (Rescorla et al., 2001)

Rescorla et al. (2001) also reported on the composition of the vocabulary of 3-year-olds who were late talkers and whose expressive vocabulary size was approximating that of normally developing 2-year-olds. These authors comment that although the children seem to acquire many of the same words as normally developing children, they also learn some different words that appear to reflect that they are older and, therefore, are experiencing different events in their environments, for example, words associated with toilet training. And, as we saw previously, children with SLI also seem to have more difficulty acquiring a wide variety of verb words than noun. These findings raise a point that we need to keep in mind. Early delays in vocabulary acquisition may well result in children with SLI having qualitatively different as well as quantitatively different vocabularies. This possibility has important implications for what we might be able to assume about their continuity of language development compared to that of children without language problems, about what concepts and world knowledge these young children are building up along their developmental path, and about what the cumulative effects might be that somewhat unusual concepts and knowledge might have on later academic and language learning.

As we saw earlier in this text, when words and their meanings join with other words and their meanings in multiword utterances, composite meanings evolve. Similar to their delay in early vocabulary, young children with SLI are typically slower to begin to use two-word semantic relations. Trauner et al. (1995) reported that the children with SLI in their study did not begin to use two-word combinations until about 3 years of age, which compares to normally developing children beginning to use these combinations sometime between 18 and 24 months. Although children with SLI may be slower to acquire the range of semantic relations expressed in two-word combinations than normal language-learning children, they seem generally to acquire the same range expressed by their language-normal peers.

In the previous chapter, we discussed normal children's abilities to learn a lot about a word's meaning from very few and fleeting exposures to the word in context. We referred to this ability as "fast mapping" or "quick incidental learning." Young children with SLI have been found to demonstrate some abilities to fast map the meanings of words, particularly in structured learning situations, but they have been found to comprehend meanings of fewer new words when the learning task involved challenging tasks of discerning the meanings embedded in ongoing narratives. Overall, preschool children with SLI seem to learn new words more slowly than their normal-language peers (Gray, 2005) and "may need to hear a new word twice as many times as a child with [normal language] before comprehending it" (Gray, 2003b, p. 56) and may need an additional doubling in opportunities to use it while continuing to hear it before the word becomes a permanent part of their vocabulary (Gray, 2003b). This means that the SLI child will have needed quadruple the opportunities to hear the new word than a child with normal language in order to use it independently.

Even if children with SLI are successful in gleaning meanings of words, this does not necessarily result in them using the words. One suggestion for this limitation is that the children have difficulties accessing or retrieving the words for production rather than a failure in storing the words in memory. Another reason proposes that difficulties using words that seem to be known in the lexicon are a result of knowing only incomplete or partial meanings of the words. McGregor and her colleagues (e.g., McGregor, Newman, Reilly, & Capone, 2002; McGregor, Oleson, Bahnsen, & Duff, 2013; Sheng & McGregor 2010a, 2010b) suggest that the children may have a mental representation of a word, but it may not be a fully developed representation and may therefore be fragile. As McGregor, Friedman, Reilly, and Newman (2002) write, the fragileness of the meaning makes the word more susceptible to "retrieval failure" (p. 332).

The observation that many children with language problems have difficulties in retrieving known words (word-finding problems) is not new (e.g., German, 1979; Kail, Hale, Leonard, & Nippold, 1984; MacLachlan & Chapman, 1988). In fact, many children with SLI are described as having word-finding problems, with most children having deficits with a number of other language skills as well (Dockrell & Messer, 2007). The word-finding difficulties can show up when children are asked to name pictures, particularly in timed naming tasks, and in their connected speech (German, 2000; McGregor, 1997). What is not clear is if the word-finding problems children exhibit are due to less complete and stable mental representations of the words, an indication of reduced speed of processing proposed as one of the possible information processing deficits seen in children with SLI, or both factors. The connected speech of children with language problems is also often characterized by hesitations, dysfluencies, reformulations, word substitutions, and fillers, features that are regularly interpreted as being related to difficulties generating language, including possible word retrieval difficulties. Additionally, the children may use a substantially higher number of words without clear referents, such as *thing, this, that, here*, and *there*.

It does not appear that children with SLI have semantic difficulties in the absence of problems with other aspects of language. In describing the children they had followed from 2½ to 5 years of age, Scarborough and Dobrich (1990) have written that when the children reached age 5, "no child ever showed a purely lexical deficit. Instead, residual phonological and syntactic problems, in combination and in isolation, were seen in most cases" (p. 80). To the extent that these findings are correct, we suspect that most if not all children with SLI with semantic difficulties will also have deficits with syntax and morphology, and we suspect that the children will have comprehension problems as well.

Syntax and Morphology

As we saw earlier in this chapter in the discussion of possible clinical markers of SLI, these children are known to have inordinate difficulty with the morphosyntactic aspect of language, and it is doubtful that any child with SLI escapes at least some problems in this area.

Deficit syntactic and morphologic skills are almost "classic" characteristics of preschoolers with language impairments (e.g., Leonard, 2014; Menyuk, 1964; Riches, 2016). Lahey's (1988) insightful comment of several years ago continues to describe accurately young children with SLI, stating that "by far the most outstanding characteristic of this group of children and one that they all share, is late and slow development of form with better development of content and use interactions" (pp. 59–60).

Not withstanding Hadley and Short's (2005) findings documenting the emergence of verb tense marking in children between 2 and 3 years of age, it is generally at about 2 ½ to 3 years of age that evidence of syntactic and/or morphological problems can be more confidently identified, as children's MLUs, sentence complexity, and use of morphological markers are expected to increase greatly. As examples of the difficulties that are observed in these children in the preschool years, we tend to see the following:

- Shorter length of utterances (MLU) than same-age peers
- Syntactically simpler sentences, including limitations in the types of transformations used and limited use of subordination
- Omissions and/or confusions of grammatically obligatory elements, such as articles and noun plural morphemes
- Subject case marking problems, as in *him* for *he* and *her* for *she* when the pronouns are to serve as subjects of sentences
- Failure to consistently mark verbs for tense and number, with particular difficulties with both regular and irregular past-tense marking

Table 3.5 provides a list of some of the common problematic morphemes for children with SLI.

Because, as we have seen, verb morphology is particularly vexing for children with SLI, their abilities in this area have been the subject of considerable study. One consistent but frustrating observation about the morphosyntactic performances of these children is the inconsistency in their use of morphological markers (e.g., Leonard et al., 2003; Miller & Leonard, 1998; Rice, Wexler, & Cleave, 1995). Their inconsistency means that sometimes they treat a finite verb (one that needs to carry tense and number, such as "The girl run<u>s</u>" or "The boy jump<u>ed</u>") as a nonfinite verb (an infinitive form or bare stem form, such as "The girl run" or "The boy jump"). Overall, however, they make many more verb morphological errors than their typically developing peers. Other patterns with regard to their use of grammatical

TABLE 3.5 | Some Troublesome Grammatical Morphemes for Children with SLI

Morpheme	Examples
Plural -<u>s</u>	boy<u>s</u>; coat<u>s</u>
Possessive -<u>'s</u>	baby<u>'s</u>; cat<u>'s</u>
Regular past -<u>ed</u>	play<u>ed</u>; lik<u>ed</u>
Third-person singular -<u>s</u>	play<u>s</u>; like<u>s</u>
Articles <u>a</u> and <u>the</u>	<u>a</u> boy; <u>the</u> cat
Copula	The baby <u>is</u> big
<u>On</u>	<u>on</u> the floor; put <u>on</u> the coat
Auxiliary <u>be</u>	The baby <u>is</u> crying; The girls <u>are</u> playing
Irregular past tense	ate; went; drank
Complementizer <u>to</u>	I'm going <u>to</u> (go); gon<u>na</u> (go)

Source: Leonard, McGregor, and Allen (1992).

markers for verbs have also been observed. These, along with the pattern of inconsistent use, are shown in Table 3.6.

Two alternative explanations for why these children demonstrate inordinate difficulties with verb morphology have featured prominently in the literature. One is referred to as the *surface account* (e.g., Leonard, Eyer, Bedore, & Grela, 1997; Leonard, McGregor, et al., 1992) because it focuses on the phonetic features, that is, the morphophonological characteristics

TABLE 3.6 | Patterns of Verb Morphological Problems of Children with SLI

Patterns	Descriptions and Examples
Inconsistent errors	Bare stem verbs ("The girl run") used frequently but not always Sometimes verb marked correctly ("The girl runs")
Errors of omission common	Likely to omit grammatical markers ("Baby sleeps" or "Baby sleeping") Likely to omit auxiliaries, which mark the number and tense ("Baby sleeping")
Errors of commission infrequent	When verbs marked for tense and number, they tend to be marked correctly ("Baby is sleeping," not "Baby are sleeping")
Regular past-tense verbs problematic	Inconsistent use of finite or infinitive (bare stem) verb when finite form required ("[yesterday] Boys jump" instead of "Boys jumped") Perform at level worse than younger normal children matched for overall language level
Irregular past-tense verbs problematic	Frequently overgeneralized ("Kitty runned" instead of "Kitty ran") Bare stem used ("Kitty run" instead of "Kitty ran") Perform at levels similar to younger normal children matched for overall language level when percent correct versus percent incorrect metric used ("Kitty run" correct vs. "Kitty runned" incorrect) Perform at levels similar to those for regular past tense (i.e., worse than younger, language-matched children) when percent correct marking for knowledge of past tense used as the metric (percent correct for finiteness) ("Kitty runned" credited as correct for knowledge of need to mark tense) More likely than CA-matched peers to judge bare stem forms as correct ("[yesterday] Birdie fly off" deemed okay) More likely than CA-matched peers to judge overgeneralized forms as correct ("[yesterday] Birdie flied off")
Case marking on pronouns related to verb marking	***An early suggestion:*** ▪ A potential developmental link between verb form acquisition and pronoun case development ***More recent suggestions:*** ▪ Incorrect use of objective case pronouns (***him, her, them***) as subjects (***he, she, they***) related to occurrence of verb tense marking ▪ Greater likelihood of objective case when verb unmarked for tense/number ("Her jump" more likely than "Her jumps") or auxiliary omitted ("Her jumping" more likely than "Her is jumping")
Inclusion of auxiliary verbs potentially susceptible to structural priming effects	▪ Likely to include rather than omit auxiliary if child used an auxiliary in immediately preceding utterance ("Mommy is sleeping" instead of "Mommy sleeping" if previous sentence included auxiliary, e.g., "Babies are crying")

Sources: Bishop (1994); Connell (1986); Leonard, Bortolini, Caselli, McGregor, and Sabbadini (1992); Leonard, Eyer, Bedore, and Grela (1997); Leonard, Miller et al. (2002); Loeb and Leonard (1991); Marchman, Wulfeck, and Ellis Weismer (1999); Montgomery and Leonard (1998); Oetting and Horohov (1997); Rice and Wexler (1996); Rice et al. (1995, 1998); Wexler, Schütze, and Rice (1998).

of the problematic grammatical morphemes. Leonard and his fellow researchers (Leonard, McGregor, et al., 1992) point out that these morphemes have "low phonetic substance" (p. 1077). The morphemes have shorter durations in connected speech than adjacent morphemes. They are also unstressed, nonsyllabic segments. Some of them also have lower fundamental frequencies and amplitude, meaning that they may seem to be lower pitched and less loud. These features mean that they may be auditorily less salient than surrounding morphemes. This account suggested by Leonard et al. (1997) "assumes a general processing capacity limitation in children with SLI but assumes also that, in the case of English, this will have an especially profound impact on the joint operations of perceiving grammatical morphemes and hypothesizing their grammatical function" (p. 743). That is, the children with SLI have inefficient processing mechanisms that interfere with their abilities to take in these particularly brief, often faint elements of the language and analyze them fast enough during the ongoing flow of language and environmental activity in order to figure out what they mean and what the patterns and rules are in order to use them. We encountered some of the discussion about processing capacity limitations earlier in this chapter. The surface account does not explain why children with SLI might have processing limitations that lead them to have difficulty acquiring verb morphology that typically developing children do not exhibit.

The second, the *extended optional infinitive account* (e.g., Rice, 2013; Rice & Wexler, 1996; Rice et al., 1998; Rice, Wexler, Marquis, & Hershberger, 2000), is a knowledge-based account. According to this account, children with SLI, like very young normal children, do not know that marking verb tense and number is obligatory and treat it as a rule of language that is optional to use. Where children with SLI differ from their normal counterparts is that they continue to treat verb marking as optional for an extended period of time, whereas normal children by about the age of 5 years figure out that they need always to mark tense and number on finite verbs (main verbs in clauses) rather than treat them as infinitives (bare stem verbs). While children with SLI know about finiteness of verbs and the concepts of present and past tense, they do not know they are obligated to mark tense on verbs in main clauses. We also know that by 8 years of age, while the frequency of failure to apply verb marking has declined considerably, children with SLI still are inconsistent—some suggesting about 10 to 15 percent of the time (Rice et al., 1998)—whereas normal children achieve this level of consistency at 5 years of age and by age 8 almost always use appropriate verb marking. We also know that older children and adolescents with language impairments continue to have more difficulty with verb morphology than their peers (e.g., Leonard et al., 2009; Miller, Leonard, & Finneran, 2008; Reed, Conrad, & Patchell, 2006; Reed & Patchell, 2010; Reed, Patchell, & Conrad, 2006; Rice, Hoffman, & Wexler, 2009). With regard to the reasons for the verb morphological difficulties of children with SLI, brain development with genetic bases that govern timing for acquiring finite verb marking, as discussed previously in this chapter, has been suggested (cf. Rice, 2012, 2013). There are several other accounts of the reasons children with SLI have such inordinate difficulties with grammatical morphology and verb morphology in particular. One of these accounts is based on limited linguistic knowledge. This account proposes that children have difficulty abstracting the implicit rules that govern grammatical morphology (Gopnik, 1990; Ullman & Gopnik, 1994), hence the term *implicit rule deficit account* (Leonard et al., 1997). A variation on this account suggests that children with SLI learn the rules about verb marking but have difficulties accessing them (Connell & Stone, 1992). While this account has less empirical support than the surface or extended optional infinitive accounts as far as verb morphology is concerned (Leonard et al., 1997), it is still considered among the various possible reasons children with SLI have language-learning difficulties more generally.

It is conceivable that these three accounts are not mutually exclusive. If a child has processing limitations for auditorily less perceptual and salient features of language, the child might not be able to acquire sufficient representations and knowledge regarding the features in order to manage the quite complex and thorny features of English such as regular and irregular verb forms. This incomplete knowledge might manifest both as slowed acquisition of this morphological feature and as inconsistent use of verb forms and verb tense marking that extends beyond the developmental periods shown by normally developing children.

Children with SLI may not achieve the same level of automatic verb form use that their peers achieve and might continue to show struggles and hesitations in their language when they attempt to tense mark verbs.

Two other accounts, the *dual mechanism account* (Oetting & Horohov, 1997) and the *connectionist account* (Marchman et al., 1999), have also been proposed. However, these have been subjected to comparatively less empirical study in trying to explain the grammatical morpheme problems—and in particular the verb morphological difficulties—of children with SLI.

One question that has been raised is that if children with SLI have weaknesses in their verb vocabularies, as we have noted previously, then it might be possible that their difficulties with verb morphology relate to their vocabulary. The work of Watkins and Rice (1991) explored, in part, one aspect of a possible relationship between vocabulary and verb morphology in their study of verb particles and prepositions. Certain prepositions (e.g., *in, up*) also occur as part of a verb (e.g., a multiword construction that functions as a verb, such as *climb up*), that is, a verb particle. These authors proposed that since the same word (the preposition) in these two different grammatical functions has the same meaning and carries similar levels of auditory salience (phonetic substance), any differences in children's acquisition should be primarily grammatically or morphosyntactically based. In their study, children with SLI did, in fact, have more difficulty with verb particles than prepositions, leading these authors (Watkins & Rice, 1991) to suggest that "multiple sources of vulnerability for mastery of grammatical form classes" (p. 1139) may be involved. Leonard, Miller, and Gerber (1999) took a different approach to the question of the relationship between verb vocabulary and verb morphology and looked at what children with SLI did with verb marking as a function of their lexical diversity. The findings suggested that even with greater verb vocabularies, the children's ability to deal with the grammatical marking of verbs did not keep pace, in contrast to the pattern seen for normally developing children. The findings led these authors (Leonard et al., 1999) to comment that "the lag in finite-verb morphology use in children with SLI may become more striking as vocabulary expands" (p. 687). The findings also indicated that the problems the children had with their verb morphology were "not a matter of having an inadequate number of lexical items . . . but they were simply not making use of the associated grammatical morphology" (p. 687). It appears, therefore, that children's verb morphological problems cannot be attributed wholly to vocabulary deficits.

Pragmatics and Conversational Interactions

Many children with SLI have difficulties with pragmatic and conversational aspects of language. It is not clear whether these are the result of the children's problems with morphosyntax and possibly semantics or whether these difficulties are problems in their own right and represent another area of deficit for some of these children. There are several possibilities about how pragmatic and/or conversational problems relate to other aspects of language. Among these are the following:

- Pragmatic and/or conversational problems are discrete but interacting aspects of SLI, like problems with morphosyntax, phonology, and semantics.
- Children with pragmatic and/or conversational problems form a particular subgroup of children with SLI or possibly a separate group of children (Ash & Redmond, 2014; Tomblin, 2014), which in the latter case may be referred to as a semantic–pragmatic disorder (Bishop, 2000).
- The pragmatic and/or conversational problems exhibited by children with SLI represent difficulties that are part of an autism spectrum disorder.
- The pragmatic and/or conversational difficulties that children with SLI demonstrate are the result of their unfortunate adaptations to their failures in trying to use a deficit language system to communicate and establish relationships with others.

Regardless of how pragmatic and conversational problems should be conceptualized with regard to the language problems of children with SLI, we know that children with SLI typically have problems with their relationships with others and in using language with others for expressing and understanding various functions and intentions. They can also demonstrate issues with their conversational skills, and as we will see later in this chapter and in subsequent chapters, in effectively using different discourse genres, such as narrative and exposition.

Study of the pragmatic abilities of young children with language impairments has slowed somewhat in recent years with the surge in interest in their morphosyntactic problems, but the 1980s, prompted by some work in the mid- and late 1970s, was a particularly fruitful decade for learning about the various aspects of these children's pragmatic characteristics. This is particularly true for explorations into the functions and intentions used by these children and, somewhat later, looking at the conversational patterns of children with SLI. A number of these findings is summarized in Table 3.7.

TABLE 3.7 | A Summary of Pragmatic Difficulties of Children with SLI Compared to Typically Developing Children

Areas of Pragmatics	Features

Functions and Intentions	■ Fewer occurrences of communicative initiations, including gestural and vocalized initiations
	■ Fewer occurrences of functions that initiate (child initiated) than those that involve responding
	■ Greater uses of the answering function
	■ Fewer uses of the following:
	  ■ Declarative and imperative functions
	  ■ Statement functions involving naming
	  ■ Descriptive functions
	  ■ Acknowledging functions
	  ■ Joint attention or comment

Conversation and Discourse	

Initiating Verbal Interactions	■ Initiate conversations
	  ■ With inappropriate/ineffective methods to gain listener's attention
	  ■ At the wrong times
	■ Difficulty gaining access to existing conversation

Responding to Others' Verbal Interactions	■ Less responsive to peers' attempts to initiate conversations
Sustaining Verbal Interactions	Difficulties sustaining topics over several conversational turns, in part due to ■ Problems timing turns and interrupting ■ Inserting noncontingent, irrelevant comments ■ Switching topics abruptly
Clarifying and Repairing	Frequent breakdowns in conversational interactions, in part due to above conversational behaviors In seeking clarifications: ■ Tend not to indicate lack of comprehension overtly and/or with verbal/vocal signals ■ Eye-contact behavior may signal degree of comprehension; may look at interactant's face rather than other stimuli when a message is not understood ■ Tend not to ask for clarification even though may recognize lack of comprehension In making repairs: ■ Tend to revise previous utterances when not understood ■ Use more limited repertoire of revision strategies ■ Rarely use revisions involving substitutions of one syntactic or semantic element for an equivalent

(Continued)

TABLE 3.7 | *Continued*

Areas of Pragmatics	Features
Adapting Messages/Code Switching	Problems seen in ■ Not verbally encoding the most informative elements of messages ■ Conveying both uninformative and informative elements of messages equally ■ Interpreting and using polite devices (indirect requests with and without *please*) Evidence of some ability to adapt by attempts to ■ Modify messages on basis of interactant's age ■ Revise messages to better suit interactant's language ability

When we look at the pattern reflected in the intentions and functions section of Table 3.7, it seems not only that youngsters with SLI demonstrate differences in their use of functions when compared to normal language-learning children but also that their differences suggest a passivity in their interactions. Paul (1991) has commented that the toddlers with language problems that she examined simply appeared to be "less interested in interacting with others, even nonverbally" (p. 6). The information in Table 3.7 also suggests that children with SLI may not respond as readily as normally developing children to the initiation attempts of others. Hadley and Rice (1991) found that in the peer interactions of the preschool children in their study, the children with SLI were less likely to respond to their normal language-learning peers' initiations.

Fey's (1986) interactionist approach might be a useful way to think about what we see as pragmatic patterns for these children. Fey (1986) has proposed two continua related to conversational variables. One continuum deals with children's degrees of *assertiveness* in conversation, that is, the degree to which they initiate conversational acts or turns. The second refers to the degree of children's *responsiveness* to their conversational partners' needs. For both of these continua, children can be high (+) or low (–) on the variable, depending on the pattern they display in their interactions with others. Four patterns arise:

1. + assertiveness and + responsiveness, or children who are active conversationalists
2. + assertiveness and – responsiveness, or children who are verbal noncommunicators
3. – assertiveness and + responsiveness, or children who are passive conversationalists
4. – assertiveness and – responsiveness, or children who are inactive communicators

The characteristics in Table 3.7 suggest that youngsters with SLI are more like the group described in #3 or #4, that is, passive conversationalists who are nonassertive in initiating but may respond if others do the initiating or inactive communicators who neither initiate readily nor respond easily.

Breakdowns in the conversational interactions of children with SLI are, unfortunately, common. Rice, Sell, and Hadley (1991) found that preschoolers with SLI tended to address their communicative attempts to adults more than to their peers in a preschool classroom, possibly because of their histories of unsuccessful communicative interactions with their peers and/or because of their histories of having had their communicative initiations ignored by their peers. Another finding of the Hadley and Rice (1991) study was that normally developing preschoolers were less likely to respond to the attempts at initiation of their classmates with SLI, a finding similar to that of Craig and Gallagher (1986). The preschoolers with SLI tended also not to be nominated by their normal-language counterparts as favored playmates and not to have, among their classmates, a friend without language difficulties (Gertner et al., 1994). Of particular note was that the children with receptive language involvement in addition to their expressive language problems fared worse in their peer relationships compared to the children with only expressive language problems. Rice et al. (1991) suggest that "children are sensitive to their relative communicative competence, or incompetence, at an early age" and that "as young as 3 years of age, children adjust their social interactions to take into account their communication abilities relative to those of others" (p. 1304). According to Hadley and Rice (1991), the early breakdowns in communicative interactions may be the beginning "of a negative interactive spiral generated by a child's history of communicative failure wherein a child becomes less likely to respond as he or she experiences failure in peer interactions and peers become less likely to attend to the child's initiations" (p. 1315). The long-standing failures in and problems with peer interactions that have been well documented for language-impaired children, adolescents, and adults (e.g., Asher & Gazelle, 1999; Beitchman, Wilson, Brownlie, Walters, Inglis, et al., 1996; Brinton & Fujiki, 2014; Clegg et al., 2005; Fujiki, Brinton, Hart, & Fitzgerald, 1999; Jerome, Fujiki, Brinton, & James, 2002) seem to have their roots in early childhood.

Findings about the friendships of preschoolers who have *not* been identified as language impaired provide some support for this proposition. Communicative characteristics of preschoolers less well liked and/or rejected by their young peers include the following (Black & Hazen, 1990; Black & Logan, 1995; Hazen & Black, 1989):

- Making more irrelevant comments
- Making fewer contingent responses
- Being less responsive to peers
- Taking longer turns in conversations
- Interrupting more
- Engaging in more talking over or talking simultaneously

These characteristics sound remarkably similar to the problematic pragmatic characteristics of children with SLI listed in Table 3.7, and the discussion provides a good transition to the next topic.

Socialization and Psychosocial Factors

Recall that at the beginning of the previous section on pragmatic characteristics, we noted that we could not be certain whether pragmatic problems are the result of children's linguistically based deficits or whether they are separate components. Similarly, it is difficult to separate pragmatic difficulties from socialization and psychosocial factors that are associated with SLI and to know "what's what" when we look at how youngsters with SLI behave. Although SLI has been described as occurring in the absence of *severe* emotional disturbances, there has been, for quite some time, a recognition of a relationship between some degree of psychosocial involvement and language impairment (e.g., Baltaxe & Simmons, 1988; Beitchman, Wilson, Brownlie, Walters, Inglis, et al., 1996; Beitchman, Wilson, Johnson, et al, 2001; Mack & Warr-Leeper, 1992; Prizant et al., 1990). Examples of findings from some of the older well-known research studies illustrate this point:

- Of 40 consecutive admissions to a child psychiatric unit, 50 percent of the children had language problems (Gualtieri et al., 1983).
- Of approximately 300 successive intakes of children to a community-based speech and language clinic, 95 percent of the children with expressive language problems had some form of psychosocial difficulties according to 1980 criteria used by the American Psychiatric Association (Baker & Cantwell, 1982).
- Sixty-seven percent of the children consecutively admitted because of behavioral/ emotional problems to an inpatient facility failed a speech and language screening (Prizant et al., 1990).

In some respects we may have a "chicken-and-egg" dilemma. Communicative failures may result in psychosocial difficulties, psychosocial difficulties may be a part of the syndrome of SLI, or early psychosocial difficulties may manifest themselves in terms of language problems. We would, at least, suspect a reciprocal, if not a cyclical, relationship. As Rice et al. (1991) write,

> To the extent that experiencing success in social interactions is central to a child's sense of self-esteem and social role, children with communication limitations are at risk for the development of social competencies. Limited social interactions would in turn limit their opportunities to learn communication skills from their peers, especially in the development of discourse skills. (p. 1305)

Findings from several studies may shed some light on the issue. Rescorla, Ross, and McClure (2007) found that language delay in children between ages 18 and 35 months was not associated with behavioral/emotional problems. Similarly, in Rescorla's research with Achenbach (Rescorla & Achenbach, 2002), no significant association was found between toddlers about 2 years old who were evincing slow expressive language learning (i.e., fewer than 50 single words or no two-word combinations) and scores in the problematic range on a parent-rating protocol of their child's behavior, the Child Behavior Checklist for Ages 2–3 (Achenbach, 1992), leading the authors to conclude "no link between expressive language delays and behavioral/emotional problem" (p. 742). These authors suggest that "significant behavioral/emotional problems may be more likely when children have been delayed in language for many months (i.e., after 36 months)" (p. 742). Redmond and Rice (1998) might agree with the view that behavioral/emotional problems of children with SLI are likely to emerge after children have lived with language impairment for some time. Redmond and Rice propose a social adaptation explanation of psychosocial difficulties exhibited by these children based on the findings of their study. The children with SLI in the study were rated as being within the normal range on the Child Behavior Checklist (Achenbach, 1991a) by their parents and by their teachers on the Teacher Report Form (Achenbach, 1991b), but the children's ratings were significantly poorer than those of their age-matched peers without language impairment. Teachers tended to identify more behavioral/emotional problems in the children than parents did, which the authors attributed to the situations in which the children were observed. According to the researchers (Redmond & Rice, 1998), a social adaptation model would expect "differences between teacher and parent ratings of sociobehaviors when children with SLI go to kindergarten and are experiencing the extensive social adjustments that appear at the time" (p. 696). The social and emotional behaviors reflect an overlay associated with their struggles with their language skills. Paul (2000), in reporting on the outcomes of the 2-year-olds with SELD when they were in second grade, noted that the children with histories of early language delay were significantly more shy than their normal counterparts, a finding basically consistent with that of Fujiki et al. (1999) in their investigation of withdrawn and sociable behaviors of children with SLI. Withdrawn behavior was also the one aspect of behavioral/emotional behavior that emerged as possibly associated with language delay in the toddlers in the Rescorla et al. (2007) study. Although not part of any of these studies, one wonders, assuming that a social adaptation model is accurate, if preschool experiences for these children in which they need to interact regularly with their typically developing peers might accelerate an onset of an overlay of psychosocial issues, a thought not wholly disassociated from a position raised in a somewhat different way by Paul (2000) and Paul et al. (1996). It is also possible that, with additional research, withdrawn behavior may indeed prove to be a commonly observed socioemotional characteristic of children with SLI.

Together, these studies hint at one possible scenario, one in which children with SELD or SLI begin life with their socioemotional systems basically intact but their difficult and/or negative experiences trying to use their deficient language system to interact with their environments and others in their environment lead them to adopt less than positive social behaviors and to acquire negative emotional responses. The relationship between socioemotional development and language impairment is complex, and this is, admittedly, a simplistic scenario. It fails to consider the many other important factors that affect development, such as children's basic temperaments, heterogeneity across children, or levels of language comprehension. For example, the children in the Rescorla and Achenbach (2002) study had only documented expressive language problems, whereas the children in the Redmond and Rice (1998) study had both receptive and expressive language deficits. Keep in mind that children with documented receptive language impairments seem not to fare as well as those for whom only expressive language has been documented deficient (e.g., Beitchman, Wilson, Brownlie, Walters, Inglis, et al., 1996; Beitchman, Wilson, Brownlie, Walters, & Lancee, 1996; Gertner et al., 1994). It also does not consider research on how children's emotional reactions to situations might be able to be mediated through teaching and modeling.

Studies of self-esteem and emotion regulation in school-age children with SLI (e.g., Fujiki, Brinton, & Clarke, 2002; Jerome et al., 2002) shed some light on what children with SLI face as they mature. In a preliminary study, teachers' ratings of elementary school children with SLI indicated that these children demonstrated behaviors consistent with less sophisticated management of their emotions than their typically developing counterparts (Fujiki et al., 2002). Results of another study suggested that the self-esteem of children with SLI declines with age. Younger children (6 to 9 years) with and without SLI were found not to differ in how they perceived themselves with regard to social acceptance, behavioral conduct, and academic ability. In contrast, older children (10 to 13 years) with SLI perceived themselves more negatively than their peers in each of these areas. Although the subjects in these studies were school-aged children, the findings can help us understand what might be longer-term psychosocial issues for preschool children with SLI as well the possibility that psychosocial problems likely escalate for these children as they mature. In subsequent chapters, we will see more about psychosocial issues. Baker and Cantwell (1983) summarize the discussion well for us:

> Since language is a uniquely human quality, it is therefore not unexpected that a disorder in language development might have far reaching consequences for other areas of early childhood development. (p. 51)

Narratives

We have already seen that skill in relating understandable, complete narratives is an important factor in school achievement, and children with language problems frequently have difficulty in telling good narratives. We know that preschoolers engage in early forms of narration, and by the time children enter school, their narratives usually include most of the elements of a basic narrative, e.g., setting, resolution, although there may be only one or two episodes included. They relate rudimentary accounts about things that have happened to them, and they retell favorite stories from children's books that they have been read.

We have already learned that toddlers with SELD have been shown to have problems with narrative skills in the kindergarten years (Girolametto et al., 2001), and preschoolers with SLI often demonstrate difficulties with narrative skills. The narratives of children with SLI tend to contain less information than those of preschoolers with normal language skills and, according to Applebee's (1978) narrative stages, are less mature (Paul, 1996; Paul & Smith, 1993). One explanation for youngsters' limitations on the information they encode may relate to the linguistic features the children are able to bring to the task. An efficient method to encode more than one proposition per utterance is complex sentence usage. Children whose language is limited to simple sentences or even to compound sentences are not efficient in their expression of multiple pieces of information. Contrast "When he hit the water, he started to sink so he closed his mouth" with "He hit the water. He started to go down in the water. He closed his mouth." Good, tightly composed narratives also depend on the use of high-content words with appropriate semantic choices to signal old and new information. Children with difficulties with certain abstract words, such as temporal words and deictic words, or children who have difficulties retrieving words quickly and who instead use low-content words (e.g., *thing*) will also encounter problems in producing narratives.

Production of narratives challenges most aspects of a language-impaired child's language system at the same time so that difficulties with one aspect of language may overload the child in such a way that other aspects of language break down or the whole system breaks down. Children with weak language skills have considerable difficulty juggling the multiple linguistic demands of narratives, including even the demands of those stories the children know well. For this reason, preschoolers who to the "naked ear" may appear to have adequate conversational language skills or who score within normal limits on norm-referenced language tests may evidence even quite concerning language problems when they are asked to relate narratives.

IMPLICATIONS FOR INTERVENTION

Assessment

SLI in toddlers and preschoolers appears to be manifested in different ways at different times. It follows, therefore, that assessment considerations may need to differ at different times. Additionally, many of the issues and the characteristics of young children with SLI that we have discussed in previous sections of this chapter lead to logical implications for assessment, which readers will see in the next several sections.

Toddlers

Predictive and Risk Factors in Assessment. Previously in this chapter, we reviewed several of the factors that can place infants and toddlers at risk for language impairment and those that can place a toddler with slow expressive language development (SELD) at risk for continuing language problems (Table 3.3). These factors need to be considered as part of an assessment process, in particular, (1) socialization; (2) phonological composition of vocalizations and babbling as well as verbalizations; (3) use of gestures, particularly symbolic play gestures expressing script routines and those gestures and behaviors associated with joint attention; (4) behavior; and (5) nonword repetition abilities now that there are a few tasks that appear appropriate for use with older toddlers. Assessment of toddlers needs to be multifaceted.

The increasing evidence about comprehension abilities leads us to conclude that comprehension skills need to be included as an important part of an assessment process. The evidence suggests that expressive language deficits probably do not exist in the absence of disruptions to receptive/comprehension/processing abilities (Leonard, 2009; Tomblin et al., 2007; Tomblin & Zhang, 2006) and that a substantial number of toddlers with expressive language problems have comprehension problems even though on superficial observation they may appear to understand quite well. Information about a toddler's comprehension skills can help inform about possible long-term language and learning outcomes, is important in planning intervention, and can provide additional assessment documentation of language problems.

Young children's uses of communicative intentions produced through gestures and vocalizations can be assessed even before they use their first words. Coggins (1991) provides ideas about how to manipulate the assessment environment to identify children's uses of linguistic and nonlinguistic communicative intentions. He suggests that the children's performance should be assessed under conditions of both minimal and maximal support for producing intentions:

1. Cuing (linguistic): Manipulate for minimal support using indirect model; manipulate for maximal support using elicited imitation
2. Activities (nonlinguistic): Manipulate for minimal support using novel activities; manipulate for maximal support using known event routines and scripts
3. Interactor (nonlinguistic): Manipulate for minimal support using clinician; manipulate for maximal support using mother/caregiver
4. Materials (nonlinguistic): Manipulate for minimal support using no toys or props; manipulate for maximal support using familiar objects/toys and those with thematic base (e.g., doll, bottle, and/or diaper)
5. Interaction (nonlinguistic): Manipulate for minimal support using naturalistic child-adult interactions; manipulate for maximal support using contrived tasks (e.g., desired food item in transparent, tightly sealed container)

Differences in the children's performances under these conditions can be identified, with differences possibly indicating the children's potential for change (Coggins, 1991;

Olswang & Bain, 1996; Platt & Coggins, 1990). A toddler's ability to modify communicative behavior relatively quickly under various conditions of support often has prognostic value, as we know from dynamic assessment practices, discussed more fully in Chapter 13, and can provide valuable insights about strategies that might be included in intervention plans.

Early Language Milestones. Early language developmental milestones provide additional guidelines for assessment. Many of these were highlighted in the previous chapter and even in earlier parts of this chapter. Of particular import for assessing toddlers are milestones related to prelinguistic developmental behaviors, early expressive vocabulary development, early and later multiword utterances, early emerging grammatical morphemes, and early sentences.

Tracking toddlers' progress from single-word to multiword utterances requires assessment measures that are sensitive in picking up what are important developmental patterns. Of particular importance is knowing that toddlers are moving toward productive, rule-based combinations so that these become generative in order that novel utterances using the rules can be produced as context and meaning warrant. A normally developing toddler takes about 4 to 5 months to move from the emergence of the first two-word combination to the use of many new and unique word combinations (Ingram, 1989). Ingram's (1989) work indicates that during these months, when the toddler manages to have produced about 100 novel two-word utterances, the child is likely to demonstrate a "syntactic spurt," suggesting that the child has learned about grammatical productivity, that is, the generative basis of syntax. This typically happens at about 2 years of age. At this point the toddler is, in essence, "off and running" with regard to syntax and grammar. Two assessment procedures can be particularly helpful in tracking toddlers' progress toward their use of productive two-word utterances. Long, Olswang, Brian, and Dale (1997) developed a procedure to observe and analyze the generative productivity of the types of two-word utterances showing up in young children's language as they move from using single-word utterances to word combinations, that is, MLUs slightly over 1.00.[3] Their procedure looked at "utterance level productivity (ULP), which reflects general positional rules for word combinations; and grammatic level productivity (GLP), which reflects specific rules based on semantic consistency" (p. 36). These authors (Long et al., 1997) reported that the children with SELD in their study who achieved grammatic-level productivity as a result of intervention were the ones who showed greater progress. Hadley's (1999) approach was to analyze the spontaneous language of children with MLUs between 1.00 and 2.00 (Brown's Stage I) over time for changes in the number of *unique syntactic types* the children use. A unique syntactic type is "a combination of two or more words with syntactic status that could fit into the phrase structure of a more grammatically complete adult utterance" (p. 263). Hadley (1999) found that her procedure was highly correlated with children's performances on the Index of Productive Syntax (Scarborough, 1990) and their MLUs. As Hadley (1999) states, the procedure was designed for "tracking the progress of children in this early stage of grammatical development" (p. 269). Both of these procedures appear to help professionals more precisely distinguish between toddlers who are displaying progress toward using generative, productive multiword combinations and those whose word combinations seem stalled and/or nonproductive for expansion.

Another aspect of early language development that needs to be assessed—and one that is related both to the ideas noted here about tracking toddlers' early acquisition of grammatical features and to those associated with verb morphology as a possible clinical marker—is children's acquisition of early verb morphemes between 2 and 3 years of age (Hadley & Short, 2005). Probes can be developed to explore children's use of these forms, and a comprehensive language sample that includes analyses of children's verb forms is an essential aspect of assessment for toddlers. Additional information about language sampling is included in Chapter 13.

3. Recall that an MLU of 1.00 means only single words without any grammatical morphemes attached, whereas an MLU of 1.50 suggests single words with grammatical morphemes and/or equal numbers of single-word utterances with no grammatical morphemes and two-word combinations with no grammatical morphemes.

Assessment Instruments and Parental Report. A number of developmental instruments has been available for several years to assess infants and toddlers. Among these are the Bayley Scales of Infant and Toddler Development—III (Bayley, 2006), The Capute Scales: Cognitive Adaptive Test and Clinical Linguistic and Auditory Milestone Scales (Accardo et al., 2005), and the Vineland Adaptive Behavior Scales—III (Sparrow, Cicchetti, & Saulnier, 2016). This list is by no means complete, and new instruments are regularly developed and existing ones updated. These instruments examine a range of developmental areas (e.g., gross motor, fine motor, personal-social), including items that address communication skills. In addition to these more general assessment tools, several instruments that focus on communication skills are available for professionals to use during assessment sessions with toddlers. Space precludes providing a comprehensive list of these, and such a list would be outdated as soon as it were compiled. However, some of the more commonly used instruments over the years are The Rossetti Infant-Toddler Language Scale (Rossetti, 2006), the Early Language Milestone Scale (ELMS - 2) (Coplan, 1993); Communication and Symbolic Behavior Scales - Normed Edition (CSBS - Normed) (Wetherby & Prizant, 2003) and its shortened version, the Communication and Symbolic Behavior Scales—Developmental Profile (CSBS - DP) (Wetherby & Prizant, 2002); the Sequenced Inventory of Communication Development—Revised (Hedrick et al., 1984); the Preschool Language Scale—5 (PLS - 5) (Zimmerman, Steiner, & Pond, 2011); the Receptive-Expressive Emergent Language Test—Third Edition (REEL - 3) (Bzoch, League, & Brown, 2003); and the Test of Early Language Development - 3 (TELD - 3) (Hresko, Reid, & Hammill, 1999). The procedures for a number of these instruments include some degree of parental report as well as direct professional–child interaction.

The use of parental reports of young children's communicative behaviors is an invaluable tool as a means of assessing toddlers' language abilities. Although there were initial concerns about validity and reliability when instruments based on parental reports were first developed, findings from subsequent research have allayed many of the concerns. Parental report has several inherent features that make it an attractive method of assessment. These include that (1) the parents have had more opportunities to observe their children's language, so they typically know more about what the children do with their communication than a professional can learn in an assessment session; (2) parental report can be obtained prior to professionals seeing the children and can, therefore, help professionals plan assessment sessions; and (3) it is cost effective.

Parental report procedures can be systematized, standardized, and structured, reducing some of the problem about accuracy of the procedure. A common approach, therefore, is a recognition format that presents parents with communicative behaviors and asks them to identify those that apply to their children. Two such parental report instruments using this technique that are designed specifically to tap toddlers' communication skills are the Language Development Survey (LDS) (Rescorla, 1989) and the MacArthur-Bates Communicative Development Inventories - 2 (CDI - 2) (Fenson et al., 2007). Of the two instruments, the latter is the more extensive, taking parents about 30 minutes to complete. In contrast, the LDS, according to its author (Rescorla, 1991), was designed "as a quick and efficient . . . screening tool for the identification of language delay in 2-year-old children" (p. 17). The LDS takes about 10 minutes for parents to complete. Both instruments provide parents with a list of vocabulary items (or phrases) and ask them to indicate which of the words their children use. Both have been used in the early identification of toddlers with language delays and have demonstrated good validity and reliability in assessment.

A slightly different approach to parent report was taken by Girolametto (1997) in his development of a parent report measure to profile the conversational skills of children between the ages of 1 and 3 years. This protocol is based on Fey's (1986) assertiveness-responsiveness continua used to describe children's conversational interactive style, which was discussed previously in this chapter. It asks parents to rate the degree to which each of 25 statements, reflecting various responsive or assertive conversational behaviors, describes their child. Advantages of the tool are its ease of administration and speed of completion and its ecological and social validity. According to Girolametto (1997), "The rating scale profiles the strengths and weaknesses of individual children and provides unique information that is unavailable from other assessment sources" (p. 32).

General aspects of assessing children's language and factors involved in selecting and using standardized instruments are discussed in Chapter 13.

Parent/Caregiver–Child Interactions. An important part of assessment involves the interactions between primary caregivers and their children. As we know, parents'/caregivers' interactions with their language-impaired children are, for the most part, not terribly different from the interactions of other parents/caregivers with younger normal language-learning children. That is, the parents/caregivers seem to respond more to the child's language level than the child's chronological age. The few problematic areas that have sometimes been noted generally relate to (1) the degree of directiveness in the parents'/caregivers' interactions, with parents/caregivers of language-impaired children tending to use more directive language to their children, such as commands, rather than responses to their children's initiations, and (2) the frequency with which parents/caregivers provide semantically contingent responses (recasts) to their children's utterances. Somewhat related to this latter factor is the quickness with which parents/caregivers respond. Roth (1987) has suggested that a 1-second interval between a child's production and the parent's/caregiver's response is the time frame in which a 1-year-old child can pick up on the contingency of the parent's/caregiver's response.

There need to be caveats on interpreting these findings. Recall we have indicated that a child's language behavior itself may modify an adult's mode of communicative interaction so that interactions may be less appropriate and stimulating. The communicative interactions likely have reciprocal effects. However, some of these adult behaviors, once established possibly because of previous adult–child interactions, may maintain slowed language development in a child. The purpose of assessing parent/caregiver–child interactions is not to judge the adult. Rather, it is to identify possible factors in the interactions that can be modified or included in interactive routines to enhance and facilitate a child's language learning.

Preschoolers

General Guidelines. For preschoolers, many more norm-referenced language instruments are available. It is also easier to obtain reliable assessment results from preschoolers than from toddlers. However, professionals still need to be alert to the fact that considerable variability can occur in preschoolers' communicative performance. As with toddlers, it is also important with preschoolers to assess caregiver–child interactions and a variety of behaviors. Language developmental milestones continue to be important guidelines, although as preschoolers mature much beyond 3 years of age, MLU may no longer be a consistently reliable indicator of language growth (e.g., Eisenberg, Fersko, & Lundgren, 2001). Additionally, gross measures of expressive vocabulary size may be less reliable indicators of language skill with preschoolers than with toddlers. Recall that we previously suggested that delays in expressive vocabulary acquisition may appear to resolve during the later preschool years. This is not to say that expressive vocabulary should not constitute part of the assessment process. Care should be taken to ensure that procedures include assessing: (1) a child's use of words with more abstract meanings and (2) the size and diversity of the growth of the verb vocabularies of children transitioning from toddlerhood to preschooler status (i.e., about 2 years of age). With regard to the latter, recall there is emerging evidence that characteristics of young children's verb vocabularies may be predictive of their levels of grammatical development in later preschool years (Hadley et al., 2016).

Language comprehension abilities would also be essential aspects of language behavior that need to be assessed. Assessment of comprehension needs to extend beyond just assessment of single-word receptive vocabulary, and any assessment of single-word receptive vocabulary needs to include abstract vocabulary words. Comprehension assessment needs to examine understanding whole units of language (not just individual words) and understanding across multiple utterances, that is, comprehension of discourse, and examine a child's ability to infer meaning.

Because syntax and morphology are especially troublesome areas for preschoolers with SLI, children's performances in these areas should be thoroughly assessed. Of particular importance are children's uses of complex sentences and the emergence of grammatical morphemes, especially their use of verb tense grammatical marking. Children's developing skills with both micro and macro aspects of narrative production are also major parts of assessment. These areas for assessment are consistent with our previous discussions in this chapter, so none of this should be surprising. However, all measures need to be fine grained rather than global and general. Chapter 13 has information that applies to the assessment of preschool children.

An area of assessment of preschool children that is particularly important is their ability in areas associated with literacy development, given our understanding of the relationship between children's early language levels and their learning to read and write. Catts (1997) suggests that many of the problems associated with reading disabilities can be observed in children before they begin formal reading instruction. This means that, in addition to preschoolers' language and their abilities with narratives and phonological processing, as discussed below, their knowledge about letter names, print concepts including being able to write their first names (Cabell, Justice, Zucker, & McGinty, 2009), literacy terms, and rhyme need to be assessed. Results can assist in identifying those children at risk for reading difficulties so that early intervention aimed at reducing the odds of reading failure can be provided.

Illusory Recovery. If preschoolers can appear to recover from deficits in certain aspects of language behavior at different times, this has implications for assessment. Language performance needs to be assessed in such a way that overcomes the possibility of obtaining *false negative* results—that is, results indicating that no problem exists when, in fact, it does.

One way to address the problem of illusory recovery is to ensure that assessment is comprehensive, that is, that many aspects of communication are assessed, as well as behavioral aspects known to be associated with SLI. Table 3.3 provides a guide to areas that would be included in a comprehensive assessment. Comprehension abilities are a major clue to whether a child's expressive abilities are demonstrating an illusion of recovery or whether a language impairment continues to be present. It may also be appropriate to assess over several sessions and in a variety of settings, including in a child's home and in situations where the child interacts with other children (Hadley & Schuele, 1998).

Another way to address the problem is to stress or challenge the child's language performance. It is not enough to know what a child *does* with language. We need to know what a child *can do* with language. Earlier we indicated that narrative production particularly challenges a child's language performance. Asking a child to relate a narrative should probably be a standard part of a preschooler's language assessment not only to stress the system but for its predictive value as well. However, professionals should avoid basing any decisions about a child's language abilities only on production of stereotyped narratives such as fairy tales. These may be "rehearsed" narratives for a child because they have occurred frequently in the child's environment. Rather, novel narratives should be elicited using one or more of the several ways described in Chapter 13 and considering the various advantages and disadvantages of the various methods.

Previously in this chapter, we discussed the possible clinical markers of SLI—nonword repetition, use of verb tense morphology, and sentence recall. We indicated that for toddlers, there was information that permitted assessment of these areas of performance. For preschoolers, we are more confident in our assessment of these abilities. These are areas that are essential to include in assessment and to be assessed thoroughly. Findings can help to overcome some of the issues related to illusory recovery. Preschoolers' performances in these areas may have value in predicting which children are likely to have SLI and/or are at risk for continuing language deficits. Various formal and informal methods available to assess children's abilities in these areas are presented in Chapter 13.

Social Communicative Interaction. Part of assessing language performance involves assessing children's communication in social, interactive situations. For preschoolers, this goes beyond assessment only with the primary caregiver. Ideally, children should be assessed as they interact in a group with other children, some of whom are normal language-learning children. As Rice, Sell, and Hadley (1990) point out, however, most systems designed to measure children's social communicative interactions are inordinately complex and cumbersome to render them impractical for routine assessment.

To provide "a quick way of obtaining clinically relevant information about the use of language in natural settings along the social dimension" (p. 7), Rice et al. (1990) developed the Social Interactive Coding System (SICS). This instrument focuses on Fey's (1986) assertiveness/passiveness conversational dimension and examines a child's interactions with peers during a variety of activities that typically occur in preschools, such as art, dramatic/symbolic play, and free play with toys. Each turn a child takes in an interaction, the nature of each turn (e.g., initiation, response—verbal, response—nonverbal, ignore), and the number of turns in the interaction are recorded on a standardized protocol that also allows for the addressee of the child's interactions to be recorded. The tool incorporates a real time observational technique in which the professional records all of the child's interactions in a 5-minute period and then takes a 5-minute break to update notations on the protocol. The "5-minutes-on/5-minutes-off" procedure is repeated three times for a total of four observational segments. The advantages of the SICS include that (1) it can be completed in the classroom, (2) it is easy to learn, (3) minimal equipment is necessary, and (4) results are immediately available for interpretation. The authors caution, however, that the SICS should be used not as a sole assessment procedure but rather as a supplement to other forms of assessment.

Chapter 13 provides additional information about assessment of children's language in general. The information in that chapter is relevant to language assessment of toddlers and preschoolers and should be used in conjunction with the information presented here.

Intervention

Decisions about Intervention. The issue of predicting which toddlers and preschoolers will outgrow their early delays in acquiring language without assistance and which will not leads to a main consideration for intervention. That is, under what conditions is intervention recommended, when is intervention recommended, and what is the nature of the intervention—monitoring, indirect intervention, or direct intervention carried out by a professional? There are no hard-and-fast answers to these. The philosophical and theoretical positions of the professional, the philosophical and procedural positions of the organization in which the professional works, and the attitudes and wishes of the caregivers affect the decision. Professionals' decisions are influenced by information about identification of language impairment and standards to which a child's language performance is being compared, predictive and risk factors relevant to a specific child, and the long-term implications of unresolved language impairments. To this, information about a child's potential for language change and the factors important in facilitating the change are added.

A word of caution is warranted. The quality of input into decision making about recommending or not recommending intervention, whether it is the professionals' or parents' input, is only as good as the information and understanding that these individuals have about associations among language, literacy, and socialization. Whether to intervene or not seems more related to what professionals observe in the expressive language of behaviors of young children rather than what abilities the children have with regard to language comprehension. As Zhang and Tomblin (2000) write in describing the findings of their study that "intervention receipt was more closely related to expressive language than to receptive language" (p. 352) and that the "aspect that is most available to the listener has the greatest effect on the child's receipt of clinical services" (p. 354). In contrast, language problems had the greater negative effect on academic and social variables compared to speech sound production problems. These results indicate that professionals need to be alert to what factors of children's communication abilities they are judging with regard to intervention recommendations. The results also indicate that professionals need to provide individuals who have had fewer opportunities to know about the potential impact of language ability on other areas of children's development and achievement with the information they need to participate in deciding what to recommend about intervention.

An important principle is that, whatever initial decision is made, it is reassessed regularly as a child's behavior does or does not change. If direct intervention administered by a professional is not recommended initially, it is possible to implement indirect methods, such as parent training and/or preschool enrollment, and monitor the child's progress. If the anticipated progress is not seen in a specified period of time, a decision to intervene directly can be made. If direct intervention is the initial decision, the child's progress is also monitored regularly. If progress is rapid, the professional and parents may decide to discontinue direct intervention, implement indirect intervention programs to maintain the level of progress, and monitor the child's behaviors at regular intervals. If progress is not continued, direct intervention can be reinstated. Ongoing monitoring, regular measurements of a child's language performance across many parameters, consistent follow-up, and flexibility in moving from one form of intervention to another are critical in providing effective intervention.

Indirect Intervention. As indicated above, one aspect of intervention is deciding on the way in which services for a specific toddler or preschooler are delivered, that is, direct intervention provided by a professional interacting with the child or indirect intervention provided through consultation and collaboration with others. Both methods may also be employed either simultaneously or consecutively. The decision will differ for each child. No one service delivery model is suitable for all youngsters with SLI or SELD. However, parents/caregivers play a large role in the early language learning of toddlers and preschoolers, and their participation in intervention is essential. Furthermore, a common recommendation for youngsters with SLI is placement in a preschool program.

Parents/Caregivers. Toddlers and preschoolers spend most of their time interacting with parents/caregivers. Therefore, these adults are potentially powerful sources of change in children's communicative behavior. Involving parents/caregivers in intervention not only is mandated by federal education laws but generally makes good sense as well. As Olswang and Bain (1991) point out, the "question is not should the parent be involved in the intervention process, but how" (p. 77). The "how" usually takes one of two approaches. The parents/caregivers can augment, expand, and supplement the intervention provided directly by a professional, who is the primary agent of change, or they can serve as the primary agents of change, with the professional serving to develop the initial directions and methods for change and to monitor both the process and the progress. Whichever strategy is chosen for an individual child, the parents/caregivers need education and training. This generally focuses on two objectives: (1) creating or enhancing the child's environment to facilitate change in the child's language and (2) responding within that environment in a manner that optimally facilitates language change.

At least two primary aspects are involved with regard to changing or enhancing the child's language-learning environment. One aspect focuses on helping the parents/caregivers recognize and take advantage of language-learning opportunities that occur in a child's daily activities. This approach stresses seizing opportunities and capitalizing on language-teaching moments. These moments can occur during dressing, interactive play, meal or snack time, story time, or any other time during a day when the child's attention is focused on a specific action, object, or event. The parents/caregivers are shown how to identify these moments and how to structure their language and gestural input accordingly. The second aspect involves creating opportunities for language learning. The parents/caregivers are shown how to set up moments in the environment to facilitate a child's use of specific language behaviors and how to encourage the child to use these behaviors during those periods. These moments may or may not be specified, allocated periods. In some instances, the parents/caregivers may be able to observe a situation and know that if they make an immediate and sometimes small change, they will be able to facilitate a desired language behavior. In other instances, short periods may actually be set aside for creating the opportunities to facilitate certain communicative behaviors in the child. As with the "opportunistic" approach, the parents/caregivers are shown how to structure their communicative behavior so as to enhance the child's learning.

In helping parents/caregivers respond to the children in ways that best promote language learning, it is important to remember that the aim is likely to help them do more of some things they already do and perhaps less of others. In most instances, it may simply be a matter of changing the frequency of certain behaviors, such as increasing how often they use expansions and recasts of the children's utterances and encourage imitation. These are language-facilitating techniques described in Chapter 14, where more specific information about intervention is presented.

Earlier we indicated that most parents/caregivers of children with SLI provide language interactions that are similar to those of parents of normally developing children, but there may be two or perhaps three adult behaviors that are worthy of particular attention. One may involve helping the parents/caregivers reduce the frequency with which they use directive speech acts, including commands and demands for responses from the children, and increase their use of (1) responsive speech acts, (2) information-seeking questions for which the information presumably is not known to the adult, (3) confirmation requests that are used to affirm that the adult understood the child correctly, and (4) simple recasts and expansions of the child's utterances that serve to maintain the content of the child's utterances but do so in a form that modifies slightly that used by the child. Both Fey and his colleagues (Cleave & Fey, 1997; Fey, Cleave, Long, & Hughes, 1993; Fey, Krulik, Loeb, & Proctor-Williams, 1999) and Girolametto and his colleagues (Girolametto et al., 1996; Girolametto, Weitzman, Wiigs, & Pearce, 1999) describe parent-training programs that teach parents how to engage in these behaviors with their children. Both groups of researchers have reported positive effects of their programs in helping to advance the language of toddlers and preschoolers with SELD and/or SLI.

Another area in which parents/caregivers may be able to facilitate children's language learning is to increase the frequency with which they respond to what the child says and to do so with semantically contingent statements (Girolametto et al., 1996). These responses again maintain the content of the child's utterances and serve as comments about the content of the child's utterance. For example, to the child's utterance "big doggie," the adult might say, "Yes, it is a big doggie." A third possibility for enhancing further a child's language learning may focus on helping parents/caregivers provide quicker responses to the children's utterances, that is, reduce latencies in parents'/caregivers' responses.

Preschools. Preschool experiences are often recommended for youngsters with SLI in order to provide a stimulating language-learning environment and opportunities for social communicative interactions for the children. Peers have been shown to be able to facilitate the language development and social interaction skills of children with SLI or SELD (e.g., DeKroon, Kyte, & Johnson, 2002; Robertson & Ellis Weismer, 1997). However, the simple presence of normal language-learning children in a preschool does not guarantee that these children will be effective facilitators for children with SLI. Special attention may have to be given to how the aims of such an approach can be achieved.

One problem that has been observed is that normal and language-impaired youngsters together in preschools do not particularly spend very much of their time in communicative interactions with each other (Hadley & Rice, 1991; Hadley & Schuele, 1998; Rice et al., 1991; Weiss & Nakamura, 1992). As Hadley and Rice (1991) point out in their study on the conversational interactions of normal and language-impaired preschoolers,

> The implications for intervention are somewhat sobering. It seems that placement of these children [with SLI] in an integrated setting, even one in which adults are highly responsive to and encourage the children's initiation attempts, does not necessarily ensure peer interactions. . . . Preschoolers behave as if they know who talks well and who doesn't, and they prefer to interact with those who do. Therefore, placement of communicatively impaired children in an integrated setting, with normal-language peers and facilitative adults, will not in and of itself establish successful peer interactions in spontaneous interactions. (p. 1315)

It seems, therefore, that the facilitative adults in these settings need to develop strategies that specifically target encouraging successful peer interactions. It cannot be assumed that these will occur without professionals' direct attention and planning.

These adults, too, might benefit from assistance in how to make their interactions more facilitating for children's language learning. Girolametto's research team (Girolametto & Weitzman, 2002; Girolametto, Weitzman, van Lieshout, & Duff, 2000) examined the degree of responsiveness and directiveness in the language of daycare teachers with training in early childhood education. To track, categorize, and analyze teachers' interactions, the researchers used the Teacher Interaction and Language Rating Scale (Girolametto, Weitzman, & Greenberg, 2000). Results indicated that although many of the teachers' interactions with the children were characterized by language-facilitating behaviors and demonstrated some sensitivity to children's different language levels, there were aspects of their verbal interactions that the researchers identified as directive and less language facilitating. Different instructional contexts (e.g., book reading, play dough activity) resulted in different levels of directiveness. The researchers suggested that training to help teachers reduce some types of directiveness where it is not necessary for direct instruction might enhance children's language learning (Girolametto, Weitzman, van Lieshout et al., 2000).

A final note relates to the involvement of parents/caregivers as part of children's preschool experiences. Marvin and Privratsky (1999) found that, when preschool children left school at the end of a day with "remnants from recent school events, toys, or child-produced art products" (p. 231), the children's talk with their parents in the car on the way home or when they arrived home contained more references to events that had transpired at preschool than when no materials were sent home with the children. These authors suggest that sending child-centered materials home with children at the end of a preschool day may help facilitate their ability with what is a more difficult discourse situation, that is, to talk about events in the past in situations where there is no shared knowledge between narrator (the child) and listener (the parent). In developing preschool plans, part of the routine might be regular child-centered "take-home" materials that parents realize are important to talk about with their children. Another part of involving parents in their children's preschool or day care experience considers the advantages of including parent training in conjunction with their children's attendance at preschool. For example, in one study (Roberts et al., 1989), children who attended a preschool that included regular parent/caregiver education achieved better conversational skills by 5 years of age than either children who did not attend preschool but whose parents/caregivers did receive education or children who neither attended preschool nor whose parents/caregivers received education. This finding suggests that the combination of parent/caregiver education and preschool programs provides more powerful opportunities for enhancing children's language performances than parent/caregiver education alone.

Direct Intervention. Direct intervention for youngsters with SLI can be conducted individually with a child, via group sessions, or a combination of both. However, much of what is discussed in the literature describes group intervention, with or without adjunct individual sessions. Consistent with our discussion, groups have a greater potential to facilitate children's peer interactions, assist them to use language appropriately in social interaction, and provide opportunities for generalization of language skills, and they tend to have more naturalistic environments for language use and are likely to include more events and experiences to talk about and more people with whom to talk. When it comes to characterizing group intervention for toddlers and preschoolers, there are many variations on the theme. Some of these are the following:

- Some programs have smaller numbers of children in them (e.g., four) (Robertson & Ellis Weismer, 1999); others are larger, with as many as 18 to 20 (Bunce, 1995; Rice & Wilcox, 1995).
- Some consist only of children with language delays or impairment (Cleave & Fey, 1997; Robertson & Ellis Weismer, 1999); others have a mix of children with and without language problems (Bunce, 1995; Rice & Wilcox, 1995).
- Some place greater emphasis on acquisition of grammatical forms (Cleave & Fey, 1997), others on vocabulary and early word combinations (Robertson & Ellis Weismer, 1999), and others on a wide variety of aspects of language based on individual children's needs (Bunce, 1995; Rice & Wilcox, 1995).
- As indicated above, some include individual intervention sessions with children as part of the total intervention program (Cleave & Fey, 1997); others use group sessions exclusively (Robertson & Ellis Weismer, 1999).

Despite these variations, there seem to be some commonalities. One is that most of the programs recognized the importance of peer interaction and socialization for the children and addressed these in varying degrees in the intervention programs. Another was the inclusion of routine events and scripts to help children scaffold their language and reduce processing demands for them.

One point that came through from the results of the study by Long et al. (1997) and Hadley's (1999) work was the need to be alert to what particular types of word combinations toddlers are and are not acquiring. Recall that a positive indication is acquisition of word combinations that reflect generative, rule-based, grammatical principles. When facilitating the acquisition of word combinations is a goal of intervention for children, Long et al. (1997) recommend that specific grammatical rules that carry "syntactic status" and can "fit into the phrase structure of a more grammatically complete adult utterance" (Hadley, 1999, p. 269) be targeted directly. These can be equally targeted in group or individual intervention sessions.

SUMMARY

In this chapter we have seen that

- Characterization and understanding of SLI as a condition is far from complete; nevertheless, SLI should probably best be thought of as a lifelong disability since it does not go away, even though intervention can moderate its effects.
- There is doubt about the existence of expressive language impairment without some degree of receptive language/comprehension/language processing involvement; comprehension is an important part of thinking about SLI in young children.
- Several different labels to describe these children have been used; SLI has gained acceptance.
- Causal factors remain elusive, but information processing, neurological factors, and genetics are promising candidates; these may not be independent causal factors but rather interrelated factors.
- Some children outgrow early delays in acquiring language; others do not. Predicting who will and who will not catch up is an important area of research. Issues related to possible "illusory recovery" need to be addressed. Issues of illusory recovery and prediction impact on assessment strategies and intervention decisions.
- Three aspects of performance, morphology related to verb tense marking, sentence recall, and nonword repetition, are possible clinical markers of SLI.
- Children with SLI can exhibit different combinations of communication problems that can involve some or all parameters of language. One common feature is difficulty with syntax and morphology and, in particular, verb morphology.
- Parental/caregiver involvement is important in obtaining assessment information, and parental/caregiver education is an important aspect of intervention.
- Placement of children in preschools will not necessarily ensure successful social communicative interactions unless these are specifically addressed within the preschool situation.
- A number of different intervention models are available, and which model is used should depend on the needs of individual children and their parents.
- Intervention is a process of ongoing monitoring, regular measurements of the children's language performances, consistent follow-up, and flexibility in moving from direct to indirect intervention modes and vice versa.

There is no question that toddlers and preschoolers with SLI are at risk for academic failure when they begin school. They are also at risk for early social failure. Proper and early identification and intervention are critical if a potential cycle of social and academic failure is to be thwarted.

4

Language and School-Age Children with Learning Disabilities

Geraldine P. Wallach

LEARNING OBJECTIVES

After reading this chapter, you should be able to

- Explain the relationship between language impairment and learning disabilities
- Describe matches and mismatches between language and academic expectations for school-age children with specific learning disabilities
- Discuss the implications for intervention for school-age children with specific learning disabilities

Medical models of clinical practice suggest that one must have a diagnosis to ensure appropriate and effective treatment. This may be a relevant and applicable approach for many conditions, but language learning and academic problems often fail to fit into neat diagnostic categories. Because the various diagnostic designations (i.e., labels) associated with language learning and academic problems represent heterogeneous groups of children and because the children's problems change over time, "one size fits all" approaches to helping the children require careful consideration. That is, intervention plans that attempt to "match" children's labels need to be evaluated with skeptical, judicious, and critical eyes. Further, the "real world" of schools is steeped in processes defined by federal and state mandates for providing services for children who are struggling in their classrooms (IDEA, 2004). Assessment and intervention for school-age children become further complicated by these mandates, which affect students' eligibility for services and decisions about settings in which they receive services. Of particular relevance for this chapter is the reality that students with diagnostic labels of *language* impairment and those with diagnostic labels of *learning* disabilities overlap for periods during their academic progression but also separate during different periods, thus creating a pattern of intertwining and untwining in nonlinear ways across time (e.g., Catts, Bridges, Little, & Tomblin, 2008; Silliman & Berninger, 2011). To complicate further already complicated issues related to identification and educational placement for children in schools, professionals' perceptions and interpretations of what it means to have a language and/or learning disability may be as diverse as the children who have them.

THE RELATIONSHIP BETWEEN LANGUAGE IMPAIRMENT AND LEARNING DISABILITIES

To provide readers with a reference point, a review of terminology related to both language impairment and learning disabilities follows. This section begins with a review of the definition of *specific language impairment* (SLI) presented in Chapter 3. It continues with additional definitions of language impairment that appear in the literature and in federal mandates. Finally, definitions of learning disabilities and related terms and conditions are explored. The underlying themes addressed in the section are: (1) the overlapping nature of definitions, (2) the primacy of language in many of the definitions and in learning and academic success, and (3) the challenges facing professionals who must operationalize these definitions in practice.

Language Disorders/Impairment Terminology

Revisiting SLI Definitions. The term SLI is often used more frequently *before* children enter school. As noted in the previous chapter, SLI describes the population of children who have language impairment in the absence of other concomitant primary disorders, for example, autism spectrum disorder, intellectual disability, hearing impairment, and oral structural or oral motor abnormalities (Kaderavek, 2015; Leonard, 1991). Kaderavek (2015) addressed the exclusionary criteria attached to SLI. The term, exclusionary criteria, refers to the absence of many of the possible conditions, such as those mentioned in the previous sentence, before a child can be diagnosed as SLI. We will see that the definitions of *specific learning disabilities (SLD)* as well as definitions of *dyslexia* (or *specific reading impairment*) that follow in this section will start to sound very similar to definitions of SLI due to their use of exclusionary criteria as well as their *language focus*. In her landmark treatise on identification issues in language disorders, Lahey's (1990) question raised in Chapter 3, "Who shall be called language disordered?" remains a current one. Decades ago, she encouraged professionals to review their practices, including two that involve the labeling of heterogeneous populations and the assessment of language abilities separate from the situations and contexts (e.g., classrooms) in which children are having difficulties (Sun & Wallach, 2014).

A Definition from the American Speech-Language-Hearing Association (ASHA). ASHA (1993) defines language disorders as follows:

> A language disorder is impaired comprehension and/or use of spoken, written and/or other symbol systems. The disorder may involve (1) the form of language (phonology, morphology, syntax), (2) the content of language (semantics), and/or (3) the function of language in communication (pragmatics) in any combination. (doi:10.1044/policy.RP1993-00208)

This ASHA definition provides professionals with a framework that includes the three major components of language—form, content, and use—and importantly, specifies that language disorders can include comprehension and/or use of both spoken and *written* language. While highlighting the components of language, along with spoken and written domains, the ASHA definition does not reference the chronic nature of language disorders and the continuum of language disorders across time.

The Federal Definition of Language Disorders. Language disorders are covered under the category of *speech or language impairment* in federal definitions. The Individuals with Disabilities Education Act (IDEA) (2004) includes language disorder as one of several communication disorders,

> such as stuttering, impaired articulation, a language impairment, or a voice impairment, that adversely affects a child's education performance (34 C.F.R.; 300.8(c)(11)).

As can be seen, the federal definition is quite broad and offers no specific information about criteria for identifying language impairment or for differentiating speech from language impairment. Guidelines for determining which children meet particular criteria in order for them to be eligible to receive intervention services are established by state and local agencies and these may include various "cut off" points on formal tests of language that children must score at or below in order to be deemed eligible to receive services. For example, in several school systems in California eligibility requirements for students to be determined to have language impairment specify that they must score at least 1.5 standard deviations below the mean, or below the 7th percentile, for their chronological ages or developmental levels on two or more norm-referenced tests (or approved un-normed but standardized tools) in one or more of the following areas of language development: morphology, syntax, semantics, or pragmatics. By including reference to language performance needing to be below developmental level, this particular example introduces the notion of *discrepancy criteria*, which is sometimes also referred to as *cognitive referencing.*

With cognitive referencing, a child whose cognitive level is below average, such that the child is diagnosed with intellectual disability (ID), but whose language performance is tested to be consistent with the low cognitive level would not be considered as having a language impairment, even though it is also below normal. The child could, therefore, not be eligible to receive language intervention services. However, if a child's language performance is tested to be below what is a reduced cognitive level, there is a discrepancy between language and cognition so the child might be deemed to have a language impairment and deemed to be eligible for language intervention services. The use of cognitive referencing is no longer considered valid or appropriate under federal guidelines, but not all states have moved away from using cognitive referencing, or a discrepancy criteria approach, in deciding which children have a language impairment and should be eligible for language intervention services.

New models for identification and service delivery are evolving, including Response-to-Intervention (RtI) models, which will be addressed later on in this chapter, but implementation of new models is slow and inconsistent across states. And professionals are challenged by the complexity of language disorders in children and the limitations of various definitions and mandates that can drive their services for children.

A Classic Definition from the Literature. Bashir (1989) provided professionals with a definition that captures language disorders as dynamic and changing over time. His suggested definition, written over three decades ago, is as timely and relevant today as it was then. It helps professionals appreciate the underlying connection between language impairment in children and learning disabilities and crystalizes the major theme of this chapter. He writes:

> Language disorders is a term that represents a heterogeneous group of either developmental or acquired disabilities principally characterized by deficits in comprehension, production, and/or use of language. Language disorders are chronic and may persist across the lifetime of the individual. The symptoms, manifestations, effects and the severity of the problems change over time. The changes occur as a consequence of context, content, and learning tasks (p. 181).

One of the significant concepts expressed in Bashir's definition is that language disorders are pervasive and changing in their form. In addition, the notion that the changes occur "as a consequence of context, content, and learning tasks" takes us into school and classroom contexts and provides us with a reminder of the curricular demands that challenge children with language learning issues (Wallach, 2008).

Learning Disabilities Terminology

As noted in the introductory comments, professionals with diverse backgrounds and educational preparations may have different perceptions about which students have *language* impairment and which ones have *learning* disabilities (LD). These differences sometimes obscure the connections between and within groups of students; differences in professionals' perspectives also influence intervention directions. As we look to definitions that have been used to identify children with language, learning, and reading disabilities, we note both similarities and differences among them.

Two prominent definitions of learning disability are that of the National Joint Committee on Learning Disabilities (NJCLD, 1991), even though it is now several decades

TABLE 4.1 | Two Major Definitions of Learning Disabilities (LD)

NJCLD (1991)	USOE as Contained in IDEA (2004) (34 C.F.R.; 300.8(c)(10.i)
Learning disabilities is a general term that refers to a *heterogeneous group* of disorders manifested by significant difficulties in the acquisition and use of *listening, speaking, reading, writing, reasoning,* or mathematical abilities. These disorders are intrinsic to the individual, presumed to be due to central nervous system dysfunction, and may occur *across the life span*. Problems in self-regulatory behaviors, social perception, and social interaction may exist with learning disabilities but do not by themselves constitute a learning disability. Although learning disabilities may occur concomitantly with other handicapping conditions (sensory impairment, mental retardation, serious emotional disturbance) or extrinsic influences (cultural differences, insufficient or inappropriate instruction), they are *not the direct result* of those conditions of influence.	Specific learning disability means a disorder in one or more of the basic psychological processes involved in *understanding or in using language, spoken or written, that may manifest itself in an imperfect ability to listen, think, speak, read, write, spell* or to do mathematical calculations, including conditions such as perceptual disabilities, brain injury, minimal brain dysfunction, dyslexia, and developmental aphasia. *The term does not include* learning problems that are primarily the result of visual, hearing, or motor disabilities; of mental retardation; of emotional disturbance; or of environmental, cultural, or economic disadvantage.

old, and that of the United States Office of Education (USOE) as it appears in the 2004 reauthorization of the Individuals with Disabilities Education Act (IDEA, 2004). These are shown in Table 4.1. What we can note about the two definitions is, first, that they use different terms to refer to the disability. The NJCLD definition uses the term "learning disabilities," whereas the IDEA definition uses "specific learning disability" (SLD). A second, and very important, issue is that both definitions are steeped in language. Difficulties in the acquisition and use of language as demonstrated by listening, speaking, reading, and writing problems and other linguistically heavy abilities like spelling and reasoning are highlighted across definitions. Both NJCLD and federal definitions reflect an exclusionary point of view. That is, other conditions (like hearing, emotional disturbance, cognitive delays) must be eliminated before a determination of LD can be made. We have seen previously that these exclusionary criteria are also included in SLI definitions. However, the NJCLD definition helps to clarify the reality that co-existing conditions may and do appear with LD but they are not the primary cause. The NCJLD definition also reminds us of Bashir's definition of language impairment by emphasizing the heterogeneity within populations and the pervasive nature of language and learning problems across the life span. While recognizing the intrinsic nature of LD (i.e., the existence of a neurological base), both definitions in Table 4.1 fail to emphasize the idea that both language impairment and LD reside both *within* and *outside of* children's heads (Nelson, 2005), a concept implied by Bashir's (1989) notion that context, content, and learning tasks change the trajectory of language disorders. In other words, language disorders look different in the school-age years because the linguistic demands of school increase the need for intact and sophisticated language skills and raise the stakes for academic and social failure for students without these language skills. Language disorders at school-age levels often look like those difficulties highlighted in NJCLD and IDEA definitions.

Sun and Wallach (2014) developed the scenario presented in Table 4.2 to help illustrate the common relationship seen between preschool SLI and school-age SLD and the major themes in this chapter. Mom's question at the end of the scenario is a common one. Professionals and parents often think of *language* impairment and *learning* disabilities as separate or different problems. The definitions offered by federal and state mandates also confuse the issue. As we have seen, terms can overlap but often address similar elements of language and learning difficulties. A classic quote from Bashir and his colleagues (Bashir, Kuban, Kleinman, & Scavuzzo, 1984) puts the primacy of language into any discussion of learning disabilities. They ask professionals to think about Tim's problem as an ongoing problem with language, not a new problem that surfaces at an older age. They ask:

TABLE 4.2 | A Language Impairment and Learning Disability Scenario

A parent of a child who has been attending a speech-language-hearing clinic for a number of years is pleased with her child's language development. The child began his intervention journey in this particular clinic at about 2½ years old. He presented as a child with delayed language in both comprehension and expression in all areas of content, form, and use. There was a suspicion of "autism" initially (before he attended the clinic) because of his difficulty relating to people, among other misinterpreted behaviors, but he was diagnosed ultimately as a child with SLI. By second grade, he had continuing language problems, particularly with comprehending instructional language and textbook/classroom content, producing spoken and written monologues (i.e., connected text in the form of stories and expository text), and reading and writing. He had many conversational skills, no speech production problems, and was very social. He was, however, struggling to keep up academically. He also looked like a child with an "attention deficit disorder" (ADD). While continuing with his language intervention in the clinic and in school, his mom expressed concern, as did his teacher, about whether he had a "learning disability." The question asked directly by mom to his speech-language pathologist was: "Is it true that Tim [not his real name] has *another problem* on top of his language problem?"

Source: Based on Sun and Wallach (2014).

> Are we speaking about a group of children, who by virtue of learning context, are called by different names, but who in reality evidence a continuum of deficits in language learning? (p. 99)

Tim's preschool intervention team at the clinic knows that when Tim goes to school he may "look like" a child with a learning disability because his *language* problems are manifesting themselves in *academic* arenas, including the highly language-based abilities of reading and writing. They also know that as preschoolers with early language impairment get older, the challenges they face within school contexts make learning more difficult for them and bring their underlying language problems to the surface. While many of preschoolers with language impairment improve in various aspects of communication, as Tim did, they fall behind their peers quickly as the language realities of classroom and curricular requirements become more demanding (Sun & Wallach, 2014). As a preschooler, Tim's language profile included a delayed mean length of utterance (MLU), morphosyntactic errors and delays, and spoken comprehension and naming issues. By grade 2, as noted in the scenario, he was a fairly good conversationalist and his comprehension was good when contextual supports were strong (e.g., facial, gesture, picture support). By contrast, his comprehension problems were evidenced as difficulties understanding and retaining new curricular content and instructional language (i.e., dealing with unfamiliar topics couched in more complex language forms and abstract language without contextual support). While continuing to have spoken language gaps, which were not as overt as they were when he was a preschooler, Tim had difficulty learning to read and write language.

We have seen that several terms appear in the literature to refer to LD. Another often encountered term is *language learning disability (LLD).* In 1982, the ASHA Committee on Language Learning Disabilities (ASHA, 1982) suggested use of this term to acknowledge the interwoven and overlapping nature of language and learning disabilities. While not an official diagnostic category, the term appears throughout the literature and is used by many SLPs including the author of this chapter (Sun & Wallach, 2014; Wallach, 2008). The thread throughout this chapter is that *the majority of learning disabilities are a manifestation of ongoing, or newly diagnosed, language impairment.* Interwoven within this basic premise is the idea that language is the embedded curriculum of school. Likewise, becoming literate incorporates both spoken and written language.

Which terms are used are mostly a matter of preference and in some instances represent professional perspectives of the users, as is the case with ASHA's suggestion above. It seems sensible, however, at this point in the chapter to make a stab at reducing potential terminology confusion for readers. Although the author clearly embraces the strong language base of most LD and prefers the term, LLD, the term that will be used in this chapter from this point forward is *specific learning disability (SLD).* From the author's perspective, this term is more frequently used in general and special education. It also complements and parallels the term, *specific language impairment (SLI).* However, readers are encouraged to keep a language focus in the forefront of the term, SLD, throughout the chapter.

From these discussions of the various definitions of language impairment and learning disabilities readers have hopefully arrived at this key concept:

> Preschool children with specific language impairment (SLI), like Tim in our scenario, are likely the same children who get different labels (e.g., SLD) when they become school-age students because their language problems manifest themselves differently than they did in the preschool period.

A challenge some professionals may have is understanding the ongoing language needs of our students, regardless of their labels, and recognizing that spoken and written language competence underlie and influence school learning (Ehren, Murza, & Malani, 2012; Sun & Wallach, 2014). School-age language impairment may "look like" SLD "as a consequence of . . . [the changes in] . . . context, content, and learning tasks" (Bashir, 1989, p. 181).

Related Terms and Conditions

Dyslexia. When we look at the two definitions of SLD, we see that reading problems are part of both definitions. Because of the prevalence of reading difficulties in SLD—and SLI—populations, it is helpful to review an influential and widely-used definition of *dyslexia*, or specific reading disability. Lyon, Shaywitz, and Shaywitz (2003) cite the definition of the International Dyslexia Association (IDA):

> Dyslexia is a *specific learning disability* that is *neurobiological* in origin. It is characterized by difficulties with accurate and/or fluent word recognition and by poor spelling and decoding abilities. These difficulties typically result from a deficit in *the phonological component of language* that is often unexpected in relation to other cognitive abilities and the provision of effective classroom instruction. Secondary consequences may include problems in reading comprehension and reduced reading experience that can impede the growth of vocabulary and background knowledge (*emphases added*). (pp. 1–2)

In both SLD and dyslexia definitions we see again a recognition of various aspects of language. The dyslexia definition makes the case for a language base for reading problems by focusing on the role of the phonological component in the reading process. Likewise, both SLD and dyslexia perspectives suggest a central nervous system basis (intrinsic to the individual) for the difficulties. While the term, dyslexia, is used more often in medical settings, school-based professionals are more likely to categorize students as those with *specific reading disabilities* under the general label of SLD as indicated in the IDA definition (Catts & Kamhi, 2012). If readers are wondering if the populations we have been discussing—children with ongoing language impairment, children with SLD and/or those with reading disabilities/dyslexia—frequently represent overlapping populations, they are correct (Wallach, 2008). The exclusionary approach used to identify these populations (i.e., it is not cognition; it is not sensory impairment; it is not instructional impairment, etc.) and the attempts to make fine distinctions among groups (i.e., Is it language impairment? Is it SLD? Is it reading disabilities/dyslexia?) are ongoing challenges for professionals who serve these children, as well as researchers who attempt to better understand the disabilities and the children who have them.

Catts and Kamhi (2012) provide us with a framework that addresses a way to talk about reading disability subgroups functionally. They call this framework "The Simple View of Reading." They suggest looking at the interactions among word recognition and listening comprehension as a strategy for understanding poor readers. They propose four subgroups (all of which are supported by research).

- Subgroup 1: These are children with problems in word recognition alone (sometimes referred to as decoding) without concomitant listening (language) comprehension issues. They are often identified as having *dyslexia.* Again, they have difficulty decoding words phonologically and also have difficulty developing a sight-word vocabulary.
- Subgroup 2: These are children who have problems with word recognition (decoding) as well as problems with listening (language) comprehension. They have spoken and written language difficulties.

- Subgroup 3: These are children who have problems with listening (language) comprehension but who have normal or above-average word recognition (decoding) abilities. They are sometimes called children with *hyperlexia.*
- Subgroup 4: These are children with good word recognition (decoding) and listening (language) comprehension skills but who have reading comprehension problems that are unspecified or that cannot be accounted for by the Simple View model. Reading comprehension is an extremely complex process. It is heavily dependent on metalinguistic abilities, which include underlying language skills. But it involves more. Keenan's (2014) current and innovative work sheds light on the complicated nature of reading comprehension problems, indicating that world knowledge, the tools used to assess language comprehension, and the linguistic demands of different texts influence what we view as a reading comprehension problem.

By now, readers are hopefully aware that language, learning, and reading disabilities represent complex and interacting problems. Professionals can get caught in the trap of spending too much time testing and looking for clean diagnostic categories and not enough time helping students acquire and use the language and learning skills and strategies needed to survive and thrive in the classroom and in life. What professionals must, however, be alert to is not overlooking core issues with language that so many of the children have so that their needs for help with the language components of learning and reading fail to be professionally addressed. In one of the most pointed and poignant statements regarding the search for a distinct population of children who are "learning disabled," Christensen's words (1992) echo through the decades. She wrote:

> Thirty years of psychometric approaches have failed to provide satisfactory answers to the learning disabled dilemma. A continuation of such a quest . . . [for a distinct group] . . . should not be conducted without addressing the serious social, ethical, and moral issues involved in the pursuit of this select group. (pp. 276–277)

These are strong words. Christensen addresses the importance of finding a balance between testing (and labeling) and teaching children. This notion of balance is certainly evidenced in newer RtI (Response to Intervention) models of service delivery that provide several tiers of instruction and support before more formal, diagnostic testing and placement in special education occurs (e.g., Wixson, Lipson, & Valencia, 2014). Although professionals live in the real world of eligibility criteria for determining services and diagnostic categorizations of students, they need to incorporate descriptive approaches into their assessments that account for classroom and curricular demands, that is, the contexts in which students are required to use language to read and learn (Sun & Wallach, 2014; Wallach, 2008). We have seen that children change over time, as do their language and learning needs. This notion of interactive ability (and disability) leads us to a discussion of two additional terms used commonly to describe students with language and learning disabilities.

Central Auditory Processing Disorder (CAPD). The relationship between language ability and the processing of auditory information remains a topic infused with long-standing controversy. Chapter 8 provides a more comprehensive discussion of issues related to CAPD, so the discussion here will be a brief overview and give a peek at some of the issues.

As described by the American Speech-Language-Hearing Association (ASHA) Working Group on Auditory Processing Disorders (2005), auditory processing and its disorders relate to:

> the perceptual processing of auditory in the CNS . . . and the auditory mechanisms that underlie the following abilities or skills; sound localization and lateralization; auditory discrimination, auditory pattern recognition; temporal aspects of audition, including temporal integration, temporal discrimination, temporal ordering, and temporal masking; auditory performance in competing acoustic signals and auditory performance with degraded acoustic signals. (p. 2)

School psychologists, speech-language pathologists (SLPs), parents, and other professionals may recognize symptoms of what might look like an auditory processing disorder, sometimes referred to as a *[central] auditory processing disorder ([C]APD)* to distinguish this condition from a peripheral hearing impairment, in students who have difficulty with auditory sequencing, auditory figure-ground, auditory blending, and other similarly defined auditory-focused tasks. From Rees's classic article (1973) to a more recent forum in the journal, *Language, Speech, and Hearing Services in Schools,* that addressed various aspects of auditory processing (Richard, 2011), researchers and professionals have batted around the value and functionality of CAPD as a separate diagnostic category for students with language learning and academic difficulties (e.g., DeBonis, 2015). Many see CAPD as a symptom, not a cause, of broader language comprehension issues (e.g., Wallach, 2011). Professionals on this side of the argument question intervention goals and objectives that target auditory skills specifically and separate them from language comprehension goals. To further complicate the issue, there is lack of consensus about definition, assessment, and intervention routes among audiologists. Burkard (2009) reminds us to think about the following each time a diagnosis of CAPD is suggested:

> There is currently great divisiveness in the field of audiology concerning CAPD. There is no broadly accepted definition of CAPD. No one really knows what causes CAPD. Despite lofty claims to the contrary, there is no clear consensus concerning the battery of tests that lead to a diagnosis of CAPD. Similarly, there is no widely accepted auditory (re)habilitation program that has been conclusively shown to help those with CAPD. (p. vii)

Until undisputed empirical evidence answers the question posed by the debate about the relevance of CAPD as a diagnostic entity to be assessed and treated specifically (see Vermiglio, 2014), we do know that the interactions among language ability, processing accuracy, and the demands of a situation (Wallach, 2014) need to be accounted for. We also need to account for how the symptoms of a CAPD relate to authentic tasks and situations that children face.

Attention-Deficit/Hyperactivity Disorder (ADHD). In 1980, the American Psychiatric Association adopted the term *attention deficit disorder (ADD)* and described it in two forms: *attention deficit disorder with hyperactivity (ADDH)* and *attention deficit disorder without hyperactivity (ADD without H)*. In the late 1980s the distinction was dropped and the term *ADHD* was adopted (American Psychiatric Association, 2000). Recall that ADHD was introduced in the previous chapter as part of the discussion of toddlers and preschoolers with SLI.

Although there are different ADHD symptoms described along a continuum of behaviors across time, students with ADHD generally have difficulty in directing and sustaining attention and, therefore, have difficulty managing the language-heavy instructional language of the classroom and the abstract and unfamiliar content of core area subjects. They are also likely to interfere with the activities of those around them. For this reason, the American Psychiatric Association considers ADHD to be one class of disruptive behavior disorder.

Two major categories of ADHD are: (1) inattention and (2) hyperactivity/impulsivity. Children with inattention may have difficulty following through with tasks such as the details required to complete homework without mistakes, sustaining attention in the classroom (especially as the curriculum becomes more demanding), and failing to listen when spoken to directly. These children may also have difficulty organizing tasks and may be distracted easily, among other characteristics. By contrast, children with hyperactivity/impulsivity are the ones who have difficulty sitting still. They may leave their seats in the classroom at inappropriate times and have difficulty engaging in activities quietly or reflectively. They are the children who may raise their hands before instructions are completed or attempt to answer questions too soon. In some cases, turn taking is an issue for them because they cannot wait to get into the discussion or conversation. They may participate in conversations with irrelevant utterances and interruptions. Tim, our student from the earlier scenario, demonstrated attention problems related to his language comprehension difficulties that included waiting for instructions to be completed before responding, answering his teacher too soon, and interrupting his classmates.

As with CAPD, ADHD may be the tip of the iceberg (Wallach, 2011; 2014). That is, ADHD may be a symptom—part of a bigger picture. In other words, we might ask: Are attention disorders the *cause* of a student's language and learning problems or are they, at least a percentage of them, the *result* of language and learning problems (Catts & Kamhi, 2012)? We might reflect on how difficult it is to attend to an unknown language for long periods of time. Similarly, we might think about how long many of us might last listening to an advanced lecture on theoretical mathematics or metaphysics (or any other subject about which we know little)? Clearly, children who have spoken (and written) language comprehension impairments may show symptoms of ADHD because it is difficult for them to maintain attention to linguistic structures and content that are above their ability levels (Keenan, 2014). Considering the other side of the coin, however, we must also recognize reciprocity between attention and language. Children who have difficulty attending to language may create a reality that sets limits on what language they learn. Finding ways to bridge the attention-language/learning gap creates a challenge for professionals who serve these students. As we saw in Chapter 3, there are currently concerted research programs to discover the degree to which SLI and ADHD are discrete conditions and the assessment methods that might assist in differentiating between the two (e.g., Redmond, 2016a; 2016b; Redmond, Thompson, & Goldstein, 2011).

Prevalence and Who's Who

We now know that the distinction among populations (i.e., children with SLI, SLD, and/or specific reading disabilities) is not always clear. Consider these numbers:

- 50 percent of students in special education are identified as students with SLD; 80 percent of those students have primary difficulties in the *language-based skills* of reading and writing (U.S. Department of Education's [2006] estimate, as cited in Paul & Norbury, 2012); the majority of students characterized as "learning disabled" in schools are at risk for academic failure due to weak literacy foundations and various aspects of language (Mason, Meadan, Hedin, & Corso, 2006).
- A smaller portion (20 percent) of students in special education are identified as SLI (U.S. Department of Education, 2006; 2007; Moore & Montgomery, 2008); additional findings have indicated that at least about half of children with SLI populations studied have poor reading abilities and the majority read below their grade levels (e.g., Catts, Fey, Zhang, & Tomblin, 1999; McArthur, Hogben, Edwards, Heath, & Mengler, 2000); as noted in Chapter 3, there is at least a 7 percent prevalence of SLI within the kindergarten population; as a chronic and life-long challenge, children with SLI continue to have ongoing language learning needs and, as noted, may be labeled as children with SLD when their language problems manifest themselves in academic areas (Bashir et al., 1984; Sun & Wallach, 2014).
- Tomblin and his colleagues (Tomblin, Zhang, Buckwalter, & O'Brien, 2003) reported that 60 percent of their kindergarteners with SLI continued to show persistent language impairments through fourth grade; going beyond fourth grade, Stothard, Snowling, Bishop, Chipchase, and Kaplan (1998) found that children who are diagnosed with SLI at young ages (kindergarten or younger) continued to experience language and academic difficulties as adolescents *even for those whose language difficulties seem to have resolved early;* as we shall see in Chapter 5, language, literacy, and learning problems remain a persistent and lifelong challenge.

While students with language impairment improve in many areas across time, longitudinal research, both old and new, suggests strongly that children with early language disorders fail to "outgrow" these difficulties or catch up with their typically developing (TD) peers.

Prevalence numbers are dynamic and ever-changing depending upon how a problem is defined. Professionals often bring different perspectives to the identification table. McArthur and colleagues (2000) emphasized the importance of evaluating written, including reading, and spoken language skills for children regardless of whether they present as having specific reading disabilities or SLI. With an understanding of the reciprocity between spoken and written language systems, we now know that poor readers, regardless of their diagnostic designations, are doubly challenged. They are at risk for spoken language and learning difficulties without the benefit of a solid written language system, or a "reading to learn" system, and also challenged in the absence of a "learning to read again" option. The "learning to read again" option relates to the level of literacy needed to access content area subjects, such as social studies, history, science, mathematics, and language arts.

Poor writers are also at a tremendous educational disadvantage for other reasons. Writing is a primary way that students demonstrate what they know, especially as they move beyond third grade. Reciprocally, writing improves reading and helps students gain employment and communicate in multiple ways (Dockrell, 2014; Graham & Herbert, 2010; Sun & Wallach, 2014). Reminding professionals of the language learning and learning disabilities connections, Dockrell (2014) notes that many students have difficulties putting their thoughts on paper, completing homework assignments, and taking notes in class, among other writing-heavy school tasks, but these problems are exacerbated for students with SLD, likely because of the language impairment underlying their learning abilities. Writing problems are commonly reported for students with ongoing language problems, as well as for those students with so-called "resolved" language problems, per Stothard et al., 1998, findings. Dockrell (2014) hypothesizes that "written language . . . [issues] . . . can be conceptualized as a window into residual language problems" (p. 511). She adds that distinctions between SLI and SLD populations are often determined by "arbitrary cutoffs" that are "insufficient . . . to guide intervention" (p. 513).

LANGUAGE AND ACADEMIC EXPECTATIONS: MATCHES AND MISMATCHES

On Becoming Literate

Defining Literacy. We have seen that children, like Tim in our earlier scenario, who are diagnosed as SLI in the preschool period, are more likely than not to have reading and writing problems as they encounter school and to be classified as SLD. Importantly, however, SLD often leads to problems acquiring higher levels of *spoken language* comprehension and expression. Higher level spoken language comprehension and expression, such as listening to and understanding lectures and engaging in debates, are considered aspects of literacy, and acquiring competencies with these skills is considered an aspect of becoming literate (e.g., Nippold, 2007; Scott & Balthazar, 2010; Suddarth, Plante, & Vance, 2012; Ward-Lonergan & Duthie, 2012). Literacy is not just learning to read and write, and mastery of higher levels of language influences higher levels of academic success.

School learning means mastery of more formal, connected discourse abilities in spoken and written language as part of becoming literate. These linguistically based discourse abilities include things like completing formal presentations in class, interpreting the relations among events in social studies, explaining the reasons why characters in a story made certain decisions, summarizing the steps of a science experiment (e.g., Nippold & Scott, 2009; Wallach, Charlton, & Bartholomew, 2014). In addition, as children move through the grades, their performance is measured predominantly through written, not spoken, renditions (Dockrell, 2014). Academic success is clearly influenced by many factors, but understanding the language underpinnings of school tasks (Ehren, 2013) helps us to understand what is meant by SLD.

Developing three tiers of literacy. School-age students are challenged to acquire not one, but three tiers of literacy: foundational literacy, content literacy, and disciplinary literacy (e.g., Fang, Schleppegrell, & Moore, 2014). *Foundational literacies* include skills like basic reading and writing, being able to engage in conversations, and telling and writing simple stories. *Content literacies* include learning to make predictions, form inferences, and read expository text, that is, the formal language of textbooks. *Discipline-specific literacies* include those language skills needed to access curricular information (i.e., the ability to read science, history, mathematics) (e.g., Ehren, Murza et al., 2012; Shanahan & Shanahan, 2012). Thus, acquiring literacy goes way beyond decoding and reading fluency (Fang et. al., 2014). Research suggests that late-emerging poor readers who demonstrated adequate foundational literacy in the early school years may start to show reading problems around third or fourth grade when content and disciplinary literacy skills become more predominant (e.g., Catts, Compton, Tomblin, & Bridges, 2012). *This is often the period when language impairment and SLD become especially difficult to distinguish.* Thus, one of the many challenges facing special and general education professionals is to recognize the literacy-learning patterns and gaps that occur before children arrive at school as well as to evaluate the language knowledge, skills, and strategies that underlie literacy learning and academic success (Ehren, 2009; Wallach, 2008).

Using literate language styles. The demands placed on first graders are significantly different from the demands placed on fourth graders. In her now classic discussion, Westby (1994) conceptualized some of the changes in language learning demands as a continuum that moves from oral to literate styles. The continuum stretches from the most informal types of communication exchanges, like chat and conversational language, to the more formal types of communication, like planned written discourse/planned academic language. In between chat and conversational discourse and formal discourse are language events like narratives, keeping personal journals, and writing letters to friends (Wallach, 2008). Children need to master different language styles, as well as learn where and when to use them. For example, informal language might work when writing emails to close friends. On the other hand, such a language style does not work for a school report. Engaging in academic endeavors means that children must become more proficient in using and processing language that is formal, planned, impersonal, and written. Children must also shift their oral presentation styles to fit the "formality" required in school settings. They not only have to learn to read but they also need to learn to "*talk* like books" (Wallach, 2008, p. 36).

Mastering the language of textbooks. Although narratives remain a significant aspect of language learning throughout life, we saw in previous chapters that *expository discourse* is the predominant text of school; it is the language of textbooks, instructions, classroom lectures, and technical papers. Expository text is a form of nonfiction and non-narrative text that conveys information about the natural or social world (Duke, 2004) through facts, technical or content-specific vocabulary, opinion, analysis, persuasion, classification, or examples (Ness, 2011). Chapter 2 introduced readers to several classifications of expository discourse types. Another classification of the types of expository text includes: *comparison* (compare/contrast), *causation* (cause/effect), *procedural* (temporal sequence), *problem/solution, collection/description* (descriptive), and *enumeration* (Ward-Lonergan & Duthie, 2012). Children have to learn to manage the structural variations of expository text, along with all the technical and formal vocabulary and sentence structures that are part of the expository text landscape (Nippold & Scott, 2009). For example, words and phrases like *similar to, different from, except for, the cause of, as a result of, in addition to, prior to,* among many other transitional words, must become part of students' spoken and written repertoires. Transitional words often become clues to the listener or reader about which text structure is being presented (Nippold & Scott, 2009). Classroom textbooks also include many features that accompany written expository text, such as illustrations, photographs, diagrams, tables, charts, margin notes, bolded words, maps and other features such as headings, subheadings, indexes, and page numbers (Duke, 2004). These text features are provided to facilitate comprehension, but they may be distracting or confusing for students with SLD (Duke, 2004) or even not be noted by students with SLD as features designed to be helpful. The ability to comprehend informational text plays a pivotal role in academic and lifelong success (Duke, 2004; Ward-Lonergan & Duthie, 2012).

Acquiring metalinguistic ability. As we know from previous chapters, the ability to reflect upon language consciously, make judgments about language, manipulate language segments and put them back together, among other language tasks, involves metalinguistic skill, or language awareness. In her early work on metalinguistic development, van Kleeck (1994) noted that the ability to think about language and treat language as an object "frees both language and thought from the immediate context and fosters the development of abstract, decontextualized thought" (p. 53). Thus, when trying to understand children with language learning and academic problems, we need to consider the role of metalinguistic development and ability in the process. Van Kleeck reminds us to think about a two-tiered process in language learning and disorders—the spontaneous layer of language use and the meta-layer of language. In social situations, including those that involve casual conversations, listeners and speakers tend to be in spontaneous and automatic mode. They do not "stop to think" about every word and sound unless a problem (perhaps an unknown word or a heavy accent) arises. Likewise, proficient readers do not analyze every word of text, especially when they are reading familiar or less demanding text (e.g., *People* magazine). We step into meta-mode when we have to analyze or regroup linguistically. Textbook language, for example, places metalinguistic demands on students, among other demands. Many commonly used language assessment and intervention tasks, as well as classroom tasks, have metalinguistic components. Consider the following examples (adapted from Wallach, 2008):

1. Do these words sound the same or different: *rope-robe; thief-leaf; king-ring; lake-lake?*
2. Circle all the pictures that begin with the /s/ sound: *sing, ship; Sue; soda, church, star*
3. I'm going to say a word; tell me how many sounds are in the word: *bat, ship, cowboy*
4. Is this a "good" (or grammatical) sentence? *"The men is waiting for the check."*
5. Underline the sentence that tells us the main idea in the paragraph.
6. Your assignment is to write a current events report.

These tasks are familiar to special educators, SLPs, and classroom teachers. All the tasks tap into metalinguistic knowledge and skill. The first three relate to phonemic awareness (i.e., the conscious manipulation of and making judgments about sounds), the fourth example includes a grammaticality judgment, and the last two interface with higher level meta-abilities that relate to connected text. As both spoken and written text becomes more demanding, and as classroom tasks require more thinking and planning, the meta-load increases. That is, the listener/reader/learner has to analyze and evaluate language on a more conscious level. This is a reality of academic learning. While metalinguistic ability relates specifically to language awareness, another meta-component related to academic success is *metacognitive ability.* Metacognitive skills relate to the ability to think more consciously about thinking. They include self-talk, self-monitoring, and planning, among other skills (Singer & Bashir, 2012).

Summary Thoughts on Becoming Literate. Two points summarize our discussion:

- Literacy is a broad concept that goes beyond the acquisition of reading and writing (sometimes referred to as print literacy and expanded upon in our next section). Becoming literate means many things, including the ability to use formal styles of language in speaking (e.g., presenting at a conference; presenting in class) and in written reports for school.
- Students must master the intricate and interactive aspects of literacy, including foundational, content, and disciplinary literacies.

It follows that professionals working with students with SLD are challenged to evaluate the components of their assessment and intervention tools and techniques. Do they take into account broader definitions of language learning and literacy?

Longitudinal studies show individual variation among and within groups, as discussed throughout this chapter, and a recognition of various subgroups that reflect the spoken-written language relationship in different ways across time. Some children might have spoken *and* written language difficulties that "play off" one another; others might have reading and writing difficulties in what might seem like an absence of overt spoken language difficulties (Catts & Kamhi, 2012). An issue is how we examine spoken language to identify difficulties that might not be obviously explicit. Looking at word recognition only versus comprehension patterns sometimes forms a basis for differentiating subgroups, but background knowledge, metalinguistic ability, and the nature of the tasks tapping literacy-based skills must weave their way through assessment and intervention choices. In the main, however, the sobering situation is that:

- *children who are failing to read by the end of first grade almost never catch up in elementary school* (Catts, Fey, Zhang, & Tomblin, 2001), and
- *75 percent of children who are experiencing reading failure in third grade will continue to have reading problems in ninth grade* (Lyon, 1998).

These data clearly indicate the need for effective and early intervention for children who show difficulties in the foundational stages of reading (decoding and comprehending simple texts) and preparation in the very early elementary years for the skills required for "reading to learn," as well as for those skills and strategies related to "learning to read again" (Ehren, Murza et al., 2012).

In the section that follows, we will take a closer look at learning to read. The section has two major subtopics: (1) Learning to read: Making the transition from spoken to written language; this section introduces some basic challenges facing children as they advance from talking to reading; and (2) A consideration of two models of reading that provide insights into how children move from being nonreaders to readers. Again, readers of this chapter are reminded to keep broader definitions of literacy in mind as these affect our notions of what it means to be a proficient reader.

Learning to Read

Transitioning from Spoken to Written Language. While we have recognized the interplay among spoken and written language systems throughout this chapter, we also recognize that the two systems, while intimately connected across development, are not mirror images of one another. Harkening back to discussions in previous chapters and in this chapter, we know that conversational language is generally more informal and contextualized. When we speak in conversation, we use facial, gestural, and other nonlinguistic cues to get the message across. We take advantage of the physical context and listener knowledge to patch up deficiencies in vocabulary. Deictic words, such as *these* and *here,* work perfectly well in conversation, especially when they are accompanied by an appropriate gesture. In addition, spoken language is unsegmented. That is, words and sounds flow together. The unsegmented nature of spoken language is exemplified by listening to a foreign-language speaker. We often cannot figure out where one word begins and others end. Written, academic language is, by nature, more formal and decontextualized. In written language, connections cannot be made by vague words (*these, here*) accompanied by gestures. Connections are made linguistically through specific words that signal meaning. Thus, when an author uses words or phrases like *George Washington*, followed by *the general*, *he*, *the leader*, the reader has to understand that these words are connected in the text and that they refer to the same person. Deictic words, or unclear referents, cannot be used to overcome a lack of vocabulary. In conversational speech, some allowance is made for the use of vague words. We all say *thing, stuff, guy*, and *sort of* and allow others to do the same. In writing, however, more precise communication is expected. Words must be carefully evaluated for subtle differences in meaning. And since this is the expectation for writing, it follows that children will confront more sophisticated vocabulary when they read. Finally, unlike spoken language, written language is segmented. That is, there are spaces between words in sentences and letters within, which are part of the conventions of an alphabetic writing system.

In written language, the components of spoken language (phonology, morphology, semantics, syntax, and pragmatics) are represented in print. However, children learning to read must come to terms with the stylistic and functional differences between spoken and written systems. Younger and beginning readers must acquire phonemic awareness skills (i.e., those *metalinguistic skills*), including identifying letter-sound correspondences, the number of sounds in words, and segmenting and blending sounds, that relate to foundational/decoding skills required to reconcile the unsegmented and segmented differences between speech and print. Difficulties with various elements of these spoken-to-written transitions are found in children with language-learning, reading, and writing difficulties (Troia, 2014). In addition to managing speech-to-print differences (i.e., *learning to decode*), novice readers have to move from managing a contextualized form of language to managing a decontextualized one (i.e., where words and sentences create meaning in the absence of nonlinguistic cues). They also have to learn to manage syntactic forms like embedded relative clause sentences, passive sentences, other complex syntactic forms, and curricular words (e.g., *prewar, postwar, democracy*, *evidence for*) that may be less predominant in spoken language (e.g., Nippold & Scott, 2009; Scott & Balthazar, 2010). Thus, the interplay among decoding skills, word knowledge, semantic-syntactic proficiency, and connected-discourse savvy, not to mention a reader's background knowledge and experience, come together to create competent readers (e.g., Keenan, 2014).

Kamhi (2009) reminds professionals that they must consider reading processes that take into account both word recognition and comprehension. The ultimate goal of young readers, including children with SLD, is to learn to do some things with increasing automaticity so that they are able to focus on comprehending and interpreting text (Keenan, 2014; Wallach et al., 2014). Going even further, Keenan (2014) notes that

> the "click of comprehension"—the abstraction of meaning—is a multi-faceted and complex series of interactive processes that relate to both the learner and the assessment and/or instructional and intervention tools chosen to determine what that learner "knows" about a subject. (p. 469)

Keenan's last point about "what the learner knows about a subject" encourages us to separate background knowledge (prior information about a subject) from linguistic knowledge (i.e., syntactic ability, semantic ability, metalinguistic ability) when considering reading comprehension difficulties. As an example, we might think about the experiences we have had with children before and while we attempt to comprehend a chapter on child language development versus our prior experiences with quantum physics. Keenan (2014) reminds us that background knowledge, while insufficient for comprehension alone, has a significant effect upon a reader's ability to process, retain, and understand text, which is the ultimate goal of proficient reading.

Two Models of Learning to Read. There are multiple models that attempt to explain the processes involved in learning to read and how children navigate those processes. Each model reflects the theoretical perspective of its developer and none completely and fully adequately explains all aspects of what is an extraordinarily complex learned human behavior—and only humans do it. Two models are presented here. These explain many of the elements of learning to read and the challenges that children with SLD face. These models present with somewhat different perspectives, differences that are important for professionals to consider as they work with children with SLD.

Scarborough's (2003) "Reading Rope," shown in Figure 4.1, illustrates two major strands of the reading process: language comprehension and word recognition. At the bottom of the model are Word Recognition Strands. These include the awareness of sounds within words, the idea that the alphabet represents sounds, letter patterns within words, and recognition of familiar words. At the top of the model are Comprehension Strands. These include use of background knowledge, semantic and syntactic information, knowledge of connected text structures, and inferencing skills. As young readers get better at word recognition (i.e., decoding) and as word recognition becomes more automatic (as with more proficient readers), decoding words is accomplished seemingly without much energy or focus, allowing the reader to attend to comprehension and interpretation of text—the Comprehension Strands. The fluent and *integrated* execution of the two strands is reflected in the tightening of the rope as *skills become increasingly automatic* and as *comprehension becomes more strategic*, two critical concepts of reading that inform our intervention with students with SLD. In other words, one of the many challenges for professionals is to help students develop increasingly more automatic abilities (e.g., more automatic word recognition), so that they can put more attention into methods that facilitate "getting to" an author's meaning and purpose.

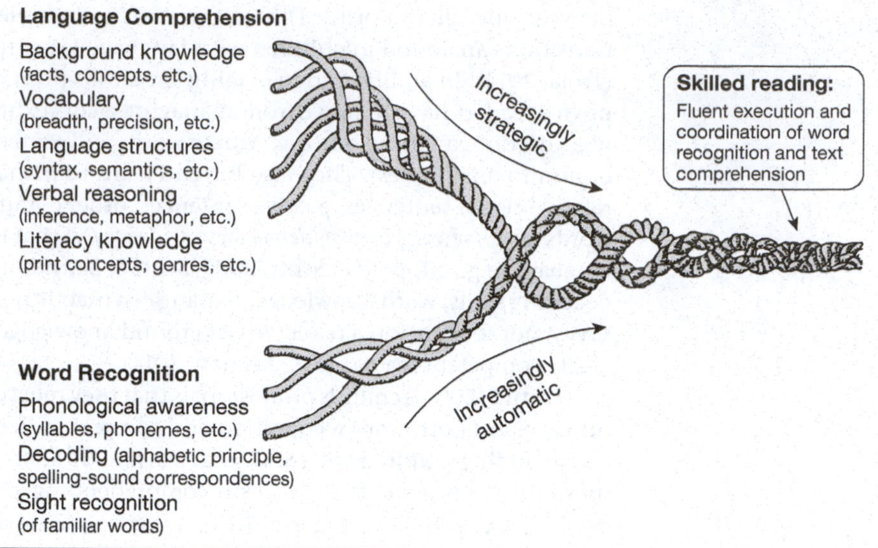

FIGURE 4.1 | The Reading Rope
Source: Scarborough (2003).

Proficient readers do many things poor readers do not do (or have difficulty doing). For example, they use background knowledge and linguistic knowledge to get to meaning. They visually scan words quickly and stop to think (e.g., being more "meta" by rereading a passage) only as needed. Indeed, they may check word recognition when facing unfamiliar words, use context to get to the meaning of words they do not know, and look up word meanings in the dictionary. Good readers use their spoken and written language knowledge—using structural cues and phrases like *by contrast, similarly*, titles, and other textual clues (like the type of expository text being used)—to comprehend text (e.g., McKeown et al., 2009). They engage in both literal and inferential comprehension strategies. Good readers also modify their approach to printed text by considering the differential demands placed upon them. For example, the energy and concentration exerted reading *People Magazine* would be different from the energy and concentration exerted, not to mention linguistic knowledge required, reading a university-level science text. Reading a language arts assignment versus reading an historical piece demand different levels of linguistic savvy (Fang et al., 2014). Indeed, proficient readers continue to "learn to read again" (ala Ehren et al., 2014) by learning to understand the requirements of a text's genre and the level of knowledge, skills, and strategies employed to successfully comprehend and interpret written text.

Owens' (2016) approach, shown in Figure 4.2, mirrors some of Scarborough's thinking about the components of reading and its processes. Owens conceptualizes "bottom up" and "top down" processes. As part of the "bottom up" processes (Scarborough's Word Recognition Strands), "reading is translating written elements into speech" (p. 364). Knowledge of both perceptual features of letters and grapheme-phoneme (letter-sound) correspondences, plus lexical access, form the word recognition subcomponents in decoding. By contrast, "top down" or problem-solving, cognitive, comprehension elements work toward formulating meaning (Scarborough's Comprehension Strands). Reiterating the complex elements of comprehension and the reader's role in interpreting text, Owens (p. 364) notes: "A reader generates hypotheses about written material based upon his or her knowledge, the content, and the syntactic structures used."

Very young, beginning readers and children with SLD have challenges on the path to automatic word recognition and, ultimately, being able to focus on comprehending an author's message. We know that pre-readers often "recognize" visual symbols in what is called the logographic stage of reading (Catts & Kamhi, 2012). They recognize holistic patterns by

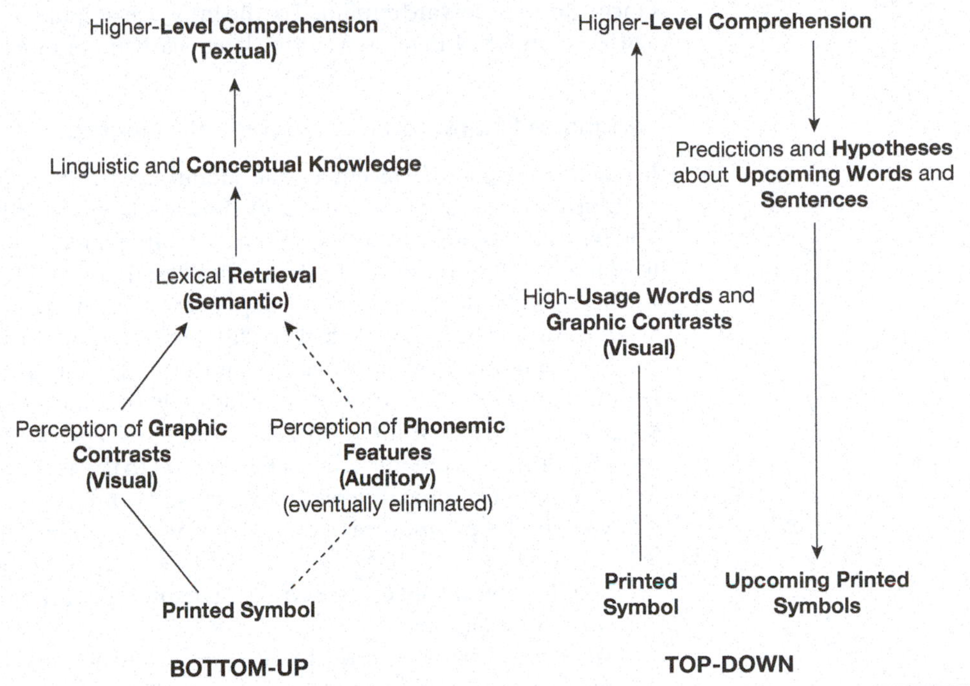

FIGURE 4.2 | Theories of Reading Processing
Source: Owens (2016).

"reading" the McDonald's sign, the "CocaCola" pattern, and like symbols that get them to meaning. Eventually, they have to use phonological awareness and phonemic segmentation and blending skills to decode words (Troia, 2014). Coltheart (2005) talked about children's dual route to learning to read aloud: the *lexical route* and the *nonlexical* route. With the lexical route, says Coltheart, familiar, printed words activate the semantic system, that is, the meaning. Similar to Owens' thinking, we sometimes call this "sight word reading." In "sight word reading," one goes "directly" from print to meaning. According to Scarborough, "sight word" reading means that automaticity has arrived. That is, there is no need to sound out the word. In Coltheart's nonlexical route, however, when faced with visually unfamiliar words (i.e., those whose printed form is not recognized automatically), children must use grapheme-phoneme correspondences (i.e., sounding out the word) to access meaning.

The relevance of both models is that they show us the multi-layered, complex nature of reading and learning to read. There is a very complicated interaction between fluent word reading and comprehension. Importantly, several processes often occur *simultaneously* in the real world, especially by the time children reach third and fourth grades. Readers must use language and conceptual knowledge, even at the word recognition stage (Owens, 2016). Indeed, a child uses "his or her knowledge to help figure out . . . [a] . . . word—much as in speech, when listening, predicting the next word, phrase, clause" (p. 365). We are also reminded to consider what Keenan (2014) wrote about "the click of comprehension" (p. 469). And Scarborough (2003) reminds us that language impairment weakens the tightness of the "Reading Rope" at different points in time, creating weaknesses in various "top down" or "bottom up" processes, to use Owens' terms. When we think about students with SLD, we need to consider their spoken language abilities, including their metalinguistic abilities, their life experiences and knowledge, and their abilities with the elements of reading described in the models.

In the next section, we outline some of the significant language patterns reported in school-age children with SLD. The components of form, content, and use are used as a conceptual framework for the discussion, in addition to considering aspects of connected text that involve an integration of many aspects of the three major dimensions of language. Once again, readers are reminded of the interface of spoken and written language at school-age levels and the interaction among language components.

Language Characteristics: A Look at Selected Patterns in Children with SLD

Research during several recent decades alone has contributed a large, cross-disciplinary body of information about the communication and language difficulties of children with SLD. The research literature is, however, unfortunately muddied by the various different terms used to refer to the children in the studies. Recall our earlier discussion of terminology. To further complicate the issue, the groups of children in the research may also be described as "reading disabled," "poor readers," or "dyslexic." Nonetheless, after we have waded through the mud of terminology and realize that these are often the same children, albeit with different labels, the body of research provides us with some broad-based information about the differences between children with SLD and their TD peers. For consistency's sake, this chapter will continue to use the term SLD, even though the authors of some of the studies referred to here might have used different terms in their work.

We must keep some ideas in mind when we are thinking about the information to come.

- Children with spoken and written language learning difficulties represent heterogeneous populations.
- Spoken-to-written and written-to spoken interactions must be kept in mind when trying to understand academic/learning disabilities.
- Macro (overall structure knowledge and skill) and micro (smaller pieces of text like sounds, words, sentences) aspects of language interact with one another.
- SLD resides inside and outside of children's heads such that we must understand communication and language problems within the context of classroom and curricular demands.

The discussion that follows integrates spoken and written language components. It is organized in this way: *form issues* related to morphosyntactic and phonological components of language; *content issues* related to "meaning making" in terms of word knowledge, naming, and the comprehension of larger units of text including a consideration of background knowledge; and *use issues* including selected social-pragmatic patterns and connected text patterns. Connected discourse, with a focus on narrative and expository text, will be discussed separately.

Form Issues. As we know from previous chapters, morphosyntactic aspects of language include both morphology and sentence structure components. Children with SLD can struggle with mastery and use of the morphological aspects of language. Some of the patterns described for preschoolers with SLI often continue to be seen in school-age children with SLD, but they generally show themselves when language becomes more complicated and demanding (e.g., requiring interpretation across sentences or clauses) and in written language. Many studies suggest that children with SLD lack sensitivity to morphologically based regularities of words. They may also lack morphological awareness or the ability to segment, evaluate, and talk consciously about suffixes, prefixes, and other word building relationships. Difficulties with command of past-tense inflections occurring with both regular and irregular forms, among other forms, are also reported to be problematic for students with SLD.

While not always apparent in simple sentences and less complicated language, problems with morphology may persist in the written language of students with SLD. Written language samples are reported to differentiate TD children from those with SLD. For example, children with SLD may show omission and/or substitution errors in the use of regular past tense, plurals, and verb-subject agreement (Scott, 2014; Windsor, Scott, & Street, 2000). Clearly, difficulties with grammatical morphology that involve decoding the meanings of morphologically complex words in spoken language (those with one root or free morpheme and one or more prefixes/suffixes or bound morphemes) have an impact upon children's written language acquisition (Carlisle & Goodwin, 2014). Nagy and Anderson's (1984) classic finding that TD children's reading materials include approximately 60 percent of morphologically complex words also emphasizes the importance of morphological development in literacy. Mastery of the science curriculum involves many linguistic skills, including understanding the derivation and categorization of words (Fang et al., 2014).

Syntactic ability is a key element of language/literacy acquisition and academic success (Nippold, 2014; Scott, 2014). Although able to demonstrate acquisition of basic syntactic forms (e.g., using grammatically correct language to engage in conversations, producing simple sentences in spoken or written reports), we know that the majority of school-age children with SLD demonstrate difficulty with multi-clausal/literate-style sentences (Scott, 2014). These students have difficulty using sentences that are generally longer and contain higher-level abstract nouns and metacognitive verbs associated with academic language (Sun & Nippold, 2012). Reminding us of the interactive nature of language components, Sun and Nippold (2012) write about the *lexicon-syntax interface*. Nippold (2014, p. 154), using a seventh grade curriculum example in Language Arts, notes that "the use of later-developing metacognitive verbs (e.g., *infer*) prompts the use of nominal clauses in complex sentences (e.g., 'The reader infers that Zeus was furious when Prometheus defied him')." Thus, word knowledge (semantics) and syntactic proficiency influence one another. Studies that have used structured communication tasks, such as describing unfamiliar objects and summarizing fictional and nonfictional videos, indicate that children with SLD in grades 2, 4, 6, and 8 produce fewer words per T-unit (one main clause with all the subordinate clauses attached to it) and fewer words per main clause than TD students at the same grade levels (e.g., Scott & Windsor, 2000).

Many studies provide information about the syntactic gaps that persist in language learning across time (e.g., Scott & Koonce, 2014) and that cut across success with comprehension and production of connected text (e.g., narrative and expository text) and content-area subjects. Syntactic difficulties in the writing styles among students with SLD are also documented widely (e.g., Dockrell, 2014). Indeed, while complex instructional language that uses sentences like those with subordinate/main clause constructions and multiply-embedded features and with passive voice is challenging for all students, "children and adolescents with . . . [specific learning disabilities] . . . struggle inordinately with these types of sentences" (Scott & Koonce, 2014, p. 287).

Phonological development and phonological disorders are aspects of language focused on the linguistic structure related to the speech sounds of language. Some children who have difficulty being understood have problems expressing language through speech because they have not accurately learned or are not applying the rules governing the phonological system of the language. Their problems are *systemic* and go beyond issues with individual sound omissions or substitutions. These types of phonological problems are considered phonological disorders and are forms of language problems. Other children have fewer, less complex "breaks" in the system that may be specific to one of two substitutions, omissions, and distortions that do not affect intelligibility to the extent that phonological disorders can and often do. These children have *articulation errors*. We refer to these children as having speech problems, rather than language problems. A discussion of this aspect of language and speech is beyond the scope of this chapter, but readers are reminded of topics in Chapter 1. We focus here on phonological and phonemic awareness.

Phonological and phonemic awareness refers to a broad set of skills that are part of evolving metalinguistic development. These skills include the ability to manipulate word, syllable, and sound segments in a conscious way. Phonological awareness sometimes refers to a more general awareness of sounds, including such abilities as rhyming, separating (or identifying) words from sentences, and identifying syllables within words. Phonemic awareness typically has a more specific reference to the segmentation, blending, and making judgments about individual sounds within words. Developmental studies and studies of children with SLD (e.g., Catts & Kamhi, 2012; Schuele & Boudreau, 2008) shed light on the importance of phonological and phonemic awareness on the acquisition of reading, as seen in the Scarborough and Owens models. Many children with SLD, including those described as poor readers and especially those who are poor decoders, have difficulties with this aspect of phonology connecting sounds to letters and reconciling speech and print differences. As noted previously in this chapter, while speech is *unsegmented* (i.e., words and sounds flow into one another), print is *segmented* (i.e., words and letters have spaces in between them). Thus, moving from spoken to written language (and back again) requires metalinguistic awareness. When we ask a child to "Tell me the first sound in *bat*," "How many sounds are in the word bat?" "Do these two words sound the same or different: *bat-cat*?" "Put the sounds together to tell me the word: /b/ . . . /ae/ . . . /t/ (bat)," we are asking the child to segment, judge, blend sounds, and manipulate the sounds of language in a direct and conscious way. This is an aspect of phonological development that requires going beyond using sounds for talking and is one of the language learning factors related to literacy success, at least in the early stages of learning to read (and write) the language (e.g., Catts & Kamhi, 2012; Troia, 2014).

Content Issues. Recall that content relates to an area of language also referred to as *semantics*. Describing the semantic skills of TD children and those with SLD is no easy task, especially when we know that helping students derive and express meaning in spoken and written form is the core of academic and life-long learning. Testing the vocabulary size of children using norm-referenced tests has been the most common method to describe the semantic skills of these children. This static measure of semantics is inadequate and can give misleading results about students' semantic abilities considering the complex nature of word learning and the broader-based nature of the comprehension and expression of meaning in sentences and connected discourse. Thus, when considering the nature of children's semantic abilities, we need to consider several interactive pieces—word meaning (and retrieval), sentence meaning, and meaning within connected text. A balance between understanding students' micro (i.e., morphosyntactic, word, and sound components) and macro-level (i.e., connected text) abilities is essential in understanding how students can learn in classrooms.

Word Level (Lexical) Considerations. Both observation and controlled experiments indicate that many children with SLD have underdeveloped lexical systems. This is reflected by their difficulties using more elaborated vocabulary in both spoken and written samples (Dockrell, 2014; Wallach, 2008). Reports on students with SLD at school-age levels frequently cite their difficulty with advanced uses of more literate-level vocabulary words (e.g., *moreover, nonetheless, imperious*) and later developing metacognitive verbs like *infer, believe* (Sun & Nippold, 2012; Nippold, 2014). Many children with SLD are commonly found to misunderstand words with multiple meanings and are less proficient at recognizing and using words that are structurally related, such as antonyms, synonyms, superordinates, and subordinates. Poor lexical knowledge is also evidenced in their inability to provide definitions of abstract nouns (e.g., *burden, gratitude, friendship*) that are precise and reflect essential meaning (Nippold, 2007). "Linguistic glue words," or smaller language units that hold complex sentences together, words like *although, except for, if,* also create problems for many students with SLD (Scott & Balthazar, 2010; Wallach et al., 2014). Likewise, the lexicon-specific items in content area subjects often interfere with comprehension. Consider words and phrases like *postwar, prewar, prior to* in history and the nominalization of words in science like *melting* (e.g., Melting is the process . . .) (Fang et al., 2014; Wallach, Charlton, & Christie, 2010; Wallach et al., 2014).

An even more problematic aspect of semantics for students with SLD is the comprehension and use of nonliteral word meanings. Figurative language, which is language that expresses meanings beyond literal meanings, cuts across word and sentence structure boundaries. This aspect of language, with its long developmental period well into adolescence, is part of metalinguistic development. Most students with SLD perform better on aspects of literal comprehension and expression and have difficulty comprehending and explaining the meanings of figurative language expressions, such as metaphors, idioms, and proverbs, than their TD peers (Abrahamsen & Sprouse, 1995; Nippold, 2007; Wallach, 2008).

The study of word finding, also known as word retrieval, in children with SLD is a complex and multifaceted one. German's (1994) landmark works, among others' works, have provided a great deal of information about the word finding problems of children with SLD.

Children's word finding difficulties are generally characterized by repetitions, filled pauses, reformulations, and circumlocutions. Some of the factors that may underlie word finding and, therefore, enhance lexical access, include the frequency of occurrence of words in the language, words that follow typical stress patterns, and words that are acquired earlier so that they are known longer (Newman & German, 2002). In both confrontation naming and spontaneous speech, children with SLD produce a range of behaviors that either are different from those of TD children or occur with greater frequency (Wiig, Zureich, & Chan, 2000).

DeKemel (2003) reminds us that there are many aspects of vocabulary ability and impairment. She talks about *conceptual* (world knowledge related to words), *semantic* (comprehension and recognition of words), and *naming* (phonological representation or production of words) components. For example, a child may know what a *cat* is because he or she has had some experiences with cats, seen cats, and knows what they look like and what they do. The child may recognize the word *cat* when hearing it; the child might be able to point to a picture of a cat after hearing the word. Finally, a child might be able to produce the name, /kaet/. Understanding students' status in terms of their word knowledge and naming and retrieval abilities can be complicated. But DeKemel's (2003) suggestions, among others, encourage us to consider semantic (comprehending words) and phonological (naming) aspects of lexical ability, in addition to conceptual foundations. Use of targeted prompting and scaffolding techniques to facilitate word retrieval is a critical aspect of exploring students' lexical proficiency or difficulty (McGregor & Windsor, 1996). And the role of written language (both reading and writing) is an essential consideration in thinking about lexical deficits in children with SLD. Vocabulary knowledge and use are enhanced by access to print (Catts & Kamhi, 2012; Sun & Wallach, 2014), that is, by spending time reading and writing, hence the importance of the reciprocal interaction between spoken and written language.

Sentence Level Considerations. The semantic challenges facing children must go beyond lexical analyses. Overlapping with some of the concepts expressed in the form section covering morphosyntactic issues, comprehending the meanings expressed via complex sentences is another aspect of language that presents difficulties for many students with SLD. Difficulties expressing meanings in writing are also evidenced in their written renditions (Dockrell, 2014; Scott, 2014). Consider this sentence from a grade 5 social studies text (Harcourt School Publishers, 2000):

> The Boston Tea Party was the colonists' response to the unfair tax instituted the prior year by the British. (p. 280).

Figuring out the who-did-what-to-whom-when is difficult for several reasons:

- the complex nature of the sentence structure; the "doers" of the action are not explicit in this passive form,
- the number of propositions (ideas in the sentence),
- the embedded nature of clauses and phrases (. . . *instituted the prior year* . . .), and
- likely a less familiar temporal word (*prior*).

Clearly, familiarity with the content, that is, knowing something about the Boston Tea Party and the Revolutionary War, is a critical aspect of "getting to meaning." The form-content interaction is an important facet of language learning difficulties in students with academic problems.

Scott (2014) reminds us to consider ways that syntactic knowledge and skill interact with semantics. She points out that many factors, including the number of clauses (and propositions) in a sentence, the number of embeddings (clauses that interrupt the flow of sentences or modify parts of sentences), and confusing order (when the who-does-what-to-whom-when is reversed) create problems for students with and without SLD. For example, when a teacher says, "Take out your math books before you start your reading assignment," the two-clause sentence, consisting of a main clause (*Take out* . . .) and a subordinate clause (*before you* . . .), is spoken in the order of the events (i.e., math books first, then reading assignment). By contrast, the sentence, "Before you take out your math books, start your reading assignment," violates the order of events and may be more confusing (Wallach, 2014). Understanding the meaning of *before* and *after* in this instructional context, as well as the placement of the subordinate clause, influences comprehension. Many structural and contextual elements interact with "meaning making" at the sentence level and present challenges for students with spoken and written language issues throughout their academic careers. We know that preschoolers with early language disorders (e.g., children with SLI), and in the school years those with SLD, not only produce shorter sentences overall but have difficulty comprehending and producing complex syntactic forms in both spoken and written modes (Dockrell, 2014; Nippold, 2014; Scott, 2014). Beyond elementary school, these measures of complex syntax across instructional and curricular materials (e.g., main/subordinate sentences, passive sentences, relative clause sentences) "continue to distinguish adolescents with and without a history of SLI through the eighth and 10th grades" (Scott, 2014, p. 287). What we need to keep in mind is that these sentence-level issues affect both "getting to meaning" and expressing meaning.

Use Issues. Problems with language use, that is, pragmatic disorders, rarely appear in a vacuum. The complex interactions among social competence (using language appropriately across contexts and individuals for various purposes), linguistic ability, and emotional growth are complex and layered (Brinton & Fujiki, 2014; Sun & Wallach, 2013). Many school-age children with SLD have been shown to have different levels of difficulty with various pragmatic language tasks including entering conversations, engaging in decision-making in group projects, negotiating with peers, and resolving conflicts via language (Brinton & Fujiki, 2014). As students with SLD move through the grades toward adolescence, pragmatic differences between them and their TD peers continue to change how they are manifested. Donahue (2014, p. 328) points out that many students with SLD show problems with perspective-taking, a pragmatic deficit that may resurface in written language comprehension tasks, and can help "to explain why some readers struggle with making inferences about characters and relationships. . . ." Brinton and Fujiki (2014) agree with Donahue, stating that "literacy emerges within social contexts and transactions" (p. 181).

Communicative ability is the core of social relationships and social interactions within and outside of classrooms. Being able to engage in both social and academic conversations and being successful at creating, maintaining, and nurturing teacher and peer relations are interactive with literacy learning and emotional growth (Brinton & Fujiki, 2014; Sun & Wallach, 2013). Students who are perceived to have problems with social skills are more likely to be rejected by their peers as well as their teachers (e.g., Bryan, Bay, Lopez-Reyna, & Donahue, 1991). As students advance in school, social relationships become more complex along with academic demands. Pragmatic functions also change along the way as written language becomes a vehicle for communication and learning. As noted by Donahue (2014) earlier, students must engage with authors and become writers themselves; they must interpret authors' intentions, for example, and make the purposes and points of their written renditions clear for readers. They must take the audience into account (Who is the audience? What are their preconceived notions, knowledge?). Students must also learn how to express their feelings and emotions to adults and peers in constructive ways (Sun & Wallach, 2013). Indeed, the long-term effects of ongoing language learning difficulties, including early identified pragmatic difficulties, are important elements to consider when trying to understand emotional issues that influence the academic and social success of students with SLD (Sun & Wallach, 2013).

Connected Discourse. One of the most important areas for academic and social success for school-age students with SLD is the comprehension and production of connected text, in both spoken and written modes. It is possible that narrative and expository savvy may be sensitive measures of the pragmatic vulnerabilities of these students (e.g., Hadley, 1998). Form (morphosyntax) and content (semantics) meet within the construction of *narrative* and *expository* text.

Narratives. We know that narrative discourse relates to stories and storytelling. Narratives contain at least two utterances, often but not always follow a temporal order about experiences and events, and incorporate specific structures related to the development of theme and plot (Boudreau, 2008). A long history of research has provided us with information about the differences in narrative proficiency between TD children and children with SLD. Boudreau (2008) provides professionals with a review of the research that includes a discussion of the importance of narrative abilities in academic success. She also summarizes the ongoing nature of narrative difficulties for students with SLD, noting that "... discourse abilities appear to represent a key area of linguistic functioning that continues to differentiate children with a history of ... [SLD] ... from TD peers after other aspects of language functioning move to age-appropriate range" (Boudreau, 2008, p. 103). Across studies, children with SLD have been shown to produce stories with limitations in both content (e.g., fewer elaborated and connected episodes with fewer characters and plot twists) and form (e.g., shorter utterances, limited grammatical complexity and accuracy). Aspects of both literal and inferential comprehension influence students' performances across the grades and across spoken and written texts (e.g., Green & Roth, 2013).

Although a significant relationship exists between some narrative performance and academic success (e.g., use of "linguistic glue" words like conjunctions, creating coherence among events, references to mental states of characters), caution is warranted. When interpreting narrative performance results, one must consider several factors that may influence results. For example, is *production* being used to measure narrative *comprehension*? Additional research is needed to understand fully the relationship between narrative comprehension and production and between spoken versus written proficiency. Likewise, clinicians are reminded to keep macro- and micro-structure elements in mind. Studies suggest that children with SLD may show more uneven patterns compared to their TD peers in content-form interactions in narratives. In other words, some children with SLD demonstrate relative strengths in content elaboration but not in grammatical accuracy; others are stronger in grammar but not content (Colozzo, Gillam, Wood, Schnell, & Johnston, 2011; Scott, 2014).

Expository text. We know that expository text is informational text, the main text of school. Unlike narratives, which have a largely chronological structure with events seen through the eyes of characters, expository text is organized based on logically connected relations, signaled by linguistic elements (Scott, 2014). There are many types of expository text (e.g., problem-solution, compare-contrast, procedural, descriptive) through which the curriculum and other formal documents are transmitted. As Scott (2014) writes, "These texts ... are less tied ... [than narratives] ... to personal experience, more often encountered in the written modality, and it takes longer for children to become fluent with them " (p. 148). Expository text challenges students for many reasons:

- it is linguistically dense in terms of its formal and less personal style,
- it is crafted with complex syntactic and literate sentences and connective words, and
- its content is often less familiar.

Studies have shown that students with SLD have difficulty with productivity in terms of number of words used, sentence complexity, and grammatical accuracy in spoken and written expository summaries when compared to their TD peers (Koutsoftas & Grey, 2012; Scott & Windsor, 2000; Ward-Lonergan, 2010). Students with SLD tend to have difficulties writing organized and cohesive paragraphs, creating complexity within paragraphs, and demonstrating grammatical accuracy (Koutsoftas & Grey, 2012; Ward-Lonergan, 2010). As the content of the curriculum becomes more abstract and linguistically heavy and as the demonstration and acquisition of knowledge occur mainly through print, students with SLD remain particularly vulnerable for academic success.

Language Impairment: Students with SLD Tackling Literacy and Curriculum

We now know that preschool children with SLI come to school with many diverse language learning issues. Their spoken language difficulties follow them into their school years and contribute to their problems performing the more advanced linguistic tasks of school, such as reading and writing curricular content and tracking and attending to complicated instructional language that appears in spoken and/or written form (Catts, Compton, Tomblin, & Bridges, 2012). Pragmatic and morphosyntactic gaps contribute to difficulties talking with their teachers appropriately, engaging in peer-peer projects effectively, interpreting the intent of a speaker or author, and making long-lasting friendships (Sun & Wallach, 2013). These aspects of school learning, among others, are steeped in linguistic and metalinguistic abilities that challenge students with SLD.

The interactions among form, content, and use across spoken and written modes of communication create reciprocal, intricate relationships that are tied intimately to academic learning. We know that spoken language and written language have a reciprocal relationship. This means that the two systems "play off" one another in different ways at different points in time. Spoken language leads the way to written language (often in the "learning to read" phase) but written language also leads the way to spoken language (especially in "the reading to learn" and "learning to read again" phases). While reading the language helps children learn more spoken language, more spoken language helps students to develop additional metacognitive skills such as using self-talk to organize their thoughts (Singer & Bashir, 2012; Westby, 2014). Clearly, the spoken-to-written and written-to-spoken relationships along the path to academic success represent a continuum of changing demands, sometimes followed by changing diagnostic labels for children struggling with the curriculum (Sun & Wallach, 2014).

As children move through the grades, they are expected to comprehend material that becomes increasingly more complex and to function more strategically and independently (Wallach et al., 2014). Kamhi (2009) helps professionals understand some of the changing demands across time by highlighting Scarborough's and Owens's notions about the learning to read process in this way:

> By late elementary school and beyond, comprehension ability accounts for almost all of the variability in reading levels. Lack of reading proficiency in the early elementary school years thus reflects difficulty learning to decode whereas lack of reading proficiency in later school years reflects difficulty understanding and interpreting words, sentences, and texts. (p. 17)

So, while difficulties start early for preschool children with SLI in acquiring *foundational literacy*, which involves the early phases of literacy learning including acquiring conversational language, early narrative abilities, and decoding skills for reading, from the time they are in kindergarten, or even younger, these children are often uninterested in shared book reading (Scarborough, 2009). They can be reluctant to read and write either with assistance or independently (Catts & Kamhi, 2012; Hall, 2012; Justice, 2006; Paul & Norbury, 2012). Children with language impairment start with low initial reading abilities and continue with lower reading achievement as they advance in grades (Catts et al., 2008; Scarborough, 2009). The obstacles these children encounter when reading include coming across countless unknown words, having gaps in background knowledge, and encountering complex syntactic forms including embedded and relative clause sentences that further contribute to reading comprehension difficulties and lack of interest in reading (Scott & Balthazar, 2010). But, not only do they spend less time reading, they often read simplified texts so that they do not have exposure to materials that further develop both spoken and written language skills. Ellis's (1997) classic work reiterates the point that the watering down of school curriculum for problem learners is depriving them of the rich language and literacy experiences needed to achieve academically. This means that while their TD peers begin to expand their background knowledge, sophisticated vocabulary, familiarity with different genre structures, complexity of morphosyntactic use, and appreciation of figurative language through independent reading, students with early language impairment find numerous obstacles in the learning-to-read process and are, therefore, often characterized as having an SLD.

Deficits in language cut across aspects of content, form and/or use. Some students with SLD acquire aspects of foundational literacy. They have conversational skills; they can tell simple stories; they can decode; they comprehend literal text. They acquire aspects of spoken and written language (i.e., foundational literacies), and to observers who are not looking closely or looking at the right things, the children might look as if they have overcome their early language impairment. Recall from Chapter 3 the problem of illusionary recovery. But the illusion of recovery means the children fall behind again as TD children have another learning spurt. In addition, the lack of or limited proficiency with written language creates a perfect storm (Sun & Wallach, 2013). Students' limited reading proficiency begins to affect their spoken language advancement in several ways we have seen.

As children with SLD advance into later elementary school the limitations on their spoken and written literacy skills lead them to struggle with content and disciplinary aspects of literacy, that is, comprehension and writing within content-area subjects (e.g., Catts et al., 1999; Dockrell, 2014; Ehren, Hatch, & Ukrainetz, 2012; Fang, Schleppegrell, & Moore, 2014; Keenan, 2014). It is evident that the language-learning gaps create a mismatch with the increasingly more advanced academic demands. Their weaknesses producing and understanding connected discourse, especially expository text, which is the predominant language of textbooks (Ehren, 2009; Ehren, Murza et al., 2012; Nippold & Scott, 2009; Scott & Balthazar, 2010; Sun & Wallach, 2014), particularly affect academic success. So, while the language problems of children with SLD show themselves as reading and writing difficulties in the early grades, these evolve to higher levels of both spoken and written language problems as they advance through the grades. In our example of the expository piece about the American Revolution from a fifth grade social studies text, students are expected to learn about its causes, purposes, key characters, battles, and outcomes and summarize the text or answer questions about it. These expectations require a coming together of background knowledge, content knowledge, and linguistic structure knowledge (Hall, 2012; McKeown, Beck, & Blake, 2009). These elements merge to make the social studies task, and other content-area subjects, exceedingly linguistically and cognitively demanding for children with SLD (Wong, Graham, Hoskyn, & Berman, 2008). The large mismatches between their language and literacy proficiency and the advancing curricular requirements result in huge challenges for students with SLD, challenges that become greater with each higher grade.

IMPLICATIONS FOR INTERVENTION

Assessment and intervention decisions for school-age students with SLD need to be made with an eye to content-area learning (Anthony Bashir, Personal Communication, 2010). This notion goes back to Nelson's idea that language impairment resides *within* and *outside of* children's heads. Thus, we look at what abilities and disabilities children come with to the task of academic learning, as well as the demands of the academic task itself. In a quote that reminds professionals who work with assessing, teaching, and intervening with students who struggle with school or are at risk for struggling, Brozo (2010, p. 278) wrote: "The typical demands of a . . . school curriculum require students to possess sophisticated language tools to explore information and content in area subjects, such as history, mathematics, science, and literature." Connecting both spoken and written language to comprehending and retaining what is seen and heard in classrooms, he added that, ". . . students . . . [can] . . . struggle to make meaning from the complex prose they are confronted with daily" (p. 278). Consequently, in looking at assessment and intervention, professionals must consider both the learner and the relevance of the tools they choose to determine, not only what a student knows (Keenan, 2014), but how the student's language proficiency will allow the student to function within the context of classrooms and the instructional demands. For those of us who are focused on understanding a student's language level and ability, we might return to Lahey's (1990) classic question, "Who shall be called 'language disordered'?" and add the question, *How does that language impairment manifest itself in academic tasks?* (Wallach et al., 2014), a question that serves as a guideline for assessment and intervention.

Assessment

Whether coming from the perspective of special education, speech-language pathology, literacy and reading, or general education, among other disciplines, professionals should ask several questions that frame the direction of their assessments (Wallach et al., 2014):

- What constitute the "sophisticated language tools" that are necessary to access the curriculum that Brozo (2010, p. 278) was referring to in his quote?
- What are the most valid ways to discover what language tools a student has and does not have to access the curriculum?
- How do we find the best route for helping the student?
- What, if any, norm-referenced assessment tools are sensitive enough to help identify ongoing language-literacy profiles and needs of our students in academic trouble or at risk for academic trouble?
- How do we integrate one-on-one assessment strategies, including formal testing, with observations within the contexts where students suspected of SLD have the most difficulty (e.g., classrooms, content-area subjects)?

We can think back to the scenario presented about Tim earlier in this chapter. We might say that he is "one of the lucky ones." This is because his language issues were identified before he entered school, so intervention is likely to be ongoing. He is less likely to be at risk for being unserved until he starts to exhibit failure in learning to read and in keeping pace with his peers. Transition of services from a clinical to school setting for him has the potential to be relatively seamless. His professional team (e.g., classroom teacher, SLP, special educator) and his parents have already realized that he is at risk for encountering academic problems so they are alert to monitoring his literacy progress. And he is likely to experience services within a prism of ongoing language learning problems. His language issues have been recognized at the fore, so the educational label of "speech and language impaired" is likely appropriate. He may also receive the educational label of "specific learning disabled," which means services of SLD and/or reading specialists could be available for Tim, in addition to services of an SLP. Importantly, however, is his receiving appropriate placement and services from all relevant professionals (classroom teacher, SLD/reading specialists, and SLP) within a Response-to-Intervention (RtI) framework, to be discussed later in this chapter.

Some children might not be as "lucky" as Tim. Entering school without having a language impairment identified could mean that a child needs to start to fail before professionals become concerned and initiate an assessment process. This can often be after the child has been unable to keep up with his peers' learning for a year or two, that is, after grade 2. When this scenario describes what a child is experiencing or has experienced, it reflects a *wait-to-fail model* rather than a *preventative model.* There is now sufficient information available to professionals for them to be good at identifying which children have language profiles that place them at risk for literacy and other academic problems. With this information professionals are in a position to implement services early in order to mitigate as many negative impacts of language impairment as early as possible. Unfortunately, a wait-to-fail model continues to reflect what children with unidentified language impairment often experience when they enter school as kindergarteners.

The results of Zhang and Tomblin's (2000) study addressed some of the factors that affect which students with language impairment receive services. These authors followed up kindergarteners, who at the time had primarily speech sound disorders, impairment of expressive language only, impairment of receptive language only, or impairment of both expressive and receptive language, when the children were in second grade in order to identify which of them had received SLP intervention. They found that the children with speech-only disorders had a greater likelihood of having had intervention between kindergarten and grade 2 than any of the language impairment groups. Of the language-impaired groups, the children who had expressive language involvement were more likely than those who had receptive language involvement to have had SLP intervention. However, when the researchers associated the academic achievement and socioemotional status of the same students with their speech or language impairments, language impairment was more strongly associated with poorer outcomes in grade 2 than speech disorder. These results suggest that students with language impairment are less likely to receive intervention than those with speech problems, even though language impairment is more likely to be negatively associated with academic and social success than speech problems. The findings have implications for early and accurate identification of children with language impairment in order to provide appropriate intervention support to stave off as many academic and social failures as possible.

Language Screening. Because identification of students with possible language impairment early in their school experiences has significant implications for the students' educational experiences, how kindergarten students are screened for the presence of language problems is particularly important. Most schools screen kindergarteners either prior to their beginning school or soon thereafter for the presence of a variety of risk factors that can affect their success. Speech and language screening is typically included in the screening programs. In light of the high risk for academic struggles language impairment has for students and given research findings such as those of Zhang and Tomblin (2000) about which children are likely to receive intervention, language screening needs to employ procedures that are sensitive enough to quickly separate children at risk for language impairment from those whose language proficiency is likely able to support their learning. Those children at risk can then be followed up with more thorough evaluations that can confirm or reject the screening results.

There are several commercially published standardized language screening tests. Their use, however, needs to be considered with healthy skepticism. A number of factors contributes to the need for a cautionary approach. One is that the norms for several of these tests lead to unacceptably high false positive and false negative results, that is, missing at-risk children or over-identification of children. (Chapter 13 discusses language-test psychometrics in more detail.) A more concerning factor is that most of the screening tests examine children's abilities by asking the children to engage in primarily decontextualized speech and language tasks, such as naming pictures to assess speech sound production and/or expressive vocabulary, pointing to pictures that represent the meaning of individual words, or repeating short sentences. Such decontextualized tasks do not adequately sample the types of synthesized language skills needed to access an academic curriculum or challenge children's language abilities, per Lahey's suggestion (1990). Another concern is that many of the tests focus more heavily on speech than language and on expressive language more than high-level language comprehension.

We know a lot about language characteristics of children with SLI and about how these different characteristics related to language performance negatively impact academic success. Of particular relevance is the discussion of risk factors and clinical markers in the previous chapter and previously in this chapter. This knowledge helps us employ strategic approaches to screening and reduce reliance on norm-referenced screening tests that might have questionable ecological and psychometric validity. Here are some of things we know that can guide our language screening approaches:

- Young children's poor performance with nonword repetition tasks (NWR) is frequently associated with the presence of SLI. Including NWR tasks as part of a language screening seems like a smart, logical, and research-supported strategy. NWR tasks are also typically quite quick to administer.
- Abilities with narrative performance are highly predictive of children's subsequent academic success. Narrative is a discourse type with which kindergarten children are expected to be familiar. Poor narrative ability, therefore, portends academic struggles. Including a narrative task, such as asking a child to tell a story while looking at a wordless storybook, seems like a smart, logical, and research-supported strategy. There is a number of narrative analysis techniques, many of which are relatively easy and quick to use. (Chapter 13 includes a list of commonly used narrative analysis approaches.)
- Kindergarten children with SLI are generally able to converse in casual conversation and to use complete sentences while doing so, albeit typically using sentences that are mostly simple or compound in syntactic structure with limited use of sentences with relative and embedded clauses, that is, use of complex sentences. To tap into possible presence of language impairment, tasks that challenge a child's language proficiency during screening, per Lahey (1990), need to be used. Telling a narrative is a type of discourse that involves connected speech that places challenges on children's language

performance; therefore, including a narrative task in language screening seems like a smart, logical, and research-supported strategy. (This gives two votes for using a narrative task!) There is a number of relatively easy and quick approaches to assess children's complex sentence use, per Chapter 13.

- Children with SLI show continuing difficulties with verb morphology, especially past tense verb morphology, long after their TD peers master these linguistic forms. Sampling children's accuracies/inaccuracies with verb morphology and particularly past tense verb morphology as part of a language screening seems like a smart, logical, and research-supported strategy. A narrative retell task encourages children to use past tense to convey the story, and stresses children's language proficiencies as well. (This gives a third vote for using a narrative task!) Again, there is a number of relatively quick and easy to use analysis methods, including a simple method of tallying opportunities for past tense verb use and tallying if use was correct or incorrect.
- Children's abilities with sentence recall tasks have shown promise in identifying those youngsters at risk for SLI. These tasks are quick and easy to administer and some commercially published, norm-referenced language tests include tasks that target sentence recall. Based on current research, including a sentence recall task as part of a screening seems like good practice. Sentence recall tasks that include some complex sentences with embedded clauses, particularly relative clauses, also provide a glimpse of children's morphosyntactic abilities. Recall that, when sentences to be repeated challenge children's language by exceeding their morphosyntactic skills, the children will use their own morphosyntactic skills rather than rotely imitating the structures in the target sentences.
- Screening for aspects of speech abilities cannot be overlooked, but the prominence of speech screening as part of overall screening procedures needs to be kept in perspective given findings such as those of Zhang and Tomblin (2000) that children with speech disorders tend to be provided intervention more than those with language impairment. A connected speech task, such as that of a storytelling task or sentence recall task, can suffice as a speech screening procedure while also providing important information about a child's language proficiency. (Here is another vote for the utility of a narrative task as a screening strategy!)

It is important to keep in mind that the purpose of screening is to raise red flags about some children's language (and speech) abilities and give "green lights" to the abilities of others, with the idea that the academic performance of the children with the "red flags" will be monitored carefully and/or the children will be provided with subsequent in-depth assessments. The purpose of screenings is *not* to confirm or reject the presence of language impairment. This purpose is left to a comprehensive evaluation that can follow.

There is another bit of knowledge that arises from the research literature that can guide our procedures and that is relevant to screening and assessing children's language. We have learned that young children's success in the early stages of learning to read is highly predictive of their later reading levels and general academic success and that language proficiency is highly predictive of children's success in learning to read. This means that if a child has language problems the child is at risk for learning to read. Therefore, such a child needs language intervention and reading support in the early grades. Waiting until a child is in third grade or later to provide services places the child at high risk for subsequent academic failure. For a child whose performance on language screening tasks is suspect, the child needs to move to a language assessment as soon as possible, and from there to intervention services (language intervention and reading support) as soon as possible if assessment results indicate language problems. This approach is consistent with a preventative strategy rather than a wait-to-fail model.

Language Assessment. Given the wealth of information available about the assessment process in other chapters, particularly Chapters 3, 5, and 13, the discussion here will focus on some of the important principles that support the three core purposes of language assessment of school-age children suspected of having SLD. These three purposes are: (1) identifying a student as having or not having a language impairment; (2) determining the eligibility of a student with language impairment for intervention services; and (3) developing, as part of an interprofessional educational team, an intervention plan for the student. We will embed discussion of issues related to these purposes as we address here several principles of assessment.

Assessment Principle 1: Understand the difference between identifying a student for services and creating and implementing an intervention program. There is a difference between identifying a student for services and developing an intervention program for the student. It is critical to be clear about the purpose of the assessment. Working toward a particular placement requires understanding federal and state mandates to make a case for a student, either to receive or not to receive services. It is equally essential to keep in mind what language impairment "looks like" at school-age levels. Implementing an intervention plan cannot be done effectively from a series of norm-referenced tests. Tests and tools may give us some clues but dynamic assessment, which is a combination of assessment and brief intervention, as discussed in Chapter 13, can help professionals make more effective intervention choices (see a classic discussion by Palincsar, Brown, & Campione, 1994).

Assessment Principle 2: Be aware of the strengths and weaknesses of tools chosen. Because professionals need to be focused toward curriculum access for students, instructional demands, and teachers' language styles, assessment tools should connect to the disciplinary literacies embedded in school curriculum and the contexts in which students must succeed. One-on-one testing is not equivalent to group learning in the classroom. However, we can glean information by going beyond what a test says it is testing. For example, results from a combination of subtests that provide information about higher levels of comprehension (e.g., figurative language, multiple meanings, inferring meaning) and expression of syntax (e.g., subordinate-main clause constructions, embedded relative clause sentences, passive sentences) may provide clues into a student's difficulty with instructional and textbook language. But it is important not to be misled by what tests or tools indicate they are testing. Tests labeled "auditory discrimination" are tapping into phonemic/metalinguistic skills related to early reading, not auditory discrimination (e.g., Schuele & Boudreau, 2008; see Wallach, 2011).

Assessment Principle 3: Stress the language system. This point has been made several times because it is such an important one. Tools and approaches that challenge students' language skills and are sensitive enough to uncover early or ongoing language impairment need to be used. In her landmark discussion about assessment, Lahey (1990) reminded us to "push" the language system to really understand what children can do with language. Tasks that are "too easy" miss underlying language impairment. We need to remember that these children typically talk in sentences and can carry on casual conversations for several dyadic turns. Using timed naming tasks or sampling beyond conversational skills, such as those involving narratives and expository discourse, should be included in assessment batteries.

Assessment Principle 4: Collect spoken and written samples. Given the reciprocity of spoken and written language, students' abilities across systems need to be considered. Discourse analysis is relevant to both spoken and written language. By collecting narrative and expository samples, starting with familiar topics and moving toward less familiar topics and by looking at spoken and written systems together, we learn more about students' metalinguistic and metacognitive abilities, as well as their linguistic knowledge. Difficulties with print referencing and other early literacy abilities need to be considered as red flags for future academic problems (Justice & Ezell, 2004). Previously in this chapter, three tiers of literacy—foundational literacy, content literacy, and disciplinary literacy—were presented. Students' abilities with these three literacy tiers should also be part of assessments.

Assessment Principle 5: Observe in the contexts in which students must survive and thrive. A significant aspect of every assessment for school-age students with potential or identified language impairment is to observe them in their classrooms. With federal and state mandates, this is now usually a required component of assessment in order to qualify a student for services. Working with general and special education teachers within a collaborative framework is another critical aspect of the assessment process. Observing students in curricular activities or subjects that are the most difficult for them is one way to begin. Evaluating

TABLE 4.3 | A Language Intervention Scenario

A group of middle school students (grades 6 and 7), who have knowledge of, and interest in, basketball, are asked to decide what a headline from a current sports section of a local newspaper means and how it could help them figure out what might be in the article. The headline reads: "Jazz Helps Lakers Become Mellow in Victory." The students, who are provided with a structured outline to follow, brainstorm about possibilities. The questions on the outline include: "What I Know," and "What I Need to Know." The clinician writes the words suggested by the students in two columns headed with the two questions. The article is then read by the SLP. The words in the two columns are checked for accuracy and completeness. A third column, "What I Learned," is added after listening to the article. Students are asked to summarize their findings orally, followed by preparing and completing a written rendition with outlines that include overall structure and sentence/word structure support. The same format, with a less predictable script, is followed using a new, but somewhat related, theme (from a current events activity related to social studies) that reads: "Rodman and Players Visit North Korea." The coin is now flipped and students take turns reading the Rodman article and then completing an outline for their peers. Outlines with helpful word/phrase choices are compared and a final rendition is created by the group.

Source: Based on Wallach (2014).

the nature of a teacher's instructional style to identify matches and mismatches between instructional language and a student's language abilities, as well as identifying instructional supports for language comprehension that are or are not provided, would be pieces of a classroom observation. Analyzing the language of textbooks and other curricular materials is also included in this aspect of the assessment process (Wallach, 2008).

Intervention

By way of introducing some of the elements of language intervention at school-age levels for students with SLD, consider another scenario, presented in Table 4.3, that highlights a portion of what Tim's intervention (recall the previous scenario) might look like at sixth or seventh grade. Although an SLP leads the students in the activity, the approaches and strategies illustrated in the scenario provide examples for others to use to scaffold students' learning. It reflects some of the elements of school-age/literacy-focused intervention that incorporate current research findings and practical applications. The language intervention includes helping students with SLD acquire the language *knowledge* (e.g., learning new words), *skills* (e.g., putting together a report), and *strategies* (e.g., figuring out what to do to complete a task) needed to access the curriculum (Ehren, 2009; Ehren, Murza et al., 2012; Ehren et al., 2014). The intervention is steeped in metalinguistic and metacognitive "practice." It integrates spoken and written language components with an eye toward facilitating language that would relate to the social studies' classroom with its inferential, predictive, and interpretive activities. The clever use of familiar content (basketball) *as a start* helps students "practice with" known content and context but with less familiar language and new strategies before they move on to more complicated, curricular-specific content (current events) and language. Taking background knowledge into consideration is a critical component of both spoken and written language comprehension and use of prior knowledge helps to reduce competing demands for resources, that is, avoiding overwhelming students with too much new information. When too many things "compete" for students' attention and memory, "something has to suffer." More sophisticated language, embedded in unfamiliar content and practiced with new strategies, creates competition for resource allocation for students with SLD. One of the several strategies employed in the scenario was the SLP's reading of the text initially to help the students focus on the comprehension and planning aspects of the activity. The scaffolds the SLP provided with visual maps and outlines and her work on macro (expository text) and micro (syntactic/word) levels are integrated within the activity. Clearly, many factors come together—student ability, SLP's choices, content, activities, sequence, timing, and dosage—to create a multidimensional and effective intervention (Wallach, 2014). The scenario illustrates how goals and objectives can be operationalized to provide *strategic* and *curriculum-relevant language intervention* for a heterogeneous group of students.

In the following sections a three-tiered framework for language intervention at school-age levels will be presented. The framework highlights some of the information currently available from research in speech-language pathology, general and special education, learning disabilities, and literacy, among many other disciplinary sources (Stone, Silliman, Ehren, & Wallach, 2014). We will also consider aspects of language intervention that go beyond working on core language deficits (Sun & Wallach, 2013), an especially important component for children and adolescents with ongoing language literacy and academic issues. We will then turn to a discussion of service models, with a particular focus on Responsiveness-to-Intervention (RtI) models and Common Core State Standards (CCSS).

A Three-Tiered Framework for Language Intervention at School-Age Levels. A number of questions help guide our intervention decisions. These reiterate a number of issues addressed in this chapter. For example:

- What language knowledge and skills does the student "bring" to the academic demands facing him/her?
- Will the goals and objectives of intervention help the student to access the curriculum?
- Will the goals and objectives of intervention improve his/her grades?
- Does the student comprehend what he/she is reading (or listening to from a lecture)?
- Does the student write reports and what are the characteristics of the reports?
- How does the student organize his/her thoughts in spoken and written text?
- Is there research to support intervention choices and where do these choices come from (Wallach et al., 2009)?

While only a sampling of questions one might ask, the focus is to keep the changing nature of students' language abilities (and disabilities) in mind within the context of changing language forms used to transmit curricular content (Ehren, Murza et al., 2012; Fang et al., 2014; Sun & Wallach, 2014).

Three overlapping components of language intervention are: (1) engaging students' background knowledge and interests into intervention choices as a starting point; (2) matching language intervention choices within the context of the specific requirements of curriculum content-area subjects; and (3) balancing content and structure knowledge in the search for meaning. A strong metalinguistic and metacognitive emphasis weaves its way throughout the discussion (Wallach et al., 2009; 2010; 2014).

Engaging Students' Background Knowledge and Interests into Intervention Choices. Helping students use their prior knowledge to express and reflect upon what they know, as well as to become aware of what they may not know and what they need to know, encourages them to be more actively involved in "attacking" (comprehending) spoken and written text (Wallach et al., 2014). Various research-based frameworks appear in the literature, including the TWA (**T**hink Before Reading, Think **W**hile Reading, Think **A**fter Reading) paradigm (Mason, Meadan, Hedin, & Corso, 2006) and various renditions of Ogle's (1986) K-W-L (What I **KNOW,** What I **WANT** to Know, What I **LEARNED**) model, and are highlighted in the intervention scenario (Wallach et al., 2010; 2014). The "What I know" element of Ogle's (1986) K-W-L model combines *before* and *during* reading (or listening) activities (McKeown, Beck, & Blake, 2009). The "What I learned" is an *after* reading (or listening) activity. A variation of the K-W-L activity has been described by Wallach et al. (2010), using "LL" as the element in the third column to represent "What I **LEARNED** about **LANGUAGE**." Table 4.4 provides an example using the Korean conflict as the curricular focus. Used as a tool to help students with SLD to develop a strong "meta" approach to tasks, the KWL/KWLL example, and others like it, demonstrates one way to facilitate students' linguistic and metalinguistic knowledge using curricular content as a backdrop (Ehren, 2013).

While there are many aspects of intervention at school-age levels that focus on specific aspects of content, form, and use components, activation of background knowledge is always a critical component. Using the K-W-LL format (Table 4.4), students are guided in their expression of "known" and "unknown" information. The students also summarize what they have learned about expository text, i.e., how to organize a cause/effect report, how/when to use selected connecting words. The final product will be the completion of a solid

TABLE 4.4 | An Example of the KWLL Model

K (What I **KNOW**)	W (What I **WANT** to Know)	LL (What I **LEARNED** about **LANGUAGE**)
■ Conflicts may cause wars. ■ The Korean War happened after World War II. ■ The country is still separated.	■ What caused this war? ■ What does it have to do with current events today? ■ What were some key battles during the war?	■ How to organize a cause/effect paragraph ■ The use of "connecting" words and phrases like *prewar, postwar, was caused by*

Source: Wallach (2008). © 2008 Geraldine P. Wallach.

current events report. This approach is not intended to "fill in" students' gaps in content knowledge, but rather to help students become active in using what they do know, identifying what they do not know, and discovering the metalinguistic and metacognitive strategies for finding their missing information in shared responsibility between general education teachers and specialists (Ehren, 2013).

Matching Language Intervention to Language Demands of Curricular Content. With school-age children an overall goal is to pair the foci of language intervention with students' curriculum content demands, as noted by Bashir in a classic chapter written in 1989. Intervention includes the meta-strategies that relate to those curriculum demands. Looking across curriculum, we see that expository text, complex and embedded syntax, and relational and abstract words and phrases predominate in textbooks and classroom instruction and influence academic success. However, it is important to keep focused on the specific language requirements of different elements of curriculum. For example, social studies and history include managing expository structure and abstract word meanings like *democracy, freedom, conflict,* in addition to understanding temporal orientation of events noted by temporal linguistic forms, evaluating sources, synthesizing information, and using prior knowledge to fully understand and retain historical information (Fang et al., 2014). Therefore, narrative discourse, with its character focus and temporally connected events, aligns more closely with language arts curricula and often with the social studies/history curricula rather than, for example, science curricula. Science involves managing a challenging quantity of technical terms and interlocking definitions and writing and thinking concisely in cause-effect and problem-solution modes (Fang et al., 2014; Wallach et al., 2014). Therefore, there is a greater alignment of science with, perhaps, procedural and/or explanatory discourse genres.

Connected Discourse (Macro structure work). Research in both narrative and expository text intervention suggests that explicit teaching of the overall structure of these genres, within a strong metalinguistic and metacognitive approach, improves their comprehension and use. Helping students understand the differences between narrative and expository text is also relevant as many students with SLD have difficulty organizing and retaining information from connected text and they have a limited understanding of "where to begin" and what is important to attend to when listening and/or writing (Boudreau, 2008; Nippold & Scott, 2009; Ward-Lonergan & Duthie, 2012). Singer and Bashir (2012) emphasize the use of guided practice and "self-talk" to help students with SLD learn to organize, comprehend, and write connected text. The use of a variety of different *graphic organizers* (Wallach, 2008; Ward-Lonergan & Duthrie, 2012; Westby, 1994) can help students to visualize the underlying structure of text while, at the same time, talking about the text. Figure 4.3 illustrates a graphic organizer for use with a historical fiction narrative. Students are taught to identify and use the story grammar elements (e.g., setting, problem) while filling in the important events from the story. The vertical arrangement provides students with a more accurate organization of a written report.

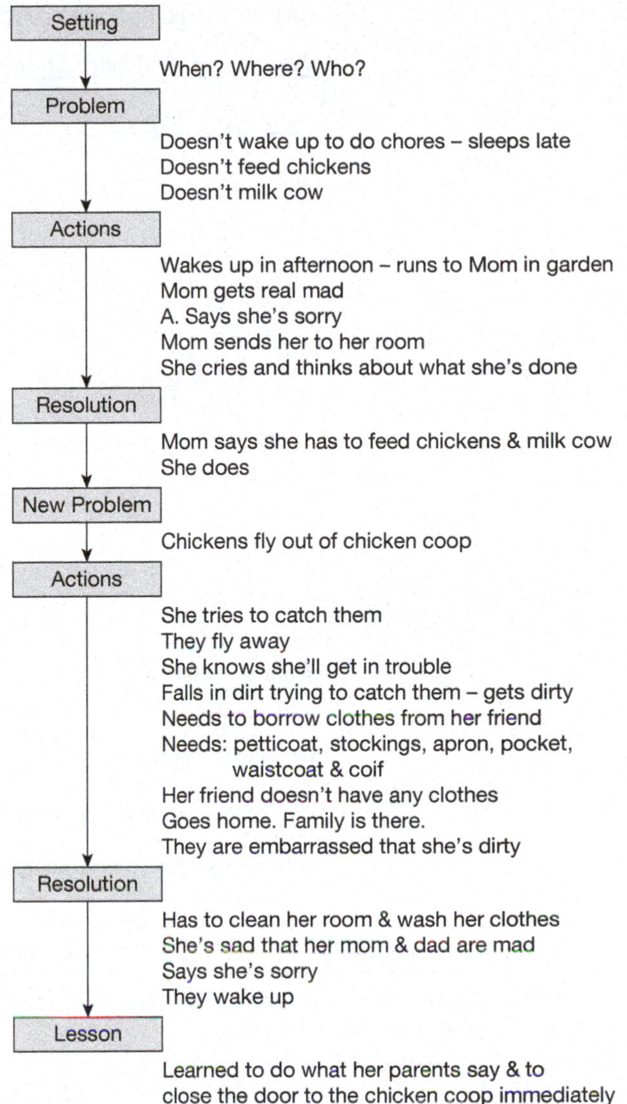

FIGURE 4.3 | A graphic organizer representing an accurate visual representation of the text structure of a narrative text.

Source: Singer and Bashir (2004).

Singer and Bashir (2004, 2012) remind us to match the appropriate graphic organizer to the activity and content-area requirements. The organizer in Figure 4.3, which is focused on story grammar for learning a historical fiction, would be inappropriate for learning about expository text. Singer and Bashir (2012) note that a vertical presentation, as opposed to using a horizontal organizer, might be a more accurate representation of what is required of the students, for example, to write a summary and book report. Singer and Bashir (2004) use a strategy they call the *EmPower* strategy to support students' writing. EmPower stands for **E**valuate, **M**ake a **P**lan, **O**rganize, **W**ork (write), **E**valuate (edit), and **R**ework and serves as a mnemonic and language scaffold to help students with SLD follow the steps needed to create summaries and reports.

Wallach (2008) used another type of graphic organizer to help fifth-grade students learn about a sub-genre of expository text, i.e., compare-contrast. Figure 4.4 shows this graphic organizer. Titles, sample sentences, and key words are highlighted, and syntactic and word level components are included in the activity that may span several weeks of work for the

SAMPLE TITLE FOR MY TOPIC:

Two wars in the United States **(Facts and Details)**

How I feel about wars **(Opinions and Feelings)**

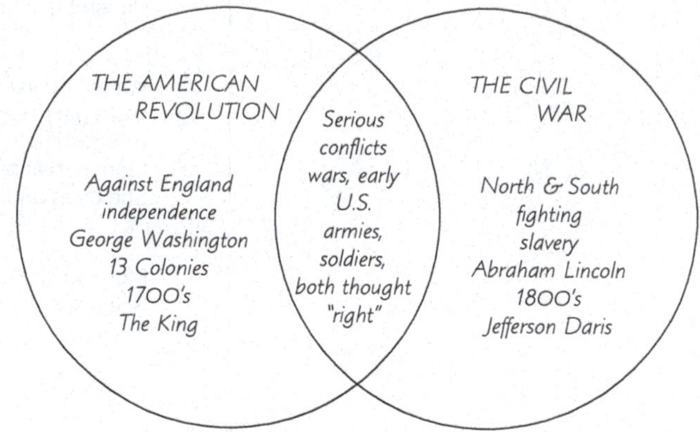

Sample Sentence: *The American Revolution and the Civil War are similar because they were serious conflicts.*

Linguistic "Glue" Words

Different, alike, although, on the other hand, compared with, rather than, same, similar, but, still, instead of . . .

A compare-contrast diagram using Grade 5 social studies as a backdrop for learning about expository text.

FIGURE 4.4 | A compare-contrast diagram using grade 5 social studies as a backdrop for learning expository text.

Source: Wallach (2008).

students. The scenario in Table 4.3 that introduced this section might start with a comparison activity, using a similar graphic organizer and having the students compare two basketball teams (e.g., the L.A. Lakers and Utah Jazz), before progressing to more complex text with less familiar content, for example, comparing the Korean War and World War II. However, we need to remember that different organizers are used for different text structures, and different tools and activities, some of which were illustrated in the intervention scenario (Table 4.3) with our sixth and seventh graders, for example, predicting what a title suggests about a text, underlining key words from passages, identifying different genres of text, and highlighting main ideas, would be chosen according to students' needs and abilities (Wallach et al., 2014).

Syntax, Words, and More (Micro structure work). In addition to macro-level abilities, intervention needs to include work on complex syntactic forms like passives and multiply embedded clausal sentences that are known to be problematic for school-age students with SLD (Scott, 2014; Scott & Koonce, 2014). Complex syntax permeates school texts and the requirements of writing as students move through the grades (Nippold, 2014), as does complex morphology. Emphasizing the importance of morphological savvy, Scott (2014) notes: "Given the status of verb morphosyntax errors as a clinical marker of young children with SLI, the tendency for these problems to surface in more complex linguistic contexts, as well as the need to relate and adjust verb markers across clauses and sentences in academic discourse, it makes a great deal of sense to target these forms in language intervention with older children and adolescents" (p. 148). She reminds us of the importance of connecting improvement of morphological ability to the demands of curricular content, not randomly choosing intervention targets from workbooks, as we shall see in our intervention section.

Recall the example previously in this chapter about the Boston Tea Party and the sentence, *The Boston Tea Party was the colonists' response to the unfair tax instituted the **prior** year by the British.* Wallach et al. (2009) provide examples of sentence combining by selecting the main propositions of the sentence (e.g., UNFAIR TAX/TEA PARTY) and using word banks to highlight key words, for example for the temporal word, *prior*, in the sentence, with choices like *before/prior, after/following, while/meanwhile,* to decide which should be used with the main propositions to unravel the who-did-what-to-whom-when in sentences. Another sentence provides an additional example: *A law was passed saying that no ship carrying colonial goods could leave Boston Harbor **until** the colonists had paid for all the tea that was destroyed.* Working again on key words (e.g., *until*) helps students understand how to deal with the who-did-what-to-whom-when challenge, but in this sentence there is also the opportunity to expand students' understanding of morphological relations (e.g., *colony, colonists, colonial*), another important element of intervention (Carlisle & Goodwin, 2014; Wallach, 2014). Scott (2014) provides a set of scaffolded interactions between clinicians/teachers and their students that serves to help students acquire higher levels of literate language forms. Although Scott addresses complex syntax, her recommendations can form a template for facilitating word and morphological awareness. Among the scaffolding interactions are:

- Discussion and illustration of the structure and meaning of a complex sentence (or target form). Modeling, reading to students, providing explicit examples, and engaging in other facilitative methods are among intervention techniques that can be used.
- Facilitation of awareness and identification. The students might read in unison and/or repeat sentences or use various computerized examples to "practice with" the targeted form.
- Active manipulation. Sentence combining tasks as above can be used in a type of "cut and paste" activity.
- Examination of text. The student searches for complex forms within a text and bolds or underlines the targeted form.

As per the scenario in Table 4.3, intervention starts with familiar topics and topics of interest and moves to curricular content once students grasp the strategic approach to making meaning.

Balancing Content and Structure Knowledge in the Search for Meaning. Language intervention for school-age students with SLD is multi-faceted and complex. It is not possible within the scope of this chapter to cover every approach and technique available. This section has emphasized selected language skills and strategies that related to content and disciplinary levels of literacy and provided a way to consider the integration of spoken and written language with meta-skills and strategies. Although young children with SLD (perhaps third grade and earlier) might need additional help with some of the foundational aspects of literacy, including developing phonological and phonemic awareness skills (Schuele & Boudreau, 2008; Troia, 2014), we need to help the students become more *actively* engaged in learning as they search to "make meaning" out of what they see and hear, regardless of where students are on the learning curve of academic success.

Clearly, developing the ability to manage connected text and acquiring advanced syntactic forms are among the linguistic underpinnings needed to unravel the complexity of unfamiliar curricular content. Likewise, having a repertoire of higher level and abstract vocabulary knowledge and naming ability, coupled with strategies for finding the meanings of unfamiliar words independently, are other elements on the intervention canvas. Because textbooks contain many relational words and phrases (e.g., *before, after, moreover, meanwhile, at a previous time*) and make high use of academic and abstract words (e.g., *evidence, method, integrate, identify, contribute*) (Lesaux, Kieffer, Faller, & Kelley, 2010), focusing intervention on these words within familiar and unfamiliar contexts and embedding them into connected texts, are additional ways to help students with SLD survive and thrive in their classrooms.

The interactions between structure (form) and content (semantics) knowledge create challenges in finding ways to balance them. McKeown and her colleagues (McKeown, Beck, & Blake, 2009) provide some insights into this complex interaction and balancing act. They divide students as "good" or "poor" readers and describe good readers as those who use background knowledge to interpret text (i.e., to figure out its meaning) and pay attention to the organization and structure of text, especially when topics are unfamiliar and informationally heavy, as those in curriculum. These and other insights (McKeown et al., 2009; Wallach, 2008) provide a picture of good readers that can help guide the focus of intervention:

- Proficient readers use linguistic information, as signaled by key words and phrases, to facilitate comprehension;
- Structural knowledge is especially important when the content is moderately or very unfamiliar to readers;
- Good readers use background knowledge when they have it, but background knowledge is most useful when a text is well structured; and
- Comprehension and retention are especially difficult if both background knowledge and structural knowledge are limited.

The efficacy research of McKeown and colleagues (2009) suggests that focusing on strategies that are directly related to the texts students are reading, i.e., social studies, science, and helping students to understand ways in which structural cues can help them get to meaning are most effective.

Beyond Core Linguistic Deficits: Keeping the Bigger Picture in Mind. We read in the previous chapter about preschoolers with SLI concerns about psychosocial issues. We will see these raised again in the next chapter, as well as here. Implied in our concerns is an underlying question: What are the ongoing effects of language impairment on social and emotional growth? We know that communicative ability is fundamental to building social relationships and social interactions. Being able to engage in both nonverbal (very early developmentally) and verbal dialogues helps to facilitate and nurture relationships with one's family, peers, and other members of the community (Sun & Wallach, 2013). Developing more nuanced aspects of language, such as discerning a speaker's intention, taking another's perspective, understanding different teachers' classroom rules, and manipulating one's language to meet the needs of the situation, are abilities that interface with socialization and the formation of peer relationships within and outside of the classroom. In a summary of longitudinal research, Brinton and Fujiki (2014) remind us that many children with early language and persistent language impairment have social and emotional problems that include, among others, trouble joining groups in play and negotiating and resolving conflicts or demonstrating anxiety or antisocial personality behaviors. On the other hand, some children with ongoing language difficulties do quite well. Nonetheless, the interactive nature of language and emotional components becomes apparent for many students within the SLD population. Consequently, Brinton and Fujiki (2014) encourage us to be mindful of the emotional components of SLD, writing that because

> . . . of this interactive relationship . . . managing the social and emotional issues associated with . . . [SLD] . . . may be as essential as managing linguistic deficits. (p. 174)

As we will see in the next chapter, these issues continue into adolescence (Wadman, Durkin, & Conti-Ramsden, 2011).

The 2001 World Health Organization's International Classification of Functioning, Disability and Health (WHO-ICF) provides a framework to think beyond the core linguistic deficits observed in school-aged children with SLD (Campbell & Skarakis-Doyle, 2007; Sun & Wallach, 2013). Implications of the WHO-ICF model point to the importance of an interprofessional team approach to planning and implementing intervention for children with SLD.

Sun and Wallach (2013) identify several guiding points for team members in implementing an interprofessional approach to intervention:

1. *Consider interpersonal interactions, relationships, and social life while assessing and providing intervention for students with SLD.* Assessment and intervention should cut across settings and intervention topics. Students might be observed across classroom, home, and other social settings. Discussions might include, not just topics that address academic content, but those that incorporate topics related to current school news, perspective taking and strategies that facilitate social competence.
2. *Observe and address environmental influences on language and social and behavioral functioning.* Similar to the above-mentioned suggestion, observation and intervention should take place in socially rich and flexible environments such as playgrounds, cafeterias, classrooms, or school clubs. Students' assessments of their own roles in social and academic situations are often helpful. Singer and Bashir's (2012) work in self-regulated learning, while not focusing specifically on social-emotional components, offer guidelines for managing more effectively interpersonal interactions.
3. *Write Individualized Education Programs (IEPs) that combine core linguistic deficits with emotional and social competence.* Information about students' linguistic abilities (e.g., form and content, discourse abilities) needs to be coupled with information about ways to manage communication breakdowns and find solutions, sometimes through language choices, for resolving social conflicts. Helping students develop effective strategies for perspective taking and recognizing their own emotional and social strengths should be weaved into core language goals and objectives.
4. *Offer a continuum of services for students with SLD that are interconnected among school-based professionals (e.g., social workers, SLPs, general and special educators, psychologists, counselors).* As suggested by Campbell and Skarakis-Doyle (2007): "Mutual exchange of knowledge and skills among team members" and "bridging boundaries between disciplines through a sharing conceptual framework and common language" (p. 526) are crucial for collaboration. Team members might share a set of socially relevant goals to provide concurrent and cohesive services to support generalization to other settings and communication partners.
5. *Recognize the role of language proficiency in expressing one's feelings and emotions.* Students with SLD often have difficulty elaborating on events, choosing words to express their feelings, or explaining their behaviors and motivations (Brinton & Fujiki, 2014). Sun and Wallach (2013, p. 62) suggest that "working on mental state verbs including metacognitive (e.g., *realize, understand, imagine*) and metalinguistic verbs (e.g., *explain, argue, agree*)," can help students come to recognize how these verbs play important roles in dealing with interpersonal interactions and improve their social and conversational understanding.

Changing Directions in Service Delivery and Educational Standards. Service delivery models provide guides that help professionals plan and implement assessment and intervention programs for children with SLD both within and outside of their classrooms. In the *traditional service delivery models,* sometimes referred to as "pullout" models, which are still used in many school settings, students leave their general education classrooms temporarily to receive services of specialists whose rooms are elsewhere in the school. Services can be provided individually to a student or to students who might be seen in small groups. In *in-class service delivery models,* sometimes called "push in" or "collaborative" models, services target groups of students within the classroom. In some cases services involve demonstrating sample language-literacy-based lessons, preferably with the classroom teacher, or team teaching during which language elements embedded in the curricular content are highlighted and disentangled. Various *consultative models,* sometimes called indirect service models, include making recommendations to teachers and other interprofessional team members. All models should be focused on providing curriculum-relevant intervention.

Two more recent ideas about serving students with SLD have emerged. These have the potential to increasingly change how students are identified for services and how the services are delivered.

Response to Intervention (RtI). The *Response to Intervention* (RtI) model has its foundations in the reauthorization of the Individuals with Disabilities Education Act (IDEA) (2004). With reauthorization, states were permitted to evaluate students' responses to scientific and research-based intervention and instruction before being tested, diagnosed, and/or streamed into special education (Wixson et al., 2014). RtI embraces a *prevention model* approach that contrasts with older models that were based upon school failure. Older models also often employed *discrepancy models,* sometimes called *cognitive referencing* models, which we know from our previous discussion in this chapter and the previous chapter, use IQ gaps between verbal and performance subtests, among other norm-referenced tools, to determine a student's eligibility for services in schools. Recall from Chapter 3 the discussion of standards of comparison. Criticism surrounds use of discrepancy models including the "disproportionate number of students from culturally and ethnically diverse groups of English language learners who are identified as learning disabled . . ." (Wixson et al., 2014, p. 637).

Ehren and Whitmire (2009) think of RtI as a framework for assisting students rather than a single model. In addition to instruction and intervention needing to be evidence based, principles and components of RtI include:

- Only qualified professionals who meet the accepted standards of their respective fields deliver the scientifically based instruction.
- Data on students' baseline performances are obtained and students are reassessed at regular intervals to determine and monitor their responses to instruction.
- Instructional approaches are modified as a result of students' progress data, and instructional approaches are implemented in increasingly intensive approaches if students do progress adequately in response to an earlier implemented instructional approach.

Ideas of "tiers" are commonly used to explain the increasingly intensive levels of instruction. RtI, in the beginning stages of implementation in many school systems, is a three-tiered system (with various modifications in different school districts) of service delivery (Moore & Montgomery, 2008; Roth & Troia, 2009; Staskowski & Rivera, 2005). Table 4.5 summarizes some of the features of each of the RtI tiers.

Common Core State Standards (CCSS). Another evolution occurring within school settings is the adoption of a new set of achievement standards across the grades that incorporate a number of specific language-based literacy milestones and expectations for students (National Governors Association Center for Best Practices and Council of Chief State School Officers, 2010). As these standards are implemented, in practice, across states, we may uncover new challenges conducting research that links evidence-based practices to our intervention choices for students with SLD (Whitmire, O'Rivers, Mele-McCarthy, & Staskowski, 2014). Because many of the standards relate to language-literacy achievement, SLPs, reading specialists, and special educators with expertise in language and literacy have primary roles as they consult with and advise general educators to create and deliver interprofessional, curriculum-relevant language-literacy intervention to students.

A brief review of selected standards demonstrates their language-loaded nature (National Governors Association Center for Best Practices and Council of Chief State School Officers, 2010). Examples include:

- First Grade Common Core State Standard related to Listening and Speaking
  Describe people, places, things, and events with relevant details, expressing ideas and feelings clearly
- Third Grade Common Core Standard related to Reading Comprehension
  Describe the relationship between a series of historical events, scientific ideas or concepts, or steps in technical procedures in text, using language that pertains to time, sequences, and cause/effect
- Fifth Grade Common Core Standard related to Morphology
  Use common grade-appropriate Greek and Latin affixes and roots as clues to the meaning of a word (e.g., photograph)

TABLE 4.5 | Features of RtI Tiers

Tiers	Features
Tier 1	■ Evidence-based practices typically delivered by general education teachers in their classrooms ■ Students are screened for their levels of performance ■ Formative assessment approaches used at frequent intervals to monitor progress ■ Forms of instruction differentiated for different students with the help of and consultation with other professionals such as speech-language pathologists ■ Language and literacy consultation re: strategies to help in the development of effective language and literacy instruction
Tier 2	■ Intervention may be implemented as a result of findings from a screening ■ Instruction focuses on each student's specific educational and language literacy needs ■ Instruction delivered by a combination of professionals, including, for example, the speech-language pathologist and/or classroom teacher ■ Instruction may occur in small groups ■ Progress is monitored frequently ■ If a student fails to respond in interventions in Tier 2, a more comprehensive assessment may be warranted
Tier 3	■ Targeted intervention and/or specialized treatment occurs in this tier for specific academic needs ■ Delivered by any appropriate specialists in consultation with general and special education teachers ■ Intervention occurs on an intensive basis often in small groups or individually ■ Team consultation continues ■ Progress monitored frequently ■ Specific language-literacy focused intervention that is curriculum relevant Some frameworks of RtI consider Tier 3 instruction as a form of special education, whereas other frameworks of RtI have special education as a fourth tier.

Sources: Moore and Montgomery (2008); Roth and Troia (2009); Staskowski and Rivera (2005); Troia (2005).

Epilogue

The road from language impairment to SLD may be a long and bumpy one for Tim (Sun & Wallach, 2014). The literature is, however, rich with information that provides us with innovative and evidenced-based techniques to improve services for students with SLD. Clearly, understanding the role that language plays in school learning and its impact upon children with SLD is critical to their success. Students with SLD with language learning problems have many challenges, especially as they move from the early grades and the task of learning to read and write to later grades where curricular content becomes more demanding and as they become more aware of their own difficulties.

Clinicians and educators have a shared responsibility on the road to understanding fully the ways that SLI and SLD interact and intersect with one another. Professionals are also challenged to interpret carefully the significance (or not) of co-existing conditions like CAPD and ADHD, and their associated behaviors, in SLI and SLD populations (Shaywitz, Fletcher, & Shaywitz, 1995). It is essential to view behaviors that often surround SLD, like attentional difficulties, impulsivity, and social-emotional problems, as part of the larger context in which they occur. As professionals in regular and special education become more familiar with the CCSS, they will see that integration of basic communicative processes (i.e., language processes and skills) is at the heart of current thinking about academic success (Haager & Vaughn, 2013; National Governors Association Center for Best Practices and Council of Chief State School Officers, 2010). Incorporating techniques into intervention that help the children become more "meta" and strategic about their choices are pieces of this complex puzzle and particularly as they progress into the secondary grades and later as they transition into the workforce (Ehren et al., 2014). Finally, we must also remember that while labels may be appropriate for shoes, dresses, and other goods, they do not reflect the complex and ever-changing nature of children and the environments in which they must learn. The children need more from intervention.

SUMMARY

In this chapter we have seen that

- Children with language impairment and learning disabilities are members of overlapping populations. While different terms have been used to refer to these children, such as *Specific Language Impairment (SLI), Specific Learning Disabilities (SLD), Dyslexic,* and *Language Learning Disabled (LLD),* among others, the primacy of language must be understood across contexts, time, and learning tasks.
- Learning disabilities emerged as a diagnostic category in the 1960s and has since been redefined several times and across different disciplines.
- Children's labels may change due to the ways language impairment manifests itself once children enter school and to school professionals' orientations and backgrounds.
- Language impairment shows itself differently across time and learning tasks, across spoken and written language, and across spontaneous and metalinguistic levels of language.
- Spoken and written language form a reciprocal relationship that influences the development of both systems and informs the direction and focus of intervention for students with SLD.
- Language assessment and intervention for school-age students with SLD should be focused on the demands of the academic environment and with emphasis on helping students acquire the language knowledge, skills, and strategies needed to access the curriculum with its changing language demands.
- The demands of different content areas (e.g., science, social studies, language arts) must be understood by specialists, general educators, and special educators so that students with SLD not only "read to learn" but they also "learn to read (again)" to manage the different linguistic requirements of each subject.
- The impact of language upon social and emotional growth and self-concept development (and vice versa) should be a component of assessment and intervention. Many children with SLD have continuing pragmatic language difficulties.
- Educational models of service delivery are evolving with RtI frameworks providing a three-tiered level of services to replace traditional discrepancy models of identification and intervention.
- Common Core State Standards are among the new directions that will drive core curricular and intervention directions with school-based professionals taking on new and exciting challenges.

5

Adolescents with Language Impairment

LEARNING OBJECTIVES

After reading this chapter, you should be able to

- Explain why adolescents with language impairment are described as an increasingly recognized yet underserved group with significant problems
- Describe characteristics of adolescents with language impairment
- Discuss issues related to assessment for adolescents with language impairment
- Discuss issues related to intervention for adolescents with language impairment

The developmental period known as adolescence is generally described as beginning at about 11 to 12 years of age and, in Western societies, continuing until 18 to 21 years of age, depending on which theory of adolescent development is being used. During these years, considerable cognitive, physiological, emotional, social, and educational changes occur. Language changes too, and the changes in language are both affected by and affect other areas of development. When an adolescent experiences a language impairment, whether the impairment is severe or whether it is less severe so that the adolescent's language is more likely to be shaky or, using Nelson's (1998) words, "almost but not quite" right (p. 223), the teenager is at risk for problems in all areas of development.

Knowledge about adolescents with language impairment remains incomplete, especially for those adolescents whose language problems exist in the absence of other conditions known to affect language, such as specific language impairment (SLI), described in Chapter 3 with regard to preschoolers. What we do know, however, is that young children with SLI mature into adolescents with SLI. As was clear in the previous two chapters, SLI is not a "curable" condition, but it is a manageable condition with appropriate intervention across ages and grades. In the previous chapter on language and learning disabilities, we made the point that many of the children considered to be learning disabled had been preschoolers with SLI (whether or not their language impairment had actually been identified) and that they continued to be SLI (and therefore have language problems) when they entered school even if the label for their problems was changed to "learning disability" or if they retained a label of "language impaired" in addition to "learning disability." These children grow up and many enter adolescence with continuing language problems and accompanying learning difficulties. In summarizing the results of her study, Rescorla (2009) writes that "slow language development at 24–31 months is associated with a weakness in language-related skills into adolescence relative to skills manifested by typically developing peers" (p. 16).

As we will see in this chapter, adolescents with language impairment do not constitute an inconsequential group, and the problems they encounter because of their language impairment are anything but inconsequential. However, many adolescents with language impairment remain unidentified or underrecognized, unserved, underserved, and/or neglected (Apel, 1999a; Joffe & Nippold, 2012; Nippold, 2010b; Vance & Clegg, 2010). In this chapter, we discuss why this group remains relatively underrecognized, problems related to language impairment in adolescence, and assessment and intervention factors that are particularly relevant to this group.

AN INCREASINGLY RECOGNIZED YET UNDERSERVED GROUP WITH SIGNIFICANT PROBLEMS

When this chapter on adolescents with language impairment first appeared about 30 years ago in the 1986 edition of this book, the amount of information in the literature about these teenagers was extremely limited compared to what was available about youngsters with language impairment. Some even believed that there was no need for the chapter! Some 30 years later, it is encouraging and refreshing to see the increase in the literature that addresses issues related to adolescents who continue to demonstrate language impairment. Indeed, Joffe and Nippold (2012, p. 438) echoed this sentiment in their prologue, entitled "Progress in Understanding Adolescent Language Disorders," which introduced the 2012 clinical forum on language and communication disorders in adolescents in the journal *Language, Speech, and Hearing Services in Schools*. In looking back, the title for this section of the current chapter has morphed over the years from the first title, "The Problem," to "The Continuing Problem" to "A Neglected Group with Significant Problems" to "An Underrecognized Group with Significant Problems" to the current title, "An Increasingly Recognized Yet Underserved Group with Significant Problems." The changes reflect this increased attention to adolescents with language impairment but also convey that we are "not there yet" in terms of the following:

- The services provided for these teenagers for whom, compared to services for elementary school students, sadly remain either underserved or unserved
- Our preparation of university students to serve, when they graduate, these adolescents—preparation which remains largely hit and miss in universities' curricula
- Our knowledge from research that helps us to fill the gaps in our understanding about the nature of the adolescents' language and related problems and how to develop and deliver evidence-based intervention programs

Even today, there may be some readers who are surprised to learn that there are adolescents with language impairment and that the extent of the problems associated with the population warrants an entire chapter devoted to this group of individuals.

The Shape of Adolescent Language Impairment

The evidence continues to mount that problems associated with language impairment, in the absence of other conditions such as hearing loss, intellectual limitations, and physical disabilities, persist into adolescence and even adulthood or can even emerge during adolescence, with just a few publications in the 1980s (e.g., Aram, Ekelman, & Nation, 1984) and numbers increasing steadily to a fairly consistent stream of publications since the millennium (e.g., Beitchman, Wilson, Johnson et al., 2001; Bryan, Garvani, Gregory, & Kilner, 2015; Mok, Pickles, Durkin, & Conti-Ramsden, 2014). The evidence now is convincing that adolescents' language problems can affect their personal relationships, academic success during junior and senior high school, choice of vocational and professional careers, and subsequent earning power. That adolescents with language impairment typically perform poorly academically should come as no surprise because, as we have seen in the previous chapter, language ability is a well-recognized factor in students acquiring basic academic skills, skills that most obviously include learning to read and literacy but that can also include mathematical abilities (Alt, Arizmendi, & Beal, 2014; Donlan, Cowan, Newton, & Lloyd, 2007; Fazio, 1994, 1996; Johnson, Beitchman, & Brownlie, 2010; Nys, Content, & Leybaerta, 2013). In extending the effects of language problems on learning, it should also come as no surprise that these problems affect what, if any, postsecondary education is undertaken (Clegg, Hollis, Mawhood, & Rutter, 2005; Durkin, Simkin, Knox, & Conti-Ramsden, 2009; Hall & Tomblin, 1978; Johnson et al., 2010) and how well an individual is able to achieve independence, to cope, and to achieve in the workplace (Conti-Ramsden & Durkin, 2008; Law, Rush, Schoon, & Parsons, 2009; Whitehouse, Watt, Line, & Bishop, 2009). Clegg and her colleagues (2009) looked at the language abilities of adolescents who were at risk for expulsion from secondary school because of behavior problems and concluded that "for a high proportion of secondary age pupils at risk of permanent school exclusion, language difficulties are a factor in their behaviour problems and school exclusion" (p. 123).

Socioemotional difficulties are a significant issue for adolescents with language impairment. In earlier chapters, we saw how problems with social interactions and even socioemotional difficulties are associated with specific language impairment in preschool years and language-learning disabilities in the earlier school years. These problems are seen in the difficulties students have in establishing and maintaining positive interpersonal relationships, as evidenced in a significant number of publications, among them Asher and Gazelle (1999), Conti-Ramsden and Botting (2004), Durkin and Conti-Ramsden (2007, 2010), Lindsay, Dockrell, and Strand (2007), and Snowling, Bishop, Stothard, Chipchase, and Kaplan (2006), as well as others shown in Table 5.1. Although behavior issues associated with externalizing characteristics (e.g., oppositional behavior, hyperactivity, conduct problems) have sometimes been reported for adolescents with language problems (Beitchman, Wilson, Brownlie, Walters, Inglis, et al., 1996; Botting & Conti-Ramsden, 2000; Clegg et al., 2009; Cohen, Farnia, & Im-Bolter, 2013). It appears that these adolescents may be more apt to demonstrate problematic behaviors related to internalizing difficulties (e.g., withdrawal behaviors, shyness, limited friendship, social phobia, and social initiation problems) (Beitchman, Wilson, Johnson et al., 2001; Conti-Ramsden & Botting, 2004; Wadman, Durkin, & Conti-Ramsden, 2008). Internalizing difficulties have been types of problems reported also in younger school-age children with SLI (Fujiki, Brinton, Isaacson, & Summers, 2001; Fujiki, Brinton, Morgan, & Hart, 1999). In their meta-analyses of research addressing emotional and behavioral outcomes later in childhood and adolescence for children with specific language impairments, Yew and O'Kearney (2013) concluded that "relative to typical children, SLI children experience clinically important increases in the severity of diverse emotional, behavioural . . . symptoms and more frequently show a clinical level of these problems" (p. 516). There are some indications that students with SLI have difficulties with emotion regulation, a psychosocial issue that could be expected to affect interpersonal relationships (Fujiki, Brinton, & Clarke, 2002), as well as other evidence that has begun to document a decline in their self-esteem as the students mature and progress in school (Jerome, Fujiki, Brinton, & James, 2002; Lindsay & Dockrell, 2012; Wadman et al., 2008). Along with language impairment, these socioemotional and behavioral issues can persist across childhood and into adolescence (St Clair, Pickles, Durkin, & Conti-Ramsden, 2011).

In an early study of the relationship between socioemotional problems and language abilities in older children and adolescents, 71 percent of the students (aged 8 to 13 years) in a school setting who had been identified as having mild/moderate behavioral disorders had language scores between one and two standard deviations (1 to 2 SD) below the means for the normative sample (Camarata, Hughes, & Ruhl, 1988). Sadly, none of the students had had language evaluations prior to the data collection for that research project. Even sadder is the reality that students exhibiting a variety of behavioral issues continue not to routinely receive language evaluations, so that their language impairment often goes unidentified (Hollo, Wehby, & Oliver, 2014). As examples, Walsh, Scullion, Burns, MacEvilly, and

TABLE 5.1 | Characteristics of Adolescents and Adults at Follow-Up Who Had Language Impairment Identified in Their Preschool or Elementary School Years

Researchers	Age(s) of First Identification of Language Impairment	Age(s) at Follow-Up Assessment	Characteristics at Follow-Up			
			Language Ability	*Reading and Academic Ability*	*Social/Emotional/Behavioral Characteristics*	*Other*
Aram et al. (1984)	3;5–6;11	13;3–16;10	90% of subjects had language scores in moderately to profoundly delayed range	—More than 50% of subjects below 25th-percentile rank on reading and spelling measures —75% received special academic assistance*	Greater prevalence of behavior problems than peers	
Hall & Tomblin (1978)	Mean ages: 6;1 language-impaired (LI) group 6;4 articulation-impaired (AI) group	Mean ages: 22;3 LI 23;0 AI	50% of LI continued to have language problems as adults; 5.5% of AI continued to have articulation problems	From grades 3 through 12, LI scored significantly lower on composite scores of academic achievement tests than AI at each grade level except grade 3		Less postsecondary education pursued/achieved by LIs than AIs
Weiner (1974) (case study)	4 years old	16 years old	—Continuing semantic delay —Continuing morphological and syntax problems	—Second-grade reading level —Placed in work-study special education program in spite of normal nonverbal IQ	Ignored/teased by teenage peers	
Beitchman, Brownlie, et al. (1996) Beitchman, Wilson, Brownlie, Walters, Inglis, et al. (1996) Beitchman, Wilson, Brownlie, Walters, & Lancee (1996)	5 years old	12;6 years old	Continued significant delays in receptive and expressive language performance	—Significantly lower educational achievement test scores than subjects without language impairment —About 50% had received special academic assistance	—Increased risk/presence of psychiatric disorder in adolescence —Less participation in extracurricular nonsports activities and organizations —Behavior difficulties more apparent in school environment than at home —Rated as less socially competent —Links to externalizing and internalizing behavior problems	

Johnson et al. (1999) Beitchman, Wilson, Johnson, et al. (2001)	5 years old	19 years old	—Continued significant delays in receptive and expressive language performance (means below –1 SD) —Only 50% had received speech/language intervention, even in early school years	Significantly poorer reading, spelling, and math test scores than subjects with no language impairment at 5 years of age	—Elevated rates of anxiety disorder (social phobia the most common anxiety disorder) —Likelihood of antisocial personality disorder	For language-impaired subjects, a decline in performance IQ with advancing age into early adulthood
Johnson et al. (2010)	5 years old	25 years old	Receptive vocabulary within normal limits but significantly lower than normal (unaffected) peers	Compared to unaffected peers, young adults with SLI —Performance IQ within normal limits but significantly lower —Reading comprehension borderline but significantly lower —Arithmetic abilities at lower end of normal and significantly lower than peers —Fewer individuals with SLI completed high school or university levels	—Early parenthood for 35% of SLI adults vs. 15% for unaffected peers —No difference in marital status or living with partner	—Lower socioeconomic status than unaffected peers —Fewer with salaries in highest income bracket —No self-perceived difference in satisfaction with quality of life
Tomblin, Freese, & Records (1992)	Mean age: 8;6	Mean age: 21;6	LI young adults significantly poorer than the young adults without early LI for —Receptive single-word vocabulary —Use of well-formed sentences —Confrontation naming speed —Sentence imitation; speaking rate	LIs significantly poorer than the young adults without early LI for —Oral and written spelling —Reading comprehension	Socioeconomic status of LI subjects' families based on their fathers' occupations lower than that of young adults without early LI	LIs significantly poorer than adults without early LI for —Auditory perception of rapid temporal information —Performance IQ

(Continued)

TABLE 5.1 | *Continued*

Researchers	Age(s) of First Identification of Language Impairment	Age(s) at Follow-Up Assessment	Characteristics at Follow-Up			
			Language Ability	*Reading and Academic Ability*	*Social/Emotional/Behavioral Characteristics*	*Other*
			—Interpreting agent–action questions for semantic acceptability —Token test performance —Word fluency			
Conti-Ramsden, Botting, Simkin, & Knox (2001)	7 years old	11 years old	—Receptive and/or expressive vocabulary and/or morphology/syntax below 16th-percentile rank —88.5% still had low language scores (below 16th-percentile rank)	—Two-thirds below the normal range on single-word reading —80% below normal on reading comprehension		About 25% showed declines in nonverbal IQ to levels below normal
Conti-Ramsden, Durkin, Simkin, & Knox (2009) Conti-Ramsden, St Clair, Pickles, & Durkin (2012) Mok et al. (2014)	7 years old	17 years old	—Expressive language scores below –1 SD —Receptive and expressive language lower than unaffected (normally developing) peers —Steady growth in language skills between ages 7 and 17 years although remaining at lower levels	—SLIs reading comprehension below –1 SD level —44% of SLIs achieved at least 1 expected qualification for secondary school credential (approximately a high school diploma); 88% of unaffected peers achieved same level —53% of SLIs achieved low or minimal level qualification compared to 11% of unaffected peers —25% of SLIs did not complete any secondary school credentialing	—About 60% had peer-relation problems beginning in childhood and persisting into adolescence or adolescent-onset peer-relation problems	—Approximately 33% of SLIs who, at age 7, had lower nonverbal IQ than other SLIs, albeit still within normal limits, showed deceleration in nonverbal IQ over 10 years to age 17 —66% of SLIs showed stable pattern of growth from ages 7 to 17

Stothard, Snowling, Bishop, Chipchase, & Kaplan (1998)	3;9–4;2 Retested at 5;6 years and groups formed, among them: —"Resolved" language delay at 5;6 years —"Persistent" language impairment at 5;6 years	15–16-year-olds	—Persistent LI group: all measures below –1 SD and several approaching –2 SD level —Significant decrease in vocabulary between 8 and 15 years of age —"Resolved" language delay group: most measures at lower end of normal range; significantly lower than control group (normal language) on four of eight measures	—Persistent LI group: 95% scored below 12-year level for reading and spelling; performances at –2 SD level; 50% received no special academic assistance, 30% tutoring, and 20% placed in special classes/ schools —"Resolved" language-delay group: 52% scored below 12-year level for reading and spelling; performances mostly at lower end of normal range		—For persistent LI group, a decline in nonverbal IQ between "normal" nonverbal IQ in preschool years to ~50% with scores below –1 SD
Clegg et al. (2005)	Mean age: 9;11	Mean age: 36;2	—11;9 age equivalent of receptive vocabulary —11;1 age equivalent of expressive vocabulary —No change in receptive and expressive language past early 20s —Significantly lower language than unaffected siblings —Sentence repetition lower than unaffected siblings —Nonword repetition lower than unaffected siblings	—Significant and severe literacy deficits —9-year age equivalency for reading and spelling compared to 14–16-year age equivalency for unaffected peers —94% of SLIs did not pass secondary school examinations at expected chronological age of 16 years or at any time thereafter; did not attain a certificate of secondary education (approximately high school diploma)	—About 50% had limited range of friendships —30% still bullied or teased —25% living with partner at follow-up; ~30% had lived as married for ±1 month —Higher scores on tests of psychiatric morbidity, especially items for social anxiety, no close friends, odd speech	—Performance IQ within normal limits; similar levels to unaffected siblings —60% employed at time of follow up but only 17% had been in continuous employment since leaving secondary school —Two-thirds had periods of unemployment of ±2 years; 18% never had any paid employment

(*Continued*)

TABLE 5.1 | *Continued*

Researchers	Age(s) of First Identification of Language Impairment	Age(s) at Follow-Up Assessment	Characteristics at Follow-Up			
			Language Ability	*Reading and Academic Ability*	*Social/Emotional/Behavioral Characteristics*	*Other*
			—Significantly impaired theory of mind**	—About 50% subsequently attended adult education course or technical/apprenticeship experience; ~50% no training/education beyond age 16 years		—41% had been dismissed from one or more jobs —40% living independently; others reliant on parents for support
Rice & Hoffman (2015)	Mean age: 6;11	21 years of age	—Receptive vocabulary (per Peabody Picture Vocabulary Test scores) lower for SLIs than unaffected peers at first measurement —SLIs' scores remained below those of unaffected peers across years —SLIs did not catch up			

*"Special academic assistance" consisted of special education services, tutoring, remedial instruction, and/or special classroom/special school placement.

** Theory of mind is a person's ability to attribute mental states to themselves and others, allowing people to predict, judge, and explain others' behavior and understand social interactions.

Brosnan (2014), in their investigation of older children and adolescents with primary diagnoses of attention deficit/hyperactivity disorder (ADHD), reported that "almost three-quarters of the study cohort had *previously undetected language difficulties* [emphasis added], with over 70% of those having both receptive and expressive language difficulties" (p. 59), and Joffe and Black (2012), reporting on the adolescents in their study, wrote that "though underperforming academically, the students' language difficulties had not previously been recognized and the students were receiving no specialist support" (p. 468).

In other reports focusing on students with problem behaviors, Kauffman (2001) has suggested that these pupils demonstrate difficulties in relating to peers and in making and keeping friends, and Marcon (1998) found that for a group of high school graduates, their kindergarten language abilities differentiated those who had been identified on leaving high school as demonstrating significant maladaptive behaviors from those showing no significant maladaptive behaviors. As expected, those adolescents with the lower early language skills fell mostly into the maladaptive group. A 50 to 70 percent co-occurrence rate of emotional or behavioral difficulties in school-age children and speech and language problems has been suggested in some of the literature (Hummel & Prizant, 1993; Prizant et al., 1990), and in one study the proportion of children who had received treatment for behavioral or emotional problems who also had language impairment ranged from 60 to 95 percent (Cohen, Davine, Horodezky, Lipsett, & Isaacson, 1993).

Not surprisingly, the problems adolescents have in establishing and maintaining positive interpersonal relationships frequently affect their relationships with their peers, teachers, and even with their parents and siblings (Durkin & Conti-Ramsden, 2007, 2010; Lindsay et al., 2007; Mok et al., 2014). Difficulties with peer relationships are particularly concerning for adolescents, for whom having conversations with friends provides important sources of support and influences identity and group affiliation (Thurlow, 2005). There is also evidence that, although the amount of time older children and adolescents spend talking with friends increases into the teenage years, this increase seems not to replace the amount of time they spend talking with family members (Raffaelli & Duckett, 1989). These results suggest that, overall, teenagers spend more time in discourse with others, meaning that conversational abilities take on greater importance as children mature into adolescents and can have increasing implications for the quality of interpersonal relationships.

Several longitudinal studies have followed children, whose language impairment was identified in their early years, into adolescence and even adulthood and reported on how these individuals have fared in their later years. As early as 1984 Aram et al. realized that "language disorders recognized in the preschool years are only the beginning of long-standing language, academic, and often behavioral problems" (p. 240). Some of the academic, language, and social, emotional, and behavioral outcomes for adolescents who were identified first as language impaired either in the preschool years or in the early school years are summarized in Table 5.1.

Parents of adolescents with SLI have expressed a number of concerns about outcomes for their teenagers (Conti-Ramsden & Botting, 2004; Conti-Ramsden, Botting, & Durkin, 2008; Hughes, Turkstra, & Wulfeck, 2009; Joffe & Black, 2012; Lindsay & Dockrell, 2004; Pratt, Botting, & Conti-Ramsden, 2006). Among the parental concerns, which are more frequently expressed or different from those of other parents, are the following:

- Relatively negative expectations for the adolescents' future and life as an adult
- Limited employment options and lack of independence
- Difficulties with social relationships and socialization
- Conduct problems
- Narrowed educational pursuits
- Limited community resources to support the adolescents in their adulthood
- The adolescents' potential vulnerability to victimization and/or experiences having been bullied

As we see above and will see in our discussion below, these parental concerns may be justified.

TABLE 5.2 | Different Types of Credentials with Which Adolescents with Speech or Language Impairments and Specific Learning Disabilities Left School, Compared to Total Students in Special Education, in 2004–2005 School Year, Excluding Students Moved into General (Regular) Education

Types of Credential on Leaving High School	Types of Disability		
	Speech or Language Impairments	*Specific Learning Disabilities*	*Total Students in Special Education*
Left with a diploma	67%	61%	57%
Left with a certificate	12%	14%	17%
Left with no credential	21%	25%	26%

Source: U.S. Department of Education (2006).

Personal and Societal Costs of Adolescent Language Impairment

While a language impairment in adolescence potentially limits opportunities for an individual's personal, vocational, and economic self-realization, the problem is not just the individual's. It is also society's problem. Undereducation and underemployment are common outcomes of a language impairment (Clegg et al., 2005; Johnson et al., 2010; Law et al., 2009; Whitehouse et al., 2009). As a result, potentially valuable human resources and contributions are wasted. In some instances, rather than contributing to society as a self-sufficient adult when the underlying potential to do so may have existed, an individual with residual language problems takes from society.

Adolescents with language impairment are at risk for leaving school before earning their full high school diploma (or equivalent), that is, dropping out (Clegg et al., 2005; Conti-Ramsden et al., 2009; Johnson et al., 2010). Table 5.2 shows data from the U.S. Department of Education (2006) indicating the percentage of adolescents with speech or language impairment in the 2004–2005 school year who left high school with a diploma or a certificate or either dropped out or otherwise left without receiving a formal credential. Because we know that a large number of adolescents labeled as having a specific learning disability have language impairment, data for this group of adolescents with a disability are also presented. As is evident, about one-third of the adolescents with speech or language impairment and a similar percent (36 percent) of those with specific learning disabilities either dropped out or otherwise left high school without receiving a formal credential or left with a certificate rather than a diploma. In Western societies, these individuals are likely to have difficulty finding long-term gainful employment, if any employment at all. Students who are at risk for dropping out or who have dropped out are more likely to be the individuals associated with juvenile delinquency, drug and alcohol abuse, and even youth suicide. Related issues involve states' efforts in the last several years to improve students' achievement scores on benchmarking tests and to reduce the number of students on the special education rolls and possible effects of Response-to-Intervention (RtI) activities that encourage assessment and trial interventions before initiating formal diagnostic testing and possible placement in special education.

A particular trend is states' moving some students from special education to general/regular education as students transition from elementary to secondary grades. This trend is notable for children who received speech or language services as elementary students. Figure 5.1 illustrates the percentage of students between 14 and 21 years of age who moved from special education to general education (regular education) in 2004–2005, the same academic year for which data on students leaving schools without diplomas were presented in Table 5.2. It is interesting to note that between 40 and 45 percent of students 14 to 21 years of age who had been classified as speech and/or language impaired for special education in previous grades were moved into regular/general education, while 10 percent of the same-age students classified as specific learning disabled in previous grades were moved into regular/general

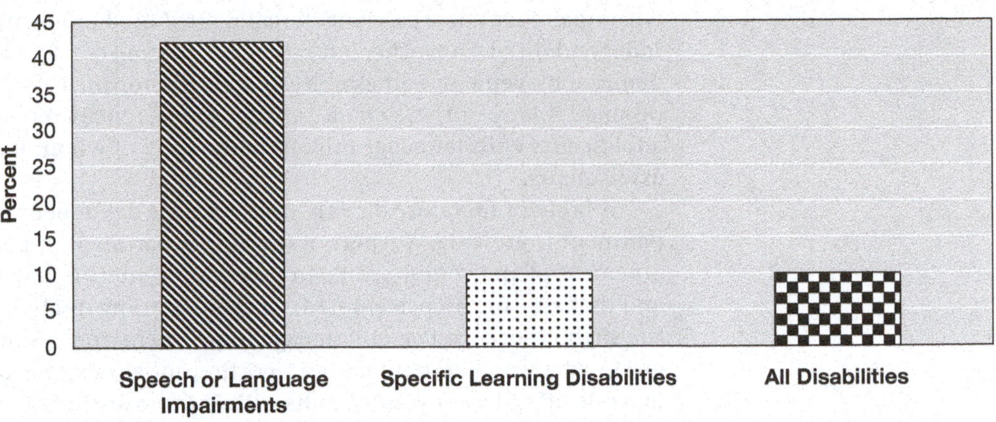

FIGURE 5.1 | Percentage of Students between 14 and 21 Years of Age Moved from Special Education to General Education (Regular Education) according to 2004–2005 Data

Source: U.S. Department of Education (2006).

education. The percentage for the total number of students 14 to 21 years of age moved from special education to regular/general education was also 10 percent. The reasons for so many adolescents with speech and/or language impairments being reclassified from special education to regular/general education are worth investigation to determine if the teenagers legitimately no longer need special education support services or if other motivations led to their being moved into regular/general education. Even considering the 2004–2005 data, a substantial percentage of adolescents with speech and/or language impairments drop out of high school, that is, leave with no credential.

In adolescence, juvenile delinquency, youth suicide, and drug and alcohol abuse have been linked to deficits in basic skills, including speaking and listening abilities. A relationship between juvenile delinquency and adolescent language impairment is beginning to be documented in the literature, even though there has been some degree of awareness of a link between communication impairment and adult prison populations for several years. A comparison of the oft-cited characteristics of adolescents at risk for juvenile delinquency or those already in detention and the characteristics commonly associated with adolescents with language impairment shows considerable overlap and correspondence. For example, some of the characteristics that have been attributed to juvenile offenders or those at risk for juvenile delinquency include difficulties with interpersonal and social relationships, problems with emotional control, poor academic achievement including reading and writing difficulties, presence of learning disabilities, specific phonological deficits, and discrepancies between verbal IQ and nonverbal IQ scores, with nonverbal scores better than verbal scores (e.g., Archwamety & Katsiyannis, 2000; Bigelow, 2000; Foley, 2001; Kirk & Reid, 2001; Snowling, Adams, Bowyer-Crane, & Tobin, 2000). According to Svensson, Lundberg, and Jacobson (2001), over 50 percent of youths in juvenile detention centers have significant reading or written-language problems. Doren, Bullis, and Benz (1996) examined what factors of students with disabilities predict their arrest. Their results indicated the following:

- Students with specific learning disabilities were almost four times more likely to be arrested than other students with disabilities.
- Students with poor social and/or personal adjustment were 2.3 times more likely to be arrested than other students with disabilities.
- Students with disabilities who left school without graduating were almost six times more likely to be arrested than other students with disabilities.

This last factor can be considered together with the information we saw in Table 5.2 about the percentages of adolescents with speech–language impairments who leave high school with no credential. The characteristics attributed to juvenile offenders are logically not independent of each other but rather are interrelated, for example, poor reading and academic achievement, verbal/nonverbal IQ discrepancies, and a diagnostic tag of learning disabled. Many of these characteristics sound remarkably like attributes of children and adolescents with language impairment, many of whom had not had previous language assessments.

A body of literature directly links juvenile delinquency and adolescent language impairment is growing. A report of the U.S. Department of Education (1999) indicated that 3 percent of the young people in detention centers had speech or language impairment and that another 45 percent had a specific learning disability, which is notable because of the high co-occurrence of language impairment and specific learning disability. Several groups of researchers have started reporting on various language abilities of male and female juvenile offenders or young adults with SLI who are involved with the legal system (Bryan et al., 2015; Davis, Sanger, & Morris-Friehe, 1991; Hopkins, Clegg, & Stackhouse, 2016; Rosta & McGregor, 2012; Sanger, 1999; Sanger, Creswell, Dworak, & Schultz, 2000; Sanger, Hux, & Belau, 1997; Sanger, Hux, & Ritzman, 1999; Sanger, Moore-Brown, Magnuson, & Svoboda, 2001; Snow & Powell, 2011; Snow, Powell, & Sanger, 2012). Their works have documented that the juvenile delinquent subjects in their studies can be characterized as follows:

- Have poorer results compared to nondelinquent adolescents or score in the language-impaired range on norm-referenced language tests
- Produce less complex language samples compared to nondelinquent adolescents
- Exhibit difficulties with sequencing ideas
- Do not comprehend meanings of words salient in legal contexts, such as *penalty* and *verify,* or the meaning of the Miranda rights statement
- Perceive themselves as having poor language and literacy skills that they believe negatively affect their self-esteem
- Show problems with pragmatic skills that include poor topic initiation and topic maintenance, inconsistent use of politeness techniques, and variable application of rules governing conversational interactions either because of deliberate intentions to violate the rules or because the language resource demands required during the flow of conversations exceed the adolescents' abilities to maintain appropriate use of rules
- Have difficulties relating cohesive narratives, which can interfere with their abilities to explain to law and judicial officials the scenarios in which they find themselves

Although there is evidence for an association between adolescent language impairment and juvenile delinquency, the evidence is not particularly well known, heeded, or utilized (Snow et al., 2012). The lack of awareness about the association of language and juvenile delinquency is demonstrated by findings, for example, that only a small proportion of incarcerated adolescents are likely to have received special education during their school years prior to their difficulties with the law and that, where services were provided, these tended to be for learning disabilities or behavioral disorders rather than language difficulties (Sanger et al., 2000, 2001). None of the juvenile delinquents in these two studies of Sanger and colleagues (2000, 2001) had received language services prior to incarceration, even though evaluation of their language skills while in juvenile detention indicated that a considerable number of them had language impairment.

Another potential personal and societal cost of adolescent language impairment that has also not been well documented or recognized is the possible relationship between language impairment in adolescence and youth suicide. Larson and McKinley (2003) reported that, of the individuals aged 10 to 14 years old involved with the Los Angeles Suicide Prevention Center, about half had learning disabilities. From our understanding of language and learning disabilities, we would justifiably suspect that most of these adolescents had language impairment. Given the socioemotional problems associated with language impairment in adolescence, a possible relationship between adolescent language impairment and youth suicide should not be particularly surprising.

Although the risk factors for youth suicide are far from delineated, agreed on, and empirically validated, a number of factors have been suggested. Among these are the following:

- Psychosocial and socioemotional disorders, including affective disorders, and social skills problems, including low social competence disorders
- Depression
- Problem-solving difficulties, learning disabilities, and the correlates of learning disabilities such as impulse behaviors and, as we know, problematic social skills
- Substance use and abuse
- Unemployment issues

These factors, like the situation with juvenile delinquency, are ones frequently associated with adolescents with language impairment. There is also some evidence of a link between suicide and juvenile delinquency. In one study, 63 percent of youths who committed suicide had a record of involvement with juvenile justice (Gray et al., 2002). Social skills difficulties and peer relationship problems that we see in adolescents with language impairment might also be implicated in the results of a study conducted by Massa and Eggert (2001), a study that was not specifically about language impairment or language ability. These investigators examined the weekly activities of adolescents at risk for suicide compared to those of non-suicide-risk peers and found that the at-risk teenagers spent more of the weekday and weekend time in solitary activities. Results such as these suggest that social isolation from peers may be a factor in youth suicide. As a possible link between teenage suicide and language problems, Asher and Gazelle (1999) suggest that youths with language impairment are at risk for experiencing loneliness as one of the "negative emotional consequences of peer relationship problems" (p. 20). Previously, we also noted emerging evidence that as schoolchildren with language impairment progress through school, their self-esteem falls. Jerome and her co-researchers (Jerome et al., 2002) found that older students with language impairment "perceived themselves more negatively in scholastic competence, social acceptance, and behavioral conduct than did children with typical language development" (p. 700). This contrasts with younger school children with and without language impairment, who did not differ in how they perceived themselves in these areas. Previously we have noted self-esteem and/or self-concept concerns for adolescents with language impairment, for example, Wadman et al. (2008).

Figure 5.2 illustrates some of these possible links between youth suicide and adolescent language impairment. While links between adolescent language impairment and youth suicide are currently tenuous, unclear, and inexact, there seem to be sufficient cues from the literature to be suspicious that stronger links might be present but yet unexplored and unidentified. It would, however, seem worth the time and energy of professionals who work with teenagers with language impairment to be alert to signs of potential self-harm.

Links between substance (drug and alcohol) abuse and adolescent language impairment are, as with youth suicide, currently tenuous links, although there are reasons to suppose an association. In the study conducted by Gray et al. (2002), 65 percent of those youths who committed suicide had a history of substance abuse. In a follow-up study of individuals at 19 years of age who had been identified as language impaired at 5 years of age, Beitchman, Wilson, Douglas, Young, and Adlaf (2001) found that those with substance use disorders (SUD) compared to those without SUD were more apt to have been diagnosed with learning disabilities at 12 years of age, and this association was even stronger in cases in which the learning disability was still apparent at age 19 years. These researchers did not find a similarly strong relationship between age 5 years language impairment and age 19 years substance use problems. However, there was, not surprisingly, a strong association between children with language impairment at 5 years of age and identification of learning disabilities at age 12 and age 19 years, thus suggesting a trend but not a direct relationship. This trend prompted Beitchman, Adlaf, Douglas et al. (2001) to adopt a more individually focused approach using cluster analysis to look at the possible relationship between language impairment and substance abuse. When the comorbidity of SUD and psychiatric disorders, such as anxiety, depression, and antisocial and personality disorders, was examined in individuals at 19 years

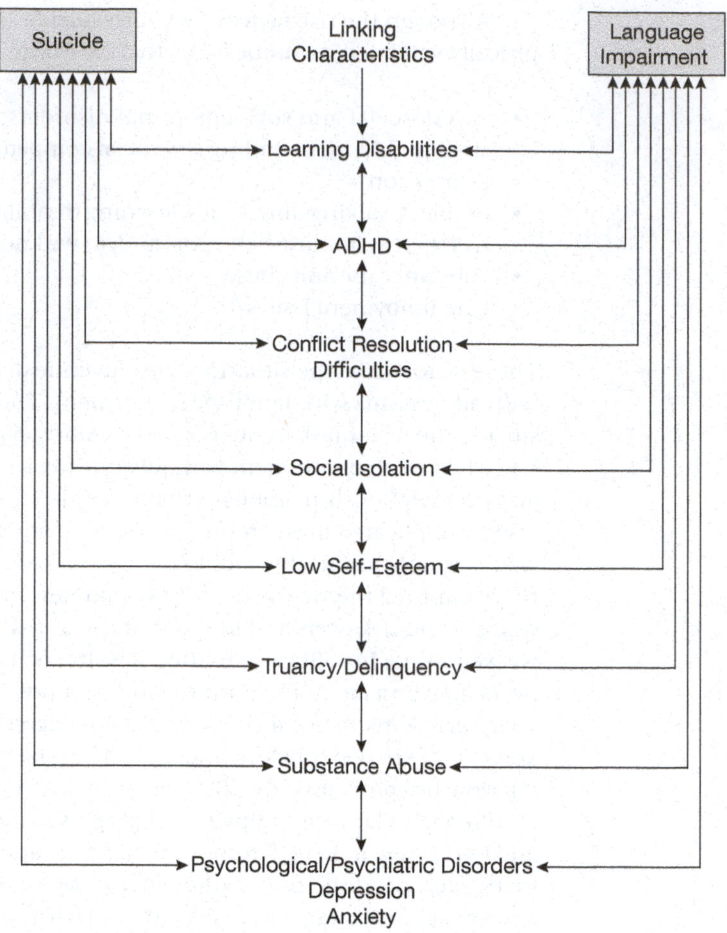

FIGURE 5.2 | Possible Links between Youth Suicide and Adolescent Language Impairment
Copyright 2002 © Vicki A. Reed, Claire Ireson, and Danielle Slack.

of age, these researchers found that a statistically significant percentage of those referred to as depressed drug abusers, as well as others referred to as having antisocial behaviors, had been identified as language impaired at 5 years of age. It may be that type of psychosocial outcome, substance abuse in adolescence and early adulthood, and language impairment recognized in early childhood are associated (Snow, 2000).

Adolescents and adults with histories of SLI have been shown to demonstrate more characteristics related to dependent-living situations and fewer independent-living characteristics (Clegg & Henderson, 1999; Clegg et al., 2005; Conti-Ramsden & Durkin, 2008; Johnson et al., 2010). Indices of dependent-living characteristics are the antitheses of those typically associated with independence, such as living outside parents' homes without parental or governmental support, holding and sustaining gainful employment without extended periods of unemployment and receipt of governmental benefits, general financial autonomy, and managing appointments and schedules without assistance. Early parenthood may also be associated with young adults with histories of SLI (Johnson et al., 2010), a factor that can, in turn, impact on types of employment and educational directions.

For most adolescents in Western societies, obtaining a driver's license signifies a passage from childhood to adulthood and a mark of increasing independent living. The language of driving instructions and both oral and written examinations for licenses contains many features that are known to be problematic for adolescents with SLI, for example, verbs, compound nouns, and abstract adjectives, such as *hazardous* (Pandolfe, Wittke, & Spaulding, 2016). It might not be surprising, therefore, that adolescents with SLI have been found to struggle with the language related to driver's licenses. They understand significantly less of the vocabulary that appears in driving manuals (Pandolfe et al., 2016). Difficulties obtaining driver's licenses potentially restrict employment and post-secondary educational options for adolescents with language impairment, as well as potentially contributing to fewer independent living conditions and undermining self-esteem and self-concept further.

A substantial proportion of children and adolescents with SLI may be at risk for bullying and other forms of victimization (Conti-Ramsden & Botting, 2004; Lindsay, Dockrell, & Mackie, 2008; Redmond, 2011). In one study, the rate with which adolescents with SLI reported that they had been the victims of bullying was more than three times that of their peers without SLI, with 36 percent of adolescents with SLI having been bullied within a week of data collection for the study (Conti-Ramsden & Botting, 2004). A particularly disturbing research finding related to victimization is that young, female adults (25 years) with a history of SLI have greater reported incidences of sexual assault than their peers without SLI (Brownlie, Jabbar, Beitchman, Vida, & Atkinson, 2007).

In the past several decades, increases in technologies have led to dramatic changes in the nature of education, communication, and work. With regard to the nature of work, there are now fewer opportunities for unskilled workers, and these types of jobs have more limited opportunities for long-term employment and advancement. Yet, the information in Table 5.1 demonstrates that adolescents and adults with histories of SLI are likely to be employed in lower-paying, more unskilled jobs. The nature of work has increasingly required employees who can problem solve, read well at high literacy levels, follow instructions, integrate information, and generalize knowledge to new situations and who possess good interpersonal skills in order to work effectively as members of teams (Casner-Lotto & Barrington, 2006; Ehren & Murza, 2010). These employee assets are ones that are typically limitations of adolescents and adults with SLI.

A particularly important change has been the widespread accessibility to computers, smart phones, the Internet, e-mail, and messaging and texting for work, educational, and personal use. On the one hand, these technologies might benefit adolescents with SLI. For example, computer-assisted teaching and computer programs might help adolescents with language disorders to learn, access information (e.g., library resources and Internet searches), and manage production of a number of educational products (e.g., report, spreadsheets, graphics, and spell and grammar checks). Smart phone use might increase opportunities for these adolescents to establish and maintain relationships with peers that their oft-cited characteristics, such as shyness and social anxiety, lead them to find difficult. For example, use of texting and e-mail may remove several of the demands of simultaneous communicative interactions that are inherent in real-time communication.

However, there may be some downsides of these technologies for adolescents with SLI. Compared to normally developing peers, SLI adolescents have been found to use texting less frequently and to be less motivated to use texting for social purposes, such as making plans and engaging friends (Conti-Ramsden, Durkin, & Simkin, 2010; Durkin, Conti-Ramsden, & Walker, 2011). Use of cell phones for calls for both normally developing peers and the SLI adolescents has been shown to be similar, with both groups of teenagers using texting more than calling. Adolescents with SLI may be in a circular situation. The researchers (Conti-Ramsden et al., 2010) have suggested that, although use of smart phones was not particularly difficult for teenagers with SLI,

> social difficulties limit the opportunities that young people with SLI have to interact with their peers, which results in less frequent exchanges of text messages. . . . Less frequent text messaging can therefore, in time, lessen the social experiences of adolescents with SLI by reducing their opportunities to develop social networks and to make arrangements to engage in social interaction with peers. (p. 206)

It is also possible that computer use by adolescents with SLI reflects unsystematic and inefficient strategies. Rather than decreasing demands for reading, literacy, and metacognitive skills, effective computer use and electronic communication modes have increased demands for reading, literacy, and problem solving. Efficient use of the computer and the Internet for communication and information acquisition requires skills such as increased reading speed and comprehension of printed material, metalinguistic and semantically based organizational abilities, and critical assessment of larger amounts of information than previously experienced, all abilities with which adolescents with SLI can struggle. According to the research of Durkin, Conti-Ramsden, Walker, and Simkin (2009), issues with language and literacy ability helped explained why, compared to normally developing adolescents, teenagers with SLI used their home computers less for educational purposes and used some personal applications less, for example, using computer-based communication such as e-mail, MSN, and blogging; making online purchases; and downloading music. In contrast, the adolescents with SLI spent more time playing off-line computer games than their peers. In commenting about their uses of their home computers, the adolescents with SLI reported

> they found information too technical, too text-bound, and difficult to comprehend. They mentioned difficulties with reading, writing and spelling; they found navigation through different applications problematic in addition to remembering information across different times of use. (p. 211)

However, consistent with Durkin and Conti-Ramsden's (2014) thinking, encouraging students' constructive computer use might have benefits for the adolescents that could assist them, for example, in promoting more positive peer interaction and supporting their educational pursuits. Nevertheless, adolescents with SLI may find that, for both their educational and personal purposes, using their home computers is generally harder than do their peers. This led Durkin and his colleagues (Durkin, Conti-Ramsden, et al., 2009) to conclude that "adolescents with SLI were likely to elect to engage less frequently as a function of perceived ease of use" (p. 211). In addition to perceived ease of use, the more limited uses of computers by adolescents with SLI may also relate to heightened anxiety related to using them Conti-Ramsden, Durkin, and Walker (2010). These researchers reported that "level of general anxiety, perceived ease of use and language ability had a direct association and were predictive of level of computer anxiety in adolescents with SLI" (p. 136).

Westby and Atencio (2002) write,

> In the 21st century, society has entered a new technological, information era. Where people once were valued for their ability to transform raw materials into products, now they are valued for the information they can possess and transmit. To be successful, individuals are expected to use technology to integrate more and more information from more and more diverse sources and communicate this information to more and more people. (p. 70)

The adolescent with a language impairment is at greater risk than ever before for being able to keep pace in educational and in vocational pursuits in what are increasing electronic communications expectations for current school and work environments and for requirements for high literacy to obtain and achieve in employment in the modern workforce.

The personal, economic, and societal costs of adolescent language impairment are huge. Failing to recognize the issues and to address adequately the educational and social needs of adolescents with specific language impairment increases these costs.

Reasons for Still Lagging Recognition and Continuing Underservice

Despite the mounting evidence that language impairments in young children persist in adolescents and that the associated personal and societal costs are staggering, adolescents with language impairment continue to be relatively underrecognized and definitely underserved professionally. Several reasons account for this. One is the emphasis that has been placed on preschoolers and elementary school children with language impairment. Early intervention to prevent or at least lessen academic and personal failures is the rationale behind this emphasis on young children. It is certainly a logical and worthwhile rationale, and it can work. However, it does not necessarily solve the problem; recall that we have characterized SLI (and even learning disabilities) as a lifelong disability that can have different manifestations at different ages and stages of life. Ongoing support is necessary. Children with SLI are not cured while they are preschoolers or in elementary school.

An example of one way in which the emphasis on young children detracts attention from adolescents with language impairment can be found in the numbers of speech–language pathologists (SLPs) who work in secondary schools compared to those working in elementary schools and preschools. At the end of 2015, of American Speech-Language-Hearing Association (ASHA) SLPs, 3.4 percent reported they worked in secondary schools, compared to 28.5 percent

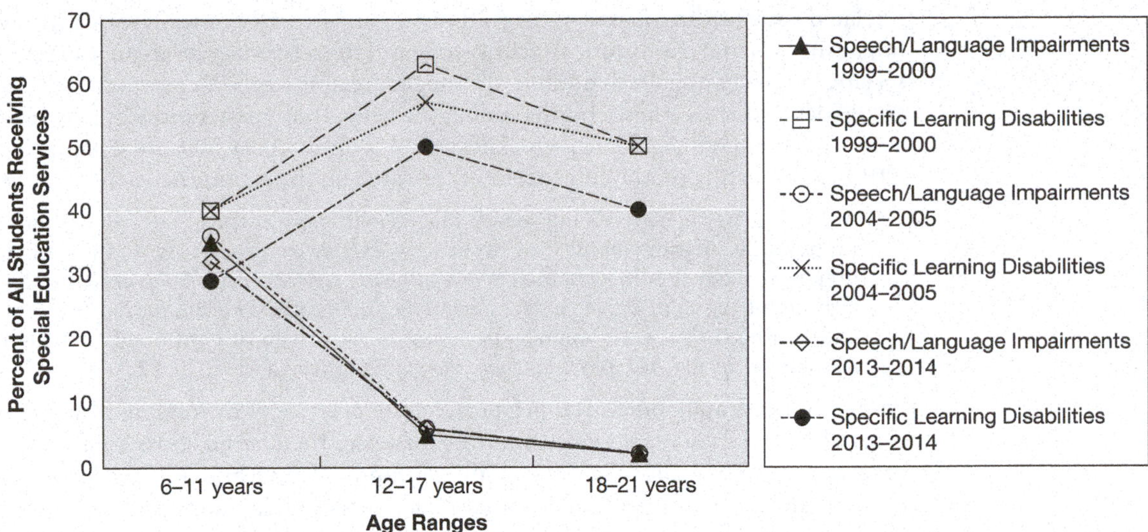

FIGURE 5.3 | Students with Speech/Language Impairments and Specific Learning Disabilities as Percentage of All Students Receiving Special Education Services in Public Schools in the 1999–2000, 2004–2005, and 2013–2014 School Years
Source: U.S. Department of Education (2001, 2006, 2015).

in elementary and preschool settings (ASHA, 2016). These workplace data can be compared to 2009. According to ASHA (2009), 34 percent of ASHA SLPs in 2009 worked in elementary schools and preschools and 3.4 percent in secondary schools. As with 2016, this represents a large difference between the 3.4 percent working in secondary schools and the 34 percent in elementary and preschools. Data from the 2002 ASHA membership (ASHA, 2002) showed that approximately 30 percent of SLPs worked in elementary and preschool settings and 2.5 percent in secondary schools. These figures suggest little increase in the proportion of SLPs serving secondary schools over the past approximate 15-year period.

The low number of SLPs serving secondary schools is consistent with the proportion of students receiving speech or language services in elementary and secondary grades. Figure 5.3 shows the 1999–2000, 2004–2005, and 2013–2014 school-year data for percentages of all students in special education who received speech or language services or specific learning disabilities services in three age groups: 6 to 11 years, 12 to 17 years, and 18 to 21 years, ages that correspond to the elementary and secondary school grades and the immediate post-secondary years. What is apparent over the 15-year period is the conspicuous increase between the elementary-school-age group and the secondary-school-age group in the percentage of students with specific learning disabilities who receive special education services compared to the dramatic decrease for students with speech or language impairments. We know that: a) it is unlikely that so many children with language impairment would have been “cured” prior to entering secondary school, b) there is a close association between language impairment and learning disabilities, and c) from the data in Figure 5.1, with the movement of students receiving speech or language services from special education rolls to general/regular education counts, many of the children with language impairment in elementary school have likely been relabeled as having specific learning disabilities on entry into secondary school or dismissed from services all together.

An obvious issue with these trends for employment of SLPs and the data for numbers of adolescents being served in the secondary schools is the following:

- If language impairment is not being identified in adolescents, then the (spurious) conclusion is that there is no population needing the services of SLPs and, therefore, no need to employ them to serve secondary schools.

However, there is inherent circularity in this scenario:

- If only very few SLPs are serving the secondary schools, who is available in these schools to identify adolescents with language impairment or to advocate for their needs?

A related issue leading to underrecognition and underservice of adolescents with language impairment is that the historical lack of services at the secondary level can lead professionals serving language-impaired children who are progressing from elementary school to secondary grades to dismiss these children under the belief that further services may not be available or further change in language skills would be limited. Recall from Chapter 3 that Rice (2013), in reporting on the children in her research on the genetic bases of SLI, wrote that

> Although they were receiving speech-language therapy at the outset of their participation in the study, ongoing monitoring of the services they were receiving . . . shows that the children were likely *to be dropped from speech pathology services by age 7–9 years* [emphasis added], although they were *likely to receive services for reading or other academic limitations* [emphasis added] after their speech-language pathology services were discontinued. . . . Thus, there was *no common approach to speech-language therapy* [emphasis added]. (p. 224)

From a professional and ethical perspective, the practice of dismissing students from services when the students need continuing support for their language issues as adolescents in order to access curricular content demands is unprofessional and probably unethical. There is a dramatic jump in curricular demands for language and literacy skills from elementary to secondary school, for example, the syntactic complexity of written texts (Scott, 2014; Scott & Balthazar, 2010), the abstract nature of vocabulary, the degree of inference involved in "reading between the lines," the shifts in teachers' language and the discipline-specific language (Fang, 2012). The practice of dismissing students with their weak language skills from intervention at the end of elementary school means that they are dismissed from services at the time they need these the most in order to survive middle and high school.

Criteria for dismissal from intervention and the tests and procedures used to determine adequacy of language functioning may result in further lack of recognition or underservice of language-impaired adolescents. Some tests may not be sensitive to the language behaviors that can cause problems for students entering secondary schools. Assessment needs to examine the high level, abstract, and figurative language abilities that are essential to drawing inferences, comprehending complex written and spoken expository discourse, and expressing integrated and cohesive information in speech and writing, that is, the language of academics in the secondary grades. An additional issue related to assessment tools is associated with notions of prevalence and, therefore, the number of adolescents who are language impaired. As we saw in Chapter 3, prevalence will be equal to what is determined to be the cutoff score for concluding that a language impairment is evident. That is, if –2 SD is the determined cutoff for determining the presence of language impairment, then automatically we know that the prevalence will be 2.5 to 3 percent (assuming a normal distribution). However, since SLI is not "cured," we might suspect that the prevalence of SLI in adolescents would be similar to that in kindergarteners, about 7 percent, using the commonly accepted prevalence based on a –1.25 SD cutoff as did Tomblin et al. (1997). A further challenge is ensuring use of assessment procedures with adequate sensitivity and specificity to enable accurate identification.

The problems surrounding dismissal criteria and assessment procedures can be exacerbated by erroneous perceptions that only insignificant language development occurs beyond late childhood and that little more can be done after late childhood to help. These reasons may account, in part, for some of the data shown in Figure 5.1 about the percentage of students with speech or language impairments who were moved from special education to regular/general education.

A failure to realize the significant, negative effects that persisting language problems have on all aspects of life is a further reason adolescents with language impairment are underrecognized or neglected. Another is the failure to understand that adolescents' academic, personal, or social difficulties may be related to language deficits, that is, the misattribution of children's academic and/or behavioral problems to conditions other than language impairment. In some cases, the nature of the elementary educational structure may have provided sufficient support to students with less severe language impairment or who are introverted and do not act out so that academic struggles might not have surfaced or been noticed. Secondary curricular demands can trigger emergence of weaknesses in language abilities. These students are at risk of having their language problems neglected because of inadequate identification or misdiagnosis. If academic problems are exhibited, the student is frequently labeled or relabeled as having a specific learning disability, as we know, and services, if any, are then likely to be provided in learning disabilities programs, evidence of which we most likely see in the data in Figure 5.3.

In light of the discussion so far, it should not be surprising to learn that we have very limited direct data on the prevalence of language impairment in adolescents, and this unquestionably adds to their underrecognition. Again, we can see how limited data can create the perception that there are no individuals with the problems. In one of the few prevalence studies (McKinley & Larson, 1989), results indicated that 7 percent of 1,028 secondary students in a regular education program failed an adolescent language screening test. In thinking about these results, we need to recall the estimated prevalence of SLI (Tomblin et al., 1997), which has been estimated at about 7 percent. Of the students in remedial English classes for grades 9 to 12, 18 percent failed the screening test, a result that underscores the relationship between deficit oral language skills and poor academic achievement. This study also highlighted the greater percentage of adolescents with language impairment in special services focused on reading/writing/literacy skills, that is, the remedial English classes mentioned above. Ehren and Lenz (1989), too, found high numbers in special services in their study. These authors reported that

> 73% of a high-risk population of middle school students, including students in compensatory education and special education, evidenced some degree of language impairment. This same study found a prevalence of language impairment of 80 percent for the group with learning disabilities. (p. 193)

As further documentation of prevalence, 45 percent of the students enrolled in special education programs in a junior high school in Arizona failed a screening test of language, as did 53 percent of the seventh-grade students (approximately 12 to 13 years of age) who had been placed in developmental reading classes because of reading problems (Despain & Simon, 1987). In this report, a disturbing finding was that only about one-half of the students in the developmental reading classes had been referred for special education services, including language intervention services. Such findings reflect "the 'happenstance' nature of identification and composition of special education caseloads at the middle school level of education" (Despain & Simon, 1987, pp. 142–143). The findings of these older studies are consistent with more recent literature. Recall we previously made the point that language impairment is not regularly identified in students labeled with other conditions or problems (e.g., Hollo et al., 2014; Joffe & Black, 2012; Walsh et al., 2014), such as ADHD, juvenile delinquency, and behavioral/emotional disorders, among others. At present, knowledge regarding normal language development during adolescence is much less complete than it is for youngsters. There is also (1) limited knowledge about effective, efficient, and comprehensive assessment procedures for use with these teenagers; (2) an increasing number but still many fewer norm-referenced tests than for younger children; and (3) a paucity of information about evidence-based intervention strategies. In these circumstances, it is no wonder that many professionals might feel that they are not being adequately prepared to work with language-impaired adolescents, a feeling that can lead to a reluctance to pursue assertively the implementation of services in the secondary schools. This is dangerous because it can lead to invisibility of adolescents with language impairment and the professionals who can serve them. As Larson and McKinley (1995) point out, "Perpetuating a lack of visibility makes professionals vulnerable to being considered an expendable service" (p. 294).

Figure 5.4 summarizes various reasons language-impaired adolescents are an underrecognized and underserved population. These reasons are not mutually exclusive but instead are interrelated. This has the danger of leading to circularity in thinking and a cycle of neglect of adolescents with language impairment. Ehren and Lenz (1989) have used the phrase "self-perpetuating cycle" (p. 194) to describe the continuing problem of identifying and serving these adolescents. However, given the relatively recent increased attention to adolescents with SLI in the literature, some of the reasons presented in the figure might be expected to change in the upcoming years. For example, the box about limited research on adolescents with language impairment might be deleted or rewritten. However, until the research information has trickled down so that we see changes, such as adequate levels of services in schools for these adolescents and increased professional preparation, the boxes in the figure will, unfortunately, need to remain.

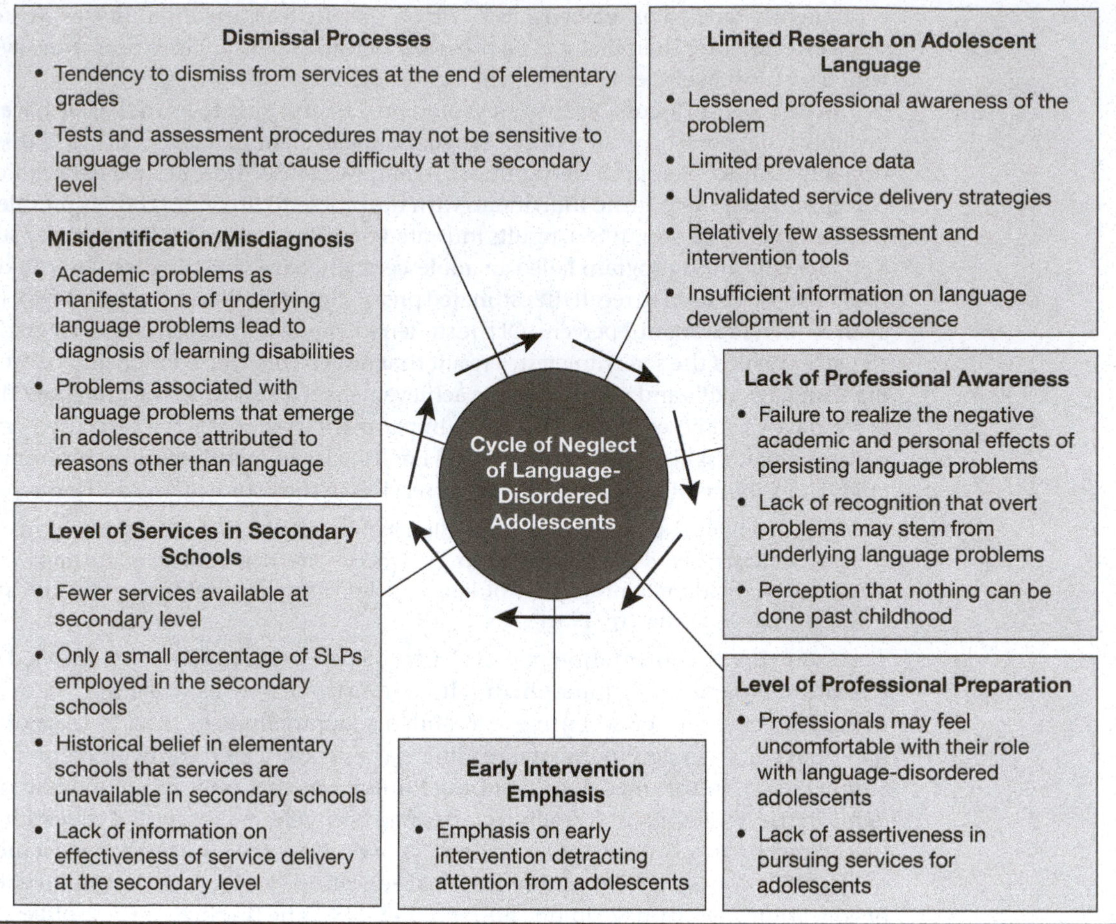

FIGURE 5.4 | The Cycle of Neglect of Adolescents with Language Impairment

It is worth noting a final but disturbing thought before moving on to other topics related to adolescents and language impairment. This thought pulls together information from Figure 5.3 and Tables 5.2 and 5.3. The data on the percentage of adolescents with language impairment who leave high school without a diploma are based on the number of adolescents who are identified in the system while they are in high school. What the information in Figure 5.3 and the discussion in this section about the underrecognition of adolescents with language impairment tell us is that there are likely many more adolescents who have not been identified and are not included in our data, except perhaps as teenagers with specific learning disabilities, but even this is not all that encouraging. It is probable that we do not have data on a considerable proportion of adolescents with language impairment. "Child Find" concepts of the Individuals with Disabilities Education Act have yet to show up as "Adolescent Find" concepts as far as language impairment is concerned.

CHARACTERISTICS OF ADOLESCENTS WITH LANGUAGE IMPAIRMENT

In Chapter 4, the language characteristics of learning-disabled school-age children were discussed. Adolescents with language impairment evince language deficits similar to those described in Chapter 4 and to younger school-aged children with language impairment. That is, language-impaired adolescents may have difficulties with words with abstract or multiple meanings or figurative language expressions, use less complex syntax, exhibit word-finding problems, have problems with morphologically complex words, and/or use nonspecific, noncontent words, such as *thing* or *stuff,* or pronouns without clear referents. And, similar to what we have seen from previous sections in this chapter as well as in previous chapters, language-impaired adolescents often experience difficulties in relationships with both their peers and adults, difficulties that have been attributed, in part, to problems in their communicative interactions. They may not adapt their communications appropriately for their listeners, or they may use inappropriate strategies, such as an aggressive or abrupt tone of voice, to deliver their messages. Their nonverbal behaviors, such as standing too close, can make their listeners uncomfortable, or these nonverbal behaviors may communicate unintentionally hostile or negative messages. Problems can exist with both expression and comprehension.

By adolescence teenagers with language problems talk in complete sentences that contain many correct syntactic and morphological features. However, some aspects of syntax and morphology may continue to be problematic for adolescents, even though errors may occur less frequently and the problems may be more subtle than in earlier years. For example, adolescents with language impairment use syntactic structures that reflect greater use of simpler, less complex forms with more errors, and the frequency with which language-impaired adolescents use the range of dependent/subordinate clause types or adverbial connectives may be less than expected of teenagers. Confirmation of these less accurate and less complex syntactic patterns (shorter utterances, less subordination, and different uses of different types of subordinate clauses) in the language of adolescents with SLI between 13 and 15 years old is evident in the findings from the research of several investigators (Nippold et al., 2008, 2009; Wetherell, Botting, & Conti-Ramsden, 2007).

The research findings regarding the persisting difficulties that preschool and school-aged children with language impairment have with verb morphology also prompt the question as to whether some problems with morphology, particularly verb form use, might continue to be evidenced by preadolescents and adolescents. Longitudinal data for children with SLI from 3 to 8 years of age (Rice, Wexler, & Hershberger, 1998) have shown that these children do not catch up with the path of increasing accuracy in marking verb tense that is demonstrated by their normally developing peers and do not reach at 8 years of age the almost 100 percent level of accuracy seen for their peers at 5 to 6 years of age. At 8 years of age, SLI children were still found to be achieving only about a 90 percent accuracy level. The difficulty is, however, that a 90 percent accuracy level might not be interpreted as an important reduction in the level of performance, an interpretation that could erroneously minimize the significance attached to this aspect of children's language performance. However, as Rice (2000) points out, morphological marking of tense in English is not optional, so that for children whose language is developing normally, "by a certain age, [use of correct] grammatical markers would show little variation" (p. 22).

For older students and adolescents, there is now a group of studies that indicates that verb problems continue to be evidenced in children and teenagers with language impairment. In a set of related studies (e.g., Reed & Patchell, 2010; Reed, Patchell, & Conrad, 2006), four groups of adolescents were asked to relate narratives from looking at a wordless picture storybook. There were two groups of younger adolescents, each group with a mean age of 13;2 years with one group having SLI and the other comprised of typically developing (TD) adolescents matched on chronological age, gender, socioeconomic status, and nonverbal IQ to the SLI adolescents. There were also two other groups of older adolescents, each with a mean age of 15;9/15;10 years, with one group also having SLI and the other normal language, again paired on the same characteristics as for the younger group. Another study (Reed & Evernden, 2001) compared verb morphologically use in narratives, also during a wordless picture book task, of 12 normally achieving students aged 8 to 12 years, age-matched peers with reading difficulties co-occurring with various degrees of language difficulties. One pattern of verb form use that emerged from these studies for the adolescents with language impairment was more errors on verb forms during the narrative task, even though the frequency of errors overall was relatively small. Recall that Rice et al. (1998) reported that the mean percent correct rate for 8-year-old children with SLI was as high as 90 percent. Figure 5.5 shows the percent of the adolescents achieving a range of percent correct verb use in the Reed & Patchell (2010) and Reed, Patchell, and Conrad (2006) studies. As can be seen, the two groups of SLI adolescents had correct rates as low as 91 and 92 percent, a result reasonably similar to the 8-year-old children with SLI in the Rice et al. (1998) study. In contrast, the lowest accuracy rate for the two groups of TD adolescents was 96 percent. Figure 5.5 also shows the trend lines for percent

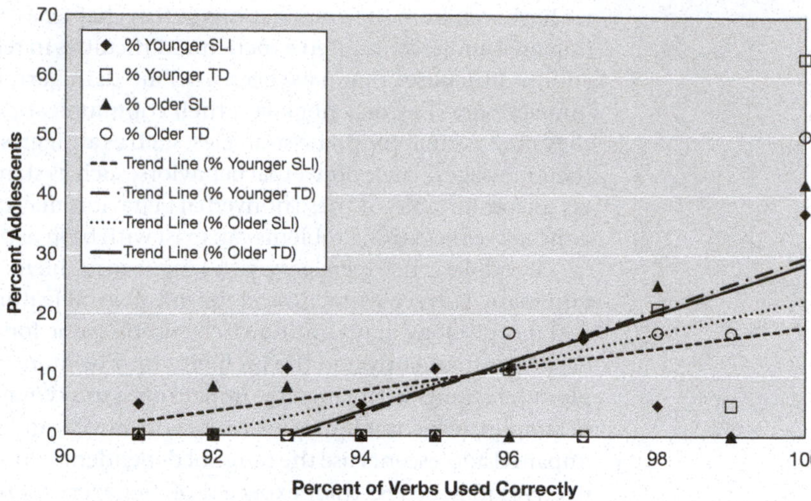

FIGURE 5.5 | Percentage of Verbs Used Correctly by Younger SLI and Typically Developing and Older SLI and Typically Developing Adolescents

Sources: Reed and Patchell (2010); Reed, Patchell, and Conrad (2006).

of verb used correctly by the younger and older SLI and TD groups. A similar result emerged in the Reed and Evernden (2001) study. As can be seen, the trend lines for the younger and older adolescents with SLI are noticeably flatter than those for both groups of the TD adolescents. The younger and older TD appeared to achieve similar accuracy rates, whereas for the SLI groups, the older language-impaired adolescents seemed to use verb forms marginally more accurately than the younger adolescents with SLI. For the younger and older TD students, 89 and 84 percent of them, respectively, performed at 98–100 percent accuracy. This contrasts with the 42 and 67 percent of younger and older SLI adolescents, respectively, who performed at the 98–100 percent accuracy rate. The language-impaired and TD groups also appeared to differ in their patterns of marking tense. As one example, the students with SLI tended to use more progressive verbs (*is running, were running* vs. *runs, ran*) than the TD students to mark tense. The unusual, greater use of progressive verb forms by SLI adolescents to convey tense (as opposed to regular and irregular past tense and third-person present) is intriguing. It might be a strategy that adolescents with SLI use to circumvent the complexities of regular and irregular verb tense marking. It might also be because the progressive grammatical morpheme is one of the earliest to be acquired by children.

Continuing verb morphological difficulties also emerged in a longitudinal study that followed up children in the earlier (Rice et al., 1998) study. Rice, Hoffman, and Wexler (2009) confirmed that verb morphological difficulties evinced in the language of young children with SLI continue to be seen when they are 15 years old in terms of their higher error rates in judgments of grammatical acceptability/unacceptability of statements in which forms of *be* and *do* verbs are or are not omitted. Sixteen-year-old teenagers with SLI have also been found to be less sensitive to omissions of verb tense and agreement inflections in statements than their normal peers (Leonard, Miller, & Finneran, 2009). The emerging evidence suggests that early verb morphological deficits associated with SLI do not resolve by adolescence, although the number of errors may not be high, and the patterns with which verb forms are used (e.g., higher progressive forms) and are detected may change with age. To the extent that verb morphology might be a clinical marker of SLI in young children, it might also be a clinical marker for SLI in adolescence.

And, there is now some evidence that these verb morphological difficulties continue into adulthood. Poll and his co-researchers (Poll, Betz, & Miller, 2010) found that tasks involving judgments of grammatical acceptability/unacceptability of statements containing verb morphological errors accurately classified young adults as having or not having SLI. Thus, it appears that verb morphological problems might continue to be effective as a clinical marker even beyond adolescence.

We might expect, however, that some language growth as a result of intervention, maturation, or both would occur between childhood and adolescence. Therefore, the language problems of adolescents may be less obvious and more difficult to identify than those of younger children. These factors can contribute to false negatives in identification (not identifying a problem when one actually exists) or even misdiagnosis.

The relative past neglect of language-impaired adolescents means that less is generally known about their specific communicative characteristics than about those of younger children with language impairment. Several authors have identified characteristics that adolescents with language problems frequently demonstrate in their conversational interactions and in their classrooms. Many of these difficulties are summarized in Table 5.3. As we can see, the problematic characteristics range across semantic, morphosyntactic, and pragmatic domains, with several of them involving metacognitive, metapragmatic, and metalinguistic skills. They also reflect high level comprehension, as well as expressive, difficulties. Larson and McKinley (1987) have suggested that problematic behaviors, such as those listed in Table 5.3, can provide starting points in determining "where a given adolescent matches or mismatches with educators', parents', or peers' expectations" (p. 15).

TABLE 5.3 | Characteristics of Adolescents with Language Impairment in Conversational Interactions and Classrooms

Adolescents with Language Impairment . . .	
Do not:	Show mastery of tense reference and subject/verb agreement
	Recall information presented in lessons
	Participate in lessons
	Appear to listen to the teacher during lessons
	Meet minimum standards for academic work
	Define words well or use them appropriately; recognize or understand meanings conveyed by bound morphemes in the form of prefixes and suffixes
	Paraphrase what is read or what others say
	Learn from other students' questions
	Get along well with peers
	Participate in group discussions
	Complete assignments on time or complete them at all
	Organize work and materials
	Prepare for class
	Work independently
	Demonstrate knowledge on tests
	Understand when directions are being given or follow directions
	Use tactful deviousness
	Sustain topics of conversation
	Consider listener's informational needs
	Recognize when a problem exists
	Develop hierarchy of ideas and thoughts for concepts
	Use a variety of complex sentences with an array of types of subordinate clauses in varying sentential positions
	Produce written connected text to communicate knowledge and meaning
	Make language categories and semantic relationships explicit
	Use language to talk about language during formal instruction
	Identify and/or understand main points; infer meaning from connected text

(Continued)

TABLE 5.3 | *Continued*

	Adolescents with Language Impairment . . .
Do:	Lack consistency in tense and number reference
	Need additional prompting to follow directions to complete tasks within their ability
	Demonstrate difficulties comprehending complex syntactic forms
	Demonstrate a negative attitude or approach to learning
	Use tactless statements
	Use concrete operations in their thinking
	Demonstrate difficulties obtaining and inferring meaning from what they hear and read
	Have a lack of awareness of communicative failure and inability to repair communicative breakdowns
	Ask irrelevant questions
	Provide irrelevant answers to questions
	Wander from conversational topics
	Use egocentric comments
	Violate the rules of conversational discourse (e.g., accessing conversations, taking turns, and closing conversations)
	Express or organize ideas illogically
	Converse in irrelevant ways with conversational partners
	Use syntactic forms that are incomplete and immature; use utterances that fail to communicate intended meaning
	Show word-finding problems; use high-frequency, low-meaning words too much
	Use messages that confuse listeners
	Have problems comprehending and using peer-appropriate slang/jargon
	Use excessive mazes and false starts
	Demonstrate poor listening skills
	Make illogical and impulsive judgments about information
	Show an abrasive communication style
	Misuse gestures/body movement and facial expressions; misuse rules related to appropriate physical distance between communicative partners
	Misunderstand cues related to gestures/body movements and facial expressions

Sources: Ehren (1994); Larson and McKinley (2003); Lenz, Bulgren, and Kissam (1995); Schmidt, Deshler, Schumaker, and Alley (1989); Simon and Holway (1991).

ASSESSMENT

A determination of match and mismatch is an essential component of assessment and intervention for language-impaired adolescents (Larson & McKinley, 1995). Each language-impaired adolescent presents a unique profile of communicative strengths and weaknesses. An objective of the assessment process is to identify each adolescent's unique profile. Summaries of problems that can characterize the communication of adolescents with language impairment, such as those in Table 5.3, can provide frameworks for assessing an adolescent's language functioning. In Chapter 4, Common Core State Standards (CCSS) for students across the range of elementary and secondary grades were introduced, with attention drawn to the number of standards that address language and literacy skills (National Governors Association Center for Best Practices and Council of Chief State School Officers, 2010). The standards relevant for the secondary grades can also serve as guidelines as to skills that need to be assessed in adolescents who may have language impairment (Whitmire, Rivers, Mele-McCarthy, & Staskowski, 2014).

Expectations are that adolescents can use all aspects of language to function effectively in their social, academic, and vocational contexts. These expectations imply, therefore, that in assessment, an adolescent's communicative performance in each of these contexts needs to be examined. If an adolescent is struggling in any or all of these contexts, then a language impairment should be suspected, and the adolescent should be more closely assessed. Because we know that language impairment is often unidentified in students with other diagnostic labels, such as ADHD, dyslexia or reading disabilities, emotional/behavioral disabilities, or specific learning disabilities, any students with these diagnoses need to have their language assessed. If language impairment is present but not being addressed, attempts with other interventions may not be as effective as they could be.

The assessment of adolescents can be divided into two parts, each serving a different function. The first part involves identifying adolescents who exhibit problematic language behaviors and who may have language impairment. The second part is a more in-depth exploration of the adolescent's language functioning to either confirm or reject the initial identification and, if the identification is confirmed, to determine the adolescent's level of functioning in a variety of areas to identify areas to be targeted in intervention and the appropriate placement for intervention and to select the appropriate service delivery format. In the following sections, we discuss aspects of both parts of the assessment process. A few norm-referenced tests are available to assist in the process. However, observations of adolescents' performances in a variety of contexts and nonstandardized assessment methods must also be included as routine parts of the assessment process.

Identification

Teacher referrals and language screening are two common methods of identifying language-impaired adolescents. These are not mutually exclusive methods. Both may—and probably should—be used.

Teacher Referrals. Referrals from general/regular education teachers, special educators, remedial teachers, and other specialists are ways of identifying adolescents with possible language problems. One critical factor in the success of this method is the degree to which these secondary school professionals understand and recognize the nature of language impairment in adolescents and know the potential sources of professional help for the adolescents. For this reason, information dissemination to these professionals is important in providing services for language-impaired adolescents (Larson & McKinley, 2003).

Information dissemination includes sharing with classroom teachers and support personnel (e.g., counselors, special educators, social workers, and principals) information about the characteristics of adolescents with language impairment, the ways in which language impairment can be manifested academically and socially, and the intervention services available. Imparting this information helps to ensure that those professionals who have daily contact with adolescents or who interact with them in a variety of situations make appropriate referrals for assessment (Ehren, 2009b; Ehren & Whitmire, 2009; Larson & McKinley, 1995). In-service presentations (Ehren & Whitmire, 2009; Reed & Miles, 1989) are one way to increase school professionals' knowledge of adolescents with language impairment and the assistance that can be provided for these teenagers and to promote referrals. Another method is to contribute to school newsletters or newsletters of educators' professional groups. McKinley and Larson (1989) used this last approach to disseminate information to secondary school principals. Another strategy is to take advantage of schools' increasing use of educators' self-developed portfolios as part of their annual evaluations. Activities that involve informing school colleagues about adolescent language and literacy can be embedded in these portfolios as performance objectives. Opportunities to inform supervisors occur as they review the portfolios and engage with the educators in discussions of the activities and the reasons for them.

Asking informed educators to complete observational/behavioral ratings scales on their students is one way to obtain referrals. Several rating scales of language and language-related skills are available for use with adolescents. Such ratings not only aid in identifying adolescents with possible language problems but also direct assessment to areas of communication most highly suspect in an adolescent and indicate those aspects of an adolescent's language functioning that most concern others.

Screening. Language screening tests are used to indicate in broad terms whether an individual's language skills are adequate or whether there is a discrepancy from normal expectations that is sufficient to warrant further assessment. Professionals disagree about the benefits of mass screenings of all students in secondary schools or if an alternative screening approach, such as screening all students in specified grades in secondary schools, such as all students in grades 7 and 10, is effective. Some suggest that a more effective approach is selective screening of students who meet certain criteria, such as students in learning disabilities programs, those who received speech–language services in earlier grades, students receiving tutoring or remedial reading services, or adolescents at risk for dropping out of school.

Only a few norm-referenced language screening tests for adolescents are commercially available. Each of these is designed to be administered individually to adolescents. The tests examine a variety of aspects of communicative functioning, and the estimated time to administer these ranges from about 2 to 15 minutes. Another approach to administering screening tests is to utilize group screening tests that can be administered to, perhaps, whole classrooms of students. Simon (1987) developed a group screening procedure, the Classroom Communication Screening Procedure for Early Adolescents, to be used primarily with students in grades 5 through 9. The procedure can be administered in the students' classrooms or in other group settings and takes about 50 minutes to complete. It is a paper-and-pencil task, although the writing is limited mostly to circling answers or writing single words so that it can be used with students who have difficulty with written language.

There are, however, several concerns with many language screening tests, and for that matter, with many diagnostic language tests for adolescents. Adolescents with language impairment generally talk in sentences, particularly in conversational contexts, and can often perform adequately on decontextualized language tasks, such as pointing to pictures that represent the meaning of words. The language struggles of adolescents may only surface in relatively demanding language tasks and when challenged with abstract, higher-level language tasks, (i.e., those required in the academic climate of secondary schools). Higher-level, abstract language tasks include those requiring comprehending complex sentences with multiple embedding of relative subordinate clauses, drawing inferences from expository discourse, or deciphering the meanings of morphologically complex words. Unless these types of tasks are major parts of screening procedures, we run the risk of missing students at risk for language impairment.

It is possible that a language sampling approach can avoid the downsides of most screening tests. For adolescents, an expository sample would tap higher-level language skills more relevant for academic performance than a narrative sample. Asking an adolescent to provide, for example, an explanation of how he or she might persuade a teacher to lift an afterschool detention is one example of a possible task. Because this is being employed as a screening task, a rating scale for characteristics of interest, e.g., use of relative clauses, literate and specific vocabulary words, appropriate nonverbal communicative behaviors, could be used to make judgments of adequacy or concern and, if concern, a follow-up, more complete assessment could be implemented. The list of characteristics could be compiled from those shown in Table 5.3. Students could also be asked to define a few printed morphologically complex words drawn from their relevant textbooks or worksheets. Other authentic, educationally relevant, but brief, tasks could be utilized, again with criterion-based rating scales to facilitate decision making about adequacy or concern needing follow-up. Such approaches can be used strategically with teacher opinions or ratings and information about students' academic and social performances in order to identify adolescents at risk for language problems.

Language Assessment

Norm-Referenced Tests. Some of the more complete language tests that are appropriate for individuals 11 years of age or older are listed in Table 5.4. Tests that examine areas of functioning closely related to language, such as phonological processing in the Comprehensive Test of Phonological Processing–2 (Wagner, Torgesen, Rashotte, & Pearson, 2013) or problem-solving abilities in the Test of Problem Solving—2 Adolescent (Bowers, Huisingh, & LoGiudice, 2007), are also included for reference. Most of the tests in the table are

TABLE 5.4 | A List of Some Adolescent* Language and Language-Related Tests

Test Name	Author(s)	Year
Clinical Evaluation of Language Fundamentals—5**B & H	Wiig, Semel, and Secord	2013
Clinical Evaluation of Language Fundamentals—5 Metalinguistics	Wiig and Secord	2014
Comprehensive Assessment of Spoken Language—2**B	Carrow-Woolfolk	2017
Comprehensive Receptive and Expressive Vocabulary Test—3	Wallace and Hammill	2013
Comprehensive Test of Phonological Processing—2	Wagner, Torgesen, Rashotte, and Pearson	2013
Detroit Tests of Learning Aptitude—4**H	Hammill	1998
Expressive One-Word Picture Vocabulary Test—4**B & H	Martin and Brownell	2011
Expressive Vocabulary Test—2**B	Williams	2007
Fullerton Language Test for Adolescents—2**H	Thorum	1986
Illinois Test of Psycholinguistic Abilities—3	Hammill, Mather, and Roberts	2001
Lindamood Auditory Conceptualization Test—3	Lindamood and Lindamood	2004
Oral and Written Language Scales—II**B	Carrow-Woolfolk	2011
Peabody Picture Vocabulary Test—4**B & H	Dunn and Dunn	2007
Receptive One-Word Picture Vocabulary Test—4**B	Martin and Brownell	2010
SCAN—3:A Tests for Auditory Processing Disorders in Adolescents and Adults	Keith	2009a
SCAN—3:C Tests for Auditory Processing Disorders for Children	Keith	2009b
Social Language Development Test Adolescent	Bowers, Huisingh, and LoGiudice	2010
Test of Adolescent and Adult Language—4	Hammill, Brown, Larsen, and Wiederholt	2007
Test of Adolescent/Adult Word Finding—2	German	2016
Test of Auditory Processing Skills—3	Martin and Brownell	2005
Test of Integrated Language and Literacy Skills	Nelson, Plante, Helm-Estabrook, and Hotz	2016
Test of Language Competence—Expanded Edition**H	Wiig and Secord	1989
Test of Language Development (Intermediate)—4th Edition	Hammill and Newcomer	2008
Test of Narrative Language	Gillam and Pearson	2004
Test of Pragmatic Language—2	Phelps-Terasaki and Phelps-Gunn	2007
Test of Problem Solving—2: Adolescent**H	Bowers, Huisingh, and LoGiudice	2007
Test of Word Finding—3	German	2015
Test of Word Knowledge**H	Wiig and Secord	1992
The Expressive Language Test	Bowers, Huisingh, LoGiudice, and Orman	2010
The Listening Comprehension Test: Adolescents	Bowers, Huisingh, and LoGiudice	2009
The Word Test—2 Adolescent**H	Bowers, Huisingh, LoGiudice, and Orman	2005
Woodcock-Muñoz Language Survey—III	Woodcock, Muñoz-Sandoval, Ruef, Alvarado, Schrank, McGrew, Wendling, and Dailey	2017

* Designed for individuals 11 years of age or older.
** Listed as among the 10 most frequently used as identified in Betz et al. (2013) (**B), or Huang et al. (1997) (**H), or both (**B & H) studies, although possibly earlier versions than those listed here.

norm referenced. Some examine skills in a variety of language areas such as syntax and semantics or listening comprehension, for example, the Oral and Written Language Scales–II (Carrow-Woolfolk, 2011), the Test of Adolescent and Adult Language–4 (Hammill, Brown, Larsen, & Wiederholt, 2007), and the Test of Integrated Language and Literacy Skills (Nelson, Plante, Helm-Estabrook, & Hotz, 2016). Others focus on one area of language such as vocabulary or pragmatics, for example, the Expressive One-Word Picture Vocabulary Test–4 (Martin & Brownell, 2011) and the Test of Pragmatic Language–2 (Phelps-Terasaki & Phelps-Gunn, 2007).

Several surveys have investigated what tests are used more frequently and what criteria of tests affect their selection for use in language assessments. For example, Betz, Eickhoff, and Sullivan (2013) asked SLPs how frequently they used 55 language and language-related tests for their assessments involving children between 5 and 9 years of age who were suspected of having SLI and compared their choices to several psychometric features of tests, such as reliability and sensitivity. In an earlier study, Huang, Hopkins, and Nippold (1997) surveyed Oregon SLPs about the language tests they used most frequently for individuals in the age range 13 to 19 years. The 10 used most often in each study are identified in Table 5.4 by double asterisks and a letter indicating the first letter of the first author's surname. In a number of cases the nominated tests in the studies were earlier versions of the ones listed in the table. Some differences in which tests were identified as being used more frequently could be expected based on the age range the SLPs were asked to consider, as well what tests were available at the time of the studies.

Norm-referenced tests allow those working with adolescents with suspected language problems to provide numbers that convey some notion about the presence and severity of an adolescent's language impairment and how an individual's language performance compares to that of TD peers. These numbers may be required by school administrators in order to qualify students for services. This is one reason that prompted Apel (1999b) to write that he is "not sure at the present time there is a way to 'beat the numbers game'" (p. 101), even though the norms and validity for a number of the tests have been questioned. However, for adolescent language assessment, it is possible that some norm-referenced tests can identify problems with some aspects of language that standardized, but generally unnormed approaches, including language sampling, might not. For example, Nippold, Mansfield, Billow, and Tomblin (2009) used both a language sampling task involving an expository discourse task about peer conflicts and two subtests (Concepts and Directions and Recalling Sentences) of the norm-referenced test Clinical Evaluation of Language Fundamentals—3 (Semel, Wiig, & Secord, 1995) to investigate the syntax abilities of adolescents with SLI. Although the language sampling task was effective in distinguishing between normally developing 15-year-olds and their same-age peers with SLI for utterance length, clause density (a measure indicating use of subordinate/dependent clauses), and noun clause use, the task was insensitive to differences for adverbial and relative clauses (Nippold et al., 2009). By comparison, the combined performance on the two subtests of the norm-referenced test clearly distinguished between the two groups of adolescents, suggesting that some norm-referenced testing may reveal language deficits that language sampling could miss. Consequently, Nippold et al. (2009) suggested that norm-referenced testing and language sampling using expository discourse tasks can complement each other. Despite the several weaknesses associated with norm-referenced tests, their use has an important place, albeit not the only place, in language assessment of adolescents.

Sensitivity (accurate identification of children with the impairment) and specificity (accurate identification of children without the impairment) of tests are major issues in deciding what to use in assessment, and these two measures of diagnostic accuracy are not always available for norm-referenced tests as professionals try to select the best tests to use. In addition, as we know, tests that are available are not always sufficiently sensitive in order to identify adolescents who struggle as a result of poor language skills. Unless skills that we know are problematic for adolescents with SLI—such as metalinguistics, abstract vocabulary, inferencing, figurative language, complex syntax with different forms of subordination, verb tense morphology, nonword repetition, and morphologically complex words—are included as part of assessment, we need to be cautious about our conclusions about the presence or absence of language impairment. A particular caution is warranted with regard to results of tests such as the Peabody Picture Vocabulary Test. It is not uncommon for adolescents with SLI to score within normal limits on this receptive, single-word vocabulary test because it tends not to be very sensitive to the semantic comprehension problems of these adolescents, which are those that create significant struggles for them in dealing with secondary school curriculum. Consequently, decisions about an adolescent's language status should not be made on the basis of such tests. In contrast, these same adolescents may score well below the cutoff for normal performance on language comprehension tests that require them to interpret figurative language expressions, make inferences, or interpret statements with ambiguities. Table 5.5 shows some examples of such higher-level language comprehension tests items that tend to be more sensitive in identifying language impairment in adolescents than more concrete, decontextualized, single-word vocabulary comprehension tests.

In comparison to the many language tests designed for use with younger children, there are fewer for adolescents. If we eliminate any of these tests because of questionable validity and sensitivity/specificity, our choices of what to use narrow even more. These are among several of the reasons that standardized, unnormed language assessments and informal observations are used and can be used so effectively with adolescents. Other reasons are that many norm-referenced tests examine only limited aspects of language behavior and usually provide for probing only small samples of any particular language skill. These alone do not yield sufficient information about patterns of language behaviors to allow us to develop

TABLE 5.5 | Examples of Higher-Level Language Comprehension Test Items

Type of Higher-level Comprehension Test Items	Examples
Ambiguous Expressions	What are two meanings of: ■ "Visiting relatives can be tiresome" ■ "The pipe is cool"
Figurative Expressions	
Proverbs	What are the meanings of the following: ■ "A rolling stone gathers no moss" ■ "A penny saved is a penny earned"
Idioms	What are the meanings of the following: ■ "It's raining cats and dogs" ■ "A house divided against itself cannot stand"
Metaphors/Similes	What are the meanings of the following: ■ "It's as light as a feather" ■ "The wind was an arrow that pierced the heart"
Inferences	Tell me who I am? ■ "I had finally gotten used to being weightless. I really enjoyed floating by the moray eels hidden in their crevices. The circling sharks, on the other hand, made me uncomfortable." Tell me what has happened? ■ "He was so dejected. He just continued to stare at the examination paper in his hands." ■ "The attorney was ecstatic. The new evidence the detectives uncovered was a game changer."

specific intervention objectives. Techniques other than norm-referenced tests are necessary when assessing the language skills of adolescents.

Unnormed Standardized Methods. In 1993, Damico advanced an argument about language assessment that continues to apply. He stated that assessment "activities used must be more *authentic,* more *functional,* and more *descriptive* than the assessment procedures previously employed with this population" (p. 29). Authentic assessment means looking at and gathering information about how an adolescent uses or cannot use his or her language in contexts that are "real" for the adolescent (e.g., in understanding what teachers say in classroom lessons, in peer interactions, in interpreting spoken and written disciplinary discourse, in trying to apply for part-time jobs, in studying for tests, or in understanding and/or explaining a movie or book). This approach to assessment is often referred to as ecological assessment (McCormick, 2003) and it attempts to assess what is important for functioning in the real world. A number of strategies are available to assist in undertaking more authentic assessment of adolescents. These include analyzing samples of an adolescent's language, creating contrived situations to elicit examples of specific language behaviors of interest, examining portfolios of the student's work, and assessing the educational system in which the student is expected to function.

Analysis of Spontaneous Language. It is impractical to attempt to analyze an adolescent's entire language behavior in any one day. However, it is important to sample language in several situations. A particularly important approach is to sample in several academic disciplines. We have seen elsewhere in this text that academic disciplines differ in how both spoken and written language is used. Therefore, one or more representative samples of spontaneous language are obtained for analysis. Specific factors related to obtaining language samples are discussed in Chapter 13. There the focus is more on the younger child than on the adolescent with a suspected language impairment. However, the principles of obtaining a sample in varying communicative situations and of audio or video recording the sample apply in all instances. Here we discuss approaches that are appropriate specifically for adolescents. For adolescents, samples of their language in dealing with increasingly complex genres are important for the assessment process, thus samples of conversation, narrative, and expository discourse are necessary. Because language characteristics vary with different academic disciplines (Ehren, Murza, & Malani, 2012; Fang, 2012; Fang & Schleppegrell, 2010; Schleppegrell, 2001), samples collected from adolescents as they deal with several different disciplines have the potential to be particularly revealing about an adolescent's language ability in ways that are directly tied to educational functioning.

With regard to conversational language samples, several analysis approaches are available. One example is Larson and McKinley's (1995) Adolescent Conversational Analysis. This analysis method provides for examination of both the listener and the speaker roles of an adolescent during conversational interactions. Listener abilities that are analyzed are understanding the speaker's vocabulary and syntax, following the speaker's main ideas, listening in a nonjudgmental way, and signaling lack of understanding. Speaker abilities are divided into four aspects: language features, paralanguage features, communication functions, and verbal and nonverbal communicational rules. Within each of these broad aspects, specific features of communicative functioning are noted and analyzed. Each of the communicative behaviors is judged as appropriate or inappropriate each time it occurs during a language sample. The tallies or frequency counts of both appropriate and inappropriate behaviors are transferred to a profile form that summarizes an adolescent's strengths and weaknesses. This profile can lead to the development of specific intervention objectives and can form part of the basis of a valid and defensible intervention plan.

As Nippold (2014b) writes, "During conversations, adolescents with typical and impaired language development produce utterances that are shorter and less complex than those they produce during other genres. . . ." (p. 41). In multiple studies (Nippold, Hesketh, Duthie, & Mansfield, 2005; Nippold, Mansfield, & Billow, 2007; Nippold, Mansfield, Billow, & Tomblin, 2008; Wetherell, Botting, & Conti-Ramsden, 2007), the language—and in particular the syntax—that adolescents with SLI used was less complex in language sampling contexts that used conversation than those that used either a narrative or an expository task, with an advantage for more complex syntax occurring in an expository task that involved adolescents talking about peer conflict resolution as opposed to one that asked adolescents to explain a game or sport. Another limitation of using only a conversational language sample with adolescents to identify language impairment and areas of language problems is that, in situations that do not require the use of particular forms, these students can avoid using aspects of language that are not well established in their repertoires or those that continue to create problems for them (Reed & Patchell, 2010; Wetherell et al., 2007). A guiding principle for examining the language of an adolescent is that we need to look for what is *not* present in the adolescent's language or what the adolescent *does not do* with language as much as looking at what an adolescent does do or use. Because a conversation task might not push or challenge an adolescent to use aspects of language that are difficult for the adolescent, we need to include in our assessment practices tasks that induce attempts at using language targets of interest so that we can find out what the adolescent is capable or not capable of. Certain types of narrative and expository discourse tasks seem to accomplish this.

As we saw in Chapter 3, a narrative task can often put sufficient demands on language ability to push or stress an individual's language performance. Problems with narrative production are also implicated in children whose early language problems persist into the adolescent years (Stothard et al., 1998). There are several types of narrative tasks, each having its advantages and disadvantages and each stressing an adolescent's language performance in different ways. In the Wetherell et al. (2007) study and those of Reed and colleagues (Reed, Conrad, & Patchell, 2006; Reed & Evernden, 2001; Reed & Patchell, 2004, 2010; Reed, Patchell, et al., 2006) that looked at verb tense, a storytelling task from a wordless picture book was used. This type of narrative task reduces demands on a student for creative story generation and the influences of variables involving degrees of previous knowledge with particular stories but does not provide an auditory model of the story so that the language used is the language of the adolescent, not that recalled from an examiner's story. Telling a story also tends to encourage the use of past-tense verbs, which means that it may trigger the appearance of verb use patterns not evident in other types of discourse, particularly those that might lead to use of present-tense verbs. A further advantage of including a language sample obtained from a narrative task is that it can provide general information about an adolescent's ability to use narrative and story structure, a particularly important genre in the adolescent years.

Nippold (2014b) has suggested that narrative elicitation approaches other than a wordless picture book be considered. Different narrative tasks may lead to different features and complexity of language elicited in the samples, an effect that has the possibility of skewing results obtained from analyses of the samples. Wetherell and colleagues (2007) compared the performance of adolescents with SLI in two narrative genre tasks, one the classic wordless picture story and the other a conversational narrative. Their findings revealed that the adolescents demonstrated more errors and difficulties in the wordless picture task, including more verb morphological errors, than with the conversational narrative elicitation task. Two other studies (Huber, Reed, Patchell, & Conrad, 2011; Taliaferro, Reed, & Patchell, 2015) compared the verb morphological patterns of younger and older adolescents with SLI and TD on two narrative elicitation methods—one, again, the classic wordless picture book task and the other a story generated from looking at a single picture. Similar to the findings of Wetherell et al. (2007), these two studies also found that the two elicitation methods yielded different patterns of verb morphology. The adolescents with SLI showed more problems, including less use of past tense verbs, with the wordless picture book elicitation approach than the single-picture elicitation method. One of Nippold's (2014b) suggested alternatives for narrative elicitation with adolescents is to use fables, which are first read to the adolescents while looking at single pictures illustrating the fables and which the adolescents then retell, with the assistance of the illustrations. Although Nippold proposes that fables can be "an effective way of eliciting complex syntax in the narrative speaking of young adolescents" (p. 50), she acknowledges that additional research is needed to validate use of fables for narrative elicitation. Such studies need to determine how the language characteristics that emerge with fable telling compare to those elicited by other methods. These comparative studies are essential in order to inform professionals in their choices about the approaches best able to identify adolescents of all ages with language impairment and indicate patterns of language able to provide directions for intervention.

Because expository discourse is such a core element of secondary-school curricula and adolescents' academic performance, it needs to be an essential element of language sampling. One problem that is exacerbated in sampling expository discourse is the amount of prior knowledge an adolescent has about the topic or task used to elicit the sample. Prior knowledge affects the complexity of language elicited by the task (Kamhi, 2009; Nippold, 2010a; Snyder & Caccamise, 2010). Therefore, in order to know that the obtained sample represents an adolescent's language skills and not topic knowledge, it is important that before selecting a particular topic, an adolescent's level of knowledge about it needs to be determined. As an alternative, Nippold (Nippold et al., 2005; Nippold et al., 2007; Nippold et al., 2009) has used several tasks that circumvent specific-content issues. She has asked adolescents to explain how to play a favorite sport or game and how to resolve a peer conflict. Both tasks elicited more complex language than a conversation task. Again, professionals need to be alert to the expository discourse tasks they choose to obtain language samples. Given the increasing interest in expository discourse problems associated with adolescents with SLI and recognition of the negative impact on their curriculum content learning, we are likely to see future research helping to provide clearer guidelines for selecting language sampling tasks to improve assessment accuracy.

Although Larson and McKinley (1995) suggested that the elements of analysis for the aspect of language features include an adolescent's use of a variety of syntactic forms, they were not specific in identifying what "variety of syntactic forms" (p. 286) should be examined as part of their conversational analysis. Several studies have measured a number of syntactic (and morphological) features such as number of utterances, length of utterances, verb morphological errors, and other morphological errors. However, given the expectations for use of complex sentences in secondary curriculum and the information about subordinate/dependent-clause development and conjunction usage in adolescence that is available (Loban, 1976; Nippold et al., 2005; Nippold et al., 2007; Reed, Griffith, & Rasmussen, 1998; Wetherell et al., 2007), an in-depth analysis of an adolescent's use of dependent/subordinate clauses is important. One such measure is known as *clausal density,* determined by dividing the number of utterances in the sample (or more usual for adolescent language samples, C-units or T-units, per Chapter 2) by the number of clauses (sum of independent and dependent/subordinate clauses). This measure provides relatively general data about adolescents' clausal use, but it does not reveal what types of dependent/subordinate clauses (i.e., adverbial, nominative, adjectival/relative) in what proportions and where the clauses are used. A finer-grained analysis of clausal usage has the potential to reveal the presence of language problems that are subtler but insidiously undermine adolescents' success with secondary curriculum content. Figure 5.6 illustrates a guide for proceeding systematically through increasingly finer-grained analyses of an adolescent's dependent/subordinate usage in a language sample. In light of findings about SLI adolescents' continuing difficulties with verb morphology (e.g., Leonard et al., 2009; Reed, Patchell, et al., 2006; Rice et al., 2009), another potentially important area to examine is an adolescent's verb form usage and detection of correct/incorrect forms, including the degree to which an adolescent evidences mastery of correct verb form use (especially past-tense verb forms) and the forms by which the adolescent marks tense.

In Chapter 13, several approaches to analysis methods for language samples are introduced. Some are more appropriate than others for adolescents and the types of samples relevant for this age group. One of the more widely used computerized language sample analysis systems (Systematic Analysis of Language Transcripts—SALT) (Miller, Andriacchi, & Nockerts, 2015) provides options for analyzing samples collected via conversation or through narrative, and more recently via procedural and persuasive expository genres. Databases that permit comparisons of an individual adolescent's analysis to TD adolescents of similar ages are provided for young adolescents whose samples were collected in conversation or narrative contexts and for young and older adolescents for procedural expository and persuasive samples.

Contrived Situations. The concepts of and push for the use of authentic forms of assessment can put professionals in a bind when assessing the language abilities of adolescents.

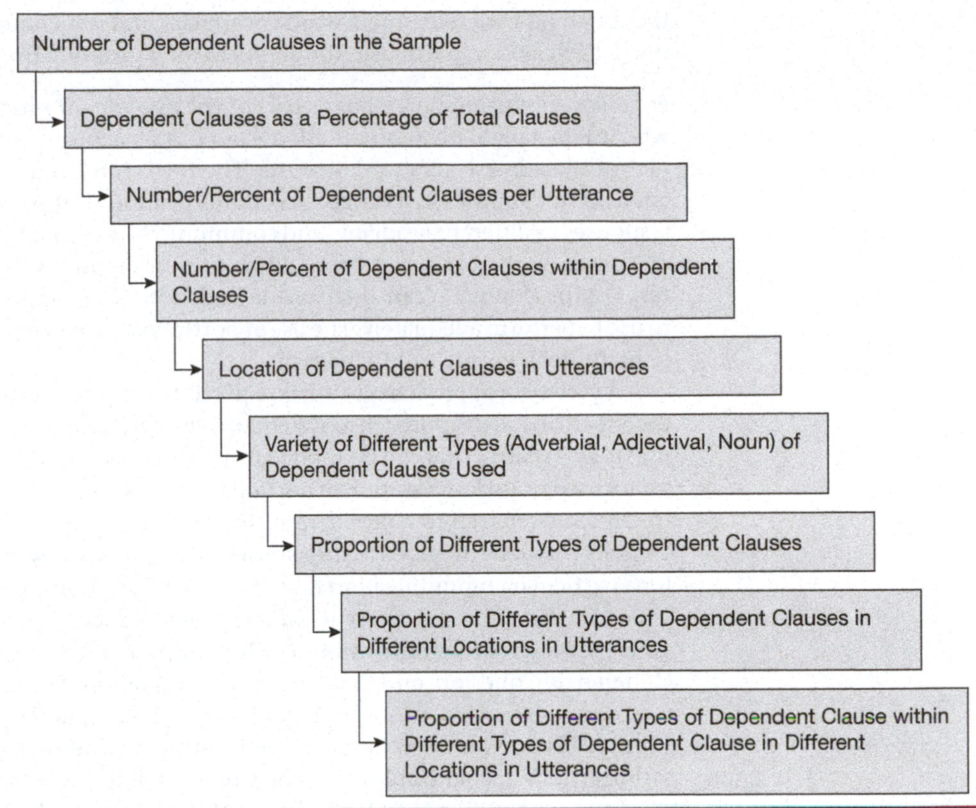

FIGURE 5.6 | Increasingly Finer-Grained Analyses of Dependent/Subordinate Clause Usage in Adolescents' Language Samples

As Nippold (1995) has indicated, "Tasks that are sensitive to later language development sometimes involve the use of language in limited or contrived contexts" (p. 320). To examine an adolescent's language performance in contrived situations seems, on the surface, to be contrary to the principles of authentic assessment. However, it may be necessary to use contrived contexts to elicit information about language abilities that are undermining a student's ability to function in authentic situations. Consequently, it might be useful to avoid considering these two approaches as mutually exclusive. Instead, using contrived situations can be helpful when additional probing of particular skills or eliciting the use of infrequently occurring language structures (e.g., adverbial connectives) is necessary or when an adolescent's ability with language needs to be stressed. Contrived situations are also helpful in assessing the degree to which an adolescent is able to learn new language behaviors and the amount of instructional effort needed from professionals to facilitate the learning, that is, dynamic assessment. Using contrived situations can also provide information about language behaviors that were not evidenced in other sample conditions and that reveal important information about an adolescent's language skills. These situations might be particularly helpful for assessing language abilities involving aspects of figurative and literate language (e.g., proverbs, word definition skills, slang, and idioms) and adverbial connectives.

Contrived situations may also be particularly helpful for examining adolescents' language comprehension abilities when norm-referenced testing for receptive language does not provide sufficient information for identification of language impairment or intervention planning. Comprehension ability is increasingly being recognized as an aspect of language performance that is often overlooked in terms of its impact on performance and outcomes from earlier language difficulties. For example, the evidence is mounting that children and adolescents who have receptive language impairment, with or without expressive language impairment, fare more poorly on measures of social adjustment and level of language abilities in adolescence. Careful assessment of an adolescent's comprehension abilities is important, and many norm-referenced receptive language tests, unfortunately, focus too much on concrete, single-word vocabulary and not enough on comprehension of connected text and, in particular, the ability to infer meaning from connected text.

Portfolios. In using portfolios as part of the assessment process, an adolescent and others who interact regularly with the adolescent (e.g., teachers and school counselors) add examples of the adolescent's work to a file. The file is intended to represent a collection of the adolescent's abilities in a variety of communication contexts and to reflect the adolescent's responses to different academic and communicative demands. A portfolio analysis of an adolescent's work from a number of different subjects and different types of communication tasks in these subjects can also provide leads as to what language the adolescent is expected to use to perform adequately. The use of portfolios as a method of assessment is seen as a particularly ecologically valid approach.

A variety of approaches to analyze portfolios of adolescents is available. Wiig (1995) has described one such approach to systematically conducting a portfolio analysis. Her approach uses a 4 × 4 matrix that can be applied in a "structured, multidimensional assessment profile for focused holistic evaluation of portfolio samples across subject areas within a curriculum" (p. 23). She referred to a profile resulting from such an assessment as an "S-MAP" (p. 23). Dimensions to be included in the assessment matrix vary by what are important dimensions for a particular communication task or context. Each dimension is then assessed on a rating scale of 1 (Good) to 4 (Unacceptable). For example, for a narrative sample, Wiig (1995) suggests that each of four dimensions (1. Organizational Structure; 2. Recall and Elaboration; 3. Coherence, Cohesion, and Conventions; 4. Evaluation, Monitoring, and Revision) be evaluated and assigned one of four ratings (1. Good; 2. Acceptable; 3. Marginal; 4. Unacceptable). Wiig (1995) provided descriptors to guide ratings within each dimension. For example, a description of "A recognizable narrative structure is followed; there is a clear beginning, middle sequence, and ending" for Organizational Structure is rated as "Good," whereas a description for Evaluation, Monitoring, and Revision of "There are many revisions or no revisions when appropriate; when there are revisions, they are abrupt and without transitions, become tangential and verbose" is rated as "Marginal" (p. 25). A matrix such as this has the potential to bring to the analysis of adolescents' portfolios a more structured and standardized approach than might otherwise occur.

Examples of students' written work can also be analyzed in ways similar to analyses used for spoken language samples. If the portfolios do not contain sufficient written samples to provide adequate work to obtain a representative picture of the students' written language abilities, contrived approaches that ask students to produce a piece of written discourse can be used. Both narrative and expository genres can be sampled. Nippold (2014b) has provided protocols for eliciting written samples of both genre types. Analyses can parallel those used for spoken language samples and include metrics derived for overall productivity, for example the number of sentences (i.e., T-units), and for syntactic complexity, for example, mean length of sentences and clausal density, as well as finer-grained analyses of dependent/subordinate clause use. Attention to the mechanics of writing, for example punctuation, paragraphing, and spelling patterns, can also be analyzed. Misspellings can often reveal information about an adolescent's phonological processing, in addition to what spelling rules might be known. The written samples can additionally be subjected to grammatical error analyses (Scott & Windsor, 2000) and use of low frequency words (*examined, surveyed*) versus high frequency general words (*looked at*).

Assessing the Educational System. Success or failure in school significantly affects all aspects of life in adolescence as well as adult life. When an adolescent suspected of having a language impairment has particular difficulty with certain subject areas, a look at the spoken and written language features of the specific discipline compared to the adolescent's language strengths and weaknesses may shed light on the reasons for the adolescent's difficulties. Larson and McKinley (2003) believe that additional analysis can include other elements of the student's educational environment, such as the student's motivation and attitude toward specific subjects and the instructional approaches used in the subjects in which the student is struggling. These authors suggest that such an assessment can help identify the source(s) of the problems.

To facilitate an educational analysis, Larson and McKinley (1995) developed the Curriculum Analysis Form. The form is divided into three parts, all of which are completed for each course an adolescent is finding especially difficult. The first section analyzes the textbook used in the course, and the second focuses on the course's organization and the student's comprehension of classroom lectures/instructions and examinations. The last section of the form asks the adolescent to answer *yes* or *no* to a list of questions designed to probe the adolescent's attitude toward the course. When the analysis is completed, it helps clarify what strategies can be employed to assist the adolescent in dealing with educational language levels.

Lunday (1996) also developed a checklist to guide assessment of what communication skills are expected for postsecondary classroom and vocational success. This form consists of six aspects of language (Vocabulary, Use, Function, Organization, Form, and Pragmatics), each of which is evaluated by answering a number of questions about expectations, for example, expected to participate in classroom discussions, expected to interpret and use nonverbal cues, and required to understand figurative expressions. The teacher's expectation for each question is ascertained (i.e., yes it's an expectation, no it's not, or not applicable). For each question, the student's success in meeting each expectation is also evaluated as being positive, negative, or somewhere in the middle (+/–). The results provide a profile of what communication skills are important for the student from a teacher's perspective and the student's degree of ability to meet those expectations. This approach is quite consistent with the match/mismatch approach to assessment advocated by Larson and McKinley (1995), and the information obtained from such an analysis helps in determining intervention objectives.

The approach employed by Lunday (1996) to assessing classroom communication expectations recognized the importance of the perspectives of the teachers in influencing what communication skills adolescents need for success. What teachers perceive to be more and less important adolescent communication skills with them can set standards for adolescents' performances and influence their students' academic and personal success. To find out what high school teachers think are important communication skills for adolescents, Reed and Spicer (2003) asked grade 10 teachers to rank the importance of 14 communication skills. The skills represented a range of what would be considered primarily skills used for managing discourse (e.g., topic maintenance, conversational clarification, and repair) and those related primarily to empathy and interpersonal relationships and considered to be addressee focused (e.g., taking a listener's perspective, comprehending vocal tone). Two metalinguistic/figurative language skills (verbal humor comprehension and appropriate slang usage) were also included among the 14 communication skills. Table 5.6 shows the teachers'

TABLE 5.6 | High School Teachers' Ranking of the Importance of Communication Skills for Adolescents' Interactions with Their Teachers, in Order from Most to Least Important

1. Relating narratives
2. Presenting differing points of view or thoughts logically
3. Employing conversational clarification and repair strategies
4. Taking a conversational partner's perspective
5. Turn taking appropriately
6. Using appropriate vocal tone
7. Establishing and maintaining appropriate eye contact
8. Selecting conversational topics
9. Comprehending nonverbal communication
10. Comprehending vocal tone
11. Conveying messages tactfully
12. Maintaining topics
13. Comprehending verbal humor
14. Using appropriate adolescent slang

Source: Reed and Spicer (2003).

ranking of the 14 communication skills from most to least important. The skills ranked as relatively high in importance were ones generally associated with discourse management strategies, while the least important skills were the two metalinguistic/figurative language skills. To identify potential areas of mismatch and, therefore, potential intervention objectives, students' degrees of ability with each of these communication skills can be compared to the relative importance attached to them by their teachers, not unlike the approach used with Lunday's (1996) checklist.

INTERVENTION

In 2008, Cirrin and Gillam published results of their systematic review of language interventions for school-age children. The authors reported that "no studies were located that focused on students in middle grades or high school" (p. S110) and of the 21 studies that met criteria for review, only two considered any intervention approaches for students age 12 years or older. This reflects in another way the underrecognition of adolescents with language impairment, but it also means that there is more limited evidence to guide intervention for adolescents with language impairment than that available for language intervention for younger children (Nippold, 2011). On a more positive note, since 2008 there is an increasing amount of literature that addresses language-impaired adolescents, which suggests that more intervention research will include adolescents. Currently, however, there are several principles that can guide intervention.

There is a general consensus among professionals working with adolescents with language impairment that these adolescents must participate in planning their own intervention, which contrasts with much of the intervention with language-impaired youngsters, who are often naive about the purposes and objectives of intervention. As early as 1985, Larson and McKinley wrote that there can be "no 'hidden agenda' when providing services for adolescents" (p. 72). The principle of no hidden agenda means the following:

- Purposes of assessments are explained and results are shared with the adolescent.
- Responsibility for identifying, establishing, and prioritizing intervention plans and objectives is a task shared among the adolescent and relevant professionals (e.g., SLPs, classroom teachers, and special educators).
- The reasons why particular skills are included in assessments and/or targeted in intervention are explained to and discussed with the adolescent.

Among the several reasons for adopting this approach are the following:

- Adolescents who recognize and accept that they have problems with communication and believe that intervention can help often begin to identify their own communicative behaviors that they wish to improve and that are important to them.
- Involvement in determining their own objectives leads the adolescents to accept responsibility for their problems, to take ownership of the problems, and to realize that they have the major role in modifying their language skills.
- Taking responsibility for their own problems and ways in which to address them means that adolescents are more likely to be motivated to improve.
- It begins to address what is a major objective of intervention with adolescents—improving their "meta" skills, that is, metalinguistics, metacognition, and metapragmatics.

Principles in Determining Intervention Objectives

Emphasize Strategies, Regularities, and the Metas. Objectives need to emphasize direct instruction that shows adolescents how to learn language (Kamhi, 2014) and how to manage language demands of learning. Adolescents need to be taught strategies, rules, and techniques that will improve their communicative performances and their abilities to use their language to learn and function socially and vocationally. These are the skills and strategies that can generalize to daily language use. The emphasis is, therefore, on using and improving metalinguistic, metacognitive, and metapragmatic abilities. Sometimes the term *executive functioning* or *self-regulation* is used to describe the focus or processes related to this strategies approach, but as Singer and Bashir (1999) point out, "both are considered 'meta' constructs" (p. 265).

Several different specific strategies approaches are described in the literature, among them the Self-Regulated Strategy Development Model (Graham & Harris, 1999), the Strategic Process Model for Strategy Development (Wiig, 1990), the Strategic Instruction Model® (SIM®) of the University of Kansas Center for Research in Learning (e.g., Deshler & Schumaker, 1988; Deshler et al., 2001), and Integrative Strategy Instruction (Ellis, 1993). What all of these have in common, according to Bray (1995), is that "students learn how to identify patterns in the information to be processed, select a plan of strategies to learn the information, implement the strategic plan, and later evaluate and monitor its effectiveness" (p. 67). This approach contrasts with intervention objectives focusing on tutoring in academic content areas. Intervention, then, includes teaching specific strategies and discussions about which of the strategies can be employed under what situations, including specific examples of other possible situations. Adolescents' conscious attempts to acquire strategies and to generate more examples of where else to apply the strategies can enhance, in very practical ways, the students' metalinguistic and metacognitive skills and facilitate generalization or bridging. Additionally, this approach stresses the pragmatic aspects of language and makes language functional for the adolescents, another guiding principle of intervention for adolescents with language impairment.

Don't Miss the Missing Language Skills Needed to Underpin Strategies. A strategy does not work if an adolescent does not have the necessary underpinning language skills. However, with adolescents the approach is not to retreat to developmental sequences, an approach often seen with younger children. First, there are no "developmental sequences," like sequential acquisition of 14 grammatical morphemes, to rely on when working with adolescents. Second, we can expect that an adolescent's language skills represent a patchy pattern, in part as a result of idiosyncratic exposures to prior interventions and as a result of academic and social successes and failures.

Intervention for any specific language skills must be determined by identifying those needed for a particular strategy for an individual to implement a strategy and those absent from the adolescent's repertoire, again the match/mismatch concept. For example, several of the strategies approaches noted previously include the strategy of teaching adolescents how to systematically implement steps to tackle paraphrasing. Thus, the adolescent is required to learn what those steps are and then to practice executing those steps, for example, knowing that the main idea of a passage needs to be identified as one of the steps. However, the process of paraphrasing and the steps within the process require multiple underpinning language skills, in this case, one of which would be access to sufficient vocabulary related directly to the topic/content of the material to be paraphrased. If an adolescent does not have a range of words to engage in paraphrasing about particular topics, an intervention objective might be to target *relevant* vocabulary. This approach to targeting vocabulary differs from an approach that involves a random selection of words and synonyms from, for example, some grade-level list of words pulled from a resource book. The first approach integrates an intervention objective directly with educationally relevant needs. It might be, however, that the adolescent has not yet learned the prefixes and suffixes relevant for the content, another underpinning skill that could be a focus of intervention. Again, however, any work on prefixes and suffixes is related to *relevant* disciplinary content rather than a random selection of prefixes and suffixes. It is also possible that the adolescent does not know the skills of how to begin deciphering morphologically complex words generally. In all cases, intervention for any of these skills would make it explicit for the adolescent as to how they relate to the paraphrasing strategy and to how they apply in other situations.

Authentic Intervention—but "Practice Makes Perfect." Just as assessment processes with adolescents need to be authentic, so does intervention. Singer and Bashir (1999) advise to

> avoid decontextualized interventions. Goals of intervention are not isolated from the day-to-day demands for communication and learning that students encounter. (pp. 271–272)

The examples above illustrate the principle of objectives having a basis in the adolescents' educational contexts.

Authentic objectives promote positive human interactions, facilitate academic success, and allow people to operate on a day-to-day basis without recurring failures. Using information about what communication skills are more and less important to adolescents and their various communication partners in different situations, such as those shown in Table 5.7 as well as Table 5.6, can be helpful in selecting intervention objectives. We see that when TD adolescents were ranking communication skills according to perceived importance in positive interactions with peers, skills more closely related to empathy and concern for communication partner tend to be ranked as more important. Figurative language skills (slang usage, verbal humor) tended to be ranked as less important. Skills related to managing discourse mostly fell into the medium important range. However, as can also be concluded from the rankings in Table 5.7, SLPs might not want to rely solely on what they believe would be important skills for adolescents because, as results of one of the studies shown in that table indicate, their opinions might differ substantially from those of adolescents, especially when adolescent peer interactions are being considered (Reed, Bradfield, & McAllister, 1998). There is also some evidence that adolescents with language impairment may perceive the relative importance of different communication skills for positive interactions with their peers differently from the relative importance perceived by TD adolescents (Reed & Brammall, 2006, 2008). For example, language-impaired adolescents have been found to rank humor comprehension and logical communication higher in importance than their TD peers and vocal tone comprehension and tact as lower in importance. When intervention centers on practical and relevant language abilities, adolescents are likely to recognize their importance and, therefore, be motivated to acquire them. This is especially true if the purposes of the objectives are explained and if real-life examples of effective and ineffective communication are provided and used as part of intervention.

It is unfortunate that for many adolescents with language impairment, their history of intervention will have been inconsistent, possibly with gaps in services, and objectives and directions of intervention may have suffered from a lack of coherence. This means that skills or strategies that might have been targets of intervention previously may not have been adequately learned in order to be stable or retained. Furthermore, these adolescents are typically inefficient learners who need additional time, repeated efforts, and more exposures than other students to learn and/or use a new skill or strategy. In contrast to their need for increased consistency and enhanced learning opportunities, their intervention has more than likely been inconsistent, with inadequate opportunities and repetitions of learning trials. This situation creates a wide gap between the learning opportunities that adolescents need to have provided for them to learn and achieve and what is often provided for them.

What is not known for adolescents is how much "practice makes perfect" or how much "more" is necessary. This translates as not knowing what the "dose" for intervention needs to be in order to be effective (Scott, 2014). And, we are not precise in what we should measure to determine effectiveness. It might be that our definitions of "effective" need to mirror the principle of "authentic objectives." That is, if an adolescent with language impairment is able to function independently or with minimal supports from general/regular educators in important learning and social environments, intervention has been effective. This approach is a departure from the idea of measuring number of correct responses for narrow intervention objectives. The former idea of "effectiveness" correlates more closely with learning, whereas the latter notion of "effectiveness" correlates more closely with performance. Drawing on the ideas of Bjork (2004), Kamhi (2014) wrote that "*Performance* is the short-term context-specific occurrence of some behavior, whereas *learning* is the long-term context-independent occurrence of the particular behavior" (p. 93).

To achieve effectiveness, Simon (1998) advised that focused practice and overlearning of strategies and their implementation are essential and that "drill is not necessarily bad" (p. 263). She added, however, that focused practice and drill need to be meaningful and to take place in context. That is, work on intervention objectives needs to be authentic, there needs to be a sufficient amount of it, and it needs to be consistent. Kamhi (2014), based on Fey (1988), comments that, in light of how much language exposure occurs for TD children to learn particular

TABLE 5.7 | Rankings of the Importance of 14 Communication Skills for Adolescents in Different Communicative Contexts, in Order from Most to Least Important

Whose Rankings:[1] TD Adolescents *Context:* In peers' communication for positive peer relationships	*Whose Rankings:*[2] TD Adolescents *Context:* In adolescent's own communication with peers for positive peer relationships	*Whose Rankings:*[2] TD Adolescents *Context:* In adolescent's own communication with teachers	*Whose Rankings:*[3] Speech–Language Pathologists *Context:* In adolescents' communication for positive peer relationships
Taking a conversational partner's perspective	Comprehending nonverbal communication	Turn taking appropriately	Initiating topics of conversation appropriately*
Comprehending vocal tone	Taking a conversational partner's perspective	Taking a conversational partner's perspective	Selecting conversational topics
Conveying messages tactfully	Comprehending vocal tone	Presenting differing points of view or thoughts logically	Employing conversational clarification and repair strategies
Turn taking appropriately	Using appropriate vocal tone	Employing conversational clarification and repair strategies	Presenting differing points of view or thoughts logically
Using appropriate vocal tone	Selecting conversational topics	Using appropriate vocal tone	Turn taking appropriately
Establishing and maintaining appropriate eye contact	Conveying messages tactfully	Conveying messages tactfully	Comprehending verbal humor
Comprehending nonverbal communication	Presenting differing points of view or thoughts logically	Comprehending vocal tone	Comprehending nonverbal communication
Employing conversational clarification and repair strategies	Turn taking appropriately	Relating narratives	Using appropriate adolescent slang
Selecting conversational topics	Employing conversational clarification and repair strategies	Establishing and maintaining appropriate eye contact	Relating narratives
Presenting differing points of view or thoughts logically	Establishing and maintaining appropriate eye contact	Selecting conversational topics	Establishing and maintaining appropriate eye contact
Relating narratives	Relating narratives	Comprehending nonverbal communication	Taking a conversational partner's perspective
Comprehending verbal humor	Comprehending verbal humor	Maintaining topics	Conveying messages tactfully
Maintaining topics	Maintaining topics	Comprehending verbal humor	Comprehending vocal tone
Using appropriate adolescent slang	Using appropriate adolescent slang	Using appropriate adolescent slang	Using appropriate vocal tone

Sources: [1]Henry, Reed, and McAllister (1995); [2]Reed, McLeod, and McAllister (1999); [3]Reed, Bradfield, et al. (1998).
*In this study, the item for topic initiation replaced the topic maintenance item in the other studies.

elements of language, providing only limited intervention time assumes that "the language learning abilities in children with language impairments are somehow better than those of typically developing children" (p. 93). We know the opposite is true about the language learning facility of language-impaired adolescents. They are not efficient language learners.

Previously in this chapter we presented data about students being dismissed from language intervention at the end of elementary school. Scott (2014) raised the question of when older children and adolescents should be dismissed from intervention. One answer may relate to the idea of "authentic" effectiveness, per above—that is, the question of how well an adolescent with a language impairment is able to function in the academic and social context of secondary school. A second answer might lie in notions of Response to Intervention (RtI) frameworks. Within these frameworks, an adolescent with language impairment could move seamlessly back and forth from special education/SLP Tier 3 intervention to supports in Tier 2 or 1 at different times within the different secondary grades, depending on language demands of the curriculum and social challenges and their match with the adolescent's skills. With this approach, there is no need to ask the question of when adolescents with language impairment should be "dismissed" from intervention. The more appropriate questions are to what degree is an adolescent still needing language-learning supports to succeed and what are the best settings with the best professionals to provide those.

Different Intervention Emphases for Adolescents at Different Stages. The period of adolescence spans 7 or more years. If thought of in terms of the changes that occur in a young child from infancy to 7 years of age, it should not be a surprising idea that the developmental stage known as adolescence needs to considered as consisting of substages, much in the same way that the 0- to 7-year period is thought of as several stages (infants, toddlers, preschoolers, and primary school age). When planning intervention, therefore, the adolescent's stage must be considered, and the strategies, activities, and objectives need to correspond to his or her social-cognitive level (Larson & McKinley, 2003).

In the early years of adolescence, teenagers with language impairment have several years of school ahead of them, so there is still opportunity to improve academic performance. Relationships with peers are beginning to take on greater importance, and there is greater expectation for appropriate interactions with a larger variety of people. For these reasons, intervention objectives with teenagers in the early years of adolescence that focus on language to improve both social and academic performance would likely be appropriate (Larson & McKinley, 2003). In contrast, teenagers in late adolescence, such as those between 16 and 18 years of age, are likely to have concerns about post-high school, i.e., vocational options, further education and training, and employment. Peer relations are more important than in the early adolescent years, and interactions with workmates take on increased importance. For these adolescents, objectives that emphasize improving language for vocational as well as social/workplace situations may be more important, whereas intervention objectives with a large focus on language to improve academic performance may carry less importance, depending on the individual adolescents. For adolescents in the years between the early and later stages of adolescence (i.e., between about 13 and 15 years), peer relationships have considerable importance, and there is still some time to take advantage of academic input. However, vocational concerns may also emerge. For these reasons, there is considerable rationale for intervention objectives with these adolescents in the middle period of development to emphasize social, vocational, and academic language skills (Larson & McKinley, 2003).

Choosing Objectives for Success. One maxim that we know well about human learning is that nothing succeeds like success; we know that success in learning leads to more success. This is a particularly important principle to consider in selecting intervention objectives for language-impaired adolescents, especially in the early stages of intervention. An adolescent with a language impairment likely has a history of academic and personal failure and may believe that he or she is not capable of learning when language is involved. It is not unusual for language-impaired adolescents to resist or avoid such learning situations, especially if they are removed from mainstream settings for their intervention. Therefore, as Bray (1995) writes, "it is important for a student to see results soon after learning and trying a strategy in order to 'buy into' the program" (p. 69). When adolescents see that they "can do it" and that it makes a difference in real ways for them, they are more apt to try to do more and to improve. Motivation problems are commonly ascribed to adolescents with language impairment. Choosing objectives that promote quick success, particularly in the early stages of intervention, can help overcome some of the problems related to motivation.

Factors in Implementing Intervention Objectives

Direct Teaching. Intervention requires direct teaching of skills and specific strategies to adolescents (Ehren, 2002) so that they actually learn these and the analysis abilities needed to apply and evaluate them, to learn to recognize when the skills and strategies should be used and which should be tried, and to learn to self-initiate applying these. Other adolescents have learned a great deal of language, a great deal about how to learn, and a great deal about how to use their language to learn, often without having been taught any of this directly; language-impaired adolescents have not, and there is little reason to believe that by the time these individuals reach adolescence, they will learn these skills without being taught directly. As an example, we know that adolescents with language impairment are likely limited in the types of complex sentences that they use, recognize in written text, and comprehend. For these reasons, expanding these adolescents' repertoire with complex sentences, and in particular those with relative clauses (adjectival clauses), is an often recommended intervention objective (Kamhi, 2014; Nippold, 2014a; Scott, 2014) that can underpin several strategies (e.g., paraphrasing, inferencing, sentence writing) and can be taught directly in intervention. Direct teaching can include, for example: a) the metalinguistic activity of discussion about what a relative clause is (syntactically and semantically) and how it functions in particular types of sentences (complex) (i.e., disambiguates a noun, describes a noun), b) an activity involving a search for relative clauses in individual sentences and subsequently in short paragraphs, c) an accompanying activity that involves discussion of what the clause "says" about the noun, and d) an activity involving combining two 1-clause sentences (simple sentences) into a 2-clause sentence with one of the clauses a relative clause. And, because an individual underpinning objective is related to strategies that it supports, activities are subsequently absorbed into the strategies and used in executing these, for example, paraphrasing the ideas in two sentences by using one complex sentence with a relative clause.

Consideration of Characteristics of Adolescents with Language Impairment. Implementing intervention objectives and, in particular, direct teaching that focuses on a strategies approach can be a bit trickier than it might seem. The things that these adolescents need to learn to do require them to use the very abilities and skills that are typically weak for them and are actually considered to be characteristics of these teenagers. This is probably why the adolescents did not acquire the strategies and skills in the first place. Table 5.8 highlights what might be incompatibilities and clashes between the requirements of learning and using language-related strategies and a number of the characteristics commonly seen in adolescents with language problems.

These adolescents have a long history—possibly as long as they are old—of "not quite having got it," "it" being whatever was in the environment to be learned at any point in time. These adolescents are also victims of the "Matthew effect" Stanovich (1986), explained as real-life examples of the second part of the proverb, "The rich get richer and the poor get poorer." Because adolescents with language impairment most likely started school with poor language skills when good language skills are required for becoming readers, they might not have learned to read fluently and well. And because reading is the greatest single source for further language acquisition and world knowledge, their poor reading skills mean that the gap between students with language problems and those able to take advantage of reading and formal education widens greatly through the early school years into adolescence. Because of the missed bits of information and the mislearning that have fed into these adolescents' concept formation and knowledge base for years, Simon (1998) suggests that "over time, a great deal of *misinformation can be acquired*" and that students' world knowledge can seem "quite weird" (p. 258). The misconceptions that adolescents with language impairment acquire mean that they attempt to build new knowledge on top of flawed, distorted, and/or incomplete information. Wiig (1995) likens this to trying to build a house on a hole instead

TABLE 5.8 | Discrepancies between Characteristics of Adolescents with Language Impairment and Requirements of Strategies Taught in Intervention

Some Characteristics of Adolescents with Language Impairment	Requirements Involved in Learning and Employing Language-Based Learning Strategies
An adolescent with a language impairment likely has weak metalinguistic and metacognitive skills.	A strategies approach requires an adolescent to analyze and think about communicative situations and language demands of a learning task, that is, metalinguistic and metacognitive skills. In essence, what this does is ask the adolescent to use what are weak metalinguistic and metacognitive skills, rather than use what might be stronger skills, to learn new strategies and apply them in new situations that, in themselves, are "meta" skills.
Many adolescents with language impairment are quite poor and inefficient information processors. Inefficient information processing abilities probably mean that an adolescent's problem-solving and task-analysis activities are slow. The educational system and interpersonal interactions expect quick responses; a language-impaired teenager may have learned over his or her many school years that adults and peers dislike incorrect responses less than delayed or no responses.	Using metalinguistic and metacognitive tasks can require that a considerable amount of information be stored in short-term or working memory long enough to be processed and mentally manipulated.
The adolescent might have figured out that if he or she guesses but is wrong, an adult will probably explain and fill in the missing parts or move on to something or somebody else so that the language-impaired adolescent is "let off the hook."	A strategies approach requires that the adolescent take time to figure out an appropriate approach to a problem and arrive at a correct answer.
To the adolescent, it may be better to respond quickly and be wrong than cause a delay or create a silence while trying to figure out a correct response. There is the possibility of a long history of a language-impaired adolescent having been provided with inadvertent positive reinforcement for quick, ill-considered responses. Adolescents with language impairment may have habituated a "guessing strategy." Response impulsivity is characteristic of many adolescents with language impairment.	Guessing is the exact opposite of what is necessary for the considered, analytical approach involved in using strategies.
Adolescents with language impairment are often concrete thinkers and concrete problem solvers. Many adolescents with language impairment are passive and dependent learners; "learned helplessness" is a term sometimes associated with adolescents with language impairment. Adolescents with language impairment often fail to self-activate or self-initiate the application of strategies even when they have learned the strategies and where to use them.	A strategies approach involves both situational analysis and performance evaluation, which are generally considered to be quite hypothetical and formal thought processes. Learning and using strategies requires that students initiate the process of analyzing a task, select one or more strategies from their repertoire, and then apply these and do so independently without needing to be prompted by another person.

of a solid foundation. A somewhat different analogy is illustrated in Figure 5.7. In this illustration, an adolescent's world knowledge is conceived of as a piece of fabric into which pellets from a shotgun have been fired and which have left randomly sized and randomly located holes in information. Concepts and knowledge that underpin the formation of new, larger, and more complex concepts are flawed, distorted, and undermined in unpredictable ways by the holes in knowledge. In working with adolescents with language impairment, professionals cannot assume that the concepts these teenagers have formed are similar to those of their normally achieving peers.

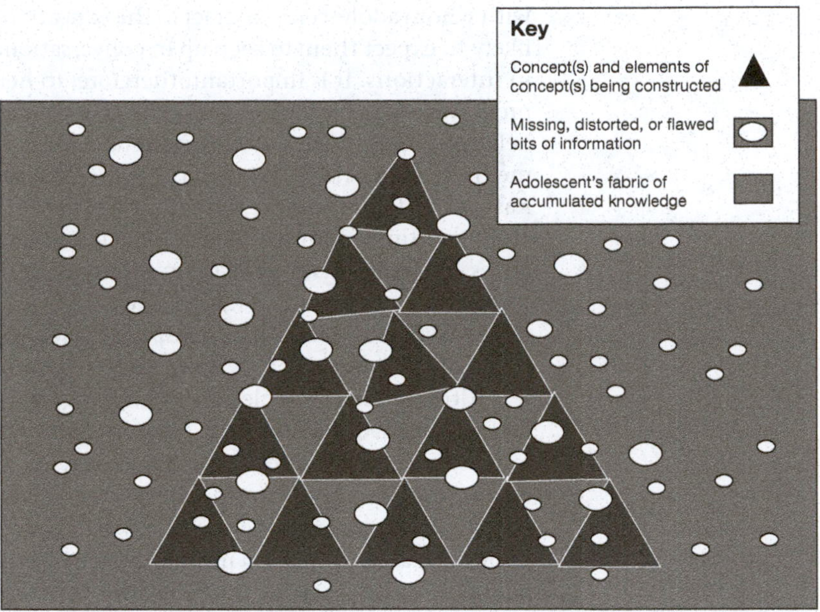

FIGURE 5.7 | A Schematic Illustration of Adolescents' Constructions of Concepts on an Incomplete Fabric of Accumulated Knowledge Flawed over Time by Missing Bits of Information as a Result of Early and Ongoing Language Impairment

© 2002 Vicki A. Reed

Intervention Approaches to Accommodate Adolescents' Language and Learning Characteristics. Although implementing intervention objectives for adolescents with language impairment might be tricky, a number of techniques and approaches can be helpful in getting around the barriers to learning raised by the language and learning characteristics exhibited by these adolescents. Among these are the following:

- Teach, expect, and reward an adolescent's self-activation and self-initiation in applying strategies and skills; stress independent learning; and identify self-activation and self-initiation as intervention objectives in their own right. This particular approach attempts to replace dependent, passive learning behaviors with those characteristic of active and independent learners and those more in line with learner expectations in the high school years.
- Ensure overlearning and stabilization, plan for and build in redundancy, and incorporate repetition in many different situations; follow up; return regularly and frequently to previously targeted objectives to review performance and ensure the skills have been maintained; and build in regular monitoring and checking of skills previously targeted that are no longer active intervention objectives. All of this is especially important in light of what has probably been an inconsistent intervention history for an adolescent and the evidence that skills and strategies often break down during periods of stress, typically when they are most needed, even when these appeared to have previously been learned quite well.
- Because speed of response is the antithesis of what is trying to be achieved by a strategies approach for these adolescents, replace habituated guessing and response impulsivity with a strategy that allows them to delay responding and provides for processing time. Increasing wait time before making responses has been found to improve the quality of the responses of school-age children with language-learning disabilities to higher-level cognitive questions involving synthesis of information and to increase their verbal fluency (i.e., reduce maze behavior) in relating the information. These findings are consistent with information from educational research involving both school-age and university students (Kaplan & Kies, 1994; Tobin, 1986, 1987). However, many of those

with whom adolescents interact in the educational system and in peer relationships are likely to expect them to keep up in conversational turn exchanges and with responses in interactions. It is important, therefore, to help these individuals to employ an appropriate wait time and for the adolescents to adopt pragmatically appropriate ways to delay responding, such as making a statement that indicates an intentional delay ("Let me think about that," "Mmmm"). For school-age children with SLI, Evans, Viele, and Kass (1997) found that the use of verbal pauses (e.g., "ah," "um") at the beginning of the children's turns during conversational interchanges predicted their use of longer utterances. Such responses mark a turn, signal awareness of the previous utterance, indicate a need for a response, and fill the space while providing time to comprehend what was to be taken in and formulate a response. Such responses need to be well rehearsed and habituated, however, if they are to be of help to adolescents.

Although many adolescents with language impairment demonstrate a pattern of ill-considered, quick responses, there are some who do not respond at all or who exhibit long, silent pauses in their utterances, leaving silences to fill the spaces where others expect responses or disrupting the flow of conversation. If the reason for the silences is that an adolescent is using these "to buy" processing time, these occurrences of unacknowledged silences, often misinterpreted by others as sullenness or obstinacy, can also be addressed by replacing the behavior with a more pragmatically appropriate delaying tactic involving a rehearsed statement or filler.

- Employ concrete, hands-on activities to work on abstract "meta" tasks. Recall that adolescents with language impairment are often at a concrete stage of cognition for learning. The idea is to use activities consistent with concrete cognitive levels—for example, sorting cards or objects, creating models, or using paper and pencil or a computer to map concepts—to facilitate development, use, and learning of various higher-level cognitive "meta"-level tasks associated with a strategies approach. For example, Scott (2014), in describing how she approaches teaching relative clauses to language-impaired school children and adolescents, uses "active manipulation" (p. 149) to combine clauses into complex sentences by cutting and pasting, via a computer, a center-embedded relative clause into an independent clause.
- Reduce information processing demands (e.g., how much information needs to be stored at a time in working memory and how much mental manipulation is involved in a task) by keeping needed information in the immediate environment. This can be accomplished by using intransient and stable stimuli (usually visual or graphic), such as lists, charts, or computer monitors, to supplement or counter transient auditory stimuli. With this technique, an adolescent can retrieve and consult bits of information in "permanent" (i.e., intransient) form that are needed to solve abstract or metatasks or needed to implement a particular problem-solving strategy. Often, the activities that address reducing information processing demands are consistent with concrete operations activities, as above.

Activities with an Authentic Focus That Integrate Aspects of Language. As we saw above, suggested techniques do not preclude the use of authentically based activities. In fact, the techniques can be ways to facilitate language-based strategies and to integrate work on several aspects of language. As an example, a science-based activity might center around a very real-life, functional ability and, therefore, quite authentic objective, such as understanding a TV weather broadcast. A small-group setting might be used to address several functional aims: (1) to understand meanings of words and roots and affixes, such as *precipitation, barometer,* and *prevailing,* as in *prevailing winds*; (2) to recognize cause–effect relationships based on the next day's forecast; (3) to identify specific differences between formal register as used in a TV broadcast and informal register inappropriate for such a communicative situation; (4) to select words, phrases, and sentences appropriate for use in a formal communicative context, such as giving a weather broadcast; (5) to prepare the script for a teleprompter; and (6) to adopt a formal communicative style to execute giving a weather report on TV. We see that these objectives encompass semantic, syntactic, morphological, and pragmatic aspects of language at both the receptive and the expressive level, yet they center on a possible curriculum-relevant activity while promoting metalinguistic and metacognitive skills across spoken and written discourse.

Service Delivery

In Chapter 4, several different models of service delivery were discussed. What we know about intervention for adolescents with language impairment is that traditional service delivery models, such as the pullout model, are not effective if used as the sole intervention approach. As early as 1983, Boyce and Larson (1983) discussed service delivery issues for adolescents and provided four reasons for the ineffectiveness of traditional models:

1. When secondary students are removed from their classrooms for short periods of time twice a week, the usual daily schedules are disrupted.
2. Secondary students who need to walk in and out of classrooms during class periods are viewed as different from their peers during a developmental period when conformity to the peer norm is important to them.
3. Intervention can be viewed as punitive because, in addition to the first two reasons, the adolescents "receive no credit for work that may be very difficult for them" (p. 23).
4. Establishing and maintaining relationships with service providers are difficult when these professionals are removed from the usual routine of the schools. Additionally, the traditional one-to-one intervention fails to promote communicative interactions and provide opportunities to practice new language skills in varied communicative contexts.

In light of the evidence that language intervention needs to have sufficient intensity and frequency with educational relevancy, service delivery models other than the traditional pullout model need to be implemented, with the pullout model reserved for only a few situations and often for only short periods of time (Ehren, 2009b; Nippold, 2012).

It is also likely that, by themselves, indirect models in which others deliver intervention are typically not sufficient to address the academic and social needs of many of these students. However, it is important to integrate the principles of this service delivery approach into more encompassing models of providing intervention for these adolescents. That is, close collaboration and consultation among all professionals who interact with an adolescent are essential for a unified and integrated intervention program. This not only is good practice but also is consistent with the legislation that guides and funds service delivery, particularly as principles of Response to Intervention (RtI), discussed in Chapter 4, that infuse both the regular/general education and special education systems, blur, appropriately, the boundaries between the two.

Although RtI models have been implemented in many elementary schools, these models have been slower to be embraced at the secondary level (Ehren, 2009b; Ehren & Whitmire, 2009). There are several reasons for the lag in RtI implementation in middle and high schools, among them the focus on students' learning content versus learning skills, general/regular secondary teachers often having less training in working with students with disabilities, the complications of secondary-school schedules, less recognition of factors affecting the learning of adolescents with language impairment, and less awareness of students with language impairment. Nevertheless, the RtI framework has potential to overcome some of the disadvantages of more traditional models of service delivery for adolescents with language impairment (Ehren, 2009b; Ehren & Whitmire, 2009). It can capitalize on consultative and consultation models and lead to language intervention support to occur more frequently within classroom settings, thus fitting more closely with educationally relevant and authentic principles. One model is for classroom teachers and specialists with expertise in language (e.g., SLP, learning disabilities teacher) to team in the students' classrooms. This model has the potential to provide curriculum-based instruction with a "lens" (Ehren, 2009a) that focuses on the language demands of curricular materials and the language of instruction. A language specialist can assist in bringing the language into focus and facilitate the adolescents to adopt language strategies that let them gain access to content in the curriculum. Helping language-impaired adolescents access curricular content is essential to their academic success, but such content access will have typically been limited previously because of their language challenges and their related issues with literacy (Ehren, 2009a).

Another service delivery model for providing direct language intervention for language-impaired adolescents is to deliver intervention in classrooms with an SLP or other language specialist as the teacher. (Larson & McKinley, 2003; Nippold, 2011; Work, Cline, Ehren, Keiser, & Wujek, 1993). In this model, existing blocks of time in the school's daily schedule are frequently utilized for intervention. Students may be seen for an entire time period on a regularly scheduled basis, sometimes as frequently as 5 days a week. As with other classes, the students are generally seen in groups, although these groups are much smaller than the usual academic class. Small-group sessions facilitate interaction and communication practice. To describe such an intervention format, supportive titles, rather than punitive ones, are recommended, such as those of Larson and McKinley (1995), that is, "Individualized Language Skills" or "Oral Communication Strategies" (p. 162). The Language Intervention Program for Secondary Students (Comkowycz, Ehren, & Hayes, 1987), implemented in Polk County Schools in Florida, selected the name Exceptional Student Education—Language Arts because the class "is taught under the rubric of a state-designed curriculum framework" (p. 204). A program in the Palo Alto Unified School District in California chose the name Language/Study Skills Class (Buttrill, Niizawa, Biemer, Takahashi, & Hearn, 1989). With this intervention format, students' efforts are recognized, intervention is not viewed as penalizing or stigmatizing, and strategies and underpinning language skills can be learned and practiced in interactive situations. The model resolves the problems of traditional service delivery formats. Furthermore, because the format fits into the daily academic schedule, intervention becomes an integrated, accepted part of the school routine.

SUMMARY

In this chapter we have seen that

- Even though we are learning more about adolescent language impairment, gaps remain in our knowledge, and this group of individuals with language impairment continues to be underrecognized and underserviced professionally.
- Gaps in our knowledge make assessment of language-impaired adolescents an especially challenging process; nevertheless, assessment must include norm-referenced procedures in combination with language sampling, observation, and other standardized, unnormed procedures.
- Fewer norm-referenced language tests have been developed for adolescents than for youngsters, and the validity, including sensitivity and specificity, of several of these adolescent tests is questionable.
- Intervention for language-impaired adolescents needs to
  - Involve the adolescents in helping to set their own intervention objectives.
  - Emphasize strategies and underpinning language skills for the strategies and improve metalinguistic, metapragmatic, and metacognitive skills.
  - Focus on functional communication skills, emphasize authentic objectives in authentic contexts, and help them acquire strategies and metaskills so that they can effectively access the content of the curriculum in their classes.
  - Consider an adolescent's developmental stage and use a variety of intervention techniques to work around the barriers to learning that an adolescent with a language impairment can exhibit.
  - Shift away from primarily using traditional service delivery models in order to accommodate the needs of these adolescents.

If only one point is to emerge from the information in this chapter, it is that language impairment negatively impacts adolescents' academic and personal successes in middle and senior high schools and limits their social, vocational, and educational opportunities as adults. Continuing to underrecognize or underserve these language-impaired adolescents would be a sad professional commentary.

6

Language and Children with Intellectual Disabilities

Stacey L. Pavelko

LEARNING OBJECTIVES

After reading this chapter, you should be able to:

- Provide an overview of intellectual disabilities
- Discuss the delay-disorder controversy associated with intellectual disabilities
- Discuss language characteristics and associated implications for intervention
- Discuss implications for intervention
- Summarize issues related to language and children with intellectual disabilities

This chapter will discuss the diverse characteristics of children with intellectual disabilities (ID). A wide range of physical conditions and behaviors exist among these children. Some children may show mild intellectual deficits and few other problems; they look like their peers, attend school, and interact well with typically developing (TD) children. They do not have seizures or other neurophysiological disorders and speak intelligibly and effectively. Other children may have more significant intellectual deficits and present a totally different picture; they have physical disabilities and attend a special school or special classroom with other severely disabled children and communicate poorly. Some children may occasionally scream and scratch themselves, others may wear a helmet to protect their head in case of falling during a seizure, and some may not communicate with speech. When reading the research on children with ID, it is important to ask several questions: What kinds of children were studied? How old were they? What did they look like? How severe was their intellectual impairment? How severe were their physical, social, and educational problems? By challenging the information in this way, readers will come to appreciate children with ID as a complex, heterogeneous group rather than falling into the trap of thinking about them as a homogeneous group of children.

AN OVERVIEW OF INTELLECTUAL DISABILITIES

Definition

Historically, the commonly used term for *intellectual disability* was *mental retardation*. The American Association on Intellectual and Developmental Disabilities (AAIDD), formerly called the American Association on Mental Retardation (AAMR), is among the more prominent professional organizations that support individuals with intellectual and developmental disabilities. It uses the term *intellectual disability* (AAIDD, 2010), which has evolved to be the more preferred term for most professionals. Schalock and colleagues (2007) provide an in-depth discussion about the shift to the term *intellectual disability*, a discussion which is beyond the scope of this chapter. What is important to understand in reading this chapter is that the term *intellectual disability* refers to the group of individuals who were previously referred to as mentally retarded in terms of number, kind, level, type, duration of disability, and the need these individuals have to access services and supports (AAIDD, 2010; Schalock et al., 2007). For the most part, in this chapter the terms *intellectual disability (ID)* and the organization name, AAIDD, will be used, unless it would be inappropriate to do so, as in a quotation, proper name, or reference citation.

An influential definition of ID is that of the AAIDD (2010):

> Intellectual disability is characterized by significant limitations both in intellectual functioning and in adaptive behavior as expressed in conceptual, social, and practical adaptive skills. This disability originates before age 18.

A diagnosis of ID requires that three criteria be met. The first criterion is a significant limitation in intellectual functioning. Intelligence refers to general mental ability and includes reasoning, planning, solving problems, thinking abstractly, comprehending complex ideas, learning quickly, and learning from experience (AAIDD, 2010). An individual's level of "intellectual functioning" is typically determined from the results of a norm-referenced test of intelligence and the AAIDD quantifies a "significant limitation" as an IQ score that is approximately two standard deviations (SDs) below the mean. However, the AAIDD cautions that professional judgment be used when interpreting the score and the test's standard error of measurement, reliability, validity, and strengths and limitations. Although each state sets its own guidelines for identifying children with ID, most states use a cutoff IQ score of 70–75, which usually equates to 2 SDs below the mean (Polloway, Smith, Patton, Lubin, & Antoine, 2009). Given the AAIDD recommended 2 SDs cutoff, approximately 2–3 percent of children will have limitations due to significant ID based on a normal distribution. From this perspective, the determination of the presence of ID can be thought of as a statistical determination as opposed to a functional one.

There is, however, another group of children to consider. These children have IQs that fall in the range of 1 to 2 SDs below the mean, or usually IQ scores of 70 to 85. This is approximately 13.5 percent of the population. The children do not fall into either the traditional ID range (70 or below) or the normal IQ range (85 or above). However, we know that they struggle both socially and academically but are often not eligible for special services in school because of the IQ cutoff of 70 to 75. When the focus of discussion about these children is language, the term *nonspecific language impairment*, has begun to be used, as we saw in Chapter 3. In Chapter 3 there is also a more complete discussion about mental age/IQ and language age comparisons in determining language performance and statistical approaches to identifying language impairment based on normal variation and normal distribution.

Several tests are used to measure intelligence, depending on the age and verbal ability of the child:

- The *Stanford-Binet Intelligence Scale—Fifth Edition* (Roid, 2003) has a long history and is still used with children of all ages.
- The *Wechsler Intelligence Scale for Children—Fifth Edition* (Wechsler, 2014) is another test used commonly with children of school age.

- As detection and intervention efforts focus increasingly on infants and younger children, the *Bayley Scales of Infant and Toddler Development—Third Edition* (Bayley, 2006) has gained popularity.
- For nonspeaking individuals, tests that do not require verbal responses are needed, such as the *Leiter International Performance Scale—Third Edition* (Roid, Miller, Pomplun, & Koch, 2013).

There are other IQ tests with specific uses and advantages. What all IQ tests have in common, however, is that they yield a mental age (MA), an estimate of an individual's level of cognitive functioning. An IQ score is derived by dividing the MA by the individual's chronological age (CA) and multiplying by 100, that is, IQ = MA/CA × 100.

Although the IQ scale is a continuous set of numbers, it is the practice of professionals in the field to describe levels of impairment for purposes of education and intervention plans and research. Until 1992, the AAIDD supported the use of descriptive labels based on IQ intervals. These labels paralleled an older set of terms that had traditionally been used in educational placement. Since 1992, there has been a shift toward describing individuals in terms of the intensity of supports they need in order to learn and function across environments. In 2010, the AAIDD proposed a multidimensional classification system, which represents a significant departure from the previous classification systems. Table 6.1 provides the older terms and new classification system. Unfortunately, states vary considerably with respect to the use of classification systems. One 2009 survey of state agencies reported that 45.1 percent of states did not use a classification system and 21.6 percent of states used a system that was consistent with the older 1983 AAMR system (Polloway et al., 2009).

The second criterion that must be met for a diagnosis of ID is a significant limitation in adaptive behavior. The AAIDD (2010) defines *adaptive behavior* as "the collection of conceptual, social, and practical skills that have been learned and are performed by people in their everyday lives" (p. 43). Adaptive skills fall into three categories (i.e., conceptual, social, practical) and include such behaviors as appropriate language, managing money, following rules, eating, dressing, and acquiring office skills. Examiners often employ norm-referenced tests, such as the *Vineland II: Vineland Adaptive Behavior Scales, Second Edition* (Sparrow, Cicchetti, & Balla, 2005) and the *Adaptive Behavior Assessment System—Third Edition* (Harrison & Oakland, 2015), that are normed on the general population to determine if an individual performs more than 2 SDs below the mean in at least one of the three categories of skills. The third criterion that must be met for a diagnosis of ID is that the limitations in intellectual functioning and adaptive behavior appear before 18 years of age, that is, during the developmental period.

TABLE 6.1 | Levels of Impairment of Individuals with Intellectual Disabilities

	AAMR/AAIDD Classification	Traditional Label	IQ Range	Percentage of Persons with ID
Previous labels	Mild	Educable	50–55 to 70	89
	Moderate	Trainable	35–40 to 50–55	7
	Severe	Custodial	20–25 to 35–40	3
	Profound	Life support	Below 20–25	1
Revised labels	Intermittent	Short-term supports, such as during an acute medical crisis		
	Limited	Supports needed regularly but briefly, such as employee assistance to remediate a job-related skill deficit		
	Extensive	Ongoing and regular assistance, such as long-term home living support		
	Pervasive	Potentially life-sustaining support, such as attendant care, skilled medical care, or help with taking medications		

In the literature on exceptional children, several other terms are used that have meanings similar to ID. *Developmental disability* is one such term. This label is used in federal law to describe mental or physical disabilities (or both) that appear before age 22 that are likely to continue indefinitely in self-care, language, learning, mobility, self-direction, capacity for independent living, and economic self-sufficiency. There is great, though not total, overlap between the categories of ID and developmental disability. The differences occur at the upper end of the impaired range (e.g., an IQ of 65), where an individual may receive a diagnosis of ID but *not* developmental disability (Grossman, 1983). There are, however, circumstances when the IQ of a child has not or cannot be determined. In these circumstances, it is common for the child to be identified by etiological category (e.g., fragile X syndrome) or labeled as *developmentally disabled* (Taylor & Kaufmann, 1991). *Autism spectrum disorder (ASD)* is another term that has substantial overlap with ID. A majority of children with ASD have IQ scores within the impaired range. Both researchers and practitioners, however, have tended to treat children with ASD as a distinct group. Therefore, a separate chapter in this text is devoted to this group of children.

Learning disability is a category of impairment that is defined in federal law. Children with ID are specifically excluded from this category. In practice, though, there is a relationship between learning disability and ID. In just the 7 years following the enactment of Public Law 94-142, a 19 percent decrease was reported in the number of children receiving special education services who were identified as intellectually disabled. In actuality, however, this decrease may have reflected a shift in labeling practices, with many of the individuals with mild intellectual disabilities being reclassified as learning disabled (Frankenberger & Harper, 1988; MacMillan & Siperstein, 2001). It is also possible that some children with IQs in the 70 to 85 range may be classified as learning disabled.

Causes and Types of Intellectual Disabilities

In the preceding discussion, test performance was used to distinguish different levels of ID. Differentiation by level of performance is important to educators and administrators because it serves to place children with ID into programs and allocate funds to those programs. Other differences related to characteristics of different children with ID are frequently more important, however, to others who are interested in uncovering the causes of ID.

Research findings from many sources suggest that there are two broad categories of ID: *biological origin*, which includes a demonstrated biological cause of the disability, and *cultural-familial origin*, which includes those individuals for whom social, behavioral, or educational risk factors predominate (AAIDD, 2010). Although this two-group distinction is useful as a shorthand way to categorize the causes of ID, the distinction is often blurred in real life. Individuals with social, behavioral, or educational risk factors may also have biomedical risk factors and vice versa. For example, a child who is born with Down syndrome (*biological origin*) may come from an impoverished environment and have *cultural-familial* risk factors such as maternal malnutrition, lack of prenatal care, and impaired child-caregiver interactions. Conversely, a child with primarily *cultural-familial* risk factors such as parental drug use and parental abandonment may also have a *biological* factor such as a single-gene disorder.

Several types of chromosomal or other genetic abnormality produce congenital syndromes associated with ID. With the completion of the Human Genome Project in 2003, a 13-year venture coordinated by the U.S. Department of Energy and the National Institutes of Health, more attention in the professional literature has been paid to the identification and diagnosis of syndromes. Although there are over 500 syndromes that can cause ID, Down syndrome (DS), fragile X syndrome (FXS), and fetal alcohol spectrum disorder are the more common syndromes (Centers for Disease Control and Prevention [CDC], 2015). DS is the most widely known genetic cause of ID (CDC, 2015) and affects approximately 1 in 700 live births. DS is most commonly caused by an extra 21st chromosome (*trisomy 21*). FXS is the most commonly known cause of inherited ID. FXS is an X-linked genetic disorder caused by a defect of the fragile X mental retardation 1 (FMR1) gene. The prevalence of FXS is reported in two ways: full mutation and permutation. The prevalence of full mutation in the general population is approximately 1 in 4,000 males and 1 in 6,000 females (Hagerman, 2006).

The prevalence of permutation in the general population is approximately 1 in 151 females and 1 in 458 males (Seltzer et al., 2012). Individuals with full mutation typically exhibit ID; in contrast, individuals with FXS permutation generally exhibit normal intelligence, but are reported to have learning disabilities, emotional difficulties, neurological deficits, and endocrine problems that further increase the chance of the FMR1 mutation in the general population (Hagerman, 2008). Males are typically more severely affected because they have only one X chromosome (Hagerman, 2008). In addition, approximately 20–50 percent of males with FXS also meet full criteria for a diagnosis of autism (using the DSM-IV diagnostic criteria) and 75 percent meet the criteria for ASD (Clifford et al., 2007; Hall, Burns, Lightbody, & Reiss, 2008; Kaufmann et al., 2004). Most of the research conducted with individuals having FXS has been with males.

Rarer genetic disorders that affect intellectual functioning are Williams syndrome (WS), Angelman syndrome (AS), and Prader-Willi syndrome. WS is caused by missing genetic material on chromosome 7, affecting approximately 1 in 10,000 to 1 in 15,000 live births (Shprintzen, 2000). This deleted genetic material includes the elastin gene (ELN), which is essential for maintaining the elasticity of fibers and connective tissue (Shprintzen, 2000). AS is a nonprogressive neurological disorder affecting approximately 1 in 10,000 to 1 in 25,000 live births that results from a deletion of genetic material from the mother's 15th chromosome (Richard & Hoge, 1999; Shprintzen, 2000). Should there be a deletion from the 15th chromosome from the father, Prader-Willi syndrome results, with occurrences ranging from 1 in 8,000 to 1 in 25,000 live births (Kleppe, Katayama, Shipley, & Foushee, 1990; Richard & Hoge, 1999; Shprintzen, 1997, 2000). Table 6.2 summarizes information pertaining to appearance, physical features, and health problems of children with some of these ID syndromes.

TABLE 6.2 | Comparison of Appearance, Physical Features, and Health Problems Associated with Children with Intellectual Disabilities Syndromes

Intellectual Disability Syndrome	Appearance/Facial Characteristics	Physical Features	Health
Angelman Syndrome	Microcephaly Large, wide, smiling mouth (*macrostomia*) with irregular spaced teeth Deep-set eyes Mandibular protrusion Hypopigmentation resulting in fair complexions A wide base and stiff-legged gait *Sources:* Richard and Hoge (1999); Shprintzen (1997, 2000)	Low tone (*hypotonia*) Hand flapping Tremors and jerky movements of the extremities Ataxia Visual problems (e.g., nystagmus, optic atrophy, strabismus, squinting, and poor acuity) *Sources:* Richard and Hoge (1999); Shprintzen (2000)	Epilepsy/seizure disorders in 80% of children Possible early failure to thrive Persistent feeding difficulties *Sources:* Richard and Hoge (1999); Shprintzen (2000)
Down Syndrome	Small head circumference Upward-slanting, oval-shaped eyes with prominent epicanthal folds Midface hypoplasia A small chin and a small nose with flattened bridge Small oral cavity with a short, high, narrow palate; possible bifid uvula or cleft	Generalized hypotonia results in gross motor delays (e.g., poor quality of movement; deficits in postural control, stability, strength, and coordination; and delayed acquisition of motor milestones, hyperreflexive)	Cardiac problems: Congenital heart defects or disease in 40% to 60% (e.g., structural malformations, pulmonary artery hypertension, and pulmonary vascular obstructive disease) Hematology concerns: Increased prevalence of leukemia or low platelet counts

(*Continued*)

TABLE 6.2 | *Continued*

Intellectual Disability Syndrome	Appearance/Facial Characteristics	Physical Features	Health
	As child develops, lips become prominent, thickened, and excessively moist Underdeveloped, protrusive jaw Malocclusion Small, short low-set ears; structure of external, middle, and/or inner ear may be abnormal *Sources:* Chamberlain and Strode (1999); Richard and Hoge (1999); Shprintzen (1997, 2000)	Low tone also results in oral-motor/feeding problems (e.g., poorly integrated suck-swallow-breathing patterns, tongue protrusion, open-mouth posture, and decreased sensory awareness and responsiveness to food placed in mouth) *Sources:* Chamberlain and Strode (1999); Richard and Hoge (1999); Shprintzen (1997, 2000) Visual problems: 40% have poor bilateral vision or amblyopia ("lazy eye"), 20% to 50% have strabismus, and 10% to 20% have nystagmus; congenital cataracts are common	*Sources:* Chamberlain and Strode (1999); Patterson and Lott (2008) Endocrine disorders: Increased likelihood of diabetes and/or thyroid problems that may lead to obesity or decreased intellectual functioning *Sources:* Chamberlain and Strode (1999); Patterson and Lott (2008) Gastrointestinal defects or blockages that may lead to nutritional problems (e.g., duodenal atresia and Hirschprung disease) *Source:* Patterson and Lott (2008) Immunodeficiencies: Low T-cell counts or T-cells that do not function adequately, contributing to increased incidence of upper respiratory infections (i.e., ear, nose, and throat infections), leukemia, and cardiac problems *Source:* Chamberlain and Strode (1999) Sleep disturbances: Sleep disorders possibly due to airway obstruction (*apnea*) 30% to 60% of children have chronic obstructive hypoventilation Difficulty regulating sleep–wake cycles due to decreased serotonin levels *Sources:* Chamberlain and Strode (1999); Patterson and Lott (2008); Shott et al. (2006); Stores (1993) Orthopedic problems: Atlantoaxial instability—increased mobility between the first and second cervical vertebrae that increases the risk of spinal cord injury; dislocation of cervical spine, hips, knees; and foot problems

TABLE 6.2 | *Continued*

Intellectual Disability Syndrome	Appearance/Facial Characteristics	Physical Features	Health
			Dementia: Unusually higher incidence Alzheimer disease type in middle age *Source:* Patterson and Lott (2008)
Fetal Alcohol Syndrome	Smooth philtrum Thin vermilion border Small palpebral fissures *Source:* Bertrand et al. (2004)	Below the 10th percentile in height and/or weight, either pre- or postnatal Small or diminished overall head circumference CNS abnormalities: structural, neurological or functional, or a combination *Source:* Bertrand et al. (2004)	
Fragile X Syndrome	Macrocephaly Prominent forehead and jaw Elongated narrow face with drooping eyelids and long ears Flattened nasal bridge High, narrow palatal arch Flat feet and small hands *Sources:* Hagerman (2002); Richard and Hoge (1999)	Hypotonia Short stature Hyperextendible finger joints Macroorchidism (large genitals) Visual problems (e.g., 8% to 30% have strabismus, nystagmus, and/or farsightedness) *Sources:* Richard and Hoge (1999); Shprintzen (1997, 2000)	Hernia Dislocated joints Mitral valve prolapse Gastroesophageal reflux in infancy Oral-motor feeding problems Seizures *Sources:* Hagerman (2002); Richard and Hoge (1999); Sterling and Warren (2008)
Prader-Willi Syndrome	Almond-shaped eyes slanting upward Narrow forehead Narrow palatal arch Micrognathia Underdeveloped chin Small hands and feet *Sources:* Richard and Hoge (1999); Shprintzen (1997, 2000)	Hypotonia and associated motor delays Short stature Hypogonadism Visual problems (e.g., strabismus and myopia) *Sources:* Burack (1990); Zigler and Balla (1982); Zigler and Hodapp (1986, 1991)	Obesity develops between ages 2 and 5 years Insatiable appetite resulting in 95% obesity *Sources:* Richard and Hoge (1999) Maladaptive behavior Sleep disturbances Self-destructive behaviors High tolerance for pain *Source:* Shprintzen (2000)

Prenatal events, such as physical injury or substance abuse, can cause injury to the fetus and lead to an ID. Fetal alcohol spectrum disorder (FASD), previously referred to as fetal alcohol syndrome (FAS), is one such condition. FASD is an umbrella term that is used to describe a range of effects caused by maternal drinking during pregnancy. It is estimated to occur in 50 per 1,000 live births (May et al., 2009) and is a leading cause of a preventable disability that can include ID (Abel & Sokol, 1987). Approximately 70–75 percent of individuals with FASD have a normal IQ, yet still demonstrate significant deficits in functional ability (O'Malley, 2007a).

The term *FASD* is not intended to be used as a clinical diagnosis. Rather, under the umbrella term, *FASD*, there are three different conditions, differentiated by the types of symptoms. Fetal alcohol syndrome (FAS) represents the severe end of FASD. A diagnosis of FAS requires three components. First, three facial anomalies must be present—a smooth ridge between the nose and upper lip, a thin upper lip, and a short distance between the inner and outer corners of the eyes. Second, impaired growth, which is defined as height or weight below the 10th percentile, either pre- or postnataly, must be documented. Third, central nervous system problems must be documented.

These can manifest as structural, neurologic, or functional (Bertrand et al., 2004). Table 6.2 includes descriptions of FAS. According to the National Organization on Fetal Alcohol Syndrome (NOFAS), individuals diagnosed with alcohol-related neurodevelopmental disorder (ARND), a second condition under the umbrella FASD, do not have the FAS facial anomalies, but may have ID and problems with learning and behavior (NOFAS, 2014). Finally, individuals with the third type of FASD, alcohol-related birth defects (ARBD), have physical defects that include heart, skeletal, kidney, ear, and/or eye malformations (NOFAS, 2014).

THE DELAY–DIFFERENCE CONTROVERSY

A fundamental issue in ID research over the years has been the *delay–difference controversy*, that is, whether the cognitive and linguistic processes of individuals with and without ID are the same. No one disputes that the *achievements* of children with ID are lower. The debate focuses on the *explanation* for that lower achievement and whether it requires us to invoke the idea of specific qualitative differences in how these children develop. To investigate the delay–difference controversy, researchers have applied the scientific method of making and testing predictions. These predictions have included the technique of matching participants with and without ID according to their CA, MA, or language age (LA) and examining their performances on a variety of tasks.

Supporters of the difference position point to three findings, any or all of which may be areas of qualitative difference in individuals with ID:

1. They suffer from a deficit in verbal mediation ability due to the inactivity of the verbal system and its dissociation from the motor system (Dulaney & Ellis, 1997).
2. They are inherently more rigid in their behavior (Dulaney & Ellis, 1997).
3. They have inadequate short-term memory (also called *working memory*) function that is necessary to perform certain cognitive tasks (Jarrold, Cowan, Hewes, & Riby, 2004; Miolo, Chapman, & Sindberg, 2005).

The notion of rigidity is hard to pin down, but it is most often illustrated by studies that show a deficit in abstract thinking. Children with DS, for example, have been found to classify objects by their common perceptual attributes (size, shape, and color) rather than by abstract categories (fruit, clothing, and furniture). They seem to have difficulty in hierarchical thinking, that is, recognizing that entities can be thought about at several levels. For example, the family pet has a proper name, *Rudy;* has a basic-level name, *dog;* has a subordinate name, *dachshund;* and has several superordinate names: *mammal, quadruped,* and *animal.* It may be hard for these children to accept that all of these names provide accurate descriptions of the same dog but at different levels of thinking.

Deficits in working memory have been offered as an explanation for a range of problems commonly seen in children with ID. It is generally believed that these children rarely employ strategies in situations that require active problem solving but can be taught to do so. However, the strategies taught for one task do not usually transfer spontaneously to other tasks. Most studies of problem solving, as well as most clinical descriptions, indicate that the performance of children with ID varies widely from one situation to the next. It has been suggested that this is due to limitations in functional working memory, which, in turn, may be the result of slowness in information processing, difficulty with simultaneous processing, and/or limitations in working memory storage capacity (Grieco, Pulsifer, Seligsohn, Skotko, & Schwartz, 2015). Research on long-term memory has reported deficits in memory consolidation and problems at the levels of encoding and retrieval, which are adversely affected by attentional deficits (Grieco et al., 2015).

In response to this evidence of differences, the delay position draws attention to the distinction between cognition and achievement. Some of the performance differences observed in familial ID may be simply due to lack of experience that results in deficits of knowledge. Other performance differences may be attributed to motivational differences in individuals with ID. Research has found persons with ID to be responsive to social reinforcement but at the same time wary of strange adults. They may be less likely to rely on their own cognitive resources and instead tend to problem solve imitatively. They may have an expectancy of failure based on experience and, therefore, be more motivated to avoid failure than to achieve success. They respond better to tangible reinforcement but often exhibit *learned helplessness,* that is, not doing things even though they know how (Bybee & Zigler, 1999). Although ID is viewed primarily as a cognitive disorder, it may have associated with it the noncognitive characteristic of *passivity,* that is, not initiating the use of certain strategies known to be available to them. It has been noted that individuals with DS, who often possess reasonably good social skills, will often use those skills in order to sidestep difficult learning situations.

There is currently no clear answer regarding the *delay-difference argument.* Proponents on both sides of the argument have offered evidence to account for the qualitative and quantitative differences found in individuals with ID. Because a multitude of factors can account for these differences, it may well be the case that a combination of both delays and differences explain the cognitive and linguistic processes of individuals with ID.

LANGUAGE CHARACTERISTICS AND ASSOCIATED IMPLICATIONS FOR INTERVENTION

All children with ID can be expected to exhibit some type of communication and/or linguistic deficit. The AAIDD specifies that one component of the adaptive behavior deficits seen in all ID is a communication disability. Consequently, professionals can expect that children with ID may need some form of language or communication intervention. This raises the age-old question of whether cognitive deficits cause the language impairment or whether both the cognitive and the language deficits result from some other deficit, generally thought to involve central nervous system functioning, and acknowledge the reciprocal and interactive effects of language and cognition. This question is difficult to answer because research investigating the complex interrelationship between language and cognition has resulted in inconsistent findings. What is important to note, however, is that in the case of ID, language impairment is in some way related to the ID. If cognition alone were the answer for determining language abilities, then the language characteristics of children with different ID syndromes would likely be very similar. However, the opposite seems to be true. Recent research suggests differing language profiles associated with various causes of ID. Language and other communication abilities may not be equally affected in children with different syndromes. The language profiles associated with Angelman syndrome, Down syndrome, fetal alcohol spectrum disorder, fragile X syndrome, Prader-Willi syndrome, and Williams syndrome, as well as specific considerations for both assessment and intervention, are discussed in the following sections.

Angelman Syndrome

Language Profile. Most children with Angelman syndrome (AS) do not acquire speech and language skills sufficient to use speech as a primary means of communication, and others may only speak a few words (Alvares & Downing, 1998; Williams, Peters, & Calculator, 2009). Although some researchers have reported children with AS demonstrate stronger abilities in comprehension when compared to production (Alvares & Downing, 1998; Jolleff & Ryan, 1993), other researchers have not found a difference (Andersen, Rasmussen, & Strømme, 2001). When children with AS do acquire some oral language, they may use it to request desired objects or to reject undesired objects, but rarely use language to label, describe, or imitate (Didden, Korzilius, Duker, & Curfs, 2004).

Children with AS may present with some clinical features such as hand-flapping, stereotypic and/or repetitive behaviors, and sensory preoccupations that overlap with some features of ASD. As a result some children with AS have been mistakenly identified as having ASD rather than AS (Williams, 2005). Several researchers have, however, reported that a percentage of children with AS do legitimately meet diagnostic criteria for ASD (Bonati et al., 2007; Moss et al., 2013).

Approximately 20–80 percent of infants with AS demonstrate feeding problems, typically stemming from sucking or swallowing disorders (Williams et al., 2009). Bottle-feeding may be easier than breastfeeding because infants often have difficulty initiating sucking and sustaining breast-feeding. Related to their sucking or swallowing problems, drooling is often a persistent problem and frequently requires the use of bibs (Williams et al., 2009). Approximately 30–50 percent of older infants evidence persistent tongue protrusion, which usually remains throughout childhood and may persist into adulthood.

Assessment Considerations. Because some children with AS have been mistakenly identified with ASD, an initial assessment of speech and language will need to provide a differential diagnosis of AS verses ASD. Because many children with AS do not develop speech and language skills sufficient to rely on speech as a primary means of communication, many children may need an augmentative and alternative (AAC) evaluation, which is discussed in Chapter 12. Finally, when evaluating infants and young children, an evaluation of feeding and swallowing behaviors may be warranted.

Intervention Considerations. Various forms of AAC systems should be considered to provide effective means of communication (Williams et al., 2009). Sign language or enhanced natural gestures may be particularly well suited for many children with AS, given the research that supports a preference for use of gestures (Calculator, 2002). AAC as an intervention approach is discussed in Chapter 12. In addition, for children with a co-morbid diagnosis of ASD, applied behavioral analysis therapy may be helpful (Williams et al., 2009). This and other intervention considerations for children with ASD are discussed in Chapter 7.

Down Syndrome

Language Profile. Children with Down syndrome (DS) typically have stronger receptive language skills than expressive language skills, with relative strengths in pragmatic skills, receptive vocabulary, and narrative skills, particularly for events, themes, and story elements (Dykens, Hodapp, & Evans, 2006; Finestack, Palmer, & Abbeduto, 2012; Miller, 1995; Roberts, Chapman, Martin, & Moskowitz, 2008). When telling stories from wordless picture books or videos, children with DS have been found to include salient events, themes, and story elements commensurate with their cognitive levels and language comprehension (Boudreau & Chapman, 2000; Miles & Chapman, 2002). Children with DS also often demonstrate a relative strength in gesture use and imitation, and these skills could be used to facilitate the use of words (Abbeduto, Warren, & Conners, 2007). In contrast, many individuals with DS demonstrate delays beyond expectations for their mental ages in phonological working memory, phonological processing, expressive vocabulary, microstructural narrative elements, and syntax, specifically with regard to production of complex syntax, grammatical morphemes, and negation (Finestack & Abbeduto, 2010; Finestack et al., 2012; Finestack, Sterling, & Abbeduto, 2013; Roberts et al., 2008). Specific areas of pragmatic skills that pose particular difficulties for children with DS have also been described. These include particular weaknesses in the ability to construct utterances that effectively convey intents and difficulty introducing topics and maintaining them (Abbeduto et al., 2006; Kumin, 2008b).

With regard to literacy, many children with DS are often able to read better than might be expected when comparing their reading skills to their other language and cognitive abilities. Children with DS typically develop emergent literacy skills and word recognition skills that are commensurate with their nonverbal development and demonstrate a relative strength in sight word reading. Decoding, phonological awareness, and writing may, however, be particularly challenging for the children.

Speech intelligibility is a particular concern for children with DS that continues into adulthood. Difficulty producing intelligible speech is likely the result of a combination of factors, including disturbances in voice, articulation, resonance, fluency, and prosody (Kent & Vorperian, 2013). Although the craniofacial anatomy of individuals with DS is characterized by an average-sized tongue with a compact mid- and lower-face bone structure and a high, often shelf-like, palate, anatomic anomalies cannot account for all aspects of the speech disorder. Studies of articulation and phonology demonstrate both delayed ("developmental") and disordered ("nondevelopmental") inconsistent error patterns (Kent & Vorperian, 2013). Many individuals with DS are also likely to demonstrate fluency disorders (Kent & Vorperian, 2013). Finally, approximately 6–10 percent of children with DS have diagnoses of ASD; these children with dual-diagnoses demonstrate distinctive patterns of unusual stereotypic behaviors, anxiety, and social withdrawal (Carter, Capone, Gray, Cox, & Kaufmann, 2007).

Because of possible structural malformations of the ear and other oral-facial structural characteristics that affect Eustachian tube function, hearing level is a concern. Approximately one-third to three-fourths of individuals with DS experience hearing loss (Roizen & Patterson, 2003).

Assessment Considerations. Because hearing loss is prevalent in children with DS and can impact language learning, hearing status needs to be closely monitored (Roberts et al., 2008). Assessment of phonological working memory using nonword repetition or memory-span tasks (American Speech-Language-Hearing Association, 2001) may provide insights into language abilities and avenues for intervention. Language and narrative samples should be obtained both with and without picture support because research has indicated significant differences in performance based on the level of visual support (Roberts et al., 2008). A thorough evaluation of writing skills will be necessary to determine whether difficulties stem from working memory deficits and/or delays in motor skills. Finally, an assessment of fluency should also be considered.

Intervention Considerations. Children with DS typically have difficulties in phonological working memory so learning might be facilitated by tasks that are broken down into different steps. They can also benefit from repeated opportunities to hear words and sentences and repeated, brief instructions (Gathercole & Alloway, 2006; Gathercole, Alloway, Willis, & Adams, 2006). In addition, picture-based storybooks may be particularly helpful (Chapman, 2003). Intervention should target use of grammatical morphemes, acquisition and use of complex vocabulary, and production of intelligible speech using developmentally sequenced goals (Roberts et al., 2008). Because of oral-motor problems that can affect speech production and intelligibility, children with DS demonstrate a relative weakness in producing intelligible speech sounds. Thus, interventions should include a focus on vocal development and producing intelligible speech (Brady, Bredin-Oja, & Warren, 2008) without necessarily aiming for speech that is free of speech sound errors. Importantly, research has demonstrated that individuals with DS continue language and literacy learning well into adolescence; thus, continued access to language and literacy support provided by a team of educators is likely beneficial for the children (Roberts et al., 2008). Because children with DS typically demonstrate a relative strength in sight word reading, intervention might be able to capitalize on this relative skill in order to use reading activities to develop improved spoken language and verbal short-term memory skills during the preschool years. In fact, some authors advocate introducing reading to these children as soon as they have comprehension vocabularies of 50–100 words (Buckley & Johnson-Glenberg, 2008). However, to address the children's potential relative difficulties in decoding printed words and phonological awareness, interventions might also include goals that promote phonological awareness, understanding and using letter-sound rules, and decoding skills (Buckley & Johnson-Glenberg, 2008).

Fetal Alcohol Spectrum Disorder

Language Profile. Most researchers have reported that children with fetal alcohol spectrum disorder (FASD) score lower on measures of language functioning when compared to control groups (Aragón et al., 2008; Janzen, Nanson, & Block, 1995; McGee, Bjorkquist, Riley, & Mattson, 2009). The children often have significant difficulties with syntactic elements of language (Carney & Chermak, 1991; Wyper & Rasmussen, 2011), but may have strengths in receptive language skills (McGee et al., 2009). Nevertheless, a consistent finding that has emerged from the research is that children with FASD typically demonstrate particular problems in using language in sophisticated social contexts (Coggins, Timler, & Olswang, 2007a; Quattlebaum & O'Connor, 2013), for example:

- understanding abstract language
- accessing peer groups
- negotiating compromises
- resolving conflicts
- maintaining friendships

Children with FASD also have difficulty with narrative language, specifically, coherence of and cohesion in narratives, with cohesive reference in nominal phrases posing a particular challenge (Coggins, Timler, & Olswang, 2007b; Thorne, Coggins, Olson, & Astley, 2007). In addition, difficulty with mental state verbs, e.g., *consider, believe,* which may be related to inadequate theory of mind, has been documented (Timler, Olswang, & Coggins, 2005a). Stevens and colleagues (2015) have suggested that deficits in both social perspective taking and empathy may underlie the children's difficulties with peer relationships. With regard to academic achievement, Adnams and colleagues (2007) have reported that children with FASD have lower scores on tests of phonological awareness, word reading, and spelling compared to their same-aged peers, and difficulties in mathematics have been well documented.

A high percentage of individuals with FASD (approximately 49–94 percent) also present with attention deficits (Mattson, Crocker, & Nguyen, 2011; Peadon & Elliott, 2010) with the proportion of individuals diagnosed with both FAS and attention deficit/hyperactivity disorder (ADHD) increasing with increasing levels of alcohol exposure. The presence of ADHD appears to be independent of IQ and likely persists into adolescence and adulthood (Bhatara, Loudenberg, & Ellis, 2006; Fryer, McGee, Matt, Riley, & Mattson, 2007; Peadon & Elliott, 2010). Because of their brain damage, infants with FASD often display a variety of behaviors such as a delayed suck reflex, poor feeding, and poor habitation to parents' natural anxiety about parenting (O'Malley, 2007b). Because of craniofacial anomalies, children with FASD are likely to demonstrate conductive hearing loss, often secondary to recurrent otitis media. Although data are limited, sensorineural hearing loss may occur with the same frequency as seen in children with DS or those with submucous cleft palate (Cone-Wesson, 2005).

Assessment Considerations. Because individuals with FASD commonly present with attentional deficits, a differential diagnosis of FASD verses ADHD is particularly important (Mattson et al., 2011). With respect to language, Thorne and colleagues (Thorne & Coggins, 2008; Thorne et al., 2007) suggest a way to evaluate one aspect of the narratives of children with FASD. Their method, the rate of nominal reference errors (rNRE), calculates errors of introduction (improper obligatory referencing of what is known verses what is new) and referential errors in tying information together. Because of craniofacial anomalies, hearing status needs to be carefully assessed and monitored, and feeding and swallowing evaluations may be warranted.

Intervention Considerations. Because children with FASD can have particular difficulties entering peer groups, resolving conflicts, maintaining friendships and negotiating compromises (Coggins et al., 2007a), intervention that includes a focus on social processing and social communication behaviors, especially those that involve mental state verbs, is often beneficial for these children. Although research regarding specific social skills interventions for children with FASD is limited, the Children's Friendship Training (CFT) procedure has some evidence to support its effectiveness (Keil, Paley, Frankel, & O'Connor, 2010; O'Connor et al., 2006). Interventions should also focus on other areas of language that are problematic for children with FASD, such as comprehension and production of complex syntax, general language competence, and production of narratives, with special emphasis on nominal cohesion (Thorne & Coggins, 2008; Timler, Olswang, & Coggins, 2005b). Although the data regarding literacy interventions for this group of children are limited, some research suggests that interventions focused on early literacy skills, such as phonological awareness, as well as narrative comprehension and retell, are effective. These skills may be appropriate intervention targets for both preschool and young school-aged children (Adnams et al., 2007).

Because infants with FASD often have issues with feeding and swallowing, therapy should focus on addressing issues of attachment that can co-occur with feeding problems. Techniques such as swaddling, feeding strategies, and sensory integration techniques have been used and suggested as being helpful (O'Malley, 2007b).

Fragile X Syndrome

Language Profile. Girls with fragile X syndrome (FXS) usually have less language delay than boys, although there is considerable variability in severity. Some research also suggests that initiating and sustaining conversations are particularly difficult for girls with FXS (Lesniak-Karpiak, Mazzocco, & Ross, 2003; Roberts et al., 2008). In contrast, boys with FXS typically demonstrate moderate to severe delays in receptive and expressive language, with greater delays noted in expressive language (Abbeduto, Brady, & Kover, 2007; Roberts, Mirrett, & Burchinal, 2001). Receptive and expressive vocabulary seems to be a relative strength for boys with FXS (Finestack et al., 2013; Roberts et al., 2008). Another relative strength may include narrative abilities, specifically those involved in providing initial settings and character details (Finestack et al., 2012). In contrast, researchers generally agree that conversational discourse skills are particularly impaired; perseveration also seems a particular challenge. This observation has led some to propose that perseveration may be a defining characteristic of FXS (Roberts et al., 2008). Additionally, pragmatic functions such as greetings, turn taking, making conversational repairs, and making requests seem especially difficult for the children. Some aspects of syntax, including production of complex clauses, complex noun phrases, and verb phrases are also particularly impaired (Finestack & Abbeduto, 2010; Price et al., 2008). With regard to literacy, children with FXS typically demonstrate difficulty with decoding and phonological awareness but strength in sight-word reading (Buckley & Johnson-Glenberg, 2008).

Speech intelligibility in conversation is a specific concern for males with FXS. Several co-morbid speech disorders, including developmental phonological errors (i.e., consonant substitutions, omissions, and distortions), voice problems, childhood apraxia of speech, and fluency disorders have all been reported in the literature (Van Borsel, Dor, & Rondal, 2008). In addition, frequent otitis media is common during the first year of life and may contribute to speech and language delays.

Many children with FASD also have a co-morbid diagnosis of ASD. Approximately 75 percent of males with FASD meet the DSM-IV criteria for ASD (Clifford et al., 2007; Hall et al., 2008; Kaufmann et al., 2004).

Assessment Considerations. The difficulty with speech intelligibility that some children with FXS present with indicates that a thorough speech evaluation, in addition to a language assessment, is a necessary element of the assessment process. For children who do not develop functional speech, AAC systems could be considered. Because many children with FXS also meet the diagnostic criteria for ASD, initial evaluations of speech and language need to carefully assess for the presence of ASD (Clifford et al., 2007; Hall et al., 2008;

Kaufmann et al., 2004). In addition, language production and comprehension in the areas of vocabulary, syntax, pragmatics, and narrative production need to be considered during assessment (Finestack et al., 2013; Martin, Losh, Estigarribia, Sideris, & Roberts, 2013). Of particular importance is documentation of the presence/absence of perseveration, especially during conversational contexts. Finally, because research has indicated a high occurrence of otitis media with associated conductive hearing loss, it is important that hearing status be carefully monitored on a regular basis.

Intervention Considerations. Children with a co-morbidity of ASD will likely have more difficulty with social and conversational language uses and may benefit from intervention strategies used for children with ASD (Roberts et al., 2008). Behavioral characteristics such as the inability to direct and sustain attention, social anxiety, and gaze aversion may interfere with conversation. Intervention should also target increasing expressive syntax, reducing perseveration during discourse tasks, and producing more complex narrative elements such as character or plot development (Finestack et al., 2012; Martin et al., 2013; Roberts et al., 2008). Narrative interventions have been shown to elicit longer utterances for children with FXS and can be used as a context for vocabulary and syntactic targets. Initial literacy interventions can use strengths in sight-word reading to build other skills; however, intensive interventions in phonological awareness are often necessary (Buckley & Johnson-Glenberg, 2008). Specific interventions to improve speech intelligibility in conversation for children with FXS have not been researched; however, Scharfenaker and colleagues (2002) suggest that reducing rate, normalizing the rhythm of speech, and improving oral-motor functioning may increase the children's speech intelligibility.

Prader-Willi Syndrome

Language Profile. Research delineating the specific language profiles of children with Prader-Willi syndrome is limited (Dimitropoulos, Ferranti, & Lemler, 2013). What is known is that many individuals with Prader-Willi syndrome demonstrate expressive language abilities that are more impaired than receptive abilities. Particular difficulties in morphosyntactic, narrative, and conversation skills, such as maintaining a topic, turn taking, and maintaining appropriate proximity to a conversational partner, have been found (Dimitropoulos et al., 2013; Lewis, Freebairn, Heeger, & Cassidy, 2002; Van Borsel, Defloor, & Curfs, 2007). Many children with Prader-Willi syndrome demonstrate oral motor impairments that significantly impact articulation and, therefore, their ability to effectively use speech to express what language they have (Lewis et al., 2002). Vowel errors and difficulty producing multisyllabic words have been shown to be particularly troublesome for these children (Lewis et al., 2002). In contrast to areas of weakness, several researchers have noted relative strengths in the areas of vocabulary and pragmatic development (Van Borsel et al., 2007).

Assessment Considerations. Because many individuals with Prader-Willi syndrome exhibit articulation difficulties, assessment needs to document the children's speech patterns, including phoneme production in multisyllabic words and vowel errors. Assessment of language needs to focus on evaluation of morphosyntactic abilities, conversational skills, and narrative abilities, including story retell, story grammar components, and story content.

Intervention Considerations. Children with Prader-Willi syndrome likely require both language intervention and intervention to address articulation errors. Research suggests that intervention approaches that follow a typical developmental course seem to be appropriate (Lewis et al., 2002).

Williams Syndrome

Language Profile. Individuals with Williams syndrome (WS) generally show strengths in the areas of phonological short-term memory, speech production, and concrete receptive vocabulary. Their difficulties with morphology and syntax are commensurate with their cognitive abilities (Brock, 2007), but they tend to have particular areas of weakness with comprehension and production of relational/conceptual vocabulary and with certain pragmatic skills, specifically, turn taking, maintaining topics, and understanding the conversational requirements of their conversational partners (Brock, 2007; Mervis, 2009). They may also tend to perseverate on personal topics (Hoffmann, Martens, Fox, Rabidoux, & Andridge, 2013). Research on the production of narratives has documented difficulty with maintaining a theme, using cognitive inferences, and employing conjunctive ties (Brock, 2007). Infants with WS often have feeding disorders due to low muscle tone, strong gag reflexes, and/or poor sucking/swallowing. Approximately 50 percent of individuals with WS experience chronic otitis media, and hyperacusis (excessive sensitivity to sound) is frequently observed in individuals with WS. Progressive sensorineural hearing loss, with mild-to-moderate high-frequency sensorineural hearing loss in adults, has also been documented (Marler, Elfenbein, Ryals, Urban, & Netzloff, 2005).

Assessment Considerations. An accurate assessment of pragmatic language is essential and needs to include an examination of discourse-level skills such as turn taking and topic maintenance. Documentation of the presence/absence of perseveration on personal topics is also necessary (Hoffmann et al., 2013). Because infants with WS can have oral motor problems, an evaluation of feeding and swallowing is an important part of the assessment process, and hearing status needs to be assessed regularly.

Intervention Considerations. Research indicates that early pragmatic delays lead to pragmatic difficulties later in life (John, Dobson, Thomas, & Mervis, 2012). Thus, intervention for pragmatic language needs to start as early as possible. Intervention for children from early intervention through early school age should, however, focus on all aspects of language and literacy. As children move into adolescence, intervention needs to include a focus on conceptual/relational language (Mervis & John, 2010). Reading instruction using a phonics-based approach appears to be an effective method for these children (Mervis & John, 2010). As intervention progresses, hearing needs to be monitored frequently because of the potential for conductive and sensorineural losses to appear.

IMPLICATIONS FOR INTERVENTION

Each child with ID presents a unique pattern of communicative strengths and weaknesses that must be identified as a result of a thorough individual assessment. There is, therefore, no single intervention prescription for children with ID. There is, however, a set of general principles and considerations that apply to all intervention efforts. As an overarching principle, intervention should comprise a comprehensive assessment and a flexible and functional intervention plan, emphasizing the child's strengths to address specific communicative–linguistic needs that are derived from case history, previous evaluations, parent feedback, and teacher input (Kumin, 2008a). The words "flexible" and "functional" are particularly central to intervention for these children. Goals and objectives of intervention need to have at their core the functional application of language, literacy, and communication. And, the goals and objectives must be sufficiently flexible to meet the individual child's functional needs, and these must be modified frequently to match the child's changing needs.

In this chapter we will discuss intervention that focuses on enhancing oral and written language. There are, however, children with ID who have significant difficulties using speech for communication. For these children, AAC approaches might be viable options. There are also other children with ID whose language development can be promoted by employing some forms of AAC. AAC as an intervention approach is discussed in Chapter 12. Chapter 14 in this text discusses language intervention principles and strategies that apply to most children with language disorders, regardless of the etiology of the disorder. Therefore, the section below on intervention implications will focus more specifically on intervention related to children with ID. It will augment the information in the previous section that introduced assessment and intervention considerations related to specific syndromes, based on the unique profiles of these children with ID. The information here is organized around four questions:

1. What is unique about children with ID that can influence intervention?
2. What are the foci and purposes of intervention for children with ID?
3. What materials are appropriate for children with ID?
4. What goals are appropriate for addressing intelligibility?

What Is Unique about Children with ID?

General language intervention approaches used with various children who have language impairments tend to be adapted to the needs of children with ID. However, four overarching considerations are particularly relevant when providing interventions for children with ID. These are: a) a need for repetition, b) intervention occurring in naturalistic environments, c) a need to plan for generalization, and d) addressing learned helplessness and poor decision making of children with ID.

As discussed in Chapter 1, the task of the language learner is to find rules and regularities from language input and experiences in order to abstract linguistic commonalities. Chapter 14 discusses that children with language impairments require multiple exposures to benefit from language interventions. When applied to children with ID, language and literacy learning opportunities and interventions need to be even more intensive and ongoing and to occur even more frequently because children with ID need many more exemplars to make these abstractions. For example, Allor and colleagues (2014) provided small-group, daily reading instruction for 40–50 minutes to children with IQs ranging from 40–80. Using their results, they estimated how long it would take a child with ID to reach an end-of-first-grade reading level. Children with IQs between 70 and 80 were predicted to require 1.5 school years; children with IQs ranging from 56–69 were predicted to require approximately 3 academic years to make the same gains. And, children with even lower IQs, 40–55, were predicted to need 3.5 years to attain the skills TD children achieve midway through first grade. As another example, Yoder and colleagues (2014) reported that daily, as compared to weekly, communication and language therapy resulted in superior spoken vocabulary outcomes after 9 months of therapy for children with DS. These results indicate that intensive, long-term intervention is necessary for children with ID to make meaningful gains in their language and literacy skills. Furthermore, children with more significant cognitive impairments require even more intense, long-term interventions.

Children with ID benefit from language and literacy interventions that use naturalistic settings and concrete examples. For example, a number of studies has documented positive effects of language and literacy interventions for children with ID when the intervention uses daily/classroom activities to enhance language-learning opportunities (Hansen, Wadsworth, Roberts, & Poole, 2014; Roberts, Kaiser, Wolfe, Bryant, & Spidalieri, 2014; Schreibman et al., 2015). One intervention method that has been shown effective for children with ID is milieu teaching (Kaiser & Roberts, 2013), which is discussed in further detail in Chapter 14. This method encourages communication partners to follow the child's lead, prompt, and model specific language skills within the context of daily routines and activities and has been used successfully to increase both language and literacy skills (Hansen et al., 2014; Kaiser & Roberts, 2013). Many children with ID, however, have significant difficulty understanding and using abstract language. Therefore, although intervention might start by focusing on enhancing concrete language that surrounds daily activities, it needs to move toward explicitly incorporating abstract language as a child acquires more language skills.

A third particular consideration is generalization. Because children with ID tend to be concrete-bound learners, many have difficulty generalizing skills targeted in direct teaching settings to environments outside the settings in which the skills were learned. Generalization is more likely to occur when language skills are targeted in a variety of settings, such as a child's home, classroom, and community. An important consideration of any intervention program is to plan explicitly for generalization by engaging caretakers, teachers, and others important in the child's home and/or classroom in providing multiple opportunities in multiple settings to practice multiple exemplars of the intention targets.

Considerable research has investigated the effectiveness of both parent and/or teacher-implemented language/literacy interventions and has reported positive, significant effects on children's language development (Rakap & Rakap, 2014; Roberts & Kaiser, 2011). Across these interventions, parents and/or teachers are given coaching and mentoring in providing language/literacy interventions in the home or classroom. Results have indicated that children make more gains when interventions were provided by both a parent and an SLP than by an SLP alone (Kaiser & Roberts, 2013). Such practices are consistent with ASHA recommendations (American Speech-Language-Hearing Association, 2005). The results of these studies also have important implications for the service delivery models used with children with ID.

Because children with ID have difficulty generalizing skills taught in one environment to other environments, the nature of service delivery models used with the children must be carefully considered. Although no one service delivery model has been proven superior over another, research suggests that classroom-based services are an effective way to provide language intervention (Cirrin et al., 2010). Furthermore, learning theory suggests skills generalize better when learned in the situations where the skills are to be applied. This means that interventions that remove children from the environments in which they need to use their communication skills are likely not the most effective for promoting increased language/literacy skills. Instead, inclusive models where children receive intervention services in their general classrooms or resource rooms may be more appropriate (Zurawski, 2014). Positive effects of language and/or literacy interventions for children with ID when the interventions are provided in classrooms have been empirically documented (Hansen et al., 2014; van der Schuit, Segers, Van Balkom, Stoep, & Verhoeven, 2010).

An unfortunate reality is that children with ID experience frequent failures. As a result, these children might adopt an approach to responding to requests or making decisions that is referred to as *learned helplessness*. They may also be reticent to initiate interactions. These characteristics reflect those of a passive communicator. Children may not do things or participate in interactions even though they know how (Bybee & Zigler, 1999). According to Jenkinson (1999), learned helplessness and poor decision making are related, and children with ID tend to make poor decisions. When making decisions, they may tend to rely on a limited number of solutions and apply those solutions to new situations inflexibly. Another issue related to decision making presents when children with ID approach multi-step processes. The limited success they tend to experience at each stage appears to result from failing to have a complete comprehension of decision situations, generating few alternative solutions, failing to anticipate the possible negative consequences of a course of action, and not selecting an appropriate course of action (Khemka & Hickson, 2006).

These failures can contribute not just to reinforcement of learned helplessness but to negative self-images, increasing resistance to trying, and a higher likelihood of being motivated by extrinsic factors, such as ease, comfort, avoidance of stress, security, health, external rewards, and avoidance of failure (Tassé & Havercamp, 2006). Therefore, in order to facilitate successful inclusion of adolescents and adults with ID in community and work environments, intervention must explicitly address decision-making skills (Khemka & Hickson, 2006), promote appropriate assertiveness and considered responses to requests, and avoid unintentionally reinforcing learned helplessness.

Although these considerations have been discussed separately, they are interconnected and interact. For children with ID to make the most gains from intervention, professionals delivering interventions need to provide appropriately intensive interventions that include multiple exemplars, provide interventions across all settings where the children need to use the targeted skills and strategies, and actively engage parents, teachers, and other caregivers in the intervention process. Finally, interventions also need to teach explicitly children with ID when and how to activate the skills and strategies taught in intervention and scaffold learning so that children become more independent and self-reliant.

What Are the Foci and Purposes of Intervention?

Like TD children, the language learning of children with DS is most rapid during the early years of life. Considering this, we may need to distinguish between early and late developmental periods and design different intervention strategies for children's several developmental stages. In the early years, a professional's role might be to facilitate language by providing and fostering greater cognitive and language stimulation. In the later years, the role might shift to teaching compensatory strategies that would help both the children and those who interact with them to communicate more functionally. For example, a program for infants and toddlers with ID might provide intensive general stimulation. As the children age, specific language forms and functions might increasingly be targeted so that ultimately, in the adolescent and adult years, communicative intervention is designed to teach abilities that improve performance in a particular school or job setting.

Early Linguistic and Preschool Stages. Research has shown that young children with ID who are at the prelinguistic stage of development use a more limited range of communicative intentions and functions than TD peers (Brady, Marquis, Fleming, & McLean, 2004; Brady, Steeples, & Fleming, 2005). However this reduced range has more to do with the children's particular levels of prelinguistic development as opposed to the disability itself. These findings suggest that an important direction for early intervention with young children who have ID might be aimed at designing situations that require them to initiate a range of speech acts (e.g., comments, requests, and protests) and prompting them to do so. Recall the previous discussion concerning the children's tendencies to be passive communicators. Therefore, encouraging a range of requesting, in addition to responding, functions is an especially important element of intervention for young children with ID.

Early intervention services are particularly important for children with ID. The overarching goal of early intervention services needs to be functional communication. Research demonstrates that parent-implemented naturalistic language interventions and milieu teaching interventions have been successful in increasing the language skills of children with ID (Parker-McGowan et al., 2014; Rakap & Rakap, 2014; Roberts & Kaiser, 2011). Therefore, early intervention services that incorporate parent training, as well as support for daycare providers and preschool teachers, represent best practices for these young children.

School-Age and Adolescent Stages. For school-age children and adolescents with ID, a curriculum-based approach, which involves collaboration between children's classroom teachers and specialists and embeds language intervention within the curriculum, provides children with functional language learning opportunities with the goal of helping the children better access curriculum content. A focus on reading and writing skills sufficient to allow the students to access literacy skills is essential. To assist these children to better grasp academic material, language intervention might include a focus on developing vocabulary and concepts from different subject areas, higher-level conversational skills such as clarification and repairs (Abbeduto & Murphy, 2004; Laws & Bishop, 2004a, 2004b), and narrative discourse skills (Kumin, 2008b). Language facilitation techniques that might be particularly helpful for the students include rehearsal, scaffolds, scripts, computer software (Kumin, 2008b), manipulative cuing systems such as *"The Story Grammar Marker"* (Moreau, 2006), and visual organizers (Voss, 2006).

Inclusion (mainstreaming) in middle school for children and teens with ID is significantly different from inclusion in elementary school. Except for those students with ID who receive most of their education in resource rooms, middle school will likely require the students to adjust to changing class schedules, and they will need to adjust to different teachers with differing expectations and teaching styles. And, as we have seen elsewhere in this text, the different content areas characteristic of secondary education have different features of the expository texts associated with them. This adds greater requirements for students' adjusting to different language demands. Individualized education plans (IEPs) that address these differing language demands for students with ID are essential.

Unfortunately, the literature on adolescents with ID is "spotty and fragmented" (Khemka & Hickson, 2006), thus providing limited guidance for intervention for these students. However, efforts during the preschool and early school years to encourage children with ID to acquire a range of both assertive and responsive communication acts (Fey, 1986) need to continue into the secondary grades in order to counter the fostering of learned helplessness behaviors, behaviors that can increase the likelihood that students with ID are targets of victimization (Garbarino & de Lara, 2002). Because individuals with ID often have difficulty making good decisions, adolescents with ID may engage in risk-taking activities, such as antisocial behavior, drug or alcohol use, and rebellious behavior (Khemka & Hickson, 2006). Therefore, interventions for adolescents with ID need to include a focus on the variety of decision-making skills they need to make effective decisions in their lives (Hickson & Khemka, 2014) and to possess and activate the assertive and responsive communication behaviors necessary to resist coercion to making risky decisions.

What Materials Are Appropriate for Children with ID?

A practical consideration in planning an intervention procedure is selecting materials that will engage children's attention and motivate them to participate in the designed activities for the selected intervention objective. In this regard, we recall that children with ID are often delayed in areas of development other than language and communication. Delays in sensory and motor development and social skills, combined with cognitive impairment, make it difficult to predict a child's interest with a particular toy or activity. Neither MA nor CA provides an unerring guide as to what will pique a child's interest. Nevertheless, a child's level of ID can provide a guide to materials and activity selection.

There may be an advantage in initially using materials that are as concrete and realistic as possible. Remembering that children with ID tend to be concrete-bound learners, real objects in real situations may be the more effective materials and activities. For example, instead of using pictures of books, real books are more likely to increase understanding of what books are for and how they are handled. Similarly, for adolescents with ID, rather than only talking about how to use public transportation, having the adolescents experience using public transportation while providing feedback and guidance on the decision-making skills involved in the process is likely more effective. The language necessary for fulfilling the activity is embedded into and practiced during repeated executions of the activity. Coaching and mentoring caregivers and teachers in materials and activity selection are also important ways to incorporate increased learning opportunities and generalization strategies into intervention plans.

What Goals Are Appropriate for Addressing Intelligibility?

Because a high percentage of children with ID also have difficulties with speech production, it is important to consider if articulatory and/or phonological impairments will hinder efforts to change other aspects of language and if improving intelligibility might allow children to display more linguistic abilities, enhance conversational interaction, and promote faster language learning. We should always keep in mind that language production teaching requires us to judge children's attempts at target forms. If those attempts are unintelligible, we are often unable to reinforce or even respond appropriately; under these circumstances, language intervention will languish.

A few interventions that have been successfully used with children who have normal IQs have also been shown to effectively increase speech intelligibility in children with ID. Phonological approaches to treatment have been widely recommended and research results have shown improved intelligibility post-treatment. Barnes and colleagues (Barnes et al., 2009) suggest the cycles approach (Hodson, 2006) and the complexity approach (Gierut, 2001, 2005). Importantly, the goal of intervention is to improve speech intelligibility, not to eliminate all errors. Following phonological/articulation intervention, children might still have some speech errors.

WRAPPING UP

There are few speech or language interventions developed specifically for children with ID; however, many interventions successfully used with TD children can also be effective for children with ID. What is unique for children with ID is how these interventions are applied. As noted previously, intervention plans must be both functional and flexible and provide the children with recurring and increased learning opportunities in naturalistic contexts. Functional communication intervention plans are ones that have at their core the application of language, literacy, and communication. Flexible plans meet individual children's functional communication needs and are frequently modified to meet children's changing needs.

SUMMARY

In this chapter we have seen that

- ID is a category of disability defined primarily by testing of intelligence and adaptive behavior.
- Major etiological categories of ID are those of *biological origin*, which include a demonstrated biological cause of the disability, and *cultural-familial origin*, which include those individuals for whom social, behavioral, or educational risk factors predominate.
- Children with ID frequently show differences in appearance and have more physical disabilities and health problems than TD children, particularly when syndromes are considered.
- Compared to their CA peers, children with ID show delays in all aspects of language (i.e., pragmatics, comprehension, semantics, syntax, and speech production); however, individual differences exist in abilities with these aspects of language, particularly where relative strengths and limitations associated with different syndromes are considered.
- Because children with ID are a heterogeneous group, there is not a single language intervention. Intervention plans should be tailored to meet individual strengths and weaknesses, be flexible, and have at their core the functional application of language, literacy, and communication.
- Intervention takes into account that children with ID tend to be concrete-bound learners who need intensive interventions that include multiple exemplars in naturalistic contexts and is explicitly planned for generalization by actively engaging parents, teachers, and other caregivers in the intervention process.

The problems of each child with ID are uniquely complex and require us to consider broad issues of personal development and quality of life. Intervention plans must be individualized to meet each child's unique needs. A professional challenge is to find resourceful solutions that extend each individual's capacity for communication and social participation, with an aim for as much individual independence as possible as an adult.

7

Language and Children with Autism Spectrum Disorder

Marsha Longerbeam • Jeff Sigafoos

LEARNING OBJECTIVES

After reading this chapter, you should be able to

- Provide an overview of children with autism spectrum disorder (ASD)
- Describe the communication of children with ASD
- Discuss implications for intervention

Professionals who serve children with language disorders are prone to change their minds. Usually these changes are relatively small: a theory might be updated to take account of new research information or a new intervention tactic might be adopted that refines previous practice. The disorder of ASD, however, has been associated with wide swings in thinking. Such significant changes cause many reactions among professionals. There is fascination with the enigmatic nature of ASD, frustration that many previous beliefs about it are eventually proven wrong, and optimism that the new ideas will improve the efficacy of treatment.

AN OVERVIEW OF CHILDREN WITH AUTISM SPECTRUM DISORDER

ASD or autism, as it has previously been referred to in the literature, was first described as a syndrome, or a unique collection of behaviors, by Kanner in 1943. The 11 individuals he studied were children of normal or near-normal intelligence but who exhibited unusual social and communicative impairments. He characterized the children as aloof and withdrawn with tendencies to communicate with repetitious or echoed utterances, fascinated by inanimate objects, and intolerant of changes in routine (Kanner, 1943). The cause of ASD was—and still is—unknown, although Kanner speculated that it is probably biological in origin. Even so, for the next three decades following Kanner's published observations, ASD was generally considered to be a type of emotional disturbance such as childhood psychosis or childhood schizophrenia. As such, it was often interpreted as resulting from psychological influences during the early years of life, in particular, from emotionally distant mothers (the "refrigerator mom" theory). Because of such perspectives, the parents of children with ASD were often and, we now know, unfairly held responsible for the condition. Intervention efforts were as likely to be concerned with changing the family as with changing the child.

Since the 1970s, several major shifts in thinking about ASD have occurred. One has been in our beliefs about the origin of the disorder. Kanner's early speculation that the origin of the disorder was biological in nature is now seen as being on the mark. We now generally accept that ASD is present from birth, is a neurodevelopmental disorder, and is a "brain disorder with a genetic basis" (Prelock & Contompasis, 2006, p. 4). More than100 genes have been implicated in the expression of ASD symptoms (Lord & Volkmar, 2002; Prelock & Contompasis, 2006). The current line of thinking is, therefore, that ASD does not stem from the actions of the parents in rearing their children but rather, in all likelihood, results from the genes they contributed in conceiving their children. Another shift has been in how the disorder is conceptualized. As reflected in the *Diagnostic and Statistical Manual of Mental Disorders*, 5th edition (DSM-5) (American Psychiatric Association [APA], 2013), ASD, with specific deficits in sociocommunication, play, and behavior, is now clearly viewed as a *developmental* rather than an *emotional* or a *psychiatric* disorder. Hence, it is more closely aligned with intellectual disability (ID) and other forms of developmental disability than with childhood schizophrenia and other types of psychotic disorders. And although many children with ASD have an intellectual disability (i.e., IQ < 70), ASD is considered distinct from ID or global developmental delay. In fact, a sizable number of children with ASD appear to be intellectually gifted. A third shift, reflected in the DSM-5 (APA, 2013), has involved collapsing what had been listed as separate sociocommunication conditions into one larger grouping—ASD—while extracting features of another particular disorder associated with a form of a sociocommunication impairment—Asperger syndrome—and recasting it as a separate category, resembling social (pragmatic) communication disorder (SPCD).

Diagnostic Criteria

ASD is characterized by two prototypical features: (a) ongoing problems in the areas of social communication and interactions in many situations, and (b) a restricted range, in combination with repetitive use, of behavioral patterns, interests, and activities (APA, 2013). The DSM-5 (APA, 2013) attaches several criteria to these two features. These are summarized in Table 7.1.

The revisions appearing in DSM–5 (APA, 2013) have continued to emphasize the developmental nature of ASD, reiterating that the symptoms must be present in the early developmental period. However, it includes the caveats that symptoms might not become fully manifested until social demands exceed a child's limited capacities or might be masked by learned strategies in later life. An additional feature addresses the functional impact of the disorder on the child's life, that is, symptoms cause clinically significant barriers to social, occupational, or other important areas of functioning. And, because there can often be confusion between and, to some degree, overlap with other developmental disabilities, the DSM–5 advises professionals that the deficits exhibited by the children suspected of having ASD are not better explained by intellectual disability (ID) or global developmental delay. However, we see in this chapter and in Chapter 6 that ID and ASD often co-occur; therefore a dual diagnosis for a child might be appropriate. For an accurate dual diagnosis of ASD and ID, a child's social communication abilities should be below those expected for the child's general developmental level, that is, the child's mental age (MA).

Although the DSM-5 carries the weight of scholarly authority, the determination of ASD might vary across different countries and in different states within the U.S. Nevertheless, professionals rely on diagnostic categories to do their work and therefore need to know how syndromes are defined and differentially diagnosed. ASD refers to a clinical syndrome that is defined by a particular set of behavioral criteria. And although ASD is a syndrome, it is a spectrum disorder, meaning that individuals with ASD can vary in terms of the severity of their syndromic symptoms (Crais, Watson, Baranek, & Reznick, 2006; Oller & Oller, 2010;

TABLE 7.1 | DSM-5 Diagnostic Criteria for ASD

Prototypical Features	Criteria
A. Social communication and social interaction deficits that are persistent in multiple contexts for all three criteria.	1. Deficits in social reciprocity—unusual social style; does not initiate or respond to conversations; one-sided conversations; does not clarify or give background information; failure to respond to name. 2. Deficits in nonverbal communication—poor eye contact; reduced facial expressions; turns away from speaker; abnormal prosody and/or volume; impairments in the use and understanding of body language and gestures. 3. Deficits in developing and maintaining relationships appropriate to developmental level—difficulties making friends; does not take another's perspective; lack of interest in peers.
B. Restricted, repetitive patterns of behaviors and interests for at least two of the criteria.	1. Repetitive or stereotyped body movements—finger flicking, body rocking, spinning, swaying; abnormal body posture; repetitive play with objects, such as lining up toys. 2. Rigid adherence to routines—specific sequences to daily routines; verbal rituals; compulsions; resistant to change; difficulty with daily transitions; rigid rule-bound behavior. 3. Fixated and/or perseverative interests—narrow range of interests such as preoccupation with numbers, letters, or symbols; perfectionistic; abnormal topics of interest; unusual fears. 4. Atypical responses to sensory input—hyper- or hyposensitivity to sounds, textures, smells, lights, movement, and/or pain.

Sources: APA (2013); Autism Speaks (2016).

Prelock, 2006). In addressing the issue of range of severity, the DSM-5 (APA, 2013) includes a severity rating scale, presented in Table 7.2. As its approach to determining level of severity, the rating scale uses the amount of support and environmental modifications that are necessary for a child with ASD to successfully function in daily activities. The rating scale is not intended to be used to determine eligibility for services for a child but rather to allow professionals to determine what levels of support might be necessary for a specific child. The DSM-5 diagnostic criteria for ASD are also designed to deal with the inherent heterogeneity of the syndrome. That is, there is explicit recognition that children with ASD present a wide range in terms of types of their social and communication impairments and in terms of their restricted, repetitive, and other aberrant behavior. For example, many, but not all, children with ASD show echolalia and/or a fascination with mechanical objects, and/or unusual motor behavior (e.g., toe walking).

An important question is whether certain behaviors are uniquely associated with ASD. This is a question of differential diagnosis. While evidence suggests that certain types of social and communicative impairment appear unique to ASD, similar social and communicative deficits and stereotypic, repetitive behaviors are seen in other conditions, such as specific language impairment (SLI), learning disabilities, ID, and attention deficit/hyperactivity disorder (Crais et al., 2006; Dahl, Cohen, & Provence, 1986; Prelock & Contompasis, 2006; Siegel, Vukicevic, Elliot, & Kraemer, 1989). Accurate early diagnosis of ASD requires identifying the presence of atypical behaviors absent in typically developing (TD) children and identifying the absence of behaviors expected of TD children (Crais et al., 2006). It is important to note that making an ASD diagnosis can be complicated. One complication arises from the fact that individuals might have social-pragmatic deficits suggestive of ASD but few of the other patterns associated with ASD. Indeed, the DSM-5 describes such individuals as having social pragmatic communication disorder (SPCD), a term introduced earlier to differentiate these tendencies from ASD. Table 7.3 describes SPCD.

TABLE 7.2 | Severity Levels for ASD

Severity Levels	Prototypical Features	
	Social Communication	*Restricted, Repetitive Behaviors*
Level 3: Requiring very substantial support	Verbal and nonverbal deficits cause severe impairments in daily functioning; very limited or no initiation and/or response to social interactions.	Rituals, repetitive, and/or preoccupations cause severe impairment in all environments; great distress is exhibited with any changes of focus or action.
Level 2: Requiring substantial support	Verbal and nonverbal deficits cause marked impairments in daily functioning; with supports in place, there is limited initiation and/or response to social interaction.	Rituals, repetitive, and/or preoccupations appear frequently and interfere with functioning in a variety of environments; frustration is obvious when others interrupt these behaviors.
Level 1: Requiring support	Verbal and nonverbal deficits cause noticeable impairments without supports in place; difficulty initiating and responding to social interactions.	Rituals, repetitive behaviors, and/or preoccupations interfere with functions in one or more environments; the child resists redirection when others interrupt these behaviors.

Sources: APA (2013); Autism Speaks (2016).

TABLE 7.3 | DSM-5 Diagnostic Criteria for Social (Pragmatic) Communication Disorder (SPCD)

Criteria	Descriptions
Deficits in social use of communication	Children with SPCD have persistent difficulties in using communication for social purposes, such as greeting others and sharing information. They also fail to use communication that is appropriate for the social context. They have difficulty changing their communication responses to match the context and/or needs of the listener. The child may use similar language with both a peer and adult and use the same level and type of language regardless of setting (e.g., playground versus classroom).
Comprehension deficit	Children with SPCD have difficulty understanding communication unless relevant points are explicitly stated. That is, they may have difficulty in making inferences and understanding idioms, humor, metaphors, and multiple meanings that depend on context for meaning.

Sources: APA (2013); Autism Speaks (2016).

Prevalence

Current estimates regarding the prevalence of ASD vary somewhat, depending on the nature of population being sampled. However, a multisite national study conducted by the Autism and Developmental Disabilities Monitoring (ADDM) Network of the Centers for Disease Control and Prevention (CDC) and reported by the CDC (2014) suggested an average prevalence of 1 in 68 for 8-year-old children. This new estimate is roughly 30 percent higher than the data surveilled in 2008 of 1 in 88, as seen in Table 7.4. The data in Table 7.4 suggest a sizable increase from rates reported in the 1970s (3.5 to 4.5 per 10,000 children) (CDC, 2014). Several explanations for the apparent increases are possible, but professionals and researchers tend to believe that most of the changes appear to reflect changes in awareness and diagnostic practices (Johnson, Myers, & Councils on Children with Disabilities, 2007; Oller & Oller, 2010; Tonge, 2002). Prevalence figures also suggest that ASD is five times

TABLE 7.4 | 2000–2010 Prevalence of ASD Among 8-Year-Old Children

Surveillance Year	Birth Year	Number of 14 Sites Reporting	Prevalence per 1,000 Children (Range)	This is about 1 in X Children
2000	1992	6	6.7 (4.5–9.9)	1 in 150
2002	1994	14	6.6 (3.3–10.6)	1 in 150
2004	1996	8	8.0 (4.6–9.8)	1 in 125
2006	1998	11	9.0 (4.2–12.1)	1 in 110
2008	2000	14	11.3 (4.8–21.2)	1 in 88
2010	2002	11	14.7 (5.7–21.9)	1 in 68

Source: CDC (2014).

more likely to occur in males than females, that is, 1 in 42 boys and 1 in 189 girls (CDC, 2014). Interestingly, in the U.S., white children are more likely to be identified as having ASD than are black or Hispanic children, potentially affecting prevalence rates for racial and ethnic groups (CDC, 2014). As well as prevalence and demographic data, the CDC (2014) report indicated that the average age at diagnosis was age four or later, even though ASD can now potentially be identified as early as about 18 months to 2 years.

Associated Problems

The core features of ASD (i.e., social impairment, communicative impairment, and repetitive and/or highly restricted behaviors) do not describe all the behaviors one is likely to find in children with ASD. Table 7.5 summarizes some of the significant comorbid conditions that are associated with ASD. Particularly noteworthy, especially because of impacts on intervention, is the high co-occurrence of ID with ASD. Recall that we saw in Chapter 6 that children who have some syndromes that result in ID have an increased likelihood of presenting with ASD as well. Largely as a result of associated problems, especially ID, individuals with ASD have been suggested to have a reduced life expectancy (Myers, Johnson, & Councils on Children with Disabilities, 2007; Shavelle, Strauss, & Pickett, 2001).

Etiology

The exact cause(s) or etiology of ASD remains unclear. Although there is a strengthening line of thought that ASD appears to be genetic in origin (Yuen et al., 2015), there are several methodological issues that make the search for the precise cause(s) difficult:

1. ASD is not a discrete disorder but affects individuals differently. There is significant variation in the types and severity of the problems manifested by individuals with ASD. Whatever is causing the disorder may be interacting with other developmental factors to produce a diverse array of behavioral profiles. And whatever the cause, it needs to account for the array of the behavioral profiles.
2. The disorder is often first manifested as a delay in communication skills observed possibly as early as 18 months of age. Even then it may not be possible to make a completely

TABLE 7.5 | Comorbid Conditions in Children with ASD

Comorbid Conditions	Descriptions
Intellectual disabilities (ID)	ASD and ID co-occur at relatively high rates, although a number of individuals with ASD can have average or above average intelligence (Bryson, Bradley, Thompson, & Wainwright, 2008; CDC, 2014; Edelson, 2006; Matson & Shoemaker, 2009).
Motor behavior deficits	Motor skill deficits are common in children with ASD, with approximately 80% exhibiting deficits in overall motor planning in both fine and gross motor skills, including oral motor planning related to speech (APA, 2013; Boutot & Myles, 2011; Dewey, Dentell, & Crawford, 2007)
Sensory processing deficits	Almost all individuals with ASD have differences in dealing with sensory input (Baranek, 2002; Myles, Trautman, & Schelvan, 2004). They can be hypersensitive (overly sensitive) or hyposensitive (hypersensitive) to sensory input. The sensory systems that can be affected are tactile (touch), auditory (hearing), visual, gustatory (taste), and proprioceptive (joint position and movement) (Bundy, Lane, & Murray, 2002). Although sensory deficits are common, they affect each individual differently.
Hearing loss	According to the Gallaudet Research Institute (2011), 1 in 53 children who are deaf are diagnosed with ASD. The Institute also noted that most children with co-occurring ASD and hearing loss are diagnosed with profound as opposed to mild or moderate hearing loss. Hearing loss of individuals with ASD presents an increased diagnostic and treatment challenge because of the nature and complexity of the communications problems observed with this group of children (Zane, Carlson, Estep, & Quinn, 2014).
Seizures	Approximately one third of all individuals with ASD develop epilepsy during early childhood or adolescence (Ballaban-Gil & Tuchman, 2000; Volkmar & Wiesner, 2004). The onset of seizures tends not to occur during middle childhood for reasons that are not understood (El Achkar & Spence, 2015).
Developmental disorders	Reported comorbid developmental diagnoses include: ADHD 21.3%, language disorders 63%, and learning disabilities 6% (Levy et al., 2010).

confident diagnosis. Consequently, researchers are unable to study the disorder until they have a confirmed diagnosis, which might not be given until age 4 (CDC, 2014). This is often the case, even though professionals are now able to provide a probable diagnosis of ASD as early as age 18 to 24 months. As a result, certain information about the origins of ASD is hidden from investigators.

3. The social and communicative impairments of children with ASD have always made developmental testing difficult, especially with young children. When the accuracy of measurements is doubted, it is hard to find support for or rule out causal factors. The data the factors are based on may be wrong.

Despite these obstacles, research on ASD has assembled an impressive amount of information and has brought many issues into focus. Although current research has proposed a number of suspected etiologies, it is now generally accepted that ASD is a brain disorder with abnormalities in brain structure and function that likely begin before birth. The cause(s) of the abnormalities has not been confirmed. However, during the past decade researchers have been investigating a number of possibilities, including heredity, genetics, and environmental toxins.

1. Postmortem studies have established that various abnormalities occur throughout the whole brain, but in particular in the limbic system, which controls emotions, memories, and arousal. Researchers have proposed that the brain of an individual with ASD has an overabundance of brain cell connections in some areas of the brain, increased

cerebral volume, and excessive cell loss in other structures. There is evidence that the brains of children with ASD grow at a different rate than those of children with TD. Their brains tend to grow too quickly, which increases head circumference that corresponds to a larger brain volume (Courchesne et al., 2001; Ha, Sohn, Kim, Hyeon, & Cheon, 2015; Minshew & Keller, 2010).

2. Imaging studies have provided evidence for brain differences in individuals with ASD. Magnetic resonance imagining (MRI), positron emission tomography (PET), and functional MRI (fMRI) studies have provided evidence of enhanced activation and connectivity as well as altered activation and connectivity in the brains of ASD individuals. This affects brain organization related to control and regulation of thinking, feeling, and behaving (Ha et al., 2015; Minshew & Keller, 2010).
3. The role of genetics has been clearly established. Evidence for a genetic contribution to ASD is found in studies of twins (Rosenberg et al., 2010). In monozygotic pairs of twins (identical) with one twin having ASD, the second twin, with the same DNA, will have ASD about 36–95 percent of the time (CDC, 2014); in dizygotic twins (fraternal) the second twin will have ASD 0–31 percent of the time (CDC, 2014). Concordance risk for non-twin siblings generally is 2–18 percent (CDC, 2014). Current literature suggests that many chromosomes, particularly chromosomes 15 and 17, are involved, and many specific genes have been mentioned, for example MECP2 (the promoter methylation gene), FMR1 (associated with fragile X syndrome), and UBE3A (associated with Angelman syndrome) (Lathe, 2006; Mullegama, Alaimo, Chen, & Elsea, 2015; Oller & Oller, 2010).
4. Environmental factors related to natal and postnatal development include, among others, early injury to the cerebellum, which processes information from the senses and coordinates movement. The injury may disrupt the development of brain connections to and between other areas of the brain. A low level of maternal folic acid (vitamin B_9) during fetal development may increase the likelihood of having a child with ASD, as well as other developmental disorders such as spina bifida and neural tube defects. However, evidence supporting such links is currently relatively weak (Lathe, 2006; Surén et al., 2013).
5. More recently, there has been a greater emphasis on studies that examine the links between environmental toxins and ASD. Some of the chemicals that have been implicated are dichlorodiphenyltrichl oroethane (DDT), polychlorinated biphenols (PCBs), lead, arsenic, toluene, tetrachloroethylene (PERC), methylmercury, fluoride, chlorypyrifos, polybrominated diphenyl ethers (PBDEs), ethanol, and manganese. These toxins do affect brain development in ways that increase ASD risk. However, the data supporting such links as primary causes are still relatively weak (Lathe, 2006; Oller & Oller, 2010).

Although many causes of ASD have been proposed from many fields of research, we continue to be uncertain of an exact cause. It is possible that there may not be one primary cause; there may be several causes, all of which negatively impact brain structure and function. This possibility raises the question that there may be multiple ASDs, all of which have some symptoms in common, but they are not identical, hence the heterogeneous nature of what we currently refer to as one entity labeled ASD. Nevertheless, two main factors continue to surface in the themes about the etiology of ASD: heredity and/or environmental influences. As we saw earlier, research has provided evidence implicating complex genetic factors, in which more than one gene might be involved to express ASD characteristics. Environmental influences continue to be suspect as well. Environmental toxins and prenatal and postnatal environments need further research. The combination of environmental toxins and genetic predispositions may also have exacerbated the increase in the reported prevalence of ASD.

COMMUNICATION IN CHILDREN WITH ASD

As we have seen, ASD is not generally recognizable in children until around 18 to 24 months. At that age, some but not all children who will eventually be diagnosed with ASD show some noticeable differences in social behaviors, such as in smiling, pointing, eye gaze, joint attention, or responding to people (Clifford & Dissanayake, 2008; Crais et al., 2006). Studies of home videos of infants have revealed that, as early as 8 to 12 months, children who go on to be diagnosed with ASD show deficits in several areas, including having less frequent eye contact, failing to orient to their names being called, lacking a pointing gesture to draw an adult's attention to aspects of the environment, and lacking a showing response (Baranek, 1999; Clifford & Dissanayake, 2008; Crais et al., 2006; Jones & Schwartz, 2004). Children with more severe symptoms tend to be diagnosed earlier.

Many of the early signs of ASD are deficiencies in a child's prelinguistic communicative behaviors that emerge prior to speech. Whereas both TD children and children with ID show a strong attraction to the sound of their mother's voice, children with ASD may show little such interest or even prefer to listen to environmental sounds (Kiln, 1991). When they are engaged in interactions with other people, children with ASD show deficiencies in joint attention (Hughes, 2008), which is a hallmark of ASD. That is, they rarely point to or show objects to others. These behaviors are frequent among preverbal children with TD, as is the use of eye contact to attract and then direct an adult's attention. Usually by their first birthdays, the absence of joint attention discriminates infants with ASD from infants with typical development (Key et al., 2015). Recall from previous chapters that joint attention is important for children to make associations between words being spoken by an adult and objects that the adult is pointing to or looking at (Baldwin, 1991; Baldwin & Moses, 2001). Children with ASD often fail to follow an adult's eye gaze or gestures despite several attempts of the adults to persuade them by using a loud voice and/or physical prompting. Therefore, children with ASD generally do not use eye gaze in order to fast map new words (Bailey, 2006).

Other early communication characteristics of ASD include deficits in synchronizing vocal patterns with caregivers, sharing emotional expressions with adults, and responding to their parents through gestures and vocalizations (Baranek, 1999; Trevarthen & Daniel, 2005). Although 8- to 10-month old children with TD respond to their names being called by turning their heads toward the sound source, infants who later end up with an ASD diagnosis do not show such orientation responses. When faced with novel situations, children with TD tend to look at the faces of their mothers and later imitate their mothers' facial expressions; children with ASD, however, often fail to do so (Dawson, Hill, Spencer, Galpert, & Watson, 1990; Grecucci et al., 2013).

Instrumental pointing (i.e., pointing to objects for the purpose of requesting them), sometimes accompanied by rudimentary verbalizations ("uh"), occurs in 12- to 14-month-old children with TD. Although some children with ASD show rudimentary forms of pointing (closing and opening of hands), they do not do so with joint attention (i.e., looking back and forth between the objects and an adult). Several months later (between 14 and 16 months), children with TD point to objects for the purpose of sharing an experience with an adult, but children with ASD tend not to engage in this type of social pointing (Johnson et al., 2007).

In later childhood, children with ASD begin to display the wide range of impairments in social interaction, communication, and imaginative play that characterize the disorder. A number of scholars has suggested that many of these diverse problems might relate to the same deficit, namely, an inability to attribute mental states to themselves or to others, or, as it is sometimes referred to, "theory of mind" (TOM) (Baron-Cohen, Leslie, & Frith, 2007; Gordon & Barker, 2007; Hughes, 2008; Sillman et al., 2003). TOM was introduced in previous chapters. The apparent inability to engage in meta-representational thinking means that children do not understand or relate to the thought processes of people with whom they interact. Obviously, this problem would significantly limit their capacity to initiate and sustain social relationships, which rely on the ability to "read" the mood, desires, and intentions of social partners. Similarly, communication requires an ability to evaluate messages according to the context in which they are produced. Part of that context is the thinking and emotional state of the speaker. We routinely relate the two in statements such as "Mommy is sad because she thought you were lost." Children with meta-representational problems are likely to be confused by this kind of sentence because they cannot imagine the emotions of the other that would result in sadness. A further consequence of a meta-representational problem is that children do not observe the subtle cues issued by their conversational partners that signal when they are expected to talk, when they should yield their turn, and when they should clarify a statement they have made. Hence, the marked deficiencies in the pragmatics of communication they often exhibit may result from meta-representational problems. These are some of the behaviors that make social deficits viewed as significant features of ASD.

Later in childhood, the social and communicative impairments observed in young children with ASD often improve. Intervention, of course, is one of the factors influencing this improvement. Some research on individuals with ASD has indicated, however, that many of them experience an aggravation of symptoms during adolescence. The ability to develop and maintain peer relationships and friendships often becomes more difficult for adolescents with ASD (Kuo, Orsmond, Coster, & Cohn, 2014) because they prefer to engage with things that interest them rather than involve themselves in activities with peers that require reciprocal social interactions.

Studies of language impairment in children with ID have frequently used the technique of matching subjects by chronological age, MA, or language age. A similar procedure has been used to study language impairments of children with ASD. In principle, this method should yield comparisons between groups of children (e.g., children with ASD, children with ID, and children who are developing typically) that are not influenced by differences in age, intelligence, or general language level. However, children with ASD are frequently difficult to match with others. Because of their tendencies to echo speech addressed to them and to produce stereotyped phrases and sentences, counts of mean length of utterance are likely to be less stable and less representative than for other children. Similarly, IQ (MA) matching is difficult for children with ASD because their performances are highly variable at different ages and with different types of intelligence tests. Additionally, much of the early communication development of children with ASD and many of their communicative behaviors are seen as so sufficiently different from those of children with TD that these are viewed as possible indicators of the impairment. In fact, several studies have suggested a profile of language skills that is generally characteristic of the disorder. In this profile, certain abilities are relatively *preserved;* that is, they appear to be commensurate or nearly commensurate with a child's intellectual level. It is important to note that these components of the child's language typically are not age-appropriate, and therefore may be a focus of clinical intervention. It is generally believed, however, that these language difficulties are secondary to intellectual impairment and, therefore, can be expected to improve as general developmental gains are made. In considering some abilities as preserved, it is also important to realize that only some aspects of the abilities seem preserved, whereas other aspects can be seen to be impaired. The picture of preserved abilities is not clear-cut or black and white.

In contrast to some abilities that seem somewhat preserved, there is a set of abilities that appear to be relatively *impaired* in children with ASD. These are the communication behaviors that are most distinctive of ASD and are frequently cited as diagnostic criteria (*see* Table 7.1). One needs to keep these factors in mind when interpreting the findings related to communication in children with ASD.

Preserved Abilities

Segmental Phonology and Syntax. One of the generalizations that can be made about the language abilities of children with ASD is that they typically do not show severe specific developmental impairment at the levels of segmental phonology (consonant and vowel production) or syntax (Stothers & Cardy, 2012). As with all generalizations, however, there remain some disagreements about phonological development in ASD (Cleland, Gibbons, Peppé, O'Hare, & Rutherford, 2010). Nevertheless, one can usually expect the following:

1. The speech the children produce will be generally intelligible in the same way that the speech of a child with TD can be understood at a young age, even though it is not yet adultlike. There is, however, some evidence that distortion errors on sounds such as /r/, /l/, and /s/ may tend to persist into adulthood in individuals with high-functioning ASD and individuals with Asperger syndrome (Shriberg et al., 2001).
2. Utterances are likely to be free of glaring syntactic problems and show a balance in structural growth, meaning that they will not have a telegraphic quality caused by limited

development of phrase structures and bound morphemes. Although the syntactic development in children with ASD is often slower than in children with TD, it follows the same developmental pattern seen in their TD peers (Tager-Flusberg, Paul, & Lord, 2005).

The presence of these abilities is a major linguistic difference between children with ASD and children with language problems due to other causes, such as ID, hearing loss, or SLI.

Lexical and Syntactic Comprehension. Many factors influence a child's understanding of language, among them the familiarity of the grammar and vocabulary, the familiarity of the topic, and the familiarity of the interactants. Under controlled conditions, it appears that children with ASD are able to comprehend the linguistic *code* at a level consistent with MA. That is, they can decode word meanings and semantic contrasts signified by changes in word order or by inflectional morphemes (Stockbridge, Happe, & White, 2014). This does not mean that a child with ASD will understand language as would a child with TD of the same age. For instance, a 5-year-old child with ASD who has an MA of 2 years will no doubt present with comprehension difficulties because of limited vocabulary and immature cognitive development. Moreover, the child is very likely to exhibit deficits in those social interactional behaviors (e.g., eye contact, joint attention) that are crucial to speech comprehension in the early years of life. High-functioning children with ASD (IQ > 85) may obtain normal scores on norm-referenced tests of vocabulary. However, they may fail to use the words in appropriate contexts and show limited use of affective or mental state words, such as *know, consider, feel*, and *remember.*

Imitation. Imitation serves as a communication tool by indicating to the communication partner that you acknowledge his or her action and that you are paying attention, and it is linked to future language development (Van der Paelt, Warreyn, & Roeyers, 2014). Unlike many children with other forms of language impairment, children with ASD *can* imitate verbal stimuli. Thus, the ability to decode, store, and encode verbal messages is present. However, the use of this ability can seem strange and sometimes even bizarre because of the children's tendency to imitate excessively and inappropriately, which we will discuss later, and it may lack obvious social intent. Therefore, imitation can also be viewed as an impaired ability for these children. Impairment in imitation and other higher level functions, such as empathy and TOM in children with ASD, has been linked to a deficit in mirror neurons, which are the neurons that fire not only while performing an action but also while observing the same action being done by someone else (Gerrans, 2009; Oberman et al., 2005).

Impaired Abilities

Nonsegmental Phonology. In contrast to their ability to master individual sound segments (consonants and vowels), children with ASD commonly display significant impairment in nonsegmental speech production, also referred to as *prosody.* Problems of this type take many forms and can vary considerably among children. Some of the most frequently reported aberrations are as follows:

1. A stereotyped rhythmic pattern, described as "singsong," that is characterized by excessive sound prolongation
2. Overly frequent and contextually inappropriate whispering
3. Unusual fluctuations in loudness
4. Limited pitch range, resulting in monotonous speech
5. Inappropriate or disfluent phrasing akin to stuttering
6. Excessive nasal resonance
7. Tonal contrasts that are inconsistent with the meanings expressed verbally, for example, sentences produced with rising intonation that clearly are not requests

Explanation of these problems is complex and incomplete because appropriate prosody has so many necessary components: perceptual–motor skill, grammatical organization, and awareness of what is socially acceptable in different circumstances (Bonneh, Levanon, Dean-Pardo, Lossos, & Adini, 2011; Shriberg et al., 2001; Tager-Flusberg et al., 2005). Paul, Augustyn, Klin, and Volkmar (2005) found that high-functioning young adults with ASD could perceive and produce prosodic emotions such as "excited" and "calm" but differentiated between the two emotions based on utterance rate alone and did not make use of other acoustic cues. Rutherford, Baron-Cohen, and Wheelwright (2002) suggested that difficulty in perception of prosody in individuals with ASD might even be attributed to impairment in TOM.

Pronoun Difficulties. Confusion and substitution of pronominal forms occur frequently in the speech of children with ASD. Some of their errors, such as confusion of gender (*he* for *she* or *it*) or case substitution (*him* for *he*), are also found in young children with TD and in children with other forms of language impairment. To some extent, therefore, the pronoun difficulties observed in ASD are merely a predictable component of the total language impairment.

The problem that appears distinct to ASD is the confusion of the person aspect of pronoun usage, that is, first-, second-, and third-person singular forms. Confusions in the use of first and second person singular pronouns is an often-cited characteristic. Children with ASD often use *you* to refer to themselves and *I* or *me* to refer to others. Perhaps as a mechanism to cope with the reversals, children with ASD may tend to use proper names instead of saying "you" or "me." A number of explanations for this phenomenon has been proposed. In years past, the problem was viewed as a failure of ego differentiation, but this idea has been abandoned along with other psychopathological accounts of ASD. Among the current explanations are the following:

1. Children with ASD are specifically impaired in their ability to understand and use certain deictic forms, that is, words whose meaning is determined by the communicative context. Because the interpretation of *I, you,* and *me* changes along with the speaker, these children find it difficult to grasp the underlying meaning of these words.
2. The problem with pronominal reference is another aspect of the difficulty children with ASD have with meta-representation, or TOM deficits. That is, they do not clearly differentiate between their own and others' mental states and attributes and, therefore, struggle with the language forms that explicitly mark this difference (Hobson, Lee, & Hobson, 2010). If this explanation is correct, one would expect pronoun use to improve as gains are made in nonverbal behaviors that direct others' attention (e.g., eye contact, gesturing) and as linguistic abilities increase.
3. Children with ASD may have attention deficits that interfere with their ability to observe pronoun use in speech between other individuals. Because they do not attend to conversation when others are speaking, they do not witness the normal shift in pronoun use. This means that they will not master pronouns as a result of incidental exposure to conversational models. According to this explanation, additional focused exposure to modeling of pronoun shifting, such as might be provided in a language intervention program, should be helpful.

There is currently no resolution, however, as to which, if any, of these explanations for the children's pronominal difficulties is accurate.

Echolalia, Formulaic Language, and Neologisms. Children with ASD display several unusual verbal behaviors that, as a group, are referred to as idiosyncratic language. The more common forms of idiosyncratic language are echolalia, formulaic language, and neologisms.

One of the most salient characteristics of children with ASD is the frequency with which they repeat utterances addressed to them. This behavior is described as echolalia when it seems to occur in an automatic and apparently unthinking way. This tendency to imitate speech too much has been described as occurring in children who frequently fail to show "social imitation" of gesture and facial expression early in development (Spengler, Bird, & Brass, 2010). Descriptions of echolalia frequently distinguish between two types: immediate echolalia, the exact repetition of a word or words directly after they are spoken, and delayed echolalia, which occurs sometime after the original utterance is produced. A third type sometimes mentioned, mitigated echolalia, refers to immediate repetitions that contain some change to the utterance.

In the past, it was often assumed that the repetitions of children with ASD were without intention and, therefore, should be regarded as pathological signs of their language disorder. At the same time, however, it has always been recognized that echolalia is not limited to children with ASD but also occurs in children with ID, children who are blind, older individuals with Alzheimer disease, and also some children with TD. A distinction between normal and pathological echolalia has been maintained on the basis of three pieces of evidence. First, the frequency of echolalia is higher in children with ASD than in those who have ID or who are developing typically. Second, echolalia continues to occur at later ages in children with ASD, while it usually disappears by the age of 2½ to 3 years in children with TD. Third, some research has suggested that imitation serves a role in facilitating the grammatical development of children with TD. It is also sometimes said that the repetitions of children with ASD are qualitatively different, usually being almost exact copies of what is said to them, whereas those of other children more frequently contain changes in certain words or inflections or in the prosodic features of the utterance. Support for this belief comes largely from published clinical observations rather than from experimental measurements and comparisons.

In recent years, echolalia has come to be viewed as less of a pathological behavior in individuals with ASD, mostly because of the pragmatic communication purposes it often serves. Careful videotape analysis has revealed that echolalia can often serve a range of interactive communicative functions, among them turn taking, self-regulation, requests, rehearsals, assertions, and affirmative answers (Sterponi & Shankey, 2014). For example, echolalia might begin when the listener's attention is diverted and persist until attention is regained; in this instance, it appears to serve a "calling" function. In another case, echolalia might be used merely to fill a conversational turn. The child is facing the listener, and it is the child's turn to talk, but there is no overt indication of communicative intent such as heightened prosody in the echolalic utterance. Different types of echolalia, immediate or delayed, might occur in response to directives or to serve to facilitate utterances addressed to the child (Sterponi & Shankey, 2014).

A limited body of research has speculated that poor comprehension skills of children with ASD may be a primary variable in causing echolalia. If this is the case, it is possible that echolalia is an adaptive response to breakdowns in comprehension. As understanding improves and other means become available for solving specific comprehension problems (e.g., requests for repetition or clarification), echolalia would be expected not to be needed any longer and should, therefore, decrease in frequency.

Interestingly, as evidence has accumulated showing that echolalia serves various pragmatic purposes for children with ASD, other research indicates that it does not seem to help in the acquisition of grammar, which contrasts with patterns we see in children with TD. Studies comparing the spontaneous and immediately imitated utterances of children with ASD have found that their echolalic utterances are less grammatically complex, with the possible exception of the early stages of acquisition.

Important aspects that can be viewed as related to echolalia are formulaicity of language and neologisms. Wray and Perkins (2000) have defined formulaicity of language as

> a sequence, continuous or discontinuous, of words or other meaning elements, which is, or appears to be, prefabricated: that is, stored and retrieved whole from memory at the time of use, rather than being subject to generation or analysis by the language grammar. (p. 1)

The formulaicity in children with ASD can include a number of different productive behaviors, such as a peculiar voice quality to reject a topic and/or use of tokens, such a yes/yeah, to indicate minimal response to a question (Dobbinson, Perkins, & Boucher, 2003). Children with ASD have a proclivity to recall certain words or phrases only in the context in which they were first learned. Thus, a child may learn a word initially (e.g., *shoe*) as a result of experiences with a particular object (sneaker) but not generalize use of the word to other stimuli (other shoes, other people's shoes, or pictures of shoes). Similarly, a word or phrase may seem to be triggered by the recurrence of the original conditions of learning, as in this example:

> Alex, when he was about 3 years old, was riding home at dusk with his mother, who told him that for supper they would have "sea scallops to eat." Just as she said this, the car ahead (Mercury-Comet, 1960 vintage) with peculiar slanting tail lights stopped and the tail lights lit up. For three or four years afterward, Alex would recite "sea scallops to eat" whenever he saw this type of tail-light on a car. (Simon, 1975, p. 1442)

A distinction is sometimes made between idiosyncratic language, in which conventional words or phrases are used with unconventional meanings, and neologisms, in which a new word or words are coined. Children with ASD produce both forms, although neologisms are far less frequent and usually consist of incorrect combinations of morphemes (e.g., *glassable* for *breakable*) rather than wholly invented strings of phonemes (e.g., *glufer*). As with echolalia, neologisms are not unique to children with ASD. They are found less frequently in the spontaneous speech of children with ID as well as that of young children who are developing typically. In children with ASD, however, neologisms are more likely to draw attention. This is because they are more frequent and because they occur in older children who are no longer given license to use language in these ways.

Idiosyncratic language varies in frequency and character among different children with ASD. This statement draws attention to the fact that, although there are similarities in how idiosyncratic language is learned or used, these children are unique in the specific words or phrases that are produced and the contexts in which they occur. In some children, the process is highly creative, so that idiosyncratic forms will appear at one time and may not reappear in other conversations. In contrast, other children make repeated use of the same word or phrase, often in contexts in which it seems meaningless. It appears unlikely that this behavior has the same function for all children who produce it. As with echolalia, the suggestion has been made that highly repeated utterances serve some form of communicative function. For example, Coggins and Frederickson (1988) studied a 9-year-old boy with ASD who frequently repeated the phrase "can I talk." By analyzing where the utterance occurred in conversational sequences, they were able to determine that it did not occur randomly but nearly always was directed to one conversational partner, the child's father. Furthermore, the utterance tended to occur in the middle of speaking exchanges and often followed adult attempts to direct activities or introduce new topics. The conclusion was that the utterance was used to force a change in whose turn it was to talk and thereby help the child to cope with conversational demands.

Communicative Functions. Even though echolalia and formulaic language may be frequent in many individuals with ASD, these do not make up their total communication system. If these are put to one side, what sort of speech acts are most commonly performed by these children? Results from different studies on this question are not easily compared because of differences in the way verbal and nonverbal behaviors are classified. However, it appears reasonably clear that children with ASD are most competent in performing instrumental communicative acts. These acts serve either to regulate the behavior of a conversational partner (e.g., by asking for an action to be performed or an object to be retrieved) or to comply with requests (e.g., by giving the partner a requested object). Children with ASD are much less competent at gaining and directing the attention of the conversational partner, which might be achieved by making eye contact, pointing, or showing objects. Compared to children with developmental language delay and children with TD matched for language level, children with ASD initiate communicative acts much less frequently. They prefer, as a rule, to follow rather than lead in a conversation and to engage their partners at a level that requires little sharing of interest and attention.

Some investigations have focused on the ability of children with ASD to change their linguistic style/register while talking with adults, children, and non-native conversational partners. A study by Volden, Magill-Evans, Goulden, and Clarke (2007) found that high-functioning children with ASD were able to change their language, depending on their conversational partner, but they were not as adept as children with TD in making these modifications. In another study (Volden & Sorenson, 2009) high-functioning children with ASD (6 to 16 years) were as skilled as age-matched controls in making "nice" and "bossy" requests to puppets. These findings are encouraging because they show that despite the "peculiar" and "irrelevant" language used by some children with ASD, others have the capacity to modify their register while having conversations with people with different characteristics.

IMPLICATIONS FOR INTERVENTION

All language disorders are complex and require careful assessment to sort out different levels of impairment. In children with ASD, this complexity is raised one or more notches because of the intricate interactions among language, cognition, and social behavior, all of which are impaired at the same time although not always to the same degrees. Faced with the enormity of the problems in this population, professionals have struggled to find effective intervention approaches. The lack of success many have experienced has resulted in an understandable tendency to abandon older methods whenever a recognizably new intervention approach comes along (McLean, 1992). Consequently, the swings in intervention have been wider in the area of ASD than with other types of childhood language impairment, with many of the intervention swings and adaptations of alternative interventions occurring in the absence of empirical evidence to support the effectiveness of the interventions (Beukelman & Mirenda, 2005; Calculator, 1999; Zane, Davis, & Rosswurm, 2008). Regardless of the specific intervention approach a professional employs, it is important to understand and observe certain general principles. These principles should be consistent with the core information about ASD reviewed to this point in the chapter. It is also important to engage in an ongoing review of intervention research to ensure that intervention is consistent with evidence and empirical approaches and to eschew fad approaches.

Assessment

Children with ASD need to be identified early on so that intervention can begin at a young age. Since ASD affects both social and communication abilities of children, professionals need to address both of these domains. Several studies indicate that both can be improved through early intervention (Kasari, Freeman, & Paparella, 2006; Landa & Holman, 2005) and that this early intervention facilitates the connections between various neural structures that are important for sensorimotor functions (Lewis, 2004). Despite the need for early identification of children with ASD, most children unfortunately continue not to be identified with ASD until between the ages of 3 and 4 years (CDC, 2014).

We know that some of the behaviors used as criteria to identify ASD are not developmentally expected in infants and toddlers; others are difficult to identify in children before 3 years of age, and some behaviors, such as repetitive behaviors that are common in ASD, are also seen in children with TD, further complicating the process of distinguishing young children with possible ASD from young children with TD (Crais et al., 2006). However, parents of children with ASD have often reported observing abnormal social interaction patterns and temperament and unusual interests in certain objects based on retrospection and review of videotapes taken of these children before the diagnosis of ASD (Clifford & Dissanayake, 2008). It seems, therefore, that it might be possible to use a list of certain undesirable behaviors. If present with any degree of regularity in infants and toddlers, these behaviors could be used to place children in an at risk category for ASD. In contrast to the undesirable behaviors that tend to be observed in the children, other important behaviors observed in children with TD are often reported as absent or limited in young children later identified as having ASD. Among these are eye gaze, joint attention, and pretend play (Clifford & Dissanayake, 2008). Since these desirable behaviors are lacking or limited, they could be used in conjunction with those undesirable behaviors that are present to form an assessment approach for young children based on a combination of what desired behaviors are not present and what undesirable ones are. The combination might indicate the degree of risk for ASD for a particular child.

To improve early identification efforts, several experts in the field (Crais et al., 2006; Prelock & Contompasis, 2006) propose using specific screening measures rather than relying just on DSM criteria. Among these measures are the Checklist for Autism in Toddlers (CHAT)

(Baron-Cohen, Allen, & Gilberg, 1992) and the Modified CHAT (Robins, Fein, Barton, & Green, 2001). The CHAT is used to screen for children with ASD at 18 months. This screening instrument assesses key factors such as eye contact, joint attention, and pretend play in children, which could be indicative of ASD (Baron-Cohen et al., 2000). Another measure is the Gilliam Autism Rating Scale-3 (GARS-3) (Gilliam, 2014), which is a norm-referenced screening for individuals ages 3 through 22. It is designed to be used by a multidisciplinary team to differentiate those individuals likely to have ASD from those who do not. The Childhood Autism Rating Scale-2 (CARS-2) (Schopler, Van Bourgondien, Wellman, & Love, 2010) has a 15-item behavioral rating scale that is grouped into four subtests: stereotyped behaviors, communication, social interaction, and development.

Assessment of children with ASD is difficult. It is unlikely to be appropriately done by nonspecialists and more likely to be done appropriately by an interprofessional assessment team. Some professionals may gravitate toward routinely using some norm-referenced tests to evaluate children. However, the nature of the social impairment in children with ASD makes most norm-referenced testing unreliable and invalid. Many of these children lack the ability to attend to stimuli presented in a fixed manner, they may have no consistent verbal or nonverbal means of responding, and the responses they produce may be contaminated by the intrusion of echolalia or idiosyncratic language. The best results may, therefore, be obtained from a standardized observation protocol, such as the Autism Diagnostic Observation Schedule-2 (ADOS-2) (Lord et al., 2012), which is considered the gold standard of diagnostic instruments (Hurwitz & Yirmiiya, 2014). In addition to the Toddler Module for children between 12 and 30 months of age, the ADOS-2 has four modules for use with individuals of varying developmental and language levels. Module 1 is used for children 31 months of age and older who do not consistently use phrases; Module 2 is for children of any age who use phrases but are not verbally fluent; Module 3 is for verbally fluent children and young adolescents; Module 4 is for verbally fluent older adolescents and adults. The protocol consists of a series of structured and semi-structured tasks that are designed to assess communication, social interaction, play, and restricted and repetitive behaviors.

Service Delivery

As we see elsewhere in this text, a pull-out model for providing intervention in the schools removes a child from the classroom and provides brief therapy sessions at another location. This model makes several assumptions about the entry-level skills and motivations of children that are questionable for many children with language disorders but is especially untenable for children with ASD. A pull-out service delivery model is designed to supplement, not replace, an academic curriculum and, therefore, presupposes a minimum level of language development, an ability to learn and generalize, and a motivation to acquire language that may not be present in a child with ASD. Because many children with ASD insist that routines be observed and become highly distressed if they are not, it is important that intervention approaches cater adequately to this need. On the other hand, programs that are too structured may not allow children to develop skills in the natural use of language. The result may be language that appears unnatural to others and does not generalize well outside of the intervention setting. Efforts at developing a collaborative service model are especially important for children with ASD.

The timing of services is another issue pertinent to intervention with children with ASD. As noted earlier in this chapter, ASD is unfortunately not often identified by infant screenings conducted during the first 18 months but is recognized in nearly all cases by 36 to 48 months of age. The implication, of course, is that one does not frequently find infant stimulation programs for children with ASD of the types that exist for other conditions (e.g., Down syndrome). On the other hand, it is not necessary—and indeed would be ill advised—to wait until a child with ASD is of school age before initiating services. Evidence is growing that some intervention approaches that focus on early, intensive intervention have positive effects on children's progress, which we will see later in this chapter.

Interprofessional approaches to intervention are increasingly being advocated as best practice for children with ASD. Based on the myriad communication and behavioral issues and therefore the intervention needs of these children, this should not be surprising. Nevertheless, there is currently limited empirical evidence of effectiveness. Many of the relevant research reports on evidence-based practices are provided separately by the various professions that serve children with ASD and are not reported on interventions delivered in truly merged interprofessional approaches. Research needs to examine interprofessional interventions for children with ASD for evidence of effectiveness in terms of accelerated and increased levels of children's development in relation to the costs for families.

Special Considerations

Children with ASD are known to have a number of associated problems (*see* Table 7.5) that may require special management during intervention. It is plain that all children must be evaluated and, if appropriate, treated for hearing loss and seizures, two conditions that appear to have elevated risk in ASD. The hypersensitivity of certain children may also dictate a change in teaching methods. Touch can be used to guide or reinforce; it is, for example, used systematically in some forms of augmentative and alternative communication, but a period of adjustment may be needed. Because many children with ASD show hypersensitivity to sound, behavioral problems may be reduced and comprehension improved by avoiding excessive speech, speaking in a clear and unexaggerated manner, and supplementing speech when necessary with gestural, visual, and/or physical prompts (Bundy et al., 2002). In a school setting, the technique of *priming,* or exposing students with ASD to school assignments before their presentation in class, has been found to reduce episodes of disruptive behavior (Koegel, Koegel, Frea, & Green-Hopkins, 2003).

Studies of the communicative functions used by children with ASD indicate that they may emerge in a different sequence than in children with TD. One might argue, therefore, that language intervention should be structured to reflect this different order of acquisition. Specifically, a child with ASD will typically use instrumental functions before those that attract or direct attention. This means that in a first stage of intervention, a goal might be to facilitate requests or protests. Procedures that often induce a communicative need for requests and protests, such as placing objects out of reach, withholding an important part of a toy, or sabotaging a play activity, are described elsewhere in this text and in other therapy texts. It is not certain, however, whether such techniques are effective for children with ASD. At a later stage of intervention, children with ASD can be encouraged to use communications that attract attention to themselves. The inherent tendency toward ritualistic behavior might be used to establish behaviors such as greeting or requesting a social routine (e.g., playing patty-cake or peekaboo). At a next stage, children might be taught functions that direct another person's attention. The earlier of these are labeling an object or commenting on an environmental event. The behaviors themselves can be introduced through various modeling approaches, which are discussed in Chapter 14. Professionals must be mindful, however, that children with ASD often begin to direct others' attention by means of echolalia. Hence, it is important to monitor children's contextual use of echolalia and evaluate whether changes in that behavior indicate the emergence of more sophisticated communicative functions.

According to Ogletree and his colleagues (Ogletree, Oren, & Fischer, 2007), effective communication in children with ASD requires interaction between three systems: "goodness of fit," "ecological systems," and "culturally competent family centeredness." Goodness of fit refers to a match between environmental demands and a child's abilities. Frequently, there is a mismatch between the two that may lead to ineffective communication in children with ASD. Therefore, in order to achieve optimal communication skills, professionals need to carefully assess present and future environmental (home, school, and community) demands and the communication abilities of children with ASD. This ecological systems approach emphasizes close relationships between the child with ASD and the people in his or her environment who can facilitate the child's development. Finally, culturally competent family centeredness refers to the central role played by parents in their intervention for children with ASD. This can potentially decrease the gap between professionals and parents and thereby increase the quality of intervention provided to children with ASD (Ogletree et al., 2007).

Intervention Approaches

As the prevalence of ASD continues to rise, the number of proposed treatments has increased. When a child is diagnosed as having ASD, families can be shocked and panicked by the diagnosis and desperate for a quick cure. Unfortunately, families are susceptible to being influenced by unsubstantiated treatment claims or fads for intervention that have no evidence base (Metz, Mulick, & Butter, 2005; Zane et al., 2008). Not only do fads and treatment approaches lacking in evidence prey upon the emotional vulnerability of families, they are fiscally costly for these families, costly for the children because they deprive them of time spent participating in evidence-based interventions, and potentially dangerous for the children. Some of the popular fads include chelation, nutritional supplements, special diets, avoidance of certain infant and child inoculations, and hyperbaric oxygen treatment. Professionals working with children with ASD and their families must keep abreast of fads and interventions being promoted without evidence and differentiate these from evidence-based practices so that they can guide families to interventions that are grounded in empirical evidence. The following sections discuss several approaches to intervention that are supported in the literature.

Theoretical Frameworks. Two theoretical frameworks have been prominent in the different approaches to intervention for ASD. Though many current intervention approaches borrow elements from these models, the distinction remains useful for understanding the fundamental frameworks of various methods.

Behaviorism. In the 1960s and 1970s, the elements of behavior modification were applied with great enthusiasm to the treatment of autism (Lovaas, 1987). Behavioral methods begin by analyzing language behaviors into a detailed series of steps and applying discrete trial training approaches. For example, to teach a child to name might require training of the following behaviors in sequence: sitting, attending to the trainer's face, nonverbal imitation, verbal imitation, labeling in response to questions, and labeling in response to other stimuli. Behavior modification has also been used to decrease self-injurious behavior and promote social interaction.

During the early stages in the development of this intervention approach, both rewards and aversive stimuli were employed to establish operant control over a behavior. In one notorious experiment, electric shock was used as a negative reinforcer (Lovaas, Schaeffer, & Simmons, 1965). Most recent behaviorist proposals, however, are strictly nonaversive. Desirable behaviors, such as the acquisition of specific gesturing and signing skills, the asking of questions, more appropriate play, or greater social interaction with peers have been taught through a sequence of prompting, fading, stimulus rotation (the systematic introduction of new targets), and positive reinforcement (Boutot & Myles, 2011; Buffington, Krantz, McClannahan, & Poulson, 1998; Gonzalez-Lopez & Kamps, 1997; Reed & Reed, 2015; Stahmer, 1999; Williams, Donley, & Keller, 2000).

Behavioral approaches have also been used to reduce undesirable behaviors, some of which are referred to as challenging behaviors (Matson & LoVullo, 2008; Matson & Nebel-Schwalm, 2007), by teaching more appropriate replacement behaviors (Buschbacher & Fox, 2003). At least two provisos to an approach that entails replacing undesirable behaviors with more appropriate behaviors may, however, be appropriate. One of these provisos is that there is some preliminary evidence that challenging behaviors of children with ASD may be maintained by nonsocial reinforcers such as self-stimulation, unlike many challenging behaviors occurring in children with other types of developmental disabilities that seem to be maintained by socially based reinforcement, either positive or negative (O'Reilly et al., 2010). To the extent that this is the case, using a behavior replacement strategy may be quite difficult because of the automatic nonsocial nature of the reinforcement that maintains the undesirable behaviors. Given the recurring theme that children with ASD frequently have difficulties with social interactions, such a finding with its implications for intervention should not be surprising. The second proviso is that some undesirable, stereotypical behaviors might be receptive to elimination or at least to a reduction in frequency when an abolishing operation, defined as "any stimulus or series of events that reduces the value of a particular reinforcer" (Lang et al., 2009, p. 889), is implemented prior to commencement of an intervention session designed to promote a new communication behavior (Lang et al., 2009). Use of a period in which a child with ASD is permitted without interruption to engage in a particular, undesirable, and stereotypical behavior (as long as there is no danger of injury) until the child shows signs that the behavior is no longer reinforcing (e.g., stopping the behavior, wanting to leave) may prepare the child to respond more appropriately to intervention strategies, at least for a period of time. Consequently, for some children in some circumstances, use of an abolishing operation may be more effective than employing a replacement behavior approach.

The first intervention outcome data published on Lovaas therapy was published by Lovaas and was highly promising. In one study, 19 children with ASD who received 40 hours of Lovaas therapy every week for 2 years were compared with two groups: those who received 10 hours of Lovaas intervention per week and those who received community support (Lovaas, 1987). The results showed that 47 percent of children in the ASD group that received 40 hours of intensive Lovaas therapy had recovered and were functioning efficiently in an inclusive classroom. A follow-up study done some several years after the initial outcome investigation revealed that eight out of the nine children from the original study were performing on par with their normal peers (McEachin, Smith, & Lovaas, 1993).

Based on behaviorist approaches, more recent investigations utilizing what is known as *applied behavioral analysis* (*ABA*) have shown that when compared with eclectic therapy approaches, ABA has led to significant gains in IQ, language, and adaptive behaviors (Eikeseth, Smith, Jahr, & Eldevik, 2002). Jones and Schwartz (2004) also found that ABA approaches that used peer and sibling models were more effective than adult models in reaching target criteria. Despite these positive findings, ABA approaches remain controversial, and some researchers have questioned whether the term *recovery* used by behavioral psychologists is accurate. Outcome studies have also been criticized for the lack of or problems with the randomized sampling methods used (Kazdin, 1993; Schopler, Short, & Mesibov, 1989; Smith, 2013). Other criticisms of this approach have included concerns about limited generalization and lack of spontaneity (Simpson, 2001).

Based on the principles of operant conditioning and ABA, early intensive behavioral intervention (EIBI) has been identified as having empirical support (Reichow, 2012; Smith, Klorman, & Mruzek, 2015) for preschool-age children with ASD. EIBI consists of highly structured and intensive treatments (15–40 hours of one-to-one teaching). An unfortunate problem with EIBI is its high cost because of the treatment intensity. Several systematic reviews and meta-analyses have concluded that cognitive, social engagement, and academic growth are accelerated by EIBI. However outcomes may vary widely across children with ASD based on the severity of the disorder (Reichow, 2012; Smith et al., 2015).

As a response to criticisms about problems with generalization and spontaneity in communication associated with ABA approaches, the *contemporary applied behavioral analysis (CABA)* was introduced. This approach combines behavioral intervention strategies with more natural methods. Unlike Lovaas therapy, the CABA approach is less adult dominated; the adult follows the child's lead and facilitates communication through behavioral strategies, such as modeling, shaping, and reinforcement (Ogletree et al., 2007). Examples of a CABA approach include the milieu approach, which incorporates techniques such as incidental teaching. An investigation by Kasari et al. (2006) with young children with ASD showed that the milieu approach led to more initiations in joint attention and an increase in symbolic play during mother-child interactions. Comparisons of incidental teaching with traditional behaviorist methods have indicated that the more natural method is just as efficient as less natural approaches in establishing new language behaviors in individuals with ASD and is more effective in promoting generalization to everyday settings and producing positive affects between parents and children (Cowan & Allen, 2007; Woods & Wetherby, 2003). The method lends itself to classroom use and can be taught effectively to classroom teachers (Dyer, Williams, & Luce, 1991).

Social Interaction Theory. In contrast to the methods that grow out of behavioral theory, social interaction theory does not recommend a specific intervention strategy. Instead, it offers a perspective on communicative interactions and suggests that some of the pragmatic deficits associated with ASD may arise when adults do not make good conversational adjustments. For example, children with ASD tend to produce more adequate responses when adults ask them yes/no questions, questions that are conceptually simple, and questions that are related to the child's topic (Curcio & Paccia, 1987; Prizant, Schuler, Wetherby, & Rydell, 1997). In an effort to help, adults often rely on a teaching mode of conversation. They consistently set the topic and use directive communication acts to elicit specific responses from the child. This, in turn, leads the child to produce a very narrow range of communicative behaviors. There is no simple solution to this problem. Attempts to be nurturing are generally ineffective with children with ASD because they tend to remain socially withdrawn (Jawaid et al., 2012). When a child does not act spontaneously, adults are thwarted from using nurturing behaviors, such as utterance expansions and responses related to the child's topic. The solution may be to (1) modify directive behaviors so that they allow more flexibility of response, for example, asking questions that have several correct answers, and (2) show nurturance by construing abnormal behaviors as normal, for example, responding to the intent of an echolalic utterance rather than its content (Stiegler, 2015).

These insights from social interaction theory can be applied to intervention in three areas:

1. Professionals can observe or record conversations between children and their parents or teachers. By coding the type of utterances produced by the adult(s) and the adequacy of the child's responses, it is possible to determine any relationships between the two. This may lead to recommendations to the adults that they increase certain behaviors and decrease others to promote more adequate language use by the child.
2. Professionals should observe themselves and carry out the same type of analysis on their own interaction with the child. Many interventionist conversations contain stimuli that are intended to be facilitating (e.g., requests for repetition or clarification), but that may have undesirable effects on a child with ASD.
3. If a child with ASD is enrolled in a classroom with children with TD, then social interaction analysis can be used to improve the effectiveness of peer-mediated intervention. In *peer-mediated programs,* children with TD are shown how to initiate social interactions with children with ASD, for example by commenting on what an impaired child is doing or offering to share a toy. Once the children with TD have been shown how to make initiations, they are verbally prompted to do so. Then, gradually, prompts are eliminated so that the behavior becomes spontaneous (Bass & Mulick, 2007; Odom & Watts, 1991; Rogers, 2000). Early analysis of how children with ASD interact with adults or with their unimpaired peers may indicate what types of gambits are most successful at stimulating social interactions. These gambits would then become the ones taught to all the children with TD involved in the intervention program.

Floor time is an intervention arising from social interaction theory. It focuses on establishing a child's connection with his or her primary caregivers. Unlike the behavioral approaches, which are adult oriented, floor time relies on a well-balanced, reciprocal interaction between the child and the adult. A primary goal of this approach is to develop warmth and intimacy between the child and the communication partners. In order to achieve this, floor time aims at fostering "attention and engagement, two-way communication, the elaboration and sharing of meanings, and the categorizing and connecting of meanings" (Greenspan, 1992, p. 443). Through both verbal and nonverbal communication, the child with ASD begins connecting with communication partners, leading to an increase in the child's interaction with the caregivers and a decrease in stereotypical behaviors (Greenspan, 1992). The term *floor time* refers to the fact that most of the interactions between the child and caregivers occur on the floor. Through formal and informal assessments, a child's processing skills, strengths, and developmental needs are evaluated. Following this, the child is asked to play, and the adult follows the child's lead and engages in social and communication interactions with the child. Initial interactions are between the child and his or her parents; later, professionals (e.g., speech-language pathologists, physical and occupational therapists, and educators) become involved with the child.

The circle of communication, which involves gestural interactions between a child and communication partners, is a key element of this approach. Communication through the use of gestures leads to a more complex linguistic communication. The goal in floor time is to achieve longer and more complex reciprocal communication interactions between the child and adults. The circle of communication can be increased by activities such as keeping a child's favorite toys or food items away from his or her reach or giving the child an incorrect item when something is requested. These actions create a communication need and lead to an increase in communication interactions. An adult can modify strategies depending on the sensitivity of the child. For example, if a child is hyposensitive, then the adult can interact with the child with high energy, and if the child is hypersensitive, then the adult can interact in a soothing and relaxed manner (Greenspan & Wieder, 2006).

Few studies examining outcomes of floor time intervention for children with ASD are available. In the one main report, 200 children with ASD who received floor time therapy were compared with 58 children with ASD who received a traditional intervention (Greenspan & Wieder, 2006). The results showed that 58 percent of the children who were treated with floor time fell within the "good to outstanding range" (compared to only 2 percent of children in the traditional therapy group), 24 percent were in the "medium range" (compared to 40 percent in the traditional group), and 17 percent had ongoing difficulties (compared to 58 percent in the traditional group). However, this outcome report is questioned on the basis of the degree to which it conforms to standards of empirical research, and more studies are needed to evaluate the effectiveness of floor time in intervening with children with ASD (Erba, 2000). Nevertheless, elements of floor time intervention are frequently seen in other intervention approaches, such as encouraging gestural reciprocal communicative interactions and following a child's lead.

Packages/Programs and Procedures/Techniques. Rather than thinking about interventions for ASD from theoretical perspectives, a somewhat different way of grouping interventions might be that suggested by Smith (2013). He, along with others (e.g., Wong et al., 2015), has proposed that there are two broad groups of ASD interventions. These can be conceptualized as intervention procedures, which generally consist of individual techniques that focus on specific skills, and intervention packages, which typically combine procedures into conceptual frameworks that guide larger and broader forms of treatment programs and that focus on core deficits of ASD. That is, a child with ASD might attend a program for children with ASD that incorporates a package consisting of several different, but likely theoretically related, procedures and that targets children's improvement across several areas of functioning.

Wong et al. (2015) identified the packages and procedures as Comprehensive Treatment Models (CTM) and Focused Intervention Practices (FIP), respectively. Odom and colleagues (Odom, Boyd, Hall, & Hume, 2010) listed 30 CTMs providing intervention programs in the U.S., most of which are associated primarily with behavioral theoretical perspectives; the others are more aligned with social interaction theories or developmental approaches. Some CTMs have been in existence over 30 years. Among the longer standing CTMs are the Denver Model, the TEACCH program, and the UCLA Young Autism Program; this last CTM is now referred to as the Lovaas Institute. These programs tend to incorporate a variety of FIPs into the more comprehensive treatment program.

FIPs are typically designed to address a single goal or skill of an individual with ASD (Wong et al., 2015). Wong and her colleagues (Wong et al., 2015) identified 27 evidenced-based FIPs, 26 of which had evidence of improving communication skills of ASD children. As with the CTMs, many of these are associated with behaviorism, and in particular ABA, such as reinforcement, prompting, and discrete trial training, although there are others that are more closely associated with social learning theory and still others associated with both behavioral and social learning approaches. Table 7.6 lists each of the 26 evidence-based FIPs shown to be effective in improving communication of children with ASD. A short explanation of each procedure, its theoretical association, and the ages of children with ASD with whom the procedure has been found to be effective are provided.

TABLE 7.6 | Evidence-Based Focused Intervention Practices for Improving Communication in Children with ASD

Focused Intervention Practices	Brief Explanations/ Descriptions	Closely Associated/Used with Broad Theoretical Intervention(s)		Ages for Which Evidence is Available (in years)		
		Behaviorism	*Social Interaction*	*0–5*	*6–14*	*15–22*
1. Antecedent-Based Intervention	Changing or eliminating events that precede the occurrence of a behavior that interferes with a child's learning or production of a desired behavior.	X		X	X	X
2. Cognitive Behavior Intervention	Explicit instruction to encourage children to metacognitively reflect on thoughts, emotions, etc., that result in negative behaviors or inhibit positive behaviors to enable them to prevent the undesirable behaviors or to produce a positive response.	X	X		X	
3. Differential Reinforcement of Attentive, Incompatible, or Other Behavior	Strategic and planned delivery of positive reinforcement or desired consequences when a child is engaging in a positive behavior or is not engaging in a negative behaviors.	X			X	
4. Discrete Trial Training	Typically used in 1 to 1 teacher-child dyads in which the child is instructed/ manded to perform a target behavior and reinforced strategically for the occurrence of a desired behavior. Often used to establish isolated skills that are systematically taught in sequence to establish performance of a more complex behavior. Used to shape behaviors.	X		X	X	
5. Extinction	Reduces or eliminates an undesirable behavior by withholding or removing reinforcers for the behaviors. Often used with other behavioral approaches such as differential reinforcement, functional communication training, and functional behavior assessment.	X		X	X	X

(Continued)

TABLE 7.6 | *Continued*

Focused Intervention Practices	Brief Explanations/ Descriptions	Closely Associated/Used with Broad Theoretical Intervention(s)		Ages for Which Evidence is Available (in years)		
		Behaviorism	*Social Interaction*	*0–5*	*6–14*	*15–22*
6. Functional Behavior Assessment	Systematic collection of a negative behavior's description, identification of antecedents that trigger the behavior, and formation of a hypothesis of the behavior's function.	X			X	
7. Functional Communication Training	Replacing a negative behavior that has a communicative function with a positive communication that leads to the same communicative result.	X	X	X	X	X
8. Modeling	Fosters imitation of an appropriate behavior; may use prompting and reinforcements.	X	X	X	X	X
9. Naturalistic Intervention	Intervention strategies that occur within the natural environment of the child but are arranged to elicit and provide positive consequences to desired behaviors.	X	X	X	X	
10. Parent-Implemented Intervention	Parents are taught to deliver intervention to improve skills and reduce interfering behaviors.	X	X	X	X	
11. Peer-Mediated Instruction and Intervention	Typically developing peers are taught to interact with child with ASD to increase appropriate behavior, communication, and social skills.		X	X	X	
12. Picture Exchange Communication System	Exchange of a picture of a desired item to a communicative partner in exchange of that item, with systematic extension from nonverbal to verbal responses of increasing complexity.	X	X	X	X	
13. Pivotal Response Training	Treatment that targets "pivotal areas" (interests, motivation, responding, self-management, initiation of social interaction); play-based and child-initiated.	X	X	X	X	

TABLE 7.6 | *Continued*

Focused Intervention Practices	Brief Explanations/ Descriptions	Closely Associated/Used with Broad Theoretical Intervention(s)		Ages for Which Evidence is Available (in years)		
		Behaviorism	*Social Interaction*	*0–5*	*6–14*	*15–22*
14. Prompting	Assistance (verbal, gestural, or physical) given to child to encourage attempts at a target skill or behavior	X		X	X	
15. Reinforcement	Consequences that follow a behavior that increase the likelihood of those behaviors occurring more frequently.			X	X	X
16. Response Interruption/ Redirection	Use of a prompts, comments, or distracters to shift a child's attention away from an interfering behavior.	X		X	X	
17. Scripting	Spoken or printed descriptions of a skill/ situation that are rehearsed by a child and then transferred to use in real situations.	X	X	X	X	X
18. Self-management	Instructions to help children recognize appropriate and inappropriate behaviors, monitor their own behavior, and reward themselves.	X	X		X	
19. Social Narratives	Narratives that describe social situations important for a child; descriptions highlight cues and examples of appropriate behaviors.		X	X	X	
20. Social Skills Training	Explicit instruction in appropriate interactions with peers, adults, or individuals.		X	X	X	
21. Structured Play Group	Small group play activities around themes that include typically developing peers; adults prompt or scaffold to support their child's participation.		X		X	
22. Task Analysis	Breaking down activities or behaviors into small, discrete steps to teach a skill.	X		X	X	
23. Technology-Aided Instruction and Intervention	Technology is used as a central tool in promoting children's learning of a skill or acquiring a goal.	X	X	X	X	X

(*Continued*)

TABLE 7.6 | *Continued*

Focused Intervention Practices	Brief Explanations/ Descriptions	Closely Associated/Used with Broad Theoretical Intervention(s)		Ages for Which Evidence is Available (in years)		
		Behaviorism	*Social Interaction*	*0–5*	*6–14*	*15–22*
24. Time Delay	Within an activity, a brief delay is inserted between the stimulus and the child's response, thus allowing the child to respond without prompting; leads to fading prompts.	X		X	X	X
25. Video Modeling	Targeted behaviors are shown via video to demonstrate appropriate/expected behavior.		X	X	X	
26. Visual Supports	Visual displays remind a child to use a desired behavior or skill independent of a prompt; can include printed schedules, pictures, and printed words among others.		X	X	X	

Source: Based on Wong et al. (2015).

As Smith (2013) advises, individual FIPs or procedures are unlikely to be sufficient to remediate complex disorders, such as ASD. For this reason, there is some remedial logic in children's participation in CTMs, which typically incorporate combinations of several FIPs. However, with a combination of FIPs being used in the intervention program, it is not always clear which of the FIPs, or which combinations of these, are the ones leading to children's improved communication performance. For this reason, evaluating treatment effectiveness and efficacy is a complex and long-term endeavor, a situation that frequently frustrates professionals and caregivers.

SUMMARY

In this chapter we have seen that

- ASD is now believed to be a brain disorder that likely has a genetic basis, although environmental factors have not been ruled out.
- ASD is characterized by social, communicative, and cognitive deficits.
- Children with ASD are heterogeneous group. Consequently, the diagnostic criteria established in the DSM-5 specify a wide range of behaviors as signs of the disorder. All children diagnosed with ASD must exhibit some impairment in each of the categories.
- ASD is often associated with a number of sensory and motor deficits, although these are included among the diagnostic criteria.
- It is important to consider the absence of expected typical behaviors as well as the presence of atypical behaviors when diagnosing ASD.
- Concerning communication characteristics can be observed by 18 months of age. These include the absence of eye contact, joint attention, and appropriate responses to people.
- Some individuals with ASD will develop functional communication skills and some do not.

- Language abilities that appear to be specifically impaired in children with ASD are nonsegmental phonology (prosody) and pronoun use. These children may also produce language that is frequently idiosyncratic or echolalic in nature. Pragmatically, they may be especially impaired in their use of language to share or direct attention, and they infrequently produce communicative acts considered to be initiating.
- An underlying cognitive deficit in children with ASD may be their inability to think about and compare their own and others' mental states, that is, "theory of mind."
- Intervention for children with ASD requires special skills in assessment and intervention. Intervention approaches based on principles of behaviorism and social interaction theory have all been used successfully with some children to promote verbal language learning and reduce aberrant communication behaviors.
- All educational and intervention services must use evidence-based practices.

ASD is often described as an enigmatic disorder because of its still relatively unclear origin and the unusual behaviors that characterize it. Recent research has added to our understanding of ASD but, at the same time, has raised new questions about causes and attributes of the disorder. Our views of what ASD is and how it can be addressed seem destined to change—perhaps fundamentally—in the coming years.

8

Language and Children with Auditory Impairments

Mona R. Griffer

LEARNING OBJECTIVES

After reading this chapter, you should be able to

- Provide an overview of hearing-impaired children and hearing impairment
- Construct a historical overview of the oral language, speech, and literacy characteristics of children with hearing impairment
- Describe other auditory impairments referred to as central auditory processing disorders and auditory neuropathy spectrum disorder
- Discuss assessment and intervention issues related to children with hearing impairments

Some children are born with little, if any, hearing, or they lose it before they acquire speech and language (i.e., prelinguistic hearing impaired). These children are likely to have communicative, academic, and social difficulties that arise as consequences of their hearing loss. While specific outcomes are difficult to predict for an individual child, improvements in technology, including digital hearing aids and cochlear implants, and more effective approaches to intervention, including early identification, have led to better outcomes for many children born with a profound or total hearing loss or for those who lose their hearing before the acquisition of language. Other children are born with some hearing. For these children, there tends to be an inverse relation between language and speech outcomes and amount of hearing; that is, as hearing loss increases, outcomes tend to be poorer.

This chapter describes current knowledge and understanding about the relationship between hearing loss and language. Although hearing loss can occur in association with other disabling conditions (e.g., intellectual disabilities, cerebral palsy, cleft palate, and/or visual impairments), this chapter focuses on children for whom hearing loss is the primary or only deficit. The relationship will be explored on the basis of severity of the loss, which is partially related to *sites of lesion* (where in the auditory system the problems leading to the hearing impairments occur) and *etiologies* (the causes of the problems in the auditory system). There is a relationship between the site of lesion underlying the hearing loss, the etiology, and the severity of the loss. Most of our discussion about hearing losses will focus on problems located in the peripheral auditory mechanism or system, which we know from Chapter 1 consists of the outer, middle, and inner ear. However, this chapter also discusses two other conditions described in the literature. These are associated with difficulties in the higher levels of the auditory pathway—*central auditory processing disorders* and the currently less well known and often misunderstood *auditory neuropathy*, currently referred to as *auditory neuropathy spectrum disorder (ANSD).*

AN OVERVIEW OF HEARING-IMPAIRED CHILDREN AND HEARING IMPAIRMENT

Hearing impairment, also called hearing loss, is a general term. It refers to difficulty in hearing at the same levels and with the same discriminative powers as other people. It produces a deficit in the sensitivity of the ear that can affect both loudness and clarity and is considered to be one of the most common health concerns for children across the United States (Meinzen-Derr, Wiley, Grether, & Choo, 2011).

Hearing impairments are described in a number of ways. For example, the Individuals with Disabilities Education Act (IDEA) (U.S. Department of Education, 2004) has described hearing impairment as either a permanent or a fluctuating loss that negatively impacts a child's educational performance. Hearing impairments can also be described with reference to etiology or the site of lesion. Most commonly, they are described in terms of degree of loss, whereby the hearing deficit is quantified to give a *decibel* level. This is an average taken across some of the frequencies used in testing hearing. The hearing level obtained is then compared to a decibel range of normal hearing. Typically, what is known as the *three-frequency average* is used, which is the average across 500, 1,000, and 2,000 Hertz (Hz) in the better ear.

A number of classification systems are available, most of which carry a functional descriptor with the degree of loss. A long-standing classification system that will be used here is that of Boothroyd (1982), which is based on extensive work on the speech perception capabilities of hearing-impaired children. Table 8.1 shows this classification system.

Measures in decibels hearing level (dB HL) are those obtained when a hearing test is performed in the conventional way, using an audiometer and pure-tone signals. An audiogram is a chart for plotting hearing levels in decibels. The dB HL is weighted with a correction factor to make reporting of pure-tone audiogram results easier to understand, as the human ear is not equally sensitive at all frequencies. Decibels sound pressure level (dB SPL) is used to measure levels of speech and classroom background noise and the output of hearing aids. Measures in dB SPL do not have the correction factor to take account of the sensitivity of the ear. The differences in the two measures are not great, but information in texts on hearing impairment is often presented both in dB HL and in dB SPL.

The term *hearing impairment* includes all forms of hearing disability, ranging from mild to severe and profound. Depending on the effects of the hearing impairment, children also have been described as hard of hearing or deaf. *Audition* is the primary means by which

TABLE 8.1 | Hearing Levels and Descriptions

Group	Hearing Level (dB HL)	Description
I	0–14	Normal hearing
II	15–30	Mild impairment
III	31–60	Moderate impairment
IV	61–90	Severe impairment
V	91–120	Profound impairment
VI	121+	Total impairment

Source: Boothroyd (1982).

hard-of-hearing children acquire speech and language. It remains the modality for speech perception despite the fact that amplification is usually required. Supplementary information comes from the visual channel, as it does for normally hearing individuals. In contrast, a *deaf* or *profoundly hearing-impaired* child is one who is unable to use the auditory channel as the primary means of acquiring speech and language or to maintain oral communication without technological assistance. While children with profound and total hearing losses traditionally were labeled as *deaf* and those with mild to severe losses were labeled *hard of hearing*, this division has been recently challenged. Currently, the term *hearing impairment* is more typically used to cover all degrees of hearing loss for children who use some form of oral communication, and *deaf* is used for children who use a manual communication system, such as American Sign Language (ASL). IDEA (U.S. Department of Education, 2004) defines deafness as the most severe form of hearing impairment such that children, with or without amplification, cannot process linguistic information through audition, thus negatively impacting their educational performance. Children who are deaf rely much more on the visual and tactile channels as the primary input modalities for speech and language acquisition and maintenance (Boothroyd, 1982; DeBonis & Donohue, 2008). Later in this chapter, we discuss degrees of hearing loss in more detail.

From the point of view of intervention, the two groups of hearing-impaired children often have very different needs, as they have different primary input modalities. Attempts have been made to use an average hearing level in decibels to delineate deaf from hard-of-hearing children, and a number of different levels has been suggested, including that of Boothroyd previously introduced. Traditionally, children with hearing losses below 90 dB HL are regarded as deaf or profoundly impaired (Boothroyd, 1982; DeBonis & Donohue, 2008), whereas Ross (1982) puts the dividing line at around 95 dB HL, and Moores (1987) and Northern and Downs (1991) use 70 dB HL as the cutoff. The major problem with using an average hearing level is that the ability to understand speech cannot be predicted from a pure-tone audiogram. Therefore, it may be unwise to attempt to define a cutoff point. Generally, the greater the degree of hearing loss, the more difficulty will be experienced with speech perception, or the understanding of speech. However, a child with a severe hearing loss (61 to 90 dB HL) may experience more difficulty in understanding speech and may function more as a deaf child than one with a loss of more than 90 dB HL. Erber and Alencewicz (1976) demonstrated that it was extremely difficult to predict speech perception abilities for children with hearing losses of 85 to 100 dB HL. It is noteworthy that Brill and his colleagues, in providing a framework for the educational needs of the hearing impaired, leave out decibel dividers for the categories of deaf and hard of hearing. They prefer the use of functional descriptors (Brill, MacNeil, & Newman, 1986), which is consistent with the more recent perspective of DeBonis and Donohue (2008), who stress the importance of taking into account an individual's functional communication abilities.

Demographic studies demonstrate that far more children are hard of hearing than profoundly impaired. Moderate to profound bilateral hearing loss has been reported in 2–3 per 1,000 infants, which increased to 6 per 1,000 school-aged children (Centers for Disease Control and Prevention, 2010).

Of importance is the change in racial/ethnic background of the students making up the hearing-impaired school population over the past several decades. Between 1977 and 1984, the percentage of children in the hearing-impaired school population who were from culturally diverse backgrounds increased, with the greatest increase occurring in the Hispanic population (Schildroth, 1986). In 1984, 5,720 out of 53,184 students were reported to the Annual Survey of Deaf and Hard-of-Hearing Children and Youth (AS) as being of Hispanic origin. In 1994, 7,381 out of 47,014 hearing-impaired students were reported to the AS as being of Hispanic origin, which represented a 28 percent increase over that 10-year period. The percentage of Asian Americans has also increased from 1 percent in 1977–1978 to 4 percent in 1996–1997 (Holden-Pitt & Diaz, 1998), and in 2003–2004 the data reported in the Regional and National Summary Report from the AS suggested an even greater prevalence of hearing impairments among Hispanic/Latino Americans, African Americans, and Native Americans or Native Alaskans (Gallaudet Research Institute, 2005). Factors that have possibly contributed to this increased prevalence of hearing impairments among these culturally diverse groups include access to prenatal care and the structural facial characteristics sometimes associated with various syndromes previously discussed in Chapter 6. These factors lead to greater identification of children with hearing loss. The changing racial/ethnic demographics have implications for programs serving children and adolescents with regard to understanding communication and hearing impairments within a multicultural context.

Types and Differing Degrees of Hearing Loss and Their Effects

In this section, types and degrees of impairment and their associated common characteristics are presented. However, these must be interpreted only as guidelines because the speech and language deficits experienced by a hearing-impaired child result from a complex interaction of many different variables. Current literature testifies to the heterogeneous nature of the hearing-impaired population.

Important in understanding how hearing loss affects speech and oral language perception is some knowledge of the *frequency* (pitch) and *intensity* (loudness) of speech sounds. Therefore, prior to discussing the effects on language and speech that varying types and degrees of sound loss can have, an overview of speech acoustics is presented.

Acoustics of Speech. From Chapter 1, we know that the different speech sounds are made up of different combinations of frequencies and intensities. Frequency equates to pitch which is measured in cycles per second (Hz). Intensity equates to loudness which is measured in decibels (dB HL). The same is true for environmental sounds. For example, the pitch of a lawn mower is approximately 500 Hz and its loudness is approximately 90 dB HL, whereas the pitch of an airplane is approximately 4,000 Hz and its loudness is approximately 120 dB HL (Northern & Downs, 2002).

The average loudness of conversational speech at 4 to 6 feet from the speaker is 60 to 65 dB SPL, and the sounds of speech contain acoustic energy between 100 and 8,000 Hz. The intensity of vowels is generally greater than that of consonants, with a 30-dB spread between the weakest and strongest speech elements at a given frequency location. If a speech signal is analyzed over time, considerable fluctuation is found, reflecting the relative strengths of the different sounds.

Some speech sounds are high in frequency or pitch, such as /s/, while others are low, such as /m/. Sounds that are voiced, such as /z/ and /m/, can have both high- and low-frequency information. In contrast, /s/ has no voicing and contains only high frequencies. With regard to intensity, voiced speech sounds, which include vowels such as /i/, /a/, and /o/, and voiced consonants, such as /m/, /b/, and /g/, are generally more intense than the voiceless consonants, such as /p/, /t/, and /k/ (Raphael, Borden, & Harris, 2007).

An important aspect of understanding speech perception relates to the properties of vowels and the acoustic information that vowels provide the listener. Also recall from Chapter 1 that the passageway from the larynx consists of a series of coupled resonators—the pharynx, the mouth, and the nose. The fundamental, or voicing, frequency is low for adult males (i.e., 80 to 300 Hz) and up to 500 Hz for adult females and children. The articulators modify the fundamental frequency by changing the shapes of the cavities or resonators, thus modifying the acoustic properties of the sound that emerges. The effect of these modifications results in the concentration of acoustic energy into clearly identifiable bands of energy at certain frequencies. These concentrations are called *formants*, which are numbered beginning with formant 1 (F1). It is primarily the first and second formants (F1 and F2) that are used in the perception of vowels, and they are differentiated largely on the basis of the ratio relationship between these formant frequencies. For example, for a male voice saying the word *bee*, the /i/ has an F1 value of 300 Hz and an F2 value of 2,500 Hz. For that same male saying the word *boo*, the /u/ also has an F1 value of 300 Hz, but the F2 value is 900 Hz. While these two vowels have the same F1 value (300 Hz), they have different F2 values, making them distinguishable acoustically (Raphael et al., 2007).

In addition to the frequency information available from formants, the beginning and end of each vowel utterance reflect the transition or change in frequency from one sound to another. The F2 transition contains the most important cue for identification of consonants, particularly for identifying the place of articulation of the consonant. For example, the voiceless stops /p/, /t/, and /k/ show the same manner of articulation, but the F2 and F3 transitions from the consonant to the vowel differ, allowing the individual to distinguish between /pa/, /ta/, and /ka/ (Raphael et al., 2007).

For hearing-impaired children, the nature of their impairment may prevent them from taking advantage of these acoustic cues. Imagine a child who has usable hearing only up to 1,000 Hz. This may make it difficult for the child to distinguish between, for example, /i/ and /I/ on the basis of frequency information and to recognize the difference in length of the vowels, but the child should have no difficulty distinguishing between /i/ and /u/ on the basis of frequency information. However, he or she will be unable to hear the voiceless consonant /s/, an important linguistic marker in English.

Erber and Alencewicz (1976) used a closed response set whereby the children were forced to choose a response to a stimulus from a finite set of possible responses to assess the functional hearing abilities of the severely and profoundly hearing impaired in an effort to establish which children could discriminate between segmental features or individual sounds and which children could discriminate only between the suprasegmental features of loudness, duration, and pitch. The majority of the children tested were able to categorize words accurately on the basis of suprasegmental features, for example, to identify a word as having one or two syllables. However, not all of these children were able to discriminate words within the same category, for example, *car/dog*, demonstrating a deficit in perceiving the segmental features that are so closely related to the acoustic patterns received by the listener. Another study (Boothroyd, 1984), using 120 children with hearing losses ranging from 55 to 123 dB HL, investigated how much of the acoustical information in the speech signal was used by children who wore hearing aids. This study required the children to distinguish between phonemic contrasts and found the hearing levels beyond which there was only chance performance. These levels were (1) 75 dB for consonant place of articulation, (2) 85 dB for initial consonant voicing, (3) 90 dB for initial consonant continuance, (4) 100 dB for vowel place, (5) 105 dB for syllabic pattern, and (6) above 115 dB for vowel height. The variable that most affected performance was the ability to discriminate monosyllabic words such as *pen*, *cat*, and *shoe*. Note that in these words, suprasegmental cues cannot be used to differentiate them. Rather, discrimination of frequency differences is required.

In the next sections, we discuss the effects of types and varying degrees of hearing loss. It is important to remember, for example, that a child with a flat hearing loss across the 30-dB level would not hear the sounds produced at frequencies between 250 and 4,000 cycles per second above 30 db HL, such as words containing the consonants "z, v, p, f, s" and "th" and some the environmental sounds, such as dripping water and birds chirping.

Most hearing losses, however, are not the same in all frequencies, which is important to remember as we look at the effects of varying degrees of loss. We also need to keep in mind the different frequency characteristics of speech sounds from the preceding discussion of the acoustics of speech and relate this information to the degree of loss. It is also important to keep in mind that poor acoustic environments can contribute to the distortion of the acoustic signal, making it more challenging for individuals with hearing impairments to understand incoming speech and linguistic messages (DeBonis & Donohue, 2008).

Site of Lesion and Types of Hearing Loss. The site of the lesion, that is, the location of the damage to the hearing mechanism that causes the hearing loss, will have an impact on the hearing status of the child. Hearing losses are generally divided into two types, depending on the site of the lesion.

Conductive hearing loss is the type caused by damage in the external ear canal, the eardrum, or the middle ear. Damage to these parts of the ear generally affects the mechanical aspects of hearing, that is, how sound waves are transferred to the inner part of the ear, specifically the cochlea. The hearing deficit consists of a loss of intensity such that sounds do not sound loud enough. Generally, an audiogram for a conductive loss depicts approximately equal hearing loss at each frequency, resulting in a flat contour (Martin & Clark, 2006). However, there is no loss in discriminative ability, so clarity is not impaired. Therefore, intervention for a child with a conductive hearing loss should be quite effective, and the child should be able to use oral language to communicate.

Conductive hearing losses are the most common type of hearing loss found in children and are typically caused by either impacted wax in the external ear canal (easily observed and remedied) or infection (otitis media [OM]) in the middle ear often with a residual of fluid (effusion [OME]) in the middle-ear cavity. While approximately 70 percent of children will have at least one episode of otitis media before 3 years of age, many children will experience recurrent middle-ear infections (Roush, 2001). Of the children who experience an isolated episode of OME, approximately 50 percent will temporarily have a mild hearing loss, while approximately 5 to 10 percent will experience a moderate one (Roberts, Hunter, et al., 2002). Children suffering long-term middle-ear disease can have either a sustained hearing loss or one that fluctuates over time, even returning to normal hearing for extended periods of time. Most of episodes of OME will repair spontaneously, but a substantial proportion may require some form of medical intervention. In the majority of cases, the hearing loss can be treated medically or surgically. This intervention consists of either antibiotics or surgery to drain the infected ear and insert ventilation tubes to aerate the middle ear. Medical intervention is undertaken to alleviate the pain caused by the acute otitis media, to ensure that infection does not spread to brain areas (meninges), and to restore normal hearing. In certain populations (e.g., Native Americans and Aboriginal Australians), the prevalence and effects of OME are much greater and warrant particular professional vigilance to monitor children's hearing levels.

There is a hypothesized relationship between the occurrence of otitis media in early childhood and language disorders such that a history of OME with or without associated hearing loss may lead to deficits in language and literacy (Friel-Patti & Finitzo, 1990). Findings from studies investigating this proposed relationship are varied. Holm and Kunze (1969), although criticized for flawed methodology had a significant impact on the beliefs held by professionals about conductive hearing loss, influencing later research, because their showed that a group of children with a history of OM (reported retrospectively) had minor performance differences on a range of educational achievement and language measures. Both retrospective studies of children with OM or studies testing for the effects of OM carried out during active OM episodes suggested a strong association between almost any OM event and a later language disorder (Howie, 1975; Needleman, 1977). In a later study, Winskel (2006) found that an early history of OM negatively affected the performance of 6- to 8-year-old Australian children, matched for chronological age, gender, and socioeconomic status, with non-OM children on measures of phonological awareness, expressive vocabulary, word definitions, and literacy skills. In contrast, Roberts, Burchinal, and Zeisel (2002) found no relationship between a history of OME or associated hearing loss on academic achievement in school-age children. They reported that children in their study who experienced more frequent episodes of OME and hearing loss during early childhood initially scored lower on math and language measures but caught up with their non-OME peers by second grade. Similar results were found by Johnson, McCormick, and Baldwin (2008), who reported that young children with a history of OME were at no risk for language delays during the early elementary school years based on performance scores from multiple measures of general language, articulation, and phonological skills.

There are at least two issues that need to be considered in determining the relationship between OME and language development in children. The first relates to persistent OME. In special populations of children, such as those with various developmental disabilities, OME is highly prevalent and persistent and produces greater negative effects on hearing levels over a long period of time (Zeisel & Roberts, 2003). In the absence of reinstatement of near normal hearing (either by medical or technological intervention), any child with protracted middle-ear problems is likely to experience a significant impact on language, which can then impact dramatically on academic performance. The same would be true if a child with a bilateral sensorineural hearing loss were left unaided for an extended length of time during critical periods for language development.

The second issue, which is more controversial, relates to the contribution of mild, fluctuating hearing loss during the language development period. If middle-ear infections are common in individual children and remain untreated for substantial periods of time, then they clearly will have an effect, per our discussion above. However, it is the actual extent and duration of hearing loss that accompanies OME that is probably the main determinant of language development outcomes. The simple occurrence of a bout of OME (given its very prevalent nature) is unlikely to cause problems in itself. Haggard, Birkin, and Pringle (1994) reviewed 13 major studies that had investigated the effects of OME on language outcomes. These authors were very critical of the design of most of the studies, and even when effects were statistically significant, effects were very small. However, 9 of the 13 studies did report adverse effects of OME on language development. The effects occurred only between the ages of 2 and 4 years and were not consistent across different language skills. Overall, Haggard et al. (1994) concluded that there is an effect of OME on language development, but it varied depending on age of onset, length of duration of episodes, and number of bouts of OME. In contrast, a prospective study conducted by Roberts, Burchinal, Davis, Collier, and Henderson (1991) found no relationship between OME and language development in children between 4½ and 6 years of age from lower- or middle-socioeconomic backgrounds. In a review of research investigating the relationship between OME and speech–language development/ academic achievement and speech perception in noise, Roberts, Hunter, et al. (2002) cautioned that most studies looked at the effects of OME, not hearing loss, on development/academic success and did not control for probable confounding factors, such as socioeconomic status. This is consistent with the previous analysis indicating that, if the OME affects hearing levels for relatively protracted periods during critical language development periods, then it may have the same effects as unmanaged mild/moderate sensorineural hearing loss (approximately 30 db HL). Because average hearing levels in OME are rarely poorer than 30 dB HL, there could be subtle effects on speech input and perception.

Young children require louder levels to perceive speech with the same performance as older children (Mackie & Dermody, 1986). Therefore, it is possible that speech perception scores might be poorer in young children with even mild hearing losses. There is some evidence for the effects of OME on speech perception. For example, Clarkson, Eimas, and Marean (1989) reported results of children with a history of OME and matched controls. Two OME groups were included: one with OME history and language delay and one with OME history and no language delay. The children in the OME-without-language-delay group performed more poorly than those in the control group consisting of children without OME and language delay. The children in the OME-with-language-delay group, in turn, performed more poorly than those in the OME-without-language-delay group. Other studies indicate that speech perception in noise, which more closely approximates normal environment listening conditions, is also impaired in OME groups relative to controls (Gravel & Wallace, 1992; Jerger & Jerger, 1983).

The role of either the hearing loss due to transient OME or its effect on speech perception as the basis for later language disorders remains controversial. Ventry (1983) was the first to point out the methodological issues related to studies in this area. Despite the early availability of a set of criteria, most subsequent studies have failed to provide prospective designs, standardized measures for evaluation of language effects, and appropriate statistical analyses of differences and, most critically, have used OME itself for prediction of effect on language rather than the presence of a hearing loss associated with the OME. As a result, there remains some uncertainty as to the actual effects that can be attributed to OME on language during early stages of development. As such, strong links between hearing loss with OME and language outcomes, based on empirical evidence, cannot be made at this time. However, DeBonis and Donohue (2008) recommend that the management of persistent conductive hearing loss in children be given careful attention, particularly in regard to classroom performance, because of the potential risk to their academic performance and speech–language development.

Sensorineural hearing loss is caused by damage to the inner ear, specifically to hair cells located in the cochlea and/or the auditory (eighth) nerve or in the auditory neurological pathways to the brain. There are numerous pre-, peri-, and postnatal causes for cochlear hearing loss (Martin & Clark, 2006). Severity of the loss depends on the extent of the damage to the hair cells. The hearing deficit typically causes both a loss of intensity and a loss of clarity so that a child has difficulty discriminating speech. Sounds can be intensified through the use of appropriate amplification, but they are not necessarily made any clearer. Another problem for many children with sensorineural impairments is abnormal sensitivity to loud sounds, or recruitment. With this deficit, the range between the point at which a sound is just heard and where it becomes uncomfortably or even painfully loud is reduced. This means that the child may have a very restricted range of usable hearing (reduced dynamic range), with soft sounds unable to be heard and loud sounds unable to be tolerated. As a result, the successful fitting of hearing aids and the perception of speech are severely compromised in some children. It is important to bear in mind that for all people, whether hearing impaired or not and whether suffering from recruitment or not, there is a maximum loudness limit above which sound becomes uncomfortable and then painful.

The degree of sensorineural impairment varies across all categories, from mild to profound (*see* Table 8.1). Sensorineural hearing loss is usually irreversible and generally is not amenable to medical intervention. Management efforts have traditionally involved the use of hearing aids/amplification (DeBonis & Donohue, 2008). More recently, however, some surgical intervention has become possible with the development of cochlear implants. An electrode is surgically implanted into the cochlea to stimulate the auditory nerve directly. However, this intervention is generally available only to individuals with more severe impairments who meet strict selection criteria. Outcomes for children receiving cochlear implants are discussed later in this chapter.

Some children experience what is called a *mixed hearing loss*, that is, a loss that has both a conductive and a sensorineural element. The loss may have one or more causes, and the particular difficulties experienced will depend on the configuration of the loss. By configuration, we mean the particular frequencies affected by the loss and the extent to which each frequency is affected.

Other children present with what is termed *central auditory processing disorders.* These children may show no evidence of hearing loss; rather, there are varying degrees of difficulty with auditory processing that result in comprehension and speech perception deficits that are believed by some to interfere with language development. Still other children can present with a condition known as *auditory neuropathy spectrum disorder (ANSD).* These children typically have hearing losses and show evidence of a neural disturbance in the auditory pathway/auditory brain stem despite normal cochlear function. Because these topics are both complicated and controversial, they are covered in more detail in separate sections later in this chapter.

Degrees of Hearing Loss. In addition to describing hearing loss by type and site of lesion, another important way of characterizing hearing loss is by degree of loss. Besides the term *normal*, a review of Table 8.1 shows the five terms used to identify differing degrees of loss. These are mild, moderate, severe, profound, and total. Following is a description of differing degrees of hearing loss and a general discussion of the speech, language, and communication characteristics associated with each degree of loss.

Mild Hearing Loss (15 to 30 dB HL). Children with this degree of hearing loss generally develop speech and language spontaneously. Traditionally, mild losses have been considered to cause only minimal difficulty for the child, with the main problem involving hearing faint speech. However, because these children are not always in advantageous listening conditions, they often miss essential auditory information. This can result in problems with language development not so much because of the extent of the effects that the loss produces on receptive communication but because the mild effects are often not identified until a child is older, by which time mild disruptions in language can turn into significant effects on academic achievement (Teasdale & Sorenson, 2007; Wake & Poulakis, 2004). The past few decades have produced research findings that have considerably increased our awareness of the effects of mild impairments on speech and language development and academic achievement.

Children with mild hearing loss are less likely to be identified in early screening programs, and their apparent inattentive behavior is often not associated with hearing loss until their poor academic achievement is investigated with routine vision and hearing tests (Yoshinaga-Itano, 1998). Another issue for children, particularly adolescents, with mild hearing losses is that they tend to resist wearing hearing aids because the advantage they get from personal amplification does not balance the disadvantage of being stigmatized by the wearing of a technology aid, thereby associating them with a group that in most communication circumstances they do not resemble. As a result, the main developmental problem this group experiences is academic underachievement. Although subtle expressive and receptive language problems will be present in the child with mild hearing loss, as the loss reaches the borderline between mild and moderate loss, the more the receptive capacity and behavior of children will mirror those of children with moderate degrees of loss (particularly for spoken language elements requiring more high-frequency sound information, such as morphology for tenses). This continuum of deficit is, however, not discrete in that some children with a mild loss can also show quite poor receptive communication skills, again emphasizing the need to both identify and monitor communication abilities in all children with hearing loss. Therefore, professionals can no longer discount the negative impact that mild hearing losses can have on children.

Minimal intervention for children with mild permanent hearing losses consists of fitting them with hearing aids, encouraging the use of visual as well as auditory cues, and providing preferential seating. With early and appropriate intervention, any language delay these children might experience should be successfully remediated. The problems faced by children with fluctuating and/or temporary hearing losses, as opposed to mild permanent losses, are discussed further in a later section.

Moderate Hearing Loss (31 to 60 dB HL). Children with this degree of hearing loss definitely benefit from the fitting of hearing aids as soon as possible following diagnosis because without amplification, conversational speech is not completely audible. Children at the lower end of this range often rely on a visual supplement to the auditory signal. Many of these children have delayed language skills and speech problems, particularly with consonants. Generally, voice can be monitored adequately, and vocal quality is normal. Without appropriate intervention, these children will not develop to their full capacity in speech, language, or academics. They may remain at an educational disadvantage throughout the school period. With appropriate amplification and intervention, they can have good audibility and speech perception as well as reasonable potential to develop normal or nearly normal speech and language skills. These children are typically in mainstreamed classes with preferential seating.

In an early but still relevant study, Davis, Elfenbein, Schum, and Bentler (1986) investigated the relationship between hearing loss, educational achievement, language development, and personality development in a group of 40 children, aged 5 to 18 years, with mild and moderate sensorineural hearing losses as well as children with severe hearing losses. These researchers found that language development and academic success could not be predicted by hearing loss or age, again reminding us that degree of hearing loss by itself is not a good simple predictor of behavioral functioning. Many of the children, however, did demonstrate aggressive tendencies and expressed more somatic complaints than their hearing peers. Parents reported experiencing more behavioral difficulties in social and school situations. These findings underscore the importance of considering all aspects of the development of children with hearing loss regardless of the severity of the losses.

Research has shown that when children with mild to moderate hearing losses are provided with early use of appropriate amplification devices and speech and language delays are addressed in intervention early, their difficulties with speech and language are likely to be limited to mild to moderate problems (Elfenbein, Hardin-Jones, & Davis, 1994). When these conditions have not occurred, their difficulties can be more serious. As with all hearing-impaired children, it is important to evaluate each child to determine the degree of intervention required and understand that moderate hearing impairment can result in significant language problems for some children (Davis, 1990). Children with mild and moderate hearing impairment often present with the following language characteristics: (1) poor vocabulary development (probably as the result of limited exposure to different alternatives for expressing concepts and difficulties dealing with metalinguistic features of vocabulary and figurative language expressions); (2) deficits in the use of morphological markers, particularly those requiring high-frequency sounds, (e.g., plurals, third-person present tense, and regular past tense) for English; and (3) delays in the development of functional words, such as prepositions and articles.

Severe Hearing Loss (61 to 90 dB HL). Children with this degree of hearing loss demonstrate the greatest variation in speech and language skills and have considerable difficulty hearing conversational speech sufficiently well for discrimination unless they wear amplification. Regardless of the level of loss, deficits in speech and language skills exist. Those with the most severe impairments respond only to sounds that are high in intensity and at close range, even with amplification. Some may have poor auditory discrimination skills. Even with amplification, there is frequently a delay in developing language. Speech will also be delayed, with consonant, vowel, and diphthong errors. Some children in this group may show an abnormal voice quality. Other factors also play a significant part, and the range of spoken language abilities is varied. The outcome for these children depends largely on how early the hearing loss is detected and when intervention begins. Audition should be the main input modality for these children but with increased reliance on visual cues, particularly in poor acoustic conditions and especially for those children at the bottom of the hearing range. Good results can be achieved with early amplification and appropriate speech, language, and educational intervention.

Every hearing loss, even if in the mild range, produces significant barriers to easy communication in environments with background noise, including school classrooms (Northern & Downs, 2002). The communication skills of children who have a severe hearing impairment particularly need to be understood in terms of the extra concentration and attention required to communicate. These difficulties are exacerbated by the effects that even mild expressive and receptive communication problems can have not only on academic achievement but also on self-identity. This can become a particular issue in adolescence for teenagers already differentiated by having to wear a technology aid. Some of these children may function in a regular classroom, but many will need special educational assistance and perhaps even special placement. Counseling about these issues is often made difficult because of the communication deficits these children experience. Educational programs need to provide information as well as emotional support that consider each child's individual, unique needs. Speech and language evaluations of children with severe hearing impairments can be critical in providing a clear picture on which to base other interventions that may be required.

Profound Hearing Loss (91 to 120 dB HL). Children with this degree of hearing loss are the ones least likely to benefit from auditory input, and many of them will rely heavily on tactile and visual cues. This degree of loss significantly impacts on speech, language, and communicative development and psychosocial adjustment. Amplified auditory input with hearing aids will give them information about environmental sounds and the suprasegmental features of speech. However, in most cases, it will not provide them with sufficient information to discriminate speech. Accordingly, the development of adequate oral language is difficult for these children, and many need to use total communication or manual communication (discussed later in the chapter) in order to communicate. In recent years, cochlear implants have begun to change descriptions of speech and language profiles of children with profound losses, as we will see later in this chapter.

A very small number of children in this group may actually have no measurable hearing levels. They are generally reported as having "hearing levels" of about 120 dB, probably because they feel the test stimuli in the lower frequencies. Such children have speech and language skills below those of their peers who have only slightly better hearing. This is a powerful demonstration of what can be achieved with just a small amount of residual hearing (Levitt, McGarr, & Geffner, 1987).

Total Hearing Loss (121+ dB HL). Children with this degree of hearing loss do not hear even with hearing aids. It appears that they feel rather than hear sounds. In the absence of cochlear implantation, vision is the primary modality through which they acquire language. The situation for many children with total hearing loss has improved recently as the result of increased resources for education and improved technology (including cochlear implants and tactile aids). However, the challenge for many is still considerable. In a qualitative research study published in the mid-1980s and before the current prominence of cochlear implantation, Sainsbury (1986) provided a graphic report on the difficulties faced in society by those with practically no intelligible speech or useful hearing. Her subjects were 171 hearing-impaired adults, including those who were born with a total hearing loss, those who had acquired their loss before 2 years of age, and those who were completely dependent on manual sign language (British Sign Language). Sainsbury noted that the problems these adults faced in making themselves understood and in being able to make hearing family and friends understand their difficulties were almost insurmountable. This group typically had low literacy levels, reducing even further their communication and integration options. At that time, either television with teletext (a closed-caption system of subtitling developed for television or movie viewers who cannot follow the spoken dialogue) was unaffordable (because of the considerably lower education levels achieved by many adults with total hearing loss that resulted in lower earning potential) or the message was often misunderstood because of their slow reading and poor language comprehension, resulting in only partial understanding of information, at best. Sainsbury also found that while a family member who could act as an intermediary between the person with total hearing loss and society is a critical source of information about the wider world, such an intermediary often had limited time and might not be as empathetic as necessary.

These findings have significant bearing on issues related to the integration of children with total hearing loss within normal hearing environments and the role of a Deaf culture within society. Children with little or no hearing experience markedly fewer problematic communications and interactions within the deaf community compared to their interactions with normally hearing individuals in the hearing world. While informal communication networks may be well developed, the person with little or no hearing remains highly dependent on the communicative functions of the formal network of both government and voluntary service providers, who must themselves provide the necessary intermediary communicative function to overcome the significant language barrier.

While studies of both expressive and receptive language capabilities have been conducted with adults with total hearing loss, the results are highly individual and depend on amplification interventions that may or may not have been experienced. Generally, however, results do not show well-developed language skills unless successful management of a technology aid has been available to the person and the individual has been exposed to sign language and an ambient environment of competent sign language users from a very early age. Cochlear implants can produce results for some individuals with total hearing loss equivalent to those achieved for individuals with less severe losses, but there is substantial variability in the results. It is important to remember that the fitting of a cochlear implant does not, in itself, guarantee easy transition to the hearing world if that is the desired goal for the family of a child with a total hearing loss.

Unilateral Hearing Loss. Unilateral hearing loss (hearing loss in one ear only) has a reasonably large prevalence, with estimates ranging from 3 to 13 per 1,000 (Northern & Downs, 2002). Total unilateral deafness is most commonly due to mumps experienced in very early childhood. As with mild hearing loss, the child and parents may be unaware of the problem until it begins to affect specialized communication requirements (e.g., telephone use), interpersonal communication, or academic achievement.

The traditional thinking was that children with a unilateral loss but normal hearing in the other ear would develop normally. This view was, however, questioned in the 1980s (Bess, Klee, & Culbertson, 1986; Bess & Tharpe, 1988; Oyler, Oyler, & Matkin, 1987, 1988). Bess and Tharpe (1988) and Bess et al. (1986) showed that at least one third of a group of children with unilateral hearing loss had delayed academic progress and that 50 percent of the group needed special resource support in their educational programs. This has similarities to the effects of mild bilateral hearing loss.

These data indicate that children with unilateral hearing loss are at risk for academic difficulties, but not all children with unilateral loss will have these problems if early intervention is provided. A study by Kiese-Himmel (2002) supports this perspective, reporting that children who were identified early and managed appropriately (e.g., fitted with hearing aids and monitored educationally) performed similarly on standardized linguistic tasks as did normally hearing children.

Age of Onset of Hearing Loss and Its Effects

Hearing loss can also be described in terms of the age at which it occurred. It has been the custom to divide losses into congenital loss, which is present at birth or occurs in the immediate postnatal period, and acquired loss, which occurs after birth, when the child has had some exposure to language through audition. As the age of onset of loss is an important factor in determining the linguistic outcome, there has been a recent trend to refer to congenital losses and those that occur shortly after birth as prelingual hearing losses and those that occur after the child has been exposed to a considerable amount of conversational language as postlingual hearing impairments. There is no agreed-on age level that is used to divide these two groups, and some would argue that, as language development begins at birth, the distinction is meaningless (Osberger & Hesketh, 1988). However, there are differences in linguistic performance between the two groups, and 2 years of age is generally used as the dividing line. The earlier a hearing impairment occurs, the more likely it is to have a deleterious effect on speech and language development. In addition, the more severe the loss, generally the more severe the linguistic impairment.

Congenital, or prelingual, losses have many different causes. Genetic factors (heredity) and meningitis (inflammation of the membranes covering the brain and/or spinal cord) in the immediate postnatal period are two common causes. Genetic hearing loss may occur alone or in conjunction with other conditions (DeBonis & Donohue, 2008; Martin & Clark, 2006), such as some of the syndromes previously discussed in Chapter 6. Other causes are prematurity and maternal rubella, with the latter declining as a cause (Martin & Clark, 2006). Acquired losses also have many different causes, and again the more common causes are meningitis and genetic factors. Other causes are severe viral infections, including influenza, mumps, and cytomegalovirus, or trauma that results in injury to the skull and blood clots in the vessels supplying the inner ear (Martin & Clark, 2006; Schildroth, 1986; Tye-Murray, 2009). Another common cause of postlingual hearing loss is due to middle-ear infections, or OME, as previously discussed.

It is important to distinguish between congenital and genetic losses. As is obvious from the preceding discussion, not all congenital losses are genetic in origin, and not all genetic losses are congenital. Genetic losses can develop in the prelingual period, but some may not develop until early adulthood.

Stability of Hearing Loss

Some hearing losses are not stable over time. Losses classified according to a stability factor are stable, progressive, and fluctuating. In a stable hearing loss, a child has access to the same quality of auditory signals across time. This consistency of auditory signals permits a child to incorporate sounds into perceptual development. In a progressive hearing loss, the hearing deteriorates over time, requiring the child to adapt to poorer and poorer auditory information. In a fluctuating hearing loss, as the loss varies, a child experiences inconsistency in the auditory signal received. This can cause difficulties particularly when the child responds to sounds on some occasions and not on others. The variation in attending to auditory stimuli is sometimes viewed as willfully inconsistent behavior. It may also be that sound is not integrated into the child's perceptual development and is not given priority as a means of learning. The effects of fluctuating losses, particularly in the early language development period, may be far reaching and may lead to problems with auditory attention even after hearing has returned to normal. As previously discussed, children with OM, or middle-ear disease, frequently experience fluctuating hearing loss (Northern & Downs, 2002).

Other Contributing Factors and Their Effects

Factors other than age of onset and degree, type, and stability of loss can influence the performance of hearing-impaired children. It is frequently difficult to assess the precise impact that these factors have on an individual child's performance. However, as they can significantly influence performance, it is important that they be considered.

Parental Hearing Status. One important factor is the hearing status of the parents. It has been suggested that normally hearing parents of hearing-impaired children can undergo periods of psychological and emotional stress on learning of their child's impairment and that this stress can interfere with their ability to relate to their child. This can have a bearing on the way they relate to their child through the use of language and auditory stimulation. Normally hearing parents of hearing-impaired children have been shown to have more rigid and negative interactions, be less emotionally available, be more physically manipulative, be more verbally dominant, yet have fewer communicative interactions and be less likely to allow the child-directed discourse that usually occurs with young normally hearing children (Pipp-Siegel & Biringen, 2000). In addition, there is sometimes a decrease of verbal input to the child in the initial period after the diagnosis (Cross, Johnson-Morris, & Nienhuys, 1980). The child, therefore, does not receive the necessary verbal input for language development. Through counseling and support, parents are usually able to improve their communicative interactions by increasing the amount and type of auditory input to their child, thereby returning to a dyadic interaction style more similar to what the normally hearing child experiences (English, 2007b; Kenworthy, 1986).

Deaf parents, on the other hand, may view their child's hearing impairment with less distress and are able to communicate effectively with their child either through the use of audition or through a manual system of communication (i.e., sign language). These children are typically emerged in an environment with adults' highly developed language abilities, albeit often communication via a manual system, increasing the odds that the children will acquire language competency. In their early years, the children of deaf parents are more likely to have relatively good receptive and expressive language skills but poor speech skills. In contrast, children of hearing parents are more likely to have superior speech skills (White & White, 1987).

Early Identification. Early identification and intervention of hearing loss is a major key to a child's development. The prevalence of hearing loss in newborns has been estimated in a number of studies to range from 1.5 to 6 per 1,000 live births (National Institutes of Health, 2006; Parving, Hauch, & Christensen, 2003; van Straaten, Tibosch, Dorrepaal, & Kok, 2001). These figures are higher than the historical figure of 1 per 1,000 live births. The increase is due to improved detection as a result of new technologies such as otoacoustic emissions (OAEs) and automated auditory brain stem response (AABR) to identify all degrees of hearing loss, including unilateral hearing loss. Left undetected, hearing loss in infants can result in serious lifelong disabilities, such as deficits in speech, language, and communication development as well as delays in cognitive and social-emotional development, all of which can interfere with successful academic performance, often resulting in limited employment success (Cunningham, Cox, & The Committee on Practice and Ambulatory Medicine: The Section on Otolaryngology and Brochoesophagology, 2003; Declau, Boudewyns, Van den Ende, Peeters, & van den Heyning, 2008; Joint Committee on Infant Hearing [JCIH], American Academy of Audiology, American Academy of Pediatrics, & ASHA Directors of Speech and Hearing Programs in State Health and Welfare Agencies, 2000; Yoshinaga-Itano, Coulter, & Thomson, 2000).

Through early identification and intervention, these problems can be ameliorated or prevented. Early identification traditionally relied on the use of high-risk registers whereby a child with risk factors for hearing loss was screened before discharge from the hospital after birth or within the first 3 months (JCIH, 1995). Although these risk factors enabled the identification of high-risk infants, several studies (Mauk, White, & Mortensen, 1991; Mehl & Thomson, 1998) reported that only 50 percent of children with hearing loss have any high-risk indicators. The JCIH (1995) argued that while high-risk registers provide important help in the early identification of hearing loss, the goal needed to be universal infant hearing screening. In 2000 the JCIH, in collaboration with other related organizations (JCIH, 2000; JCIH et al., 2000), released a position statement advocating the introduction of universal hearing screening using a physiologic measure, such as OAEs or AABR, for all infants by 3 months of age. If possible hearing loss is detected, a full diagnostic evaluation and referral for intervention by 6 months of age is also recommended (JCIH et al., 2000). In 2002, Northern and Downs (2002) reported that over 20 states in the United States had passed legislation for statewide universal infant hearing screening programs. In 2007, the JCIH, in an effort to continue the success of early hearing detection and intervention, modified its position to one advocating that all infants receive a hearing screening by 1 month of age, with those who fail being referred for comprehensive audiological testing by 3 months. If a hearing loss is confirmed, appropriate intervention should commence no later than 6 months. The JCIH also reported that in 2005, all states in the United States had implemented newborn hearing screening programs and that 95 percent of infants are now screened before being discharged from the hospital (JCIH, 2007). The U.S. Preventive Services Task Force (2008), a group that makes recommendations for preventive care based on systematic review of evidence of the benefits and harm for a given service, also recommends universal infant hearing screening.

Concomitant Deficits. Another significant factor that may affect children's outcomes is the presence of other handicapping conditions, such as developmental delay, cerebral palsy, craniofacial anomalies, visual deficits, or behavioral disturbances. The impact that other conditions have on the child's perceptual and linguistic performances vary considerably, but these conditions need to be taken into account both during the intervention process and when assessing the outcome of intervention (Levitt et al., 1987; Tye-Murray, 2009).

Background Noise. An important problem for hearing-impaired children is background noise. Background noise is affected by the level of noise in a room, the acoustics of the room, and the distance between the talker and the listener. The first two variables produce what is known as room reverberation. A room with highly reverberant surfaces, such as glass and wood, will produce a relatively high level of background noise and hamper the listener in perceiving a speech signal.

Normally hearing people have difficulty understanding speech if the background noise is too high; hearing-impaired individuals have even more difficulty because every hearing loss, even those in the mild range, produces significant barriers to easy communication in environments with background noise, including school classrooms (Northern & Downs, 2002). Classrooms with high levels of background noise cause significant difficulties for hearing-impaired children (Anderson, 2004; Berg, 1987; English, 2007a; Siebein, Gold, Siebein, & Ermann, 2000; Tye-Murray, 2009). Profoundly hearing-impaired children, in particular, have severely hampered speech perception with even low levels of background noise.

Signal-to-noise ratio is used to describe the relationship of the signal that a child needs to hear (usually speech) to the level of background noise that is present. A signal-to-noise ratio of 0 dB means that the signal and noise are at the same level, a very difficult listening condition. A signal-to-noise ratio of +20 dB (where the signal is 20 dB greater than the noise) is generally suitable for normally hearing children. Hard-of-hearing and deaf children need a signal-to-noise ratio of at least +30 dB (Berg, 1987).

Unfortunately, many classrooms do not have favorable signal-to-noise ratios, particularly those with highly reflective surfaces, such as hardwood or vinyl floors and windows without coverings. In fact, at times some classrooms have a negative signal-to-noise ratio, in which the signal is less intense than the background noise. In a survey of 45 classrooms where hearing-impaired children were mainstreamed, a third of the rooms recorded background noise levels in excess of 70 dB SPL (Ross, Brackett, & Maxon, 1991).

ORAL LANGUAGE, SPEECH, AND LITERACY CHARACTERISTICS: A HISTORICAL OVERVIEW

This section provides a brief overview of the speech and language characteristics of hearing-impaired children that have appeared for many years in the literature. The overview is a summary of findings on children prior to three significant developments that have had and will continue to have major implications for the language and speech outcomes for children with hearing impairments. One of these developments is the implementation of universal infant hearing testing, as discussed above. The known benefits of early identification and intervention include improved speech–language, communication, and social-emotional development that typically leads to successful academic performance (Farrell, 2009; Tye-Murray, 2009; Yoshinaga-Itano & Gravel, 2001). The second significant development is the cochlear implant. Evidence of the benefits of cochlear implants for children now appearing in more recent research is discussed later. Hence, the information presented in this section is from research findings primarily in the 1970s, 1980s, and early 1990s prior to these two significant events. The third development is that of the advent of digital hearing aids, though this is not quite as significant a development as the other two.

Syntax and Morphology

With regard to the development of syntax and morphology, longitudinal and cross-sectional studies reported in the 1970s and 1980s, most of which focused on older hearing-impaired children, identified considerable delay that varied widely and was generally related to the severity of hearing loss (Davis & Hardick, 1981; Engen & Engen, 1983; Levitt, 1987; Quigley, 1969; Russell, Power, & Quigley, 1976). In some cases, morphological delays as much as 5 to 6 years were reported for children having mild to moderate hearing losses (Brown, 1984). Table 8.2 summarizes a number of the syntactic and morphological characteristics reported in the earlier literature.

Although many of these patterns can be seen in the language development of young, normally hearing children, as you may recall from Chapter 2, hearing-impaired children were reported to use them for much longer periods of time, with many never acquiring adult-level competency. These significant delays in syntax and morphology were reported as impacting the academic success of the children because many of the linguistic structures that are most challenging for the hearing-impaired children are found in second-grade reading primers (Ross, 1982). Many of the children were also placed in regular education classes, which often have high levels of background noise.

Semantics

Children with all degrees of hearing loss were reported as showing vocabulary deficits that were described as both quantitatively and qualitatively different from those of normally hearing children. Children with profound hearing losses were found to be delayed as much as 4 to 5 years (Markides, 1970), while children with mild losses experienced delays of 1 to 3 years (Davis et al., 1986). One of the reasons espoused for their vocabulary delays was that hearing-impaired children needed to rely on being taught new vocabulary, and many were dependent on the visual channel for input, whereas normally hearing children are able to learn words incidentally from their ambient environments. Their poor language skills also hindered them in figuring out meanings from linguistic contexts. Table 8.2 also shows some of the semantic features reported for the language of hearing-impaired children.

As the children matured, the evidence showed that their semantic delays widened compared to their normally hearing peers (Davis, 1974; Templin, 1966), with the likelihood that they would not achieve age-appropriate language comprehension skills. With regard to academic success, the effects of the children's semantic deficits were described as extremely detrimental, as the children were unable to understand the language used in specific academic disciplines and the language used in textbooks (Brenta, Kricos, & Lasky, 1981), with particular difficulties retaining academic vocabularies (Ross, 1982).

TABLE 8.2 | Summary of Oral Language and Literacy Characteristics of Hearing-Impaired Children as Reported in the Literature before the Development of the Cochlear Implant

Syntax and Morphology	Semantics	Pragmatics	Reading and Writing	Speech

■ Considerable delay, varying widely, generally related to severity of loss
■ Morphological delays approximating 5½ years in some children having mild to moderate hearing losses
■ Overuse of nouns and verbs
■ Excessive use of simple sentence structure
■ Inaccurate use of main verb forms:
  ■ Difficulty with past-tense markers and the third-person singular present tense (e.g., "runs") and more
  ■ Omission of auxiliary verbs
  ■ More difficulty with present perfect (e.g., "have spoken") and the negative passive (e.g., "The candy was not found by the girls.")
■ Omission of function words, such as the articles "a," "the," and "an"; prepositions (e.g., "to," "of"); demonstrative pronouns; and connectives
■ Telegraphic characteristic to connected speech
	■ Reduced word content
	■ General difficulty comprehending and understanding word meanings
	■ More specific difficulty understanding abstract, figurative expressions, such as "I ran like the wind," and multiple meaning words, such as "bear" the animal and "bear" meaning the ability to tolerate something
	■ Expressive vocabulary profile can be described as concrete and literal and used in limited ways, with few synonyms
	■ Stilted manner, as they do not have a variety of words to denote shades of meaning
	■ Semantic concept development is also delayed
	■ Concepts such as size and space, which are more easily perceived through vision, are learned earlier and more easily than other concepts, such as time
		■ Hard-of-hearing and deaf children between 6 and 36 months can be characterized as follows:
		  ■ Use comparable number of nonverbal language functions
		  ■ Number of functions increases with age
		  ■ Hard-of-hearing children use verbal functions more than deaf counterparts
		■ Most common intentions of young children with severe or profound hearing losses: commenting, requesting, acknowledging, and calling attention to an action/object (similar to those used by very young children with normal hearing)
		■ More pragmatic difficulty encountered by hearing-impaired preschoolers when required to respond to their partners; give inappropriate and ambiguous responses to utterances of greater linguistic complexity
			■ As many as 30% of hearing-impaired 16-year-olds reported as functionally illiterate; 60% reading at levels below grade 6; only 5% reading at the grade 10 level or better
			■ Widening gap as hearing-impaired children mature:
			  ■ At age of 9, read 1.5 grades below normally hearing children
			  ■ At age 14, read 5+ grades below hearing peers
			■ From 9 to 16 years, highest level of reading comprehension comparable to grade 4
			■ Less difficulty with punctuation and spelling in writing
			■ More difficulty in writing with various aspects of language:
			  ■ Syntactic complexity
			  ■ Lexical cohesion
			  ■ Organizing ideas to include sufficient detail in stories
				■ Segmental errors:
				  ■ Consonant errors are more frequent than vowel errors
				  ■ Consonants produced in the middle of the mouth most likely to be deleted
				  ■ Voiced sounds often substituted for voiceless ones
				  ■ Greater production of nasal consonants
				  ■ Vowel production more neutralized and a schwa (ə) quality
				■ Suprasegmental errors and voice and resonance deviations:
				  ■ Voice characterized as breathy, labored, arrhythmic
				  ■ Nasal quality
				  ■ Little control over pitch change; inappropriate pitch
				  ■ Inappropriate loudness

(Continued)

TABLE 8.2 | *Continued*

Syntax and Morphology	Semantics	Pragmatics	Reading and Writing	Speech
■ Difficulty with noun morphology: ■ Problems with plural markers, such as "two pig" for "two pigs" ■ Apply regular rules to irregular plural nouns ("mices") and to collective nouns ("sheeps") ■ Use irregular plural forms as singular nouns ("The men was hot.") ■ These morphological markers are typically: ■ Formed with /s/ (high frequency, low intensity); unstressed ■ Lower in intensity ■ Less visible in lipreading pattern ■ Masked by the background noise ■ Difficulty understanding medially embedded clauses ("The man who has the limp caught the bus.") ■ Likely to interpret sentences based on word order, thereby imposing the simple subject-verb-object rule on complex sentences	■ Rely on being taught new vocabulary, whereas normally hearing children learn words incidentally ■ Dependent on the visual channel for word learning		■ Written language described as follows: ■ "Choppy" and "rigid" ■ Less structurally complex with frequent omission of grammatical elements ■ Lacking in contextual discourse rules	

Sources: Anita, Reed, and Kreimeyer (2005); Brannon (1968); Brenta et al. (1981); Brown (1984); Curtiss, Prutting, and Lowell (1979); Davis (1974); Davis and Blasdell (1975); Davis and Hardick (1981); Davis et al. (1986); Engen and Engen (1983); Geffner and Freeman (1980); Gold and Levitt (1975); Kent, Osberger, Netsell, and Hustedde (1987); Levitt (1987); Markides (1970); Marschark, Mouradian, and Halas (1994); Maxwell and Falick (1992); McCaffrey (1999); McClure (1966); McKirdy and Blank (1982); Moeller, McConkey, and Osberger (1983); Musselman and Szanto (1998); Nicholas and Geers (2003a); Osberger (1986); Presnell (1973); Quigley (1969); Russell et al. (1976); Seyfried and Kricos (1996); Taylor (1969); Templin (1966); Trybus and Karchmer (1977); Tye-Murray and Kirk (1993); Wilcox and Tobin (1974); Yoshinaga-Itano and Stredler-Brown (1992); Yoshinaga-Itano, Snyder, and Mayberry (1996a, 1996b); Yoshinaga-Itano (1998).

Pragmatics

The relatively few studies that addressed the pragmatic development in children with the hearing impairments indicated that many hearing-impaired children failed to learn the rules that govern conversation, such as turn taking, repair strategies, clarification, and topic negotiation. Duchan's (1988) review of the limited research showed that these children often faced challenges with conversational management skills, such as turn taking and topic initiation and maintenance. The children's lack of mastery of syntax might have accounted for some of these difficulties. For example, failure to follow the rules for turn taking may be related to difficulties with question formation. However, the problems might have also resulted from the way in which many hearing-impaired children learned language. For these children, linguistic principles and rules were generally taught as a series of exercises in the classroom or clinic, but the children did not know how to incorporate the learned skills into everyday conversational settings, and frequently instruction did not provide the skills necessary to do this (Kretschmer & Kretschmer, 1980). Other pragmatic characteristics of children with hearing impairment that were reported in earlier literature are summarized in Table 8.2.

Reading and Writing

For hearing-impaired children, learning to read often involved a two-step process: learning the language used in printed material and learning to read (Davis & Hardick, 1981). Many hearing-impaired children did not have an adequate base in auditory–oral language on which to build their reading skills, and their reading performance historically has been reported as poor, as shown in Table 8.2. A significantly unfortunate trend reported for these children was that their reading levels generally did not develop beyond the grade 4 level. These children have also traditionally been described as having significantly more difficulty with written language than their normally hearing peers. However, most of the research on writing for children with hearing impairments focused on individuals who experienced severe or profound losses, with little attention having been paid to those with milder degrees of loss (Anita et al., 2005).

The reported poor literacy acquisition for these children could have been due to a number of problems related to the degree hearing loss. These included limited access to auditory–verbal information in language acquisition, less acquired experience and world knowledge, and the type of instruction received, which might have been based on a phonics approach using a sound system to which children with hearing impairment historically had limited access (Tye-Murray, 1998).

Speech Production and Intelligibility

Speech production in hearing-impaired children is most affected by the degree of their loss and the frequencies involved in their loss. Overall intelligibility, segmental errors (consonants and vowels), and suprasegmental errors (errors in timing, intonation, stress, and prosody) can be involved. Generally, the greater the hearing loss, the more likely speech production errors extend from consonants and vowels to errors in stress, pitch, timing, speaking rate, voicing, breath control, and intensity (Tye-Murray, 1998). The difficulties hearing-impaired children have in producing vowels and consonants result from a combination of factors. Many of the consonants are low in intensity and high in frequency, making their accurate perception difficult. In addition, many hearing-impaired children have poor discrimination abilities, even if the sounds are made intense enough for them. Because greater hearing losses tend to affect suprasegmental aspects of speech more than lesser losses, most reports on these features centered on profoundly hearing-impaired children (Osberger & McGarr, 1982), who have been described as having a distinctive voice quality. In contrast, the speech of hard-of-hearing children have been reported as less likely to contain suprasegmental errors, as the nature of their hearing loss usually permitted adequate monitoring of their voices (Markides, 1970). However, intelligibility has regularly been reported as problematic for hearing-impaired children, with intelligibility to listeners decreasing as children's degrees of hearing losses increase (Markides, 1983; Svirsky, Chin, Miyamoto, Sloan, & Cadwell, 2002). One study reported that over half of children with significant hearing losses had speech that was unintelligible to listeners (Cole & Paterson, 1984).

Without early amplification, infants with profound hearing losses show differences in the normal pattern of development from a very early age (McCaffrey, 1999). Their babbling has been reported as consisting of separate consonants and vowels rather than consonant-vowel syllables (Oller & Eilers, 1988; Stoel-Gammon, 1988). Their canonical babbling emerged later than usual for the children, and some infants did not achieve it, or its production was delayed by between 15 and 18 months (Oller & Eilers, 1988). Hearing-impaired infants were reported to produce fewer consonants, with qualitative differences including more labial than alveolar productions (Stoel-Gammon, 1988), which was more pronounced as the severity of the loss increased (Yoshinaga-Itano, Stredler-Brown, & Jancosek, 1992). This could arise because although alveolars are more frequent in English, they are less visible and therefore are not as accessible as labial productions are to children with hearing impairment (Osberger & McGarr, 1982; Stoel-Gammon & Kehoe, 1994).

In summary, this section has looked at what have been the historical, long-standing, and generally concerning communicative and literacy profiles of children with hearing impairments, particularly those with severe and profound hearing losses. A more current profile of the communication and literacy outcomes for children with severe and profound hearing losses is presented later in this chapter.

OTHER AUDITORY IMPAIRMENTS: CENTRAL AUDITORY PROCESSING DISORDERS AND AUDITORY NEUROPATHY SPECTRUM DISORDER

Central Auditory Processing Disorders

Definition and Nature of Central Auditory Processing Disorders: Historical and Current Perspectives. A challenging group of children with auditory impairments is those who show no evidence of hearing loss but have language disorders and academic difficulties that some purport are due to poor auditory processing. Although descriptions of children that are compatible with auditory processing problems are found as far back as the turn of the 20th century, the idea of auditory processing disorders began to take root in the literature during the 1970s, where it met with considerable controversy; it remains a controversial issue today with regard to how best to define and conceptualize the disorder, the nature of the disorder, the best measures to diagnose the disorder, and evidence to support the best intervention approaches (Dawes, Bishop, Sirimanna, & Bamiou, 2008; Lucker, 2013; McFarland & Cacace, 2006; Moore, 2006). One ongoing controversy involves the various diagnostic terms that have been used to identify this group of children: childhood aphasia, central auditory processing disorders (CAPD), or auditory processing disorders (APD). The term *central* is used to emphasize the distinction between peripheral hearing and the perceiving and "deciphering" of auditory stimuli (i.e., processing) more centrally in the auditory system of the brain. Several researchers (Chermak & Musiek, 1997; Jutras et al., 2007) have estimated the prevalence of CAPD to between 2 and 3 percent, while others estimated between 0.5 and 1.0 percent (Hind et al., 2011), although Geffner (2013) has suggested it may be as high as 20 percent. However, the validity of these prevalence data is questionable because, as we shall see, there is no agreed-on diagnostic criteria for CAPD, and if norm-referenced tests are used in identifying the presence of auditory processing problems, then statistically 2 to 3 percent of the children would be expected to receive scores at or greater than two standard deviations below the mean on the test.

Another controversial issue concerns the fundamental notion of auditory processing difficulties, in the absence of hearing loss, as a cause of language problems. The line of thought goes something like the following. Children believed to have CAPD have, for the most part, been first identified as having language deficits, which is why they were referred for further testing, including auditory testing. Although these children are then typically found to have normal hearing, they demonstrate poorer performance when tested on a range of complex auditory perception or speech processing tasks when compared with age-related peers. Therefore, it is plausible that the auditory processing disorder is causing the language disorder in the same way that hearing loss can cause language disorders. This idea had begun to gain considerable momentum (Eisenson, 1972; Myklebust, 1954) when Rees (1973) published an influential paper suggesting that despite the evidence showing poor auditory/speech task processing performance in clinical groups of children with language disorders, the evidence for demonstrating that auditory processing disorders caused the language disorders was weak in part because the notion of auditory processing is used in two very different ways (Rees, 1973, 1981). One perspective is used by neuroaudiologists who are interested in applying behavioral and electrophysiological tests to diagnose central auditory dysfunction. The other is used by professionals interested in providing intervention for language disorders. These professionals have adopted the notion that complex language behavior, as Rees (1981) wrote, "is composed of a finite number of sub-skills that can be reduced even further to fundamental perceptual-motor abilities" (p. 94), for example, auditory discrimination, auditory sequencing, auditory memory, and identifying speech in noise (figure–ground perception). An underlying argument for the intervention perspective is that, if children demonstrate poor performance on these types of auditory skills, then with remediation these skills would improve and be correlated with improvements in their language development.

There are several weaknesses, as Rees (1981) suggested, with this basic hypothesis. One is that there is no coherent or unified theory of basic auditory skills. Therefore, each test battery can include a different range of tasks, response requirements, and suppositions about their relation to intervention. Tasks can range from those as simple as a digit span task in which a child repeats a randomly ordered series of digits presented by an examiner to tasks requiring manipulation of acoustic stimuli that degrades the signal in some way (filtered, time compressed, or with noise added at different signal-to-noise ratios) while requiring a child to respond to syllables, to words, or to sentences. A key question is why so many children with language disorders have difficulty with these tasks. It is possible that they have trouble because their auditory processing problems result in their language disorders, their language deficits lead to poor performance on these tasks, or both their poor language performance and poor performance on these auditory tasks stem from some other condition. The problems of interpreting poorer auditory skills as causally related to language disorders was emphasized by Leonard (1979) in support of Rees's analysis. He suggested that the auditory processing tasks themselves frequently confounded aspects of the disordered language performance (for which the child had already been identified).

At about the same time as these criticisms regarding the relationship of auditory processing deficits to children's language disorders were occurring, the issue of auditory processing problems as underlying factors in language disorders, as well as in reading deficits, received significant attention because of a series of studies by Tallal and her colleagues (Tallal, 1975, 1976, 1980; Tallal & Piercy, 1973a, 1973b, 1974, 1975; Tallal, Stark, & Curtiss, 1976). The researchers tested a group of well-defined children with language disorders by altering critical perceptual elements of the speech, in particular the speed of transition between consecutive speech sounds. Included among their findings was that the group of children with language disorders who had trouble identifying the speech sounds when presented with normal transition times between the sounds improved when the transition time was lengthened. Similarly, the children could only identify the order of two sounds when the duration between them was extended. These results appeared to demonstrate the presence of a specific auditory processing problem, possibly temporally based, in the children with language disorders. Evidence for specific auditory processing problems can also be found in other studies involving children with well-defined reading problems (Dermody, Katsch, & Mackie, 1983; Dermody, Mackie, & Katsch, 1983). Considering children with reading problems is relevant because of the well-recognized overlap of language disorders and poor reading performances.

Different perspectives and controversies continue to exist with regard to the relationship between CAPD and specific language and learning disorders. Jerger (1998) argued that there was converging evidence in support of auditory perceptual disorders, but subsequently, several researchers again refuted some of the earlier findings regarding language disorders and/or reading problems and poor auditory temporal processing (Breier, Fletcher, Foorman, Klaas, & Gray, 2003; McAnally, Castles, & Bannister, 2004; Troia, 2003). One issue revolves around the nature of auditory stimuli (e.g., words vs. acoustic stimuli) used with participants in investigations. Cacace and McFarland (1998) have claimed that because most investigators use only acoustic stimuli with their participants it is not possible to validate the theory that auditory processing deficits underlie language and learning disorders. Nevertheless, Katz et al. (2002) have suggested a possible causal relationship between auditory processing problems and speech–language deficits, dyslexia, and attention deficit disorder, in contrast to Jerger and Musiek (2000, 2002) and the ASHA (2005) that have suggested that language (or reading) disorders and auditory processing deficits may coexist, but a causal link is not proposed. After reviewing the work of McAnally et al. (2004), Breier et al. (2003), Rosen (2003), Watson et al. (2003), and Musiek, Bellis, and Chermak (2005), DeBonis and Moncrieff (2008) concluded that any direct or indirect relationship between auditory processing difficulties or, for that matter, any specific deficit in any type of auditory processing skill would be very difficult to associate with a specific language, learning, or reading disability.

Several groups have attempted to arrive at some consensus about this ongoing controversial issue but in doing so may have added to the controversy. One group participating in the Consensus Conference on the Diagnosis of Auditory Processing Disorders in School-Aged Children defined the condition as a deficit in the processing of information that is specific to the auditory system (Jerger & Musiek, 2000) and, therefore, proposed a name change from CAPD to APD because the former term did not accurately refer to anatomical loci, was not adequately operationalized, and did not represent the possible peripheral and central interactions (DeBonis & Moncrieff, 2008). ASHA (1996, 2005) also attempted to address the controversy by convening several task forces to develop—and later revise on the basis of newer research findings—a consensus statement for the profession. According to the ASHA (2005) technical report, CAPD involves "difficulties in the perceptual processing of auditory information in the CNS as demonstrated by poor performance in one or more of the [following] skills" (p. 2): sound localization and lateralization, auditory discrimination, auditory pattern recognition, temporal aspects of audition, auditory performance in competing acoustic signals, and auditory performance with degraded acoustic signals. Although the ASHA (2005) technical report mentions the confusion created by changing the term, it recommended the continued use of the term *CAPD* but stated that the two terms could be used interchangeably (DeBonis & Moncrieff, 2008).

Other researches propose yet a different perspective. Bellis (2014) reported that based on the research of Moore and colleagues (2010), the British Society of Audiology suggested that the definition of CAPD "purported to represent a more general cognitive and/or developmental disorder rather than a bottom-up, auditory deficit per se" (p. 215). Research conducted by Dawes and Bishop (2009), Watson and Kidd (2009), and Moore and colleagues (2010, 2011) provided evidence that "poor listening is not primarily associated with poor thresholds on tests of basic auditory processing" (Moore, 2011), but rather it is "associated with variable performance on those tests" (p. 303). Moore (2011) reported that "our evidence suggests that most listening problems for children are due to poor attention or working memory" (p. 303).

Moore (2006) emphasized that although the underlying problem remains unclear, CAPD should be viewed as distinct from a language disorder, although in some cases it may coexist or be linked to those deficits. Moore and colleagues (2011) stressed the importance that future directions in research should focus on determining whether or not these cognitive problems, which often contribute to language deficits, are rooted in the auditory mechanism.

Assessment. Given the conceptual issues involved in controversies about CAPD, we can expect similar controversies with regard to clinical assessment for CAPD. CAPD is typically identified by audiologists based on school-age children's failure on a number of behavioral auditory processing measures related to norm-related performance (e.g., auditory discrimination tasks, auditory pattern recognition tests, dichotic speech tests, and monaural low-frequency speech tests) (Bellis, 2003, 2006; DeBonis & Moncrieff, 2008). The children's failure, however, may be due to specific dysfunction of the auditory system mechanisms or to more general cognitive processes such as attention problems or even language impairments. Not surprisingly, there are also myriad clinical issues, some related to those raised by Rees (1973, 1981), with regard to CAPD assessment, such as the lack of diagnostic criteria, lack of appropriate norms, and confounds with language, attention, motivation, and memory factors (DeBonis & Moncrieff, 2008; Moore, 2011). As a result, there remain significant problems with the consensus viewpoints, which, as pointed out by Jerger (1998), simply listed the kinds of performance deficits reported in the literature. As a response to some of this, a test battery approach for CAPD has been advocated as the main method of choice of assessment (Musiek, 1999), although it, too, has been questioned as to whether it is diagnostically superior to that of individual tests (Turner, Robinette, & Bauch, 1999). To date, there is no gold standard assessment measure or test battery for diagnosing CAPD (Dawes et al., 2008); however, Moore (2011) recommended the use of valid questionnaires that identify listening difficulties and measures that assess memory and attention that clearly differentiate auditory from other cognitive factors.

Cacace and McFarland (1998, 2005, 2006) asserted that CAPD is a modality-specific perceptual dysfunction in the absence of peripheral hearing loss. McFarland and Cacace (2009) explain that modality specificity refers to the idea that various characteristics, for example, "perception, attention, motivation, language abilities, decision processes, motor skills, and so forth" (p. 200), must be considered as factors with regard to any individual's test performance. As Cacace and McFarland (2005) pointed out, because current approaches tend to be unimodal, children are often misdiagnosed. Therefore, these authors (Cacace & McFarland, 2005; McFarland & Cacace, 2009) advocate for modality specification as a diagnostic criterion (DeBonis & Moncrieff, 2008) and for a multimodal approach to testing. Other researchers who stress the notion of auditory-specific processing deficits (e.g., Moncrieff, 2006) argue for multidisciplinary approaches whereby professionals from related disciplines (e.g., education, speech–language pathology, and neuropsychology) offer additional information regarding attention, motivation, language, and cognition to enhance auditory findings (Musiek et al., 2005). There also continues to be controversy regarding whether electrophysiological and electroacoustic measures should be used in conjunction with behavioral tests (Jerger & Musiek, 2000; Katz et al., 2002; Moore, 2006).

Although differing and unresolved conceptual, clinical, and theoretical issues continue to hamper the quest for consensus on CAPD diagnostic criteria for assessment and indeed the existence of CAPD, Keith (1999) purports that there is a general consensus surrounding the actual existence of CAPD. Despite some argument for multidisciplinary approaches to assessment, others suggest that some of the confusion surrounding CAPD can be partially attributed to different disciplines coming to assessment from their conceptual viewpoints. For example, according to Friel-Patti and Finitzo (1990), speech–language pathologists work within a network model that assumes that sound, meaning, and the intention of a message are all integrated, distributed, and processed at multiple levels throughout the nervous system, not just the central auditory nervous system. These professionals, therefore, are interested in the relationships that occur at different levels of processing. Audiologists, on the other hand, adopt a model that is based around the central auditory nervous system (Cacace & McFarland, 1998, 2005) and that assesses the integrity of various sections within that pathway and does not encompass the full language system. From a clinical perspective, an era of controversy centers around whether the disorder should be characterized as a dysfunction in an underlying mechanism that results in a unique set of behaviors or whether the disorder should be determined on the basis of performance results obtained from a test or series of tests developed to identify signs and symptoms (Friel-Patti, 1999; Northern & Downs, 1991). From a theoretical perspective, there are two main theoretical issues that also frustrate consensus and impact approaches to assessment:

- Whether an auditory-specific perceptual deficit solely exists (Cacace & McFarland, 1998, 2005; McFarland & Cacace, 1997, 2006, 2009) or whether it is actually a broader information-processing deficit that affects processing auditory stimuli as well as other sensory modalities more globally

- Whether there is a general temporal processing deficit such that there is difficulty processing a rapid succession of acoustic signals entering the nervous system (auditory–temporal deficit hypothesis) (Tallal et al., 1996) or whether it is actually a deficit specific to speech perception such that deficits result from an inability to identify phonological characteristics of phonetically similar sounds (speech-specific hypothesis) (Mody, Studdert-Kennedy, & Brady, 1997)

We can see in these points a number of issues related to information-processing accounts of specific language impairment in children and the surface account of the grammatical deficits of children with specific language impairment that were presented in Chapter 3.

Although the arguments surrounding CAPD began more than 30 years ago, they remain relevant today, and despite Rees's (1973, 1981) early significant criticisms, the area of CAPD has continued as a focus of professional and research interest. The development of auditory skills test batteries has also continued (Flowers, Costello, & Small, 1970; Katz, Curtiss, & Tallal, 1992; Keith, 1986, 1999; Willeford, 1977), and a number of professionals administer them on a regular basis. The quest for consensus, therefore, needs to be at least twofold: consensus on the conceptualization of CAPD and consensus on assessment approaches. Of course, the latter is strongly determined by the former and will come if we can integrate theoretical and clinical perspectives. Suggestions in the literature have appeared related to the need to widen our diagnostic lens to encompass phonological working memory issues in an attempt to identify the underlying, fundamental nature of processing deficits (Friel-Patti & Finitzo, 1990). A wider diagnostic lens would lead beyond a multidisciplinary approach and tackle these conceptual and clinical issues from an interdisciplinary, if not a transdisciplinary, perspective as well as from a holistic approach where children's auditory, language, literacy, and cognitive abilities are analyzed and reported. It would also require professionals and researchers to critically evaluate current assessment tools by examining the underlying processes that are required in order for children to respond to such tasks.

Intervention and Management Approaches. In terms of intervention based on findings from auditory processing testing, a range of approaches has been developed for CAPD. At about the same time as Leonard's (1979) previously discussed perspective gained attention, a review of 34 studies that attempted to determine whether intervention to improve auditory processing skills produced positive results on language showed that there was little success with such intervention approached in actually remediating the language disorders (Hammill & Larsen, 1974). Nevertheless, research findings regarding the possibility of temporal auditory processing problems underlying poor language and/or reading problems led some researchers to produce commercial programs for intervention. Two examples of such programs are *Earobics* (Cognitive Concepts Inc., 1998, 2000a, 2000b) and a British computer game system called *Phonomena* (MindWeavers Inc., 1996). There are limited peer-reviewed independent data and no real conceptual framework for indicating why these programs, which emphasize auditory discrimination skills, would lead to improvements in complex language skills.

The most well known of the commercial products is the *Fast ForWord (FFW)* program (Scientific Learning Corporation, 1997). The theoretical basis for FFW assumes that temporal processing deficits are fundamental to the nature of CAPD (the auditory–temporal deficit hypothesis) and therefore underlie the language disorders that result. Further, it assumes that by providing acoustically modified, rapid temporal sound sequences, a brain's plasticity can be modified, thus acting as a catalyst for facilitating language-learning processes (Gillam, 1999). FFW is comprised of computer games and computer-generated synthetic speech in adaptive training to improve children's abilities for identifying rapidly presented sounds and temporally altered speech. Tasks include discrimination of sounds, analysis of order of presentation, and identification of speech sounds. FFW was later developed into *Fast ForWord Language (FFW-L)* (Scientific Learning Corporation, 1998), an expensive, proprietary program that includes tasks such as phonemic awareness, language structures, and story comprehension. These changes reduced the emphasis of the program on auditory processing and increased the emphasis on language intervention.

As previously discussed, there is no direct evidence to support that temporal processing deficits underlie or actually cause language impairments. Furthermore, there is no direct evidence to support that intervention using FFW actually modifies brain plasticity with regard to enhancing temporal processing abilities in children who have language disorders. However, Tallal et al. (1996) reported that trials with around 500 children suggested significant gains in language skills after completing the training program, which involves mastering 90 percent of the computer games. Several of the unanswered questions about the effects resulting from the training have included whether the changes in language can be attributed to the systematic and incremental nature of the practice associated with completing the tasks, the amount of practice provided in the program, or fundamental improvements in processing auditory information. Gillam (1999), after reviewing a critical body of research regarding intervention for temporal processing deficits, issued a number of cautionary statements related to using FFW. He alerted professionals and parents to the fact that the tasks used in the program consisted of "massed-practice learning paradigms and speech-modification algorithms" (p. 365) designed to train discrimination between increasingly minute differences in tones, phonemes, syllables, and words. This type of discrete skill training has been criticized by practitioners and researchers because it does not capitalize on children's motivation, interest, or need to learn language, nor does it rely on their world knowledge. Gillam (1999) also criticized the two major field studies by Merzenich et al. (1996) and Tallal et al. (1996) that lent support for using FFW and called into question the efficacy of this approach due to design flaws and methodological weaknesses.

Until the early 21st century, independent studies aimed at taking a closer look at FFW as an intervention approach were sparse. Some case studies were published in a special issue of the *American Journal of Speech-Language Pathology* (Friel-Patti, Desbarres, & Thibodeau, 2001; Loeb, Stoke, & Fey, 2001). Only a few groups of independent researchers have experimentally investigated the efficacy of FFW and FFW-L in comparison with other intervention approaches with children who have language impairments. Table 8.3 provides a comparison of these studies. Taken collectively, these studies lend support for the continued controversial perspectives about FFW/FFW-L because, as previously stated, the approach does not provide sufficient support for the auditory–temporal deficit hypothesis, nor does it yield strong evidence that the training programs improve language abilities more than other language intervention approaches.

Further support for the cautionary use of computer software programs come from results of a systematic review of auditory and language interventions for children diagnosed with APD conducted by Fey and colleagues (2011). Only six studies were found that reported outcomes for auditory measures; two of which also reported on spoken or written language outcomes. Results indicated "weak evidence to suggest that intensive, short-term interventions (i.e., traditional auditory interventions, Fast ForWord, and Earobics) may be associated with improved auditory functioning among school-aged children who met the broad criteria for APD, with or without spoken language disorder. There is less evidence that these same interventions affect the spoken and written language performance of children with APD" (p. 252).

Regardless of the specific nature of auditory processing deficits, suggestions for management of the disorder recommend that a variety of interventions be used. Ferre (2006) recommends environmental modifications (e.g., reduce background noise and preferential classroom seating), use of compensatory strategies (e.g., curricular modifications), and direct intervention (e.g., activities/tasks that target discrimination skills, binaural processing and temporal patterning abilities, and auditory closure, metamemory, and speech-to-print skills). For language deficits, language intervention is important (Wallach, 2011).

The evidence to date strongly indicates that professionals need to maintain a reasonably high index of suspicion about the nature of auditory processing problems in children with language disorders, but the possibility of auditory processing problems in children with

TABLE 8.3 | A Comparison of Efficacy Studies Using Fast ForWord Intervention

Study	Characteristics of Participants	Treatment Groups	Language Measures	Procedures	Outcomes
Pokorini, Worthington, and Jamison (2004)	■ 54, 9-year-old school-age children with language impairments and reading deficits ■ 43 males; 11 females ■ Approximately 75% African American; 20% Caucasian; 5% Hispanic; 42% living below poverty level	■ Randomly assigned to one of three treatment conditions: ■ Group 1 ($n = 20$): FFW (early version) (Scientific Learning Corporation, 1999, 2000) ■ Group 2 ($n = 16$): *Earobics Step 2* (Cognitive Concepts Inc., 1998, 2000b) ■ Group 3 ($n = 18$): *Lindamood Phonemic Sequencing Program* (LiPS) (Lindamood & Lindamood, 1998)	■ Concepts and Directions, Recalling Sentences, and Listening to Paragraphs subtests of the *Clinical Evaluation of Learning Fundamentals, Third Edition* (CELF-3) (Semel, Wiig, & Secord, 1995) ■ Phoneme Blending and Phoneme Segmentation subtests of the *Phonological Awareness Test* (PAT) (Robertson & Salter, 1997) ■ Letter-Word Identification, Passage Comprehension, Word Attack, and Spelling subtests of the *Woodcock Language Proficiency Battery-Revised* (WLPB-R) (Woodcock, 1991)	■ Pretest: 4 to 6 weeks prior to intervention ■ Treatment: three 1-hour sessions for 20 days ■ Posttest: 6 to 8 weeks following completion of intervention	■ No significant improvement in performance on any of the CELF-3 subtests for any of the treatment conditions ■ A significant improvement in children receiving the LiPS intervention for blending phonemes as compared with children receiving FFW or Earobics ■ No significant improvement in performance in reading-related skills on any of the WLPB-R subtests for any of the treatment conditions ■ The researchers suggested that factors that may have contributed to the outcome of their study were the small sample size, the lack of verbal IQ scores, and the majority of participants being from lower socioeconomic backgrounds

Cohen et al. (2005)	■ 77 school-age children, ages 6 to 10 years old with severe mixed receptive–expressive specific language impairment ■ 55 males; 22 females	■ Randomized controlled trial (RCT) ■ All children received speech–language therapy at school ■ Additionally, children randomly assigned to one of three treatment conditions: ■ Group 1 ($n = 23$): home-based intervention with FFW-L (language version) (Scientific Learning Corporation, 2001) ■ Group 2 ($n = 27$): home-based intervention using commercially available, educationally based computer games designed to facilitate language but did not contain modified speech (used as a control for computer game exposure) ■ Group 3 ($n = 27$): no additional home-based intervention (control group)	■ *Clinical Evaluation of Language Fundamentals-3rd Edition UK* (CELF-3 UK) (Semel, Wiig, & Secord, 2000) ■ *Test of Language Development: Primary-3rd Edition* (TOLD: P-3) (Newcomer & Hammill, 1997) ■ *Phonological Assessment Battery* (PhAB) (Frederickson, Firth, & Reason, 1997) ■ *The British Ability Scales, 2nd Edition* (BAS II) (Elliot, 1996) ■ *Bus Story Test, 4th Edition* (Renfrew, 1997)	■ Group 1: FFW-L computer activities for approximately 90 minutes, 5 days a week, for 6 weeks, under parental supervision ■ Group 2: educationally based computer activities for approximately 30 minutes, 5 days per week, for 6 weeks ■ Group 3: no additional intervention beyond school-based therapy ■ Postintervention assessment at 9 weeks and at 6 months following completion of intervention conducted by a qualified speech–language pathologist (SLP) who was independent of the research study	■ For all children regardless of group, significant gains in performance on CELF-3 UK and other outcome measures, except for the BAS II Word Reading Scale, at both 9-week and 6-month postintervention follow-ups ■ No significant difference among groups in the amount of improvement made ■ Findings questioned the benefit of using acoustically modified speech to treat children with severe mixed receptive–expressive deficits because children who received FFW-L did not make any more gains then those receiving any other treatment approach

(*Continued*)

TABLE 8.3 | *Continued*

Study	Characteristics of Participants	Treatment Groups	Language Measures	Procedures	Outcomes
Gillam et al. (2008)	■ 216 children, ages 6 years to 8 years, 11 months, with an average age of 7 years, 6 months, with language impairments and normal nonverbal IQ ■ 136 (63%) males and 80 (37%) females ■ 100 (46%) Caucasian; 63 (29%) African American; 32 (15%) Hispanic; 21 (10%) Other	■ RCT with children assigned to one of four treatment conditions: ■ Group 1: ($n = 54$)—FFW-L (language version) (Scientific Learning Corporation, 1998) ■ Group 2: ($n = 54$)—CALI computer-assisted language intervention provided using instructional modules from Earobics (Cognitive Concepts Inc., 2000a, 2000b) and Laureate Learning Systems Software (Semel, 2000; Wilson & Fox, 1997) ■ Group 3: ($n = 54$) ILI—individualized literature-based language intervention based on the work of Gillam and Ukrainetz (2006), Norris (1989), and Strong and Hoggan (1996)	■ *Comprehensive Assessment of Spoken Language* (CASL) (Carrow-Woolfolk, 1999) ■ A computer-delivered “backward masking” task based on procedures outlined by Marler, Champlin, and Gillam (2001); Thibodeau, Friel-Patti, and Britt (2001); and Wright et al. (1997) ■ *The Token Test for Children* (DiSimoni, 1978) ■ Blending Words subtest of the *Comprehensive Test of Phonological Processing* (CTOPP) (Wagner, Torgesen, & Rashotte, 1999)	■ Pretest: prior to intervention ■ Probe: 6 weeks following pretesting ■ Treatment: all children received 1 hour and 40 minutes of intervention, 5 days per week, for 6 weeks, supervised by a qualified SLP ■ Group 1 (FFW-L): children played with 5 of 7 computer games for 20 minutes until reaching a 90% completion criterion for any five games ■ Group 2 (CALI): children played with seven instructional modules from the Earobics and Laureate software programs; when they achieved a 90% correct mastery level, the next level of exercises was presented	■ Except for one child, the children in all four treatment conditions made significant improvement on CASL, the backward masking task, and the Token Test for Children ■ Children who received the CALI and FFW-L interventions performed better on the Blending Words subtest of the CTOPP than those who received the AE and ILI interventions ■ Children with poorer backward masking scores who were randomly assigned to the FFW-L treatment condition did not demonstrate greater improvement in scores obtained from CASL when compared to peers with poorer backward masking scores who were randomly assigned to the CALI, ILI, or AE condition

	■ Group 4: ($n = 54$) AE—academic enrichment comprised of computer games designed to teach science, mathematics, and geography; examples of software include *Magic School Bus Discovers Flight* (Scholastic Inc., 2001), Coin Critters (Nordic Software Inc., 1999), and Dinosaur Adventure 3-D (Knowledge Adventure Inc., 1999) ■ The computer software used in the CALI and ILI conditions did not contain acoustically modified speech stimuli		■ Group 3 (ILL): intervention by a qualified SLP targeted semantics, syntax, narrative, and phonological awareness skills ■ Group 4 (AE): procedures shared common characteristics as the FWW-L and CALI conditions; this intervention was designed as a nonspecific intervention comparison; none of the software was specifically designed to facilitate language or develop auditory processing skills ■ Posttest: 3 and 6 months following completion of treatment	■ The researchers concluded that FFW-L was no more effective in improving language abilities or temporal processing skills than any of the other approaches investigated in this study

language disorders should not necessarily be ignored or dismissed. Approaches that assess aspects of processing auditory information essential for language learning might provide good ways to provide early identification of children at risk for language disorders, including reading problems. However, before adopting or recommending any one specific intervention approach, professionals need to review the current empirical evidence in order to make informed decisions about one or more approaches.

Auditory Neuropathy Spectrum Disorder

Auditory neuropathy spectrum disorder (ANSD), historically referred to as auditory neuropathy (AN) or auditory dys-synchrony (AD), is a form of hearing impairment first cited in the professional literature by Starr, Picton, Sininger, Hood, and Berlin (1996). It is diagnosed with a range of complex audiological tests that are used to identify the characteristics of the condition. Children and adults with this condition typically present with a hearing loss, although some individuals can exhibit normal pure-tone thresholds. The loss can range from mild to profound based on pure-tone audiometry. Other characteristics include normal middle-ear functioning but absent acoustic reflexes based on tympanometry, intact outer hair cell function in the cochlea based on otoacoustic emissions and/or cochlear microphonic recordings, and poor neural synchrony based on absent or abnormal auditory brain stem responses (ABRs) (Berlin et al., 1998; DeBonis & Donohue, 2008; Hood, 1998; Martin & Clark, 2006; Rance, 2005; Tye-Murray, 2009). Estimates of prevalence of ANSD in children, if they have a hearing loss, range from approximately 0.5 percent to a whopping 24 percent (Tang, McPherson, Yuen, Wong, & Lee, 2004). It is likely that the extraordinarily large prevalence range relates to issues of imprecise and somewhat controversial diagnostic criteria and complex assessment procedures, as we will see. Older children and adults with ANSD often report that they can hear sounds but have difficulty understanding speech.

Because ANSD usually includes involvement of the peripheral auditory system, children are often misdiagnosed as having only a peripheral hearing loss (DeBonis & Donohue, 2008; Tye-Murray, 2009). However, others think that, because many children and adults with ANSD type of hearing loss also exhibit difficulties with processing temporal cues and find auditory discrimination, localization/lateralization, and word recognition tasks particularly challenging, they make up a subset of the population with auditory processing deficits (Rance, 2013). Therefore, the administration of electrophysiological tests along with behavioral audiometry to help in the differential diagnosis of this condition is recommended (Gibson & Graham, 2008; Madden, Rutter, Hilbert, Greinwald & Choo, 2002a; Martin & Clark, 2006). Akdogan, Slecuk, Ozcan, and Dere (2008) also suggest the use of the caloric test—vestibular evoked myogenic potentials (VEMP)—to assist with differential diagnosis. The VEMP assesses the integrity of the vestibular nerve, which is often involved when cochlear types of hearing impairments are present.

The specific cause(s) of ANSD is unknown. Damage to the inner hair cells of the cochlea, demyelination of the auditory nerve, a reduced number of neurons at the level of the auditory brain stem, or a spiral ganglion cell disorder may result in the condition (Rance, 2005; Rance, McKay, & Grayden, 2004). Hood (1998) and Raveh, Buller, Badrana, and Attias (2007) speculate that there is more than a single etiology for ANSD despite the fact that all individuals display a common pattern of test results, as described above. Hood (1998) also points out that

> while any disorder of the auditory neural pathways from the VIIIth nerve to the cortex might be defined as an auditory neuropathy, the current use of the term relates specifically to more peripheral portions of the auditory pathways in the area between the outer hair cells and brainstem. Auditory neuropathy differs from other disorders affecting the VIIIth nerve, such as a vestibular Schwannoma, in that there is no space occupying lesion and radiological findings are normal. (pp. 16–17)

Not surprisingly, in light of the information above, the exact site of lesion is also unclear. Martin and Clark (2006) suggest that several possible sites might have defects: the inner hair cells; the inner hair cell–cochlear nerve juncture; the cells of the auditory nerve itself; and/or the nerve fibers of the auditory nerve. It is possible, however, that there could be multiple sites because any combination of these might be implicated in ANSD (Martin & Clark, 2006).

ANSD is often diagnosed in the at-risk infant population. This includes neonates who have a history of time spent in the neonatal intensive care unit due to prematurity and/or medical conditions such as anoxia, hyperbilirubinemia, intracranial hemorrhage, exposure to ototoxic drugs, and cerebral palsy (Berg, Spitzer, Towers, Bartosiewicz, & Diamond, 2005; Berlin, Morlet, & Hood, 2003; Dunkley, Farnsworth, Mason, Dodd, & Gibbin, 2003; Franck, Rainey, Montoya, & Gerdes, 2002; Madden et al., 2002a; Rance et al., 1999; Raveh, Buller, Badrana, & Attias, 2007; Starr, Sininger, & Pratt, 2000). Children with ANSD also frequently have a familial history of hearing loss (Akdogan et al., 2008; Raveh et al., 2007) or other familial risk factors (Sininger & Oba, 2001). Additional associated conditions with ANSD in the pediatric population include diseases such as meningitis (Rance et al., 1999) and postviral infections (Starr et al., 2000).

With regard to management of ANSD type of hearing impairment in children, several aural rehabilitative approaches have been suggested. Depending on the nature of the ANSD, some experts advocate for either traditional amplification or cochlear implants (Madden et al., 2002a; Madden, Rutter, Hilbert, Greinwald & Choo, 2002b; Rance & Barker, 2008; Rance, Barker, Sarant, & Ching, 2007; Zeng & Liu, 2006). Madden et al. (2002b) found that certain individuals benefited from the direct electrical stimulation provided by cochlear implants when there was involvement of the inner hair cells or inner hair cell–cochlear nerve juncture. Outcomes regarding the use of hearing aids are varied. Some researchers report that depending on the characteristics presented by their participants, certain individuals did well with conventional amplification (Madden et al., 2002a; Rance, Cone-Wesson, Wunderlich, & Dowell, 2002). Other experts claim conventional hearing aids often have little benefit (Berlin et al., 1998; DeBonis & Donohue, 2008; Tye-Murray, 2009; Zeng, Oba, Garde, Sininger, & Starr, 1999) because the problem lies with poor neural synchrony in the auditory nerve, not with amplification capacity of the inner ear (Zeng et al., 1999). Still others suggest that individuals demonstrate poorer performance following amplification than would be expected when compared to persons with comparable degrees of sensorineural hearing loss (Berlin, Hood, Morlet, Rose, & Brashears, 2002; Berlin et al., 2003; Rance, 2005). Because of the controversy over traditional amplification, some have proposed rehabilitation plans that include speech reading (Hood, 1998), cued speech (Cone-Wesson, Rance, & Sininger, 2001), or a combination of sign language and cued speech followed by cochlear implants and auditory–verbal intervention for children whose families want them to assimilate into a hearing world (Berlin et al., 1998; Berlin et al., 2002; DeBonis & Donohue, 2008).

There is a limited amount of information available about speech and language outcomes for children with ANSD. What is available suggests that outcomes vary depending on age of onset and amount of residual hearing. Anecdotal reports by Madden et al. (2002a) and Berlin et al. (1998) indicate that children experience expressive language delays, but to date no empirical studies have been published addressing spoken language outcomes of these children (Rance, 2005, 2007). However, one study investigated the receptive language and speech production skills in children with ANSD. Findings from Rance et al. (2007) indicated that school-age children with ANSD type of hearing loss who wore conventional hearing aids demonstrated varied yet comparable single-word vocabulary comprehension skills as measured by the *Peabody Picture Vocabulary Test* (Dunn & Dunn, 1997) when matched with children with sensorineural hearing loss. They also found comparably good articulation skills between the two groups, although considerably more variation in phoneme production was demonstrated than what would be expected from normally hearing children as measured by the *Diagnostic Evaluation of Articulation and Phonology* test (Dodd, Hua, Crosbie, Holm, & Ozanne, 2002). These researchers concluded that even though children with AN/AD develop language at a slower rate when compared to children with normal hearing, the spoken language skills of children in their study were relatively well developed, especially given the fact the population of children with ANSD often present with auditory processing deficits (Kraus et al., 2000; Michalewski, Starr, Nguyen, Kong, & Zeng, 2005; Rance et al., 2004; Starr et al., 1991; Zeng, Kong, Michalewski, & Starr, 2005; Zeng et al., 1999). According to Rance et al. (2007), possible factors influencing the results of their study included (1) that all participants were diagnosed and received early intervention prior to 1 year of age, (2) that the children tested had a good understanding of speech and performed well with amplification, and (3) that most of the children were enrolled in educational programs that exposed them to oral language as a primary mode of communication. However, one could challenge the conclusions drawn by Rance et al. (2007) with regard to relatively good spoken language outcomes because the only production measure given was a test assessing articulation and phonology skills. Future research that investigates the relationship among semantics, syntax, and pragmatics of children with ANSD type of hearing loss in interactive contexts using dynamic assessment measures is needed to obtain a more accurate picture of their overall expressive language and literacy abilities.

Most of the research regarding communication abilities with this population has focused on the children's speech perception abilities. Some literature has suggested that many children with ANSD exhibit poorer word recognition than would be expected given their pure-tone thresholds on behavioral audiograms (Berlin, 2000; Lee, McPherson, Yuen, & Wong, 2001; Simmons & Beauchaine, 2000; Starr et al., 1991; Tye-Murray, 2009). In addition to the supposed degraded quality of the neural signal received by the brain, several nonauditory factors are believed to lead to poor speech perception abilities of children with ANSD (Rance, 2005). These may include a child's age, cognitive level, speech–language developmental level, speech production skills, attention span, and lack of auditory stimulation (Rance, 2005), especially given the fact that many of these children had medical issues as neonates (Franck et al., 2002).

Given these factors as described in the ANSD literature, a question arises as to the relationship, if any, between ANSD and CAPD. As previously stated, many children with ANSD type of hearing loss are described as having auditory processing deficits (Kraus et al., 2000; Michalewski et al., 2005; Rance, 2013; Rance et al., 2004; Starr et al., 1991; Zeng et al., 2005; Zeng et al., 1999). Some have attributed the reported poor speech recognition difficulties of individuals with ANSD to severe deficits in temporal processing abilities based on results of psychophysical tests (Zeng et al., 1999). Rance et al. (2004) reported a strong relationship between temporal processing and speech discrimination abilities in children with ANSD such that the greater the difficulty with temporal processing tasks, the poorer the speech perception performance. Therefore, several researchers have alluded to a relationship between auditory processing deficits and ANSD, although the issue of presence/absence of hearing loss confounds discussions, and there are different opinions as to whether the involvement in ANSD occurs in the peripheral and/or the central auditory system (Berlin, Hood, & Rose, 2001; Kraus et al., 2000; Michalewski et al., 2005; Rance, 2013; Rance et al., 2004; Starr et al., 1991; Starr et al., 1996; Tye-Murray, 2009; Zeng et al., 2005; Zeng et al., 1999). Interestingly, Rapin and Gravel (2003) raised concern about the increased frequency with which the term *auditory neuropathy* is appearing in the professional literature to describe a group of children who present with various medical diagnoses, ages of onset, degrees of hearing loss, and test results. They discussed that ANSD is an overused diagnostic label that is often applied when involvement of the central auditory pathway from the level of the brain stem to the auditory cortex in the brain is suspected. They proposed that the term *auditory neuropathy* should be reserved only for individuals who demonstrate "documented evidence for selective involvement of either the spiral ganglion cells or their axons, or of the 8th nerve as a whole" (p. 707).

It will take several years of methodologically sound research to decipher the currently obscure boundaries between the conditions known as CAPD and ANSD in order to determine what relationship, if any, exists between the two. It will also take several more years to explicate ANSD as a disorder either separate from or as part of other hearing impairments and to refine relevant diagnostic procedures and criteria. The current picture is cloudy.

INTERVENTION AND MANAGEMENT APPROACHES

Early intervention, as discussed previously in this chapter, requires accurate and early diagnosis, fitting of appropriate amplification, early special education, and early speech and language intervention, all of which are seen as important in the development of speech, language, and academic skills of children with hearing impairments. Most children with hearing impairments continue to need intervention throughout the school-age years.

Technology Aids and Sound Amplification Systems

There are several options available for providing auditory input to children with significant degrees of hearing loss. These include hearing aids, cochlear implants, and assistive listening devices. Another option, the tactile aid, which converts sound into vibrations on the skin, is also available for children who do not respond to sound when fitted with traditional hearing aids and who are not candidates for cochlear implants.

Hearing Aids. Hearing aids provide auditory input to children with significant degrees of hearing loss, although occasionally in special circumstances aids are recommended for children with lesser hearing losses. There are six types of personal hearing aids, their names reflecting where they are worn by the user: (1) body aids, (2) behind-the-ear (BTE) aids, (3) in-the-ear (ITE) aids, (4) in-the-canal (ITC) aids, (5) completely-in-the-canal aids (CIC), and (6) eyeglass aids (Mueller, Johnson, & Carter, 2007). The most common type of hearing aid for infants and children is the BTE. Also referred to as ear-level aids, these hearing aids have their components housed in a small, crescent-shaped case that fits behind the ear of the user. Figure 8.1 illustrates a typical BTE and its components. Body aids and eyeglass aids are seldom fitted today, and manufacturers are making few technical improvements for them. ITE and ITC aids are recommended by some manufacturers; they are small and inconspicuous, and the amplified signal they deliver is good. However, a number of factors, such as frequent need for repair and the requirement for safety, make them less durable and versatile for use with children (Beauchaine, Barlow, & Stelmachowicz, 1990). With the exception of ITE, ITC, and CIC aids, in which all the components are contained in the earpiece, personal hearing aids require the use of a separate ear mold that fits into the user's ear. Ear molds are individually made for each ear from plasticlike materials. The ear mold delivers the amplified sound into the ear canal. It is essential that the ear mold fit snugly so that sound will not leak out around the sides. If this happens, the leaked sound is then fed back into the hearing aid microphone, causing a high-pitched squeal, known as feedback, which interferes with the listening of both the individual wearing the hearing aid and other people nearby. To avoid feedback, it is necessary to ensure a well-fitting mold by refitting it as the child grows. In older children, this may be

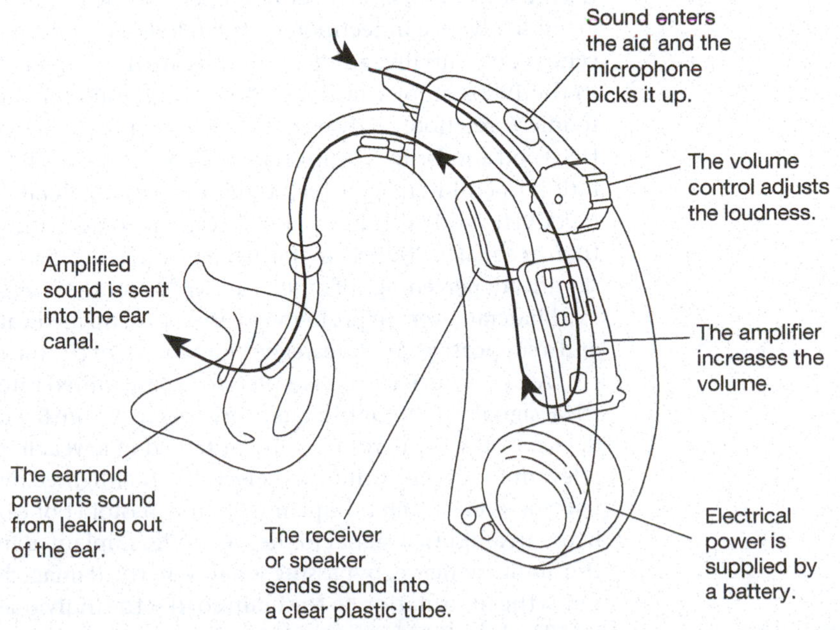
Sound enters the aid and the microphone picks it up.
The volume control adjusts the loudness.
Amplified sound is sent into the ear canal.
The amplifier increases the volume.
The earmold prevents sound from leaking out of the ear.
The receiver or speaker sends sound into a clear plastic tube.
Electrical power is supplied by a battery.

FIGURE 8.1 | An Example of a BTE Hearing Aid

every 6 to 12 months, whereas in children under the age of 4, a refit may be needed every 3 to 6 months.

The purpose of any type of hearing aid is to amplify sounds, making them louder, and to deliver them to the ear of the listener so that they are more easily detected. A personal hearing aid contains four basic components: a microphone, an amplifier, a receiver, and a battery. The microphone picks up sound waves and converts them into electrical energy. It is encased in the hearing aid itself and appears as either a small opening or a grid somewhere on the case. The amplifier then boosts the electrical signal. The receiver, which is built into the hearing aid (except for body-worn hearing aids), converts the amplified electrical energy back into sound waves, and the battery provides the power for all the other circuits. Each hearing aid has specifications for the type of battery needed, and it does not function if the battery is inserted incorrectly. Modern hearing aids not only provide amplification to make sounds loud enough to be heard but also offer sophisticated signal processing using programmable digital technology. This means the aids can be better "tuned" and adapted to hearing needs related to more specific listening environments.

One of the key factors in intervention is the selection of appropriate amplification devices. With infants and young children, much time is required for the proper selection and fitting of a hearing aid by an audiologist. The procedure can be complicated by the fact that the audiologist often works with incomplete test data because of the difficulty of testing young children and because these children provide little or no feedback on the outcome of the fitting. It is important for professionals to monitor the speech and language development of children fitted with hearing aids.

If a child is to benefit from any hearing aid, he or she and the family/caregiver(s) must know how to maintain the device so that it functions properly. Audiologists generally provide an orientation to the family or caregiver(s) that includes instructions for care and how to conduct a listening check and ongoing counseling once a hearing aid is fitted (Mueller et al., 2007; Tye-Murray, 2009). Daily monitoring should be performed by the child (if old enough) and by all adults in regular contact with the child. Either a personal ear mold or a hearing aid stethoscope is needed. After inspection of the battery and tubing, the aid is turned on and turned to the "M" (microphone) setting so that the listener can evaluate the quality of the signal, listening for static or intermittent cutout (Flexer, 1990; Osberger & Hesketh, 1988; Reichman & Healey, 1989). The American Academy of Audiology (2004) recommends regular, ongoing follow-up for all children fitted with hearing aids (Tye-Murray, 2009).

Cochlear Implants. The development of the cochlear implant (CI) represents the single greatest advance in technology for individuals with significant hearing impairments in recent years. Initially, adults, primarily with acquired significant losses, received implants. In the 1980s, implantation became a viable aid for children, initially for children in their toddler/preschool, early elementary school years, or older. The current, rather conservative U.S. Food and Drug Administration (U.S. FDA) guidelines recommend "cochlear implementation in children aged 12–23 months with bilateral profound sensorineural hearing loss (>90dBHL) and in children aged 2 years and older with severe-profound hearing loss (greater than or equal to 90dBHL in the better hearing ear" (Sarant, 2012, p. 333). CIs are also fitted to a significant percentage of infants under 12 months of age meeting candidacy guidelines, such as a bilateral severe to profound hearing loss, no medical or psychological contraindications, and a supportive family/caregiver environment (Holmes & Rodriguez, 2007).

A CI is a device that uses electrodes implanted into the cochlea, where it delivers electrical signals to the eighth (auditory) nerve. Figure 8.2 depicts the parts of a CI and how the device works. A microphone is contained in a wearable speech processor. Acoustic signals relevant to speech stimuli are selectively highlighted by the speech processor and transmitted to a receiver that is implanted in the mastoid bone behind the ear. The receiver then delivers an amplified signal to the electrodes implanted in the cochlea, which then stimulate the auditory nerve, bypassing what were the damaged hair cells. The auditory nerve then sends the information to the brain so that the individual can perceive the sound.

The benefits of improved speech perception, speech production, and language development from having cochlear implants can vary, depending on the combination of a number of variables. One of these variables is whether the CI is a single-channel or a multichannel

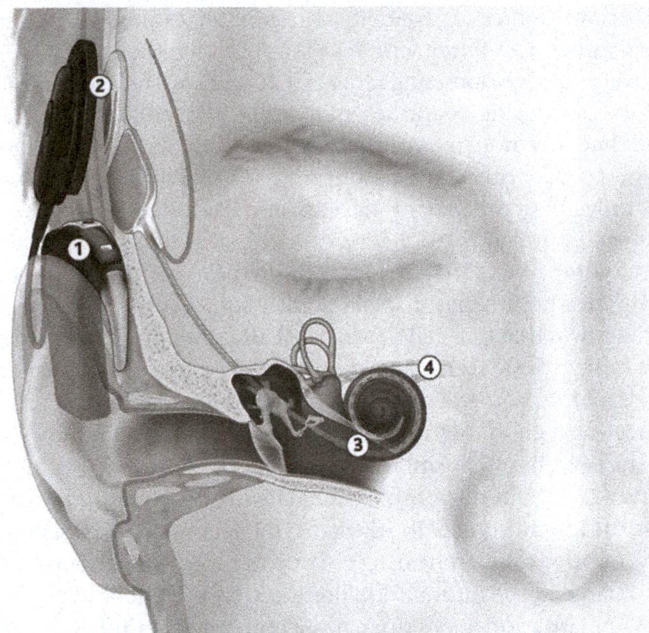

The Nucleus Cochlear Implant bypasses parts of the ear that no longer work properly by sending signals directly to the hearing nerve.

1 Microphones on the sound processor pick up sounds and the processor converts them into digital information.

2 This information is transferred through the coil to the implant just under the skin.

3 The implant sends electrical signals down the electrode into the cochlea.

4 The hearing nerve fibres in the cochlea pick up the signals and send them to the brain, giving the sensation of sound.

FIGURE 8.2 | The Parts of a Cochlear Implant and How It Works
Source: Reprinted by permission of Cochlear Ltd.

device. Multichannel devices provide information about more frequencies relevant to speech stimuli than single-channel devices. Leigh, Dettman, Dowell, and Briggs (2013) cited numerous studies that discussed factors, such as the age of onset of the hearing loss, the status of the individual's hearing mechanism, the age at which the device is acquired, the time span since acquiring the device, the amount of and type of intervention with the device, a child's family characteristics (e.g., socioeconomic status and parental support), and child characteristics (e.g., intellectual level and personality), that influence individual children's performances and outcomes.

The CI can often provide the same functionality for a child with a profound hearing impairment as hearing aids can for a child with a much less severe loss (Blamey et al., 2001). However, there is conflicting evidence in the research as to which of these variables has the greatest influence on postimplantation outcome (Gérard et al., 2010), although age at implementation and mode of communication used during intervention are thought, at least by some, to be most strongly associated with language outcomes (De Raeve & Lichert, 2012; Peterson, Pisoni, & Miyamoto, 2010). Much of the research on language and literacy outcomes for children receiving cochlear implants indicates excellent benefits in the areas of language development and literacy achievement, with some studies suggesting that children can achieve the same levels as their normally hearing peers and most reporting greater gains than peers fitted with hearing aids. Therefore, the brief speech, language, and literacy profile for hearing-impaired children that we presented earlier in this chapter has changed since the advent of CIs (hence our description of the profile as representing a historical perspective), and as more information about how children with CIs fare over time becomes available, we anticipate that the profile will continue to change.

A recurring theme regarding variables that can affect the language and literacy outcomes for children with CIs is the age at which children are implanted. From a neurobiological perspective, there are sensitive periods for brain development. Sharma and Nash (2009) suggest that the most sensitive time for central auditory development is prior to 3½ years of age so that implantation during this developmental period would result in the most encouraging outcomes. Many studies report that the sequence and rate of language development in most children who receive their CIs at an early age can be comparable to non–hearing-impaired peers (e.g., Kirk et al., 2002; Schorr, Roth, & Fox, 2008; Stephens, 2006; Svirsky, Teoh, & Neuburger, 2004). Age of implantation has, however, not always been well controlled in outcome studies and there may be a considerable source of variability in results. For example, some individual studies have looked at outcomes in children with implants between the ages of 2½ and 13, a considerable chronological and developmental range. Furthermore, the age of implantation has been subject to the historical sequence and acceptance of CIs for children as a viable intervention approach. Recall that only more recently have infants been implanted. Protocols that enabled babies under 1 year of age with significant hearing losses to be implanted have been available in Australia for only about the past 10–15 years, and in the United States even more recently following the later approval by the U.S. FDA. Certainly, one reason that availability of CIs for infants was delayed compared to that for older children was concern about the potential higher risks, including anesthesia issues, associated with surgical procedures with infants. Another reason for the delay was that hair cells, even if not already among the damaged ones that resulted in a child's hearing loss, are, in fact, destroyed as part of the surgical implantation process. There was, therefore, some reluctance to pursue such a surgery because of concern that any residual hearing a child might have would be eliminated and until relatively convincing evidence of the benefits of implantation from outcomes studies on older children were available. Recent thinking about the role of residual hearing for children with regard to CIs suggests that because the functioning of the device is not dependent on the performance of the hair cells, benefits of prior residual hearing are due to more intact neuronal connections from the cochlea to transmit the information produced by the implant.

Given the history of implantation in children, more outcome data are available for children who have been implanted postinfancy. A quick snapshot of some of these studies is presented here. The outcome data reported in the studies generally present positive results for these children. Tomblin, Spencer, Flock, Tyler, and Gantz (1999), for example, compared the language performance of children with prelingual hearing impairment who were fitted with CIs to children with hearing impairments who did not have implants. Results showed that, as a group, the children with at least 3 years of experience with implants demonstrated greater progress as compared to children not using implants and that these gains continued to increase for 5 years postimplant. Geers and Moog (1994b) reported results for a range of language domains for 13 children with CIs. These children, after 36 months with the implant and intensive auditory–oral instruction, showed greater linguistic complexity in their spontaneous language and larger expressive and receptive vocabularies and, overall, demonstrated expressive and receptive language skills above the 60th percentile relative to normally hearing children and children who wore hearing aids or tactile aids. These researchers also found that the language abilities of the children with the implants, whose hearing losses averaged 118 dB HL, closely resembled the abilities of children with hearing losses of 90 to 100 dB HL using hearing aids. With regard to vocabulary abilities, Waltzman et al. (1997) reported that the 38 children in their study who had profound hearing impairments, been implanted prior to age 5 years, had worn their implants for a minimum of 1 year, and had experience with only auditory–verbal input (except one child who was using total communication) demonstrated significant increases in their vocabulary development relative to preimplantation baselines. Over a 36-month period, expressive vocabulary increased by 48 months and receptive vocabulary by 33 months. Rattigan, Reed, and Lee (2002), in reporting their outcomes for children with prelinguistic, severe to profound hearing losses who received and wore CIs for several years and had considerable auditory–verbal intervention, indicated that, for the majority of these children, aspects of their language and phonological processing abilities fell within the normal range on norm-referenced tests. Rubinstein (2002) reported that for children who acquired a hearing loss after they had developed some language, there was a rapid improvement in speech reception (from 0 to 45 percent) as measured by speech discrimination scores after being fitted with a CI. These outcome data also showed that the rate of growth in speech perception abilities for children fitted with CIs began to match that of children with normal hearing. In a later study, Hay-McCutcheon, Kirk, Henning, Gao, and Qi (2008) found that, regardless of the communication modality used by congenitally deaf children who received implants at approximately 4½ years of age, their receptive rather than expressive language skills were good predictors of their later language performance. Schorr and colleagues (2008) compared basic and more abstract language skills of congenitally deaf children aged 5 to 14 years who wore CIs to a matched sample of normally hearing peers. Although the children with CIs in this research performed significantly lower on measures of semantics, morphology, and syntax and demonstrated poorer metaphonological skills than the normally hearing group, their performance with regard to phonological processing abilities was a relative strength, suggesting a positive implication for literacy success. When these researchers accounted for background factors, nonverbal IQ was not predictive of language performance in the CI group, a finding that contrasts with outcome data reported by Geers (2003), although it did predict language performance for the normally hearing group. Additionally, socioeconomic status predicted language performance for children in the CI group, which is similar to findings reported by Geers (2003), but it did not predict language performance in the normally hearing group. Connor, Craig, Raudenbush, Heavner, and Zwolan (2006) examined vocabulary growth in 100 school-age children, all of whom received their implants between 1 and 10 years of age. Findings suggested that significant vocabulary growth was evidenced for those children who were implanted prior to 2½ years of age; this trend dramatically decreased if children were implanted when they were older. Schorr et al. (2008), too, found that the age at which children received their CI predicted the variance in receptive vocabulary and short-term auditory memory performance. In the Schorr et al. (2008) study, the length of experience with the device predicted receptive syntactic ability. These findings with regard to the positive impact of early implantation and the beneficial effects of increased length of experience with a CI have also been supported by the recent work of Nicholas and Geers (2007).

Understandably, outcome data are more limited for very young children who have received CIs. In a longitudinal study providing a preliminary look at the language and speech development of babies with profound hearing impairment who received CIs, Wright, Purcell, and Reed (2001a, 2001b, 2002) reported that, although the infants used a range of nonverbal communicative intentions between the ages of 8 and 15 months of age prior to receiving their implants, they used no verbal communicative intentions. Approximately 3 to 4 months after implantation, verbal communicative intentions emerged regardless of the children's chronological ages, which then ranged between 11 to 12 months and 14 to 15 months of age. The types of communicative intentions used by these infants generally corresponded to patterns seen in babies without hearing loss. It should be noted that following implantation, all infants received considerable communication intervention, many of whom received mostly an auditory–verbal intervention approach (discussed later in this chapter). More recently, Tomblin, Barker, Spencer, Zhang, and Gantz (2005) reported on the expressive language growth of 29 infants and toddlers with profound bilateral sensorineural hearing losses, all of whom had received their implants between 10 and 40 months. These researchers found that the older a child was at the time of implantation, expressive language growth could plateau, a finding somewhat consistent with those of Connor et al. (2006).

Although CI technology has produced quite remarkable results for children's language development, it is important to ensure that all individuals involved in working with children with CIs, including the children themselves, adopt realistic expectations about the range of possible outcomes for the children in terms of their expressive and receptive speech and language abilities and in terms of their social inclusion. Outcomes for the children when they reach their adolescent years deserve attention. Somewhat mixed findings arise from the work of Dawson, Blamey, Dettman, Barker, and Clark (1995), who examined 13 adolescents who had been using CIs for a number of years. Although these researchers found that vocabulary scores increased significantly for the entire sample, only three of the children reached age-appropriate vocabulary levels 5 years after receiving their implant. Tooher (2002) and Tooher, Hogan, and Reed (2002a, 2002b) have reported on the language and psychosocial abilities of adolescents who used CIs for a number of years. A theme that emerged as a result of interviews with the adolescents was that some of the language, educational, and psychosocial issues associated with hearing loss do not simply disappear because they receive an implant. It is important to recognize that the technology is only part of the support the children need. The children need to engage successfully with mainstream education and intensive speech and language stimulation is essential for them if they are to acquire good oral communication skills. For example, the adolescents noted above in the Tooher et al. (2002a, 2002b) studies performed broadly within the ranges expected of teenagers without hearing impairments on measures of language as well on psychosocial measures. Moog, Geers, Gustus, and Brenner (2011) conducted a study in which 107 adolescents who received implants during the preschool years completed self-esteem questionnaires. Results indicated that these participants were confident in their social skills, had high self-esteem, and interacted with both individuals from the hearing and deaf communities.

Determining literacy outcomes for children who have received CIs has been somewhat more protracted since acquisition of reading and writing skills generally occurs later and when formal education for children commences and requires a longer longitudinal period of study. Because studies have generally demonstrated improvements in communication, language, and speech perception skills of children who receive CIs (Geers & Brenner, 2003; Geers, Nicholas, & Sedey, 2002; Kirk et al., 2002; Nicholas & Geers, 2003b, 2007; Svirsky et al., 2004), an assumption was that children who receive CIs at earlier ages and therefore had greater experience with them would demonstrate better literacy skills and thus higher academic achievement than children who were implanted at older ages or those who wore traditional hearing aids (Marschark, Rhoten, & Fabich, 2007). Outcome studies have, for the most part, supported this assumption. For example, Rattigan et al. (2002) reported that the literacy levels for the majority of the children in their study who had prelinguistic, severe to profound hearing losses; had received and worn CIs for several years; and had experienced considerable auditory–verbal intervention fell within the normal range on norm-referenced tests. Studies by Geers (2003, 2004) looked at word reading and comprehension skills in a large number of school-age children between 8 and 9 years of age, all of whom received their implants by age 5. Findings from the earlier study, which are supported by Archbold, Nikolopoulous, and O'Donaghue (2006), suggested that age of implantation and length of time with the implant were likely important factors regarding literacy achievement. Findings from the later Geers (2004) study indicated that children who had a period of normal hearing, regardless of how brief and especially during critical periods for language development, and who received their implants soon after their hearing loss was identified were more likely to demonstrate better literacy skills, a finding that is also suggested by Spencer and Oleson (2008). A study by Connor and Zwolan (2004) that investigated the possible relationship between language and reading abilities in school-age children who wore CIs found that, rather than the primary communication modality (i.e., auditory–verbal and total communication) used by these children, the most important variables in predicting literacy performance were age at implantation, vocabulary level, and family socioeconomic status. Marschark et al. (2007), reporting on studies conducted by Johnson and Goswami (2005) and Geers (2005), stated that these researchers found results that supported those of Connor and Zwolan (2004). However, Marschark et al. (2007) expressed concern that important variables that potentially affect literacy outcomes (e.g., age of implantation, language and reading abilities prior to implantation, type of implant received, and length of experience with the implant) have not consistently been controlled for in studies.

Although findings regarding the speech, language, and literacy outcomes for children with CIs are generally positive and encouraging, there is variability in results across children. Geers and Brenner (2003) have stressed that, before the effects of postimplant outcomes can be fully accepted, it is important for researchers and clinicians to account better for the numerous variables, to the extent possible, that are predictive of communication–language and literacy skills as well as academic achievement. Recommendations include controlling for children's characteristics (e.g., gender, age of onset and etiology of hearing loss, age of implantation, type of implant, experience with implant, and nonverbal intelligence), family characteristics (e.g., hearing status, ethnicity, home language, socioeconomic status, presence of both a mother and a father, size of family, parental education, and child's participation in family life), and classroom/intervention characteristics (e.g., mode of communication used, public or private setting, mainstreamed or special education class, type and amount of therapy received, experience of clinician, and family participation). Belzner and Seal (2009), therefore, suggest that researchers develop more stringent inclusion criteria for subjects, report demographic variables that might influence or confound outcome data, and be cautious about using results to make generalized statements to the larger population. As we—and the children with CIs—have more experience with the device, we would anticipate outcome data coming from more tightly controlled studies.

Tactile Aids. Vibrotactile and electrotactile devices supplement visual information and are designed for children whose hearing impairments are so profound that they are unable to benefit adequately from conventional hearing aids or CIs (Osberger, Robbins, Todd, & Riley, 1996). Vibrotactile devices, as their name implies, enable the wearer to feel vibration of sounds on the skin. A child wears something in contact with the skin that delivers an amplified, processed, tactile signal. Electrotactile devices deliver electrical pulses to the skin. They can be placed on the wrist, the fingers, the sternum (breastbone), or the abdomen.

Tactile devices are generally more effective for increasing reception and production of the suprasegmental aspects of speech. The skin is sensitive only to low-frequency sounds, with an optimal frequency range of 40 to 400 Hz; has a greatly reduced dynamic range; and cannot discriminate as finely between frequencies as can the ear. Some devices transpose high-frequency information, and the child learns to recognize, for example, high-frequency affrication from a position on the fingers. Evidence suggests that extensive training is vital if the wearer is to learn to do this (Osberger, 1990).

It is encouraging to note that a prospective study of speech perception capabilities in children using tactile aids over a 3-year period approximated the skills in groups who had used CIs over a similar period (Eilers, Cobo-Lewis, Vergara, & Oller, 1997). In addition, the language development of children using tactile aids has shown improvement over not using auditory input stimulation, at least in the early school years (Geers & Moog, 1994a; Osberger, Robbins, Berry, et al., 1991; Osberger, Robbins, Miyamoto, et al., 1991).

Assistive Listening Devices. Assistive listening devices (ALDs) are sometimes recommended for use when children with significant hearing losses are in public environments (e.g., school and recreational situations, such as restaurants, parks, and hotels) and other group conversational situations where other types of listening devices do not allow for adequate communication. In these situations, the audio signal is often presented at a distance, making the listening environment less than desirable (Mueller et al., 2007; Tye-Murray, 2009).

There are many different types of ALD systems (e.g., hardwired and wireless, such as frequency modulation [FM], infrared, induction loop, or simple amplification) all of which enable children to receive speech with a better signal-to-noise ratio (Mueller et al., 2007; Tye-Murray, 2009). For our purposes, discussion is limited to FM systems because they are most commonly used with children in educational and/or (re)habilitative settings.

Personal FM systems and sound field FM systems for group amplification have been used for the past several decades. With all FM systems, the speaker wears a small radio transmitter and a microphone close to his or her mouth. For group amplification, the amplified signal is directed into a sound field where carefully placed electronic speakers provide a better signal-to-noise ratio to all listeners (Mueller et al., 2007; Tye-Murray, 2009). For individual amplification, a child wears a radio receiver, and the signal is directed to the ear either through an earphone or through the child's personal BTE (Mueller et al., 2007; Tye-Murray, 2009). The two major advantages of FM systems are that they provide an improved signal-to-noise ratio and at the same time permit movement of both the speaker and the child around the room. They are particularly beneficial when children are in conditions with high levels of background noise, such as most classrooms.

Educational Approaches/Communication–Language Intervention

Several communication–language intervention approaches are available for children with significant hearing impairments. For hearing-impaired children of hearing-impaired parents, the issue regarding choice of approach is often clearer than for hearing-impaired children of normally hearing parents. A fundamental principle of intervention is that hearing-impaired children be given every opportunity to become proficient with a language (English, Spanish, ASL, and British Sign Language) regardless of the mode through which the language is communicated. Therefore, if the parents are fluent ASL users, the language (and communication mode) would likely be ASL. However, where there might be mismatches between the language used in interpersonal communication and the language of an educational system and that of the print medium, as there is between ASL and reading/writing in the English language, the issue is much cloudier. An added issue is that the majority of hearing-impaired children are born to parents who have normal hearing. If the parents were American, their native language would, therefore, likely be English communicated through the auditory–oral mode. In these cases, most of the children cannot acquire language solely by the auditory–oral channel. Therefore, most traditional intervention choices for the children have included manual forms of communication, such as ASL, which is a language different from English and is typically the language of choice for the U.S. deaf population; auditory–visual approaches, such as cued speech (Cornett, 1985) in which 12 hand signals used around the mouth supplement simultaneously what is available through audition and lipreading; and total communication (TC), which uses sign, finger spelling, and spoken language to convey meaning, thereby incorporating the use of the visual, manual, and auditory systems. A different approach that has deemphasized use of manual forms of communication is an auditory–verbal approach in which a child has to rely heavily on auditory input.

The selection of the best communication intervention approach to use in the education of hearing-impaired children has long been debated, and research into the outcome of different methods remains controversial. Prior to the use of TC, the intervention approach of choice was either manual (i.e., ASL) or auditory–oral. The auditory–oral approach prohibited the use of signing and finger spelling and, instead, emphasized the improvement of a child's auditory discrimination and lipreading skills. Some early studies favored programs with a manual component or found no significant difference (Montgomery, 1966; Moores, Weiss, & Goodwin, 1978; Quigley, 1969; Seewald, Ross, Giolas, & Yonovitz, 1985), while others obtained results that supported auditory–oral programs (Greenberg, 1980; Jensema & Trybus, 1978). However, the outcome of using the auditory–oral approach was disappointing when it was observed that many children had failed to develop the expected oral communication skills and become competent language users and communicators, which had a negative impact on their academic achievement. These discouraging results led, in part, to the popularity of TC. In time, however, what became clear was that the introduction of TC into programs for the hearing impaired did not result in the hoped-for improvements in language skills (Levitt et al., 1987; Osberger, 1986).

In large part, the difficulty relates to issues of native-language levels of language proficiency. Hearing parents rarely develop their sign language or TC skills to the level required so that they can interact with their child at levels equivalent to their auditory–verbal skills (Moeller & Lukete-Stahlman, 1990; Moeller et al., 1983). In employing a signed language to communicate, hearing parents may omit function words and use only three- to four-word sentences, not unlike young children in the process of learning their native language. The parents' signed vocabulary may be limited and presented in a less consistent manner than for their auditory–verbal presentation. These conditions can lead to children's slower language development in home environments than would be the case if the children could take advantage of their parents' language presented in the auditory–verbal channel or if the children were exposed to parents whose native language was a signed language, such as ASL or British Sign Language. Hearing-impaired children of hearing parents who are exposed to alternative environments where there are fluent signers (such as in bilingual programs) in their first 5 years have increased likelihoods of developing fluent sign language, whereas later acquisition of sign language results in incomplete mastery, especially of grammar (Mayberry & Eichen, 1991).

A discussion of the controversy surrounding manual versus auditory–oral communication also needs to look at the social and emotional impact that each approach may have on hearing-impaired children and their families. A frequent argument is that those who use only manual communication isolate themselves from the rest of society because they limit their interactions to only those who can sign. Furthermore, they expose themselves to societal biases due to a lack of knowledge and understanding. However, on the positive side, because this skill allows them to relate well to their hearing-impaired peers who also sign, they can share thoughts and emotions without the isolation and frustration that come from being unable to communicate. On the other hand, because the speech intelligibility of many of these children is often poor, their communicative interaction with others is limited, leaving only individuals who are close to them able to understand their spoken language. The argument that the use of sign isolates the hearing-impaired person needs to be examined with reference to the skills of those who are educated in auditory–verbal environments.

With the improved technology, particularly CIs, available for hearing-impaired children, the auditory–verbal approach, which aims to provide a systematic program for providing auditory-only stimulation for the language channel, regained popularity in the 1990s. A specific auditory–verbal approach, Auditory–Verbal Therapy (AVT) (Estabrooks, 1994), emphasizes early detection of hearing loss, early fitting with an appropriate technology aid (hearing aid or CI), ongoing diagnostic therapy, and strong support from the family and the professionals involved in the intervention process. AVT is focused on providing support for hearing-impaired children to learn to listen, process spoken language, and talk in regular learning and living environments. It is important to realize, however, that AVT, too, is not without controversy. While auditory–verbal stimulation provides a direct path toward "normality" of speech and language function, this goal can be unrealistic for some children, and it is important to monitor a child's speech and language development closely.

Regardless of the educational environment or communication intervention approach, it has long been recognized that as much language input as possible in any communication mode will improve the language development outcomes for children with hearing impairments. Geers (2002) investigated auditory, speech, language, and reading outcomes in a reasonably large sample (130) of children with prelingual profound hearing loss after they had been fitted with a multichannel CI for 4 to 6 years. Approximately 20 percent of the variance in level of performance for the variables measured was accounted for by family factors. About 24 percent of the variance was accounted for by implant results and 12 percent by educational variables. These results suggest that professional and family intervention and support are major factors in the communication–language development and academic success for children with significant hearing impairments and that specific educational/communication approaches have a significant but lesser effect on outcome.

Several types of educational environments are available to children with hearing impairments, such as public schools and private or state-sponsored institutions, which generally offer day programs or residential facilities. Classroom placements generally consist of either self-contained settings in which only children with hearing impairments are included or mainstreamed settings in which both children with and without hearing losses are included in the same class (Tye-Murray, 2009). Mainstream settings may be inclusive classrooms, which often present challenges to regular classroom teachers who are primarily responsible for educating all children in the class (Israelite, Ower, & Goldstein, 2002), or co-enrollment classrooms, which include both a regular/general education teacher and a teacher of the deaf and hard of hearing. In some mainstreamed settings, children receive their academic instruction through AVT.

This last point raises the issue of interaction among form of technology intervention, mode of communication, and type of educational placement and educational achievement. Nevins and Chute (1996) reviewed the academic achievement and speech intelligibility of hearing-impaired children who were mainstreamed and noted higher achievement and improved intelligibility in this group as compared to nonmainstreamed peers. However, this result may simply be because hearing-impaired children who can handle mainstream education do so because of their better auditory input ability in the first place. Technology aids also played a role in Nevins and Chute's findings. In their review, about 75 percent of children having 5 years of experience with a CI tended to shift their educational placement from a special school or unit to a mainstream class. Similarly, children receiving a CI at a young age tended to be mainstreamed, although all children needed varying forms of follow-up to maintain success. These trends are consistent with the findings of Geers et al. (2002), who reported that children with CIs in a total communication setting achieved better speech perception, speech intelligibility, and language scores and were more likely to move into mainstreamed educational settings if they used speech as their primary communication mode as compared to their peers who used mainly sign language or total communication.

Children with less severe hearing losses, including those with unilateral losses, mild bilateral losses, or with ongoing issues with OME, are often overlooked in discussions of intervention and management. Yet these children may constitute a larger proportion of children with hearing losses than those with more severe losses. Current prevalence data indicate that as many as 5.4 percent of school-age children may have some type of permanent mild hearing loss (Tharpe, 2007). Reporting on the recommendations of the American Academy of Audiology (2003), McKay, Gravel, and Tharpe (2008) and Tharpe (2007) indicated that which type of amplification is used—or, for that matter, whether amplification is used—with children who have unilateral or mild bilateral losses be determined on a case-by-case basis considering factors such as a child's general health, cognitive level, communication status, overall development, family and/or child preferences, and functional needs. Currently, devices for consideration include traditional hearing aids and FM systems (previously discussed). *Contralateral routing of signal* (CROS) hearing aids are options for children whose poorer ear has inadequate hearing in order to benefit from conventional hearing aids. For older children, the surgically implanted bone-conduction devices known as the bone-anchored hearing apparatus (McKay et al., 2008; Tharpe, 2007) might be an option. Whatever approach is recommended, parental/caregiver education and active family involvement are essential if the approach is to benefit the child.

SUMMARY

In this chapter we have seen that

- Hearing loss may be peripheral or central.
- Peripheral hearing loss may be either conductive (located in the external or middle ear) or sensorineural (located at the level of the cochlea or in the auditory [eighth] nerve).
- Peripheral hearing loss is categorized by degree of loss, and while all hearing loss affects speech and language development, in general the more severe the hearing loss, the greater the potential impact on the acquisition of communication skills.
- Conductive hearing loss due to otitis media affects a child's ability to hear and understand speech and language, but the impact of otitis media itself on speech and language development remains unclear.
- Hearing loss affects receptive and expressive communication abilities, literacy skills, academic achievement, and social development.
- Universal newborn hearing screening is recommended for early identification of hearing loss.
- Children with mild hearing loss and unilateral loss are at risk for language and academic difficulties unless identified early and managed appropriately.
- New developments in technology have made cochlear implants a viable choice for many children with hearing loss. These devices provide stimulation that is often superior to that of traditional hearing aids.
- Although outcome studies on speech–language and literacy skills of children with cochlear implants generally show improved performance, future research needs to consider various child, family, education, and intervention factors more consistently.
- There is no single best communication modality or educational environment for children with significant hearing losses. Outcomes are affected by many factors, such as the age of onset of hearing loss, the type of technology aid used and amount of experience a child has with it, the language environment, and individual cognitive abilities.
- The role of central auditory processing disorders in relation to language disorders continues to be debated.
- More sophisticated assessment procedures have led to the identification of children suspected to have auditory neuropathy/auditory dys-synchrony. However, more research is needed to refine assessment and identification procedures and determine the most appropriate management options for children with this type of hearing impairment.

Any degree of hearing impairment puts a child at risk for language learning and academic success. Early identification and early intervention are key factors in helping children with hearing impairments.

9

Language and Linguistically-Culturally Diverse Children

Li-Rong Lilly Cheng

LEARNING OBJECTIVES

After reading this chapter, you should be able to

- Discuss concepts related to cultural diversity
- Discuss concepts of linguistic variation
- Discuss concepts of second-language learning
- Describe the various language characteristics of linguistically-culturally diverse children
- Discuss issues of poverty in relation to linguistically-culturally diverse children
- Describe issues in assessment of linguistically-culturally diverse children
- Discuss implications for intervention related to linguistically-culturally diverse children
- Identify several emerging issues likely to affect future language services for linguistically-culturally diverse children

According to the 2010 Census (U.S. Bureau of the Census, 2010), 308.7 million people resided in the United States on April 1, 2010, of which 50.5 million (or 16 percent) were of Hispanic or Latino origin. The Hispanic population increased from 35.3 million in 2000 when this group made up 13 percent of the total population. The Asian population grew faster than any other race group in the United States between 2000 and 2010, reaching 14.7 million, which represented 4.3 percent of the U.S. population. The African American population was 27.3 million, representing 9.7 percent of the total population.

The U.S. Census Bureau projects that by 2050, about 50 percent of the U.S. population will be African American, Hispanic, or Asian. These demographic data indicate the great need for education and health care professionals to understand the culturally and linguistically diverse (CLD) populations in the United States or, for that matter, in any country that is experiencing similar linguistic and cultural demographic changes. Much of the literature uses *CLD* in reference to this population. However, in this chapter, the term *linguistically-culturally diverse* is used to maintain focus on language and linguistic diversity, as well as consideration of cultural diversity.

Many children learn a form of spoken English that differs from that used in most of America's schools and workplaces. As a result, these students are at risk for educational failure because of their language background and not because of a language impairment.

At the same time, children who grow up in linguistically and/or culturally diverse households that are ethnic, bilingual, or both are not immune from specific disabilities in language learning. Consequently, professionals must be able to distinguish between language differences, which are the result of a child's linguistic and/or cultural environment, and language disorders, which are due to an impairment of language-learning mechanisms.

CONCEPTS OF CULTURAL DIVERSITY

Cultural diversity is commonly also referred to as multiculturalism, which is a cover term for the regional, ethnic, social, racial, linguistic, and cultural variations in any society. Although there is much overlap and interaction among the factors of ethnicity, socioeconomic status, race, language, and culture, they are, in principle, separate concepts:

- *Race* is a statement about an individual's biological attributes. By itself, race is of little importance to discussions of language acquisition and language disorders. In our global village, the idea of race is not as important as ethnicity and culture. Many people are of mixed races. The world-famous golfer Tiger Woods came up with the term "Cablanasian" to indicate his multicultural background of Caucasian, Black, Native American, and Asian. In the 2000 U.S. Census, the category "Mixed Race" was used to include the hundreds of thousands of mixed race individuals who live in the United States. There are, however, some physical differences among races, which in turn can be related to variations in language learning. For example, African American children have a lower incidence of middle-ear infection because the size and angle of their eustachian tubes permit better drainage. Insofar as otitis media may be a source of language difficulties in children, this racial difference may be of some significance. In addition, African American children have the lowest incidence of cleft palate and lip.
- Most broadly, *language* refers to all the behaviors by which individuals communicate with one another. In the context of multiculturalism, however, we attend primarily to the differences in form (phonology and grammar) and lexicon that distinguish one language (e.g., English, Spanish, or Japanese) from another and one variety of the same language (e.g., standard, nonstandard, American English, or New Zealand English) from another variety. Differences in pragmatics are also viewed as aspects of multicultural communication. For example, Hispanic American speakers tend to have a small distance between them during conversation (Pajewski & Enriquez, 1996; Taylor, 1987). This appears to be true whether the speakers are monolingual (having only one language) or bilingual (sharing aspects of two languages) and, if they are bilingual, whether they are speaking Spanish, English, or a mixture of the two. Thus, the language behavior (Spanish) and the cultural behavior (standing close during conversation) are separable components of the communication of many but not all Hispanic American speakers. When we speak of language as a multicultural variable, the meaning should be restricted to those formal elements that will be learned and used by speakers.
- *Culture* is a statement about behaviors that are shared by a group of individuals. Culture is a way of life for a group of individuals who share the same values and beliefs. Culture can be both implicit and explicit. Explicit culture is defined as what can be seen, heard, bought, or used—a piece of clothing, a special food item, a language, or an artifact that is used for special occasions. Implicit culture, on the other hand, is not easy to observe because it is invisible. Philips (1983), in her book the *Invisible Culture*, described those elements of the implicit culture that are difficult to understand and to decode. Hall (1990), in his book *The Silent Language*, gives a vivid account of the difficulty in understanding the hidden/invisible/implicit part of any culture. He described a situation in the South Pacific where an American plant manager failed to understand the implicit balance of the different tribes on the island and hired a large proportion of one of the tribes. This caused many problems for the other tribes. The chiefs of the tribes met, came up with a solution, and went to tell the manager in the middle of the night. The manager thought there was a riot and called the Marines. The hidden concept of time varied in this case,

TABLE 9.1 | Some Differences in Communicative Behavior across American Cultural Groups

White Americans	African Americans	Hispanic Americans	Asian/Pacific Islander Americans	Native Americans
Touching of hair is considered a sign of affection, especially between adults and children. Uninvited touching between men and women may be considered harassing. Direct eye contact is maintained during listening but avoided during speaking. Public behavior should be emotionally restrained.	Touching of hair may be considered offensive. Direct eye contact is avoided during listening but maintained during speaking. Public behavior may be emotionally intense and demonstrative. Interruption of another speaker during conversation is acceptable.	Touching occurs commonly during conversation. Direct eye contact may be considered disrespectful. A small distance is maintained between speakers during conversation. Parent–child conversation is usually directive, not collaborative.	Touching is more acceptable between members of the same sex than between men and women. Backslapping is considered offensive. Men and women do not customarily shake hands. Children tend to wait to participate, unless otherwise requested by the teacher. Being singled out can cause distress. Many children are socialized to listen more than speak and to speak in a soft voice.	Learning through quiet observation is valued; group teaching activities that encourage each child to speak may be disfavored. "Wait time"—the amount of time speakers are given to speak and respond—is substantially longer. Individual humility and group harmony are valued; displaying knowledge in front of others may be uncomfortable.

and the natives did not feel that waking the manager up at three in the morning meant anything other than a message needed to be delivered—no emergency, no urgency, but simply a time, like any other, to deliver the message (Hall, 1990).

Many of these cultural behaviors can influence communication. Members of an ethnic group will share many cultural elements as a result of ancestral links. Four large ethnic groups in the United States—African Americans, Hispanic Americans, Native Americans, and Asian/Pacific Islander Americans (APIs)—are commonly contrasted with one another and with white Americans of mostly European descent. As shown in Table 9.1, this comparison of behaviors across groups, collected from multiple sources, reveals several differences with the potential to cause miscommunication and misinterpretation of behavior and even communication breakdown. It is important to recognize, however, that even though ethnicity cannot be changed, it does not compel an individual to follow certain cultural standards. To expect that all members of an ethnic group will behave in the same way is prejudicial and impossible since there are so many variables that will impact one's acquisition and construction of knowledge and meaning. On the other hand, to be unaware of cultural differences and their potential effects on communication is unprofessional and naive. Balance is, therefore, a key factor in serving children with linguistically-culturally diverse backgrounds.

CONCEPTS OF LINGUISTIC VARIATION

Around the world, no two individuals communicate in exactly the same manner. The communication differences among people can be described in several ways. There are more than 6,000 languages spoken in the world, but many are on the verge of extinction or do not have a written form, and some are spoken by only a handful of people. Furthermore, a single language is also not always a characteristic of a country. In Singapore, for example, people in general know three or four languages—English, Mandarin, and Malay or Tamil.

At the broadest level, we can identify nearly 1,000 different languages that are used by 10,000 or more speakers (Crystal, 1997). Many of these languages are produced in several different forms or dialects, which vary from one another in grammar, vocabulary, and/or phonology. For example, according to Crystal (1997), the world of "Englishes" comes in many different forms. Singlish is the form of English that is spoken in Singapore; Taglish is spoken in the Philippines, with a mixture of Tagalog and English. There are significant differences in articulation in these various forms of Englishes resulting in difficulty in understanding. The famous saying "You say tomato and I say tomato. You say potato and I say potato. . . ." illustrates this point well. Crystal's concept of Englishes applies to any spoken language that is used in several areas of the world, for example, Spanish or Chinese, leading to the idea of a world of "Spanishes" or "Chineses."

The term *mixed vernacular* is an important concept that has appeared in the literature in recent decades. This is when a group of people who have been using two languages mix them into a vernacular that is neither one language (L1) nor the other (L2) but a mixture of the two. Other examples are Turkish migrants in Holland who have slipped literal translations of Dutch words into their Turkish conversation (Dogruoz, 2008) and Van Riebeeck, a Dutch pioneer, who introduced Dutch into South Africa in the 1600s. This Culemborg-Utrecht variety of Dutch evolved into Afrikaans, one of the official languages of South Africa. It is clear that languages evolve and mix and often create many varieties.

Rethfeldt (2009) provided a case study from Germany that explains the complexity of this mixed vernacular phenomenon. In the 1950s, many workers from Poland, Spain, Italy, Portugal, and Turkey migrated to Germany to help rebuild the country. There are now enclaves of these ethnic communities with second, third, and fourth generations of speakers with many varieties of mixed vernaculars. These individuals present diverse linguistic backgrounds, and language assessment for children from these populations can be challenging.

A dialect is distinguished from a language in two ways:

- A dialect is assumed to be a subset of a language and therefore should share a common core of grammatical and other characteristics with all other dialects of that language.
- Speakers of different dialects should be able to understand one another, sometimes with effort, whereas speakers of different languages should not.

The common core of a language is more evident in its written form than in its spoken form. Thus, an individual who knows English will be able to read a newspaper published in Canada, the United States, England, Australia, Ireland, Singapore, New Zealand, Hong Kong, India, or any other English-speaking nation. However, the same individual, if he or she is, for example, from Kansas, may be unable to understand easily the English spoken in some parts of Scotland, Wales, Australia, India, Jamaica, New Zealand, or even Los Angeles. This calls attention to the fact that differences in pronunciation, or accent, are conspicuous features of a dialect and cause difficulty in spoken communication between two individuals using the same language. By the same token, usage of the same words may have differences in meaning in the same language, depending on the region where they are used. A *lift* in England is an *elevator* in the United States. *Grand* is an expression of *great* or *good* in Ireland, while *grand* in the United States generally means *big*. In Australia, a *long black* and a *short white* mean a large cup of black coffee and a small cup of coffee with milk, respectively. The varying use of terms can also lead to a lot of confusion, for example, in some parts of the world the "first floor" is the floor one flight above ground, making it the "second floor" in other parts of the world. Lexical items carry local flavors.

There is nothing inherently better about one dialect than another. However, within a society, factors of history, economics, and education can combine to favor a particular dialect and establish it as the standard. *Standard American English* (SAE) is the phrase used to refer to what is considered characteristic of "mainstream" speakers of American English. In Singapore, Standard Singaporean English may sound quite different from SAE. All English-speaking nations are considered to have their own standard dialects, so it is customary to use the terms *American English*, *South African English*, *British English* (Queen's English), and so on, to refer to various national standard dialects.

The concept of a standard dialect is strongly associated with the educational level of the speaker. Individuals with considerable formal education tend to speak the standard dialect of the nation in which they live. They may also speak other dialects, depending on their personal backgrounds, neighborhoods, and experiences. The most invariant feature of a standard dialect is grammar. Whereas differences in vocabulary and pronunciation are identifiable features of regional dialects, these dialects are not usually considered nonstandard unless they include grammatical variations. Thus, we would expect that educated speakers in Mississippi, New Hampshire, and Minnesota will show discernible differences in their speech, but these will be primarily at the levels of phonology and vocabulary. For example, a casserole is called a "hot dish" in Minnesota and North Dakota but is commonly called a "casserole" in other parts of the United States.

Because the standard dialect of a nation is generally the dialect of its more educated inhabitants, it is usually preferred in the classroom. The term *school English* or *Cognitive Academic Linguistic Proficiency* (*CLAP*), in contrast to the term *Basic Interpersonal Communication Skills* (*BICS*), or *conversational English* (Cummins, 2000), must be differentiated in order to have a full understanding of what is needed to be literate and required for school success. Historically, notions of what dialectal forms are preferred and/or important for school success and literacy have led some speakers to identify standard dialectal forms as correct and nonstandard dialectal forms as wrong or substandard. At one time, it was believed that nonstandard dialects were immature forms of Standard English and that speakers who produced them were less developed in their linguistic abilities. However, research by sociolinguists has shown convincingly that nonstandard and standard forms of English are equally complex and have the same cognitive and linguistic requirements as the standard dialect.

Table 9.2 summarizes four of the factors contributing to communication differences among speakers of English. Geography and membership in an ethnic group are often considered together as making up an individual's speech community. For example, speakers who are reared in Texas may produce speech that has phonological, lexical, and grammatical characteristics distinctive of that region. Collectively, these features are sometimes described as a *twang* or *drawl* (though some might restrict those terms to descriptions of the differences in pronunciation). The features of Texan speech are sufficiently distinctive to constitute a regional dialect of English. However, this regional dialect is altered to varying degrees

TABLE 9.2 | Factors Contributing to Communication Differences among Speakers

Regional Dialect	Ethnic Dialect	Register	Idiolect
Examples: Southern, Brooklyn	Examples: African American English, Spanish-influenced English	Examples: formal, informal, caretaker	Examples: every individual speaker
Produces variation in: ■ Phonology (e.g., use of vocalic /r/) ■ Rate of speech ■ Syntax (e.g., use of *y'all*) ■ Use of gestures ■ Use of specific words or idioms ■ Vocal intensity ■ Vocal quality (e.g., nasality)	Produces variation in: ■ Distance between speaker and listener ■ Morphology (e.g., use of plural marker) ■ Phonology (e.g., use of theta) ■ Rate of speech ■ Stress and intonation ■ Syntax (e.g., use of copula) ■ Use of specific words or idioms	Produces variation in: ■ Distance between speaker and listener ■ Eye contact ■ Lexical specificity ■ Rate of speech ■ Stress and intonation ■ Syntax (e.g., simple/complex) ■ Use of gestures ■ Use of specific words or idioms (e.g., formal/informal, common/uncommon) ■ Vocal intensity	Produces variation in: ■ Rate of speech ■ Stress and intonation ■ Use of gestures ■ Use of specific words or idioms ■ Vocal quality

by the ethnic background of each speaker. We are likely to find the prototypical Texas dialect among white speakers, but some African American speakers from that state might also produce African American English (AAE), an ethnic dialect used across the United States with phonological and syntactical influences from the languages of West Africa. Regional and ethnic influences can interact, so that the AAE spoken by some African Americans living in Dallas is likely to differ in some respects from the AAE produced by some African Americans living in Seattle or Cleveland.

The influence of an ethnic dialect is sometimes difficult to separate from the effect of a native language other than English. Many characteristics of the dialect spoken by some Hispanic Americans are the result of linguistic borrowing from Spanish. English words may be pronounced with a Spanish accent, Spanish vocabulary may be substituted for English words in some contexts, and English syntax may be modified in ways that make it more consistent with Spanish syntax. Some individuals speak only English but nevertheless maintain an influence from Spanish in their dialect. Others will speak both English and Spanish, though their English will likely reveal phonological characteristics of Spanish and vice versa. All immigrant groups from non-English-speaking countries can be expected to show a similar pattern. However, we tend to focus on particular ethnic dialects for social and demographic reasons. When the number of immigrants from a particular country or region becomes large, the language differences of those individuals can become a social issue, especially in education. This has occurred in the United States with both Hispanic Americans and Asian/Pacific Islander Americans; consequently, we tend to identify dialectal issues with those two groups. The large Asian/Pacific Islander and Hispanic immigration to America has also resulted in the formation of ethnic enclaves, especially in the bigger cities such as New York, Los Angeles, and Chicago. The insulation of these subcommunities (China Town, Korean Town, Little Saigon, Little India, Little Tokyo, Little Havana just like German Town and Greek Town) helps to maintain ethnic dialects by keeping native languages in use and by mitigating the influence of English-speaking culture.

Beyond the effects of geography and ethnic background, we all vary our speech and language to suit the requirements of specific social communicative events. That is, we *code switch*, a concept we first encountered in this text in Chapter 1. Speakers of nonstandard ethnic dialects who are also competent users of Standard English often adjust their use of nonstandard features to meet the expectations of a conversational partner. In a work or educational setting, the standard dialect might be used; in an ethnic social setting, the nonstandard dialect might be used. Code switching is a natural phenomenon that reflects competency with language.

Of course, not all the features of an individual's communication are determined by region, ethnicity, learning experience, life experience, or social situation. If they were, then many of us would sound far more alike than we do. What keeps us different is our uniqueness as individuals. Variation in everything from vocal tract anatomy to personal experiences provides everyone with an *idiolect*, that is, a distinctive combination of language characteristics.

Each person's idiolect can be compared to those of other individuals within a speech community. When we evaluate children for language disorders, this is what is done. Typically, a child's idiolect is first compared to the standard dialect of the nation in which the child lives. If the child's language is found to be different, then the following possibilities must be explored:

- The child is learning the standard dialect but is language disordered.
- The child is learning a nonstandard dialect.
- The child is learning a nonstandard dialect *and* is language disordered.

To evaluate either of the last two possibilities requires a knowledge of the child's nonstandard dialect or other language. Features of the child's language that differ from the standard dialect must be evaluated to determine whether they are disordered or merely dialectal variations. For example, the substitution of "f" for "th" is a common feature in AAE.

CONCEPTS OF SECOND-LANGUAGE LEARNING

In theory, the perfect bilingual speaker is one who can comprehend and use two languages with equal facility. However, apart from professional interpreters, such competence is rarely attained. There is even a challenge in defining bilingualism, with Grosjean (1982) indicating that a bilingual individual is not just two monolinguals combined into one. The far more common situations are individuals who are characterized as follows:

- Are fluent with both written and spoken forms of their first (native) language and have less proficiency with a second language.
- Have equivalent but different areas of competence in two languages and therefore prefer to use one or the other in particular circumstances (e.g., at school, during play) or while engaged in certain tasks (speaking, reading, writing), for example, a person who learned to speak Chinese around the home kitchen table, "kitchen Chinese," or another who learned to read English because the native language spoken in the home did not have a written form.

Most children who are bilingual present a variety of linguistic profiles. Table 9.3 shows different ways in which English and another language may be mixed or kept separate. A few may be quite bilingual and highly competent in both their comprehension and their production of English and the other language. Other children may have a dominant language that they are able to speak and understand well. They will naturally prefer to use this language in all situations that allow it. Another possibility is for children to know elements of both languages but lack competence and confidence in either one. These children may be able to communicate effectively only by switching back and forth between the languages and by mixing vocabularies of both. Children with such low mixed dominance are not necessarily language disordered. Often, they may know certain words in one language and other words in another language. So, when they encounter a particular item to name, they may code switch and only use one language to name it. The ability to code switch for *effective* communication is typically considered an indication of good competency with language, but the competency may not be just with a particular language. Those children who are language impaired might mix languages as a compensatory strategy but may not do it well, while those who are not language disordered might mix languages as a result of environmental influences and probably do so with relative ease. Baker's (2000) Bilingual Family Profile, which is presented later in this chapter when we discuss assessment, provides a useful guideline for better understanding bilingual families and children in bilingual families.

TABLE 9.3 | Profiles of Language Mixing and Separation

Monolingual English	Comprehends and produces English only.
Low mixed English/other language	Comprehends and produces both languages imperfectly, though English is slightly stronger. Mixes the languages in speaking.
English dominant	Comprehends and produces English well. Uses other language when required but has less proficiency with it.
Bilingual	Comprehends and produces both languages equally well. Code switches easily.
Other language dominant	Comprehends and produces other language well. Uses English when required but has less proficiency with it.
Low mixed other language/English	Comprehends and produces both languages imperfectly, though other language is slightly stronger. Mixes the languages in speaking.
Monolingual other language	Comprehends and produces other language only.

Many factors affect the process and result of second-language learning. The model environment for children is to learn two languages from birth in an optimal language-learning environment and with optimal experience (OLLEE) (Cheng, 2009). Experiences that make up children's environments are important parts of an OLLEE. These children would hear the two languages being spoken by both of their parents, as well as by their peers, other adults, and speakers on the radio and television. The children would be able to speak, read, and write both languages at school and in all other social experiences such as church, sports teams, and clubs. Of course, such an environment is not common, even in the most linguistically diverse nations. There are some exceptions in countries such as Switzerland, Belgium, and Canada.

Bilingual acquisition is influenced by every variation from the model situation we have described. Of particular influence is whether the different languages are learned sequentially or simultaneously. For example, a daughter is born to a German university professor. Although the father speaks English, he does not use it at home. When the girl is 4, the father accepts a position at an American university, and the family moves. The daughter is exposed to English through her American friends and their families, through television, and through her father, who now begins to speak it to her at home. The mother has limited knowledge of English and, therefore, speaks mostly German with the girl and with her father. In this scenario, the girl's language learning is affected by (1) the ages at which she was first exposed to German and English, (2) the switch in the language used by her father, (3) the difference in the languages used by her mother and father, and (4) the language used by her American peers and teachers. Because she learned German and English *sequentially* rather than simultaneously, the girl is less likely to mix the two languages. There will likely be differences in the speed and accuracy with which she names items in German or English (Kohnert, Bates, & Hernandez, 1999). At age 4 and beyond, she will be aware of the difference in language skills of her two parents. Not only will she expect her mother to speak German, but she may object if her mother attempts to use English with her (Volterra & Taeschner, 1978). On the other hand, the girl and her father may develop an elaborate system for code switching between German and English (Juan-Garau & Perez-Vidal, 2001). For instance, they may use German when speaking affectionately but switch to English for an instructional purpose. Discipline may be meted out in English unless the child resists or disobeys in some way. In that case, the father may switch to German to emphasize his determination.

Children who learn two languages *simultaneously* appear to go through a sorting-out process during the preschool years. How this sorting occurs has been a controversial subject (De Houwer, 1995). Under the "single system" or "fusion" hypothesis, children are supposed to traverse three stages, beginning with a system that mixes vocabulary and grammatical features from the two languages and ending with a system in which the two are clearly differentiated (Volterra & Taeschner, 1978). The fusion hypothesis gives attention to the phenomenon of code mixing, a developmental stage in which bilingual children may for a time mix vocabulary from the two languages or, at a slightly later stage, mix the grammatical systems of the two languages. For example, a child learning Spanish and English may vary the order of nouns and adjectives, thereby creating ungrammatical or unusual sentences in both languages (e.g., "It's a clown silly" or "Es un tonto payaso"). Clinically, there has been concern that such code mixing indicates a confused stage of language learning. Thus, speech-language pathologists (SLPs) and others have sometimes advised parents of a bilingual child who is slow to acquire language, that it would be best to limit the child to a single language input (De Houwer, 1999). Research indicates, however, that bilingual children can differentiate their languages very early in development (i.e., the "separate systems" hypothesis) and that code mixing represents an adaptation to other linguistic influences (e.g., Genesse, Nicoladis, & Paradis, 1995; Pearson, Fernandez, & Oller, 1995). In particular, there is evidence that most code mixing can be explained as the result of lexical gaps in one language, imperfect attempts on the part of the child to develop pragmatic skill in code switching, or the prominence of particular aspects of the culture to which the child is exposed in the two languages (Brice, 2002; Brice & Anderson, 1999; Koeppe, 1996; Nicoladis & Secco, 2000; Peña, Bedore, & Zlatic-Giunta, 2002). For example, children may call a diaper a "baby napkin" because they have not been exposed to the word "diaper" at home.

LANGUAGE CHARACTERISTICS OF LINGUISTICALLY-CULTURALLY DIVERSE CHILDREN

Although it is convenient at times to consider linguistically-culturally diverse children as a group, there are important linguistic and cultural differences among various ethnic populations. Analysis of language and culture can be done along a continuum of detail. At a broad level, we can identify four major ethnic groups in the United States, as noted previously: African Americans, Hispanic Americans, Asian/Pacific Islander Americans, and Native Americans. By 2015, these groups together were estimated to make up almost 34 percent of the U.S. population (U.S. Bureau of the Census, 2010). At a fine level of analysis, every major ethnic group can be seen to consist of multiple subgroups that often vary greatly from one another in language and culture. Thus, we could distinguish among the following:

- African Americans living in different regions of the country, some of whom are the descendants of the former slaves, some of whom are recent immigrants from the Caribbean islands, and some of whom are refugees from Africa.
- Hispanic (Latino) Americans based on their country of origin (e.g., Cuba, Mexico, El Salvador, Puerto Rico, South and Central America or Spain).
- Asian/Pacific Islander Americans who have immigrated from different nations in different regions (e.g., East Asia, such as Korea, China, or Japan; Southeast Asia, such as Vietnam, Kampuchea, Laos, Thailand, Malaysia, Singapore, or Indonesia; South Asia, such as India, Sri Lanka, Pakistan, Bhutan, or Nepal; and the Philippines and other Pacific Islands, including New Zealand and Australia). The Pacific Islands are generally divided into three groups: Polynesia (Hawaii, Tahiti, and so on), Melanesia, and Micronesia (Guam, Saipan, and so on).
- Native Americans with different tribal ancestries (e.g., Arapaho, Navajo, Hopi, or Kumeyey).

Detailed knowledge of such subgroups may be crucial in certain educational settings. For the purposes of this chapter, however, we examine only those broad linguistic and cultural differences that exist among these four groups.

Hispanic (Latino) American Children

A major factor in the English produced by Hispanic American bilingual–bicultural children is the Spanish language. A unique dialect, Spanglish, is formed as a result of the influence of and borrowing from both English and Spanish phonology, grammar, and vocabulary.

Varieties of Spanish-Influenced English. Spanish, like English, has many national standard forms as well as nonstandard forms. Individuals from Mexico, Puerto Rico, and Cuba form the predominant groups in the Hispanic population of the United States. Consequently, those national varieties of Spanish are the most influential. The last two censuses, however, have shown a significant increase in Central and South American immigration, so that groups from El Salvador, Guatemala, Colombia, and Honduras are now more numerous and will have an increasing impact on dialectal learning. Clearly, many varieties of Spanish are spoken in America, meaning that a wide range of effects on children is possible.

Language Profiles of Hispanic American Bilingual–Bicultural Children. Several variables interact to produce different language profiles among Hispanic American children. First and most important, children's relative proficiency in English and Spanish can vary greatly, depending on such factors as the following:

- The age at which they were introduced to English and its effect on simultaneous or sequential acquisition
- The bilingual fluency of the parents and other significant language models
- The bilingual requirements or opportunities of the environment in which the children live

Readers might find a review of Table 9.3 presented earlier in this chapter helpful. Some Hispanic American children may be monolingual, communicating only in English or Spanish. Obviously, children who are ethnic Hispanics and have Spanish surnames are not obligated to know the Spanish language. This situation will occur more frequently in second- and later-generation families. Because of cultural traditions the children may know a considerable number of Spanish words and idioms, but they are functionally English monolingual. In contrast, children who have recently arrived in America or have been raised in tightly knit Hispanic American communities may speak only Spanish. Like other monolingual children, they may have acquired some English vocabulary, but otherwise they are incompetent in English.

Another variable affecting Hispanic American children's language profiles is the dialect or dialects to which they are exposed. One child might learn a Puerto Rican standard form of Spanish and an AAE nonstandard form of English. Another child might combine a nonstandard form of Mexican Spanish with SAE. The possible combinations are potentially as great as the number of varieties of Spanish and English. In actuality, however, common combinations will be determined by patterns of immigration and settlement in the United States.

Individual variation in Hispanic American children's pragmatic language profiles will be largely influenced by variables such as family expectations, ethnic pride, and cultural beliefs (Brice, 2002; Brice & Anderson, 1999; Salas-Provance, Erickson, & Reed, 2002). We have noted that the Hispanic community in America is now quite diverse, making it increasingly difficult to generalize about "Hispanic culture" or "Hispanic value systems." It remains fair to say, however, that Hispanic American children often display pragmatic communicative behaviors that are different from those of white middle-class children. They may, for instance, show more reluctance to extend topics (i.e., providing more information than is requested) in conversations with adults (Pajewski & Enriquez, 1996). Extending topics, which is valued as a sign of creativity and social skill in many Anglo educational settings, may be considered disrespectful among certain Hispanic American groups.

Phonological Differences. Spanish has slightly fewer consonants than American English, about 18 versus about 24. Table 9.4 compares the two consonant systems in terms of three groups. There are several sounds that are produced identically or very nearly so. The pronunciation of these sounds presents little difficulty to bilingual or second-language learners of English. There is a smaller group of sounds that occur only in English. Speakers of Spanish will typically substitute phonetically similar Spanish sounds. For example, /s/ or /t/ will be substituted for "th," /s/ for /z/, and "ch" for "sh." Sounds in the third group in the table are ones that are sometimes or always produced differently in Spanish than in English. To the ear

TABLE 9.4 | Consonants of Spanish and English

1. Consonants pronounced alike: f, s, h, m, n, l, w, j, "ng"	
2. English consonants that do not exist in Spanish: z, "sh," "zh" (except in Argentina), /dʒ/, /θ/ (except in central Spain)	
3. Consonants pronounced differently	Explanation of Spanish pronunciation.
b, v	Pronounced the same as a voiced bilabial fricative, a sound that does not exist in English.
p, k, "ch"	Produced without the following aspiration.
t, d	Produced as dental rather than alveolar stops. In intervocalic position, /d/ is produced as a voiced interdental fricative /ð/.
g	Produced as /g/ only when it follows /n/, as in *tango*. Otherwise, it is produced as a voiced velar fricative, a sound that does not exist in English.
r	Produced either as a flap or an alveolar trill, depending on phonetic context.

Sources: Barlow (2005); Brice (2002); Butt and Benjamin (2000); Goldstein (2001); Levey (2004).

TABLE 9.5 | Vowels and Diphthongs of Spanish and English

Vowels pronounced alike: a, e, i, o, u (though they are not lengthened as in English)
Diphthongs pronounced alike: aɪ, aʊ, iu, oɪ
English vowels and diphthongs that do not exist in Spanish: ɪ, ɛ, æ, ʌ, ə, ɔ, ʊ, oʊ

Sources: Barlow (2005); Brice (2002); Butt and Benjamin (2000); Goldstein (2001); Levey (2004).

of a native English speaker, these consonants sound slightly distorted when native speakers of Spanish pronounce English words.

The Spanish vowel system also contains fewer sounds than its English counterpart, 5 as compared to 12. Table 9.5 summarizes the points of contrast. All the Spanish vowels and diphthongs also exist in English, but there are seven vowels unique to English. Speakers of Spanish tend to substitute for phonetically similar English vowels, for example, /i/ for /ɪ/ and /a/ for /ʌ/.

Another major influence on vowel production in the two languages is the difference in prosodic features. In English, the duration of vowels varies, depending on whether they occur in stressed or unstressed syllables. Thus, in the word *elephant*, the vowel in the first, stressed, syllable is /ɛ/; the vowel in the second, unstressed, syllable is /ə/. In Spanish, vowel length is nearly constant. Therefore, in the word *elefante*, the vowels in the first, second, and fourth syllables are all /ɛ/. There is a natural tendency for native speakers of Spanish to retain their habit of producing equal vowel duration when they speak English. This habit, along with the vowel substitutions mentioned earlier, yields pronunciations such as /presiden/ for *president*, /telefon/ for *telephone*, and /mekani/ for *mechanic.*

The contrasts we have drawn thus far are between the phonetic features of English and Spanish, that is, differences in which sounds are produced and how they are produced. There are also a number of phonological differences that can affect the pronunciation of bilingual children. Some of the most important ones are as follows:

- The fricative /ð/ occurs only in intervocalic position in Spanish. Thus, in speaking English, it is typically substituted for by /d/ in prevocalic (e.g., *this*) or postvocalic (e.g., *smooth*) positions.
- In several dialects of Spanish (e.g., Cuban), /s/ can be omitted in postvocalic position.
- Consonant clusters containing /s/ as the first sound such as /sp/, /st/, and /sk/ do not occur in the word-initial position in Spanish. Consequently, Spanish speakers will often insert a vowel before the cluster so that it conforms to the Spanish phonological rule, for example, /eskul/ for *school.*
- Consonant clusters containing /s/ as the last sound, such as /ps/, /ts/, and /ks/, do not occur in word-final position in Spanish. These clusters are commonly reduced in English words, for example, /βak/ for *box* or /kot/ for *coats.*
- The only word-final consonants in Spanish are /s, n, r, l, d/. All other words end in vowels. Therefore, the tendency is to omit consonants (e.g., /kæn/ for *can't*) or add vowels to the ends of words, especially when the English and Spanish words are cognates (e.g., /fruta/ for *fruit*).

It is important to be aware of phonological differences such as these because they frequently contain the key to understanding what seem to be inconsistencies in pronunciation. For example, a Hispanic American child may correctly pronounce the consonants in the words /feðo/ *feather*, /soni/ *sunny*, and /mostod/ *mustard* but have difficulty with some of the same sounds in the words /do/ *those,* /leto/ *lettuce,* and /estó/ *stove.* It is also important to remember that the different dialects of Spanish can influence pronunciation differentially and that this, too, can be a key in understanding a child's phonological characteristics (Goldstein & Iglesias, 2001).

Grammatical Differences. Comparison of English and Spanish grammar is considerably more complex than comparison of phonology because of the number of features involved.

Many differences are relevant only to the language of adults and need not concern us in our discussion of children's grammatical learning. Some of the distinctions that are most pertinent to children are these:

- The position of adjectives in the noun phrase is more flexible in Spanish. The rules determining which adjectives precede and which follow a noun are difficult to formulate (Butt & Benjamin, 2000). However, the fact that Spanish allows postmodifying adjectives makes it more likely that bilingual children will attempt to use this structure in English, for example, *car green* instead of *green car.*
- Nearly all Spanish adjectives can function as nouns if preceded by an article or demonstrative. English requires an indefinite pronoun to express the same meaning; for example, *los rojos* (literally, *the reds*) has the same meaning as *the red ones* in English.
- Indefinite articles are omitted following certain uses of the copula, certain common verbs (*have, buy, take, look for, wear*), and certain prepositions.
- In referring to parts of the body, clothing, or other personal belongings, the possessive pronoun is replaced by the definite article; for example, "Me quité los calcetines" is translated literally as "I took off the (i.e., my) socks."
- Spanish does not require the auxiliary verb *do* to support the transformation of statements into questions ("He did it" → "Did he do it?") or statements into negative commands ("Do it!" → "Don't do it!"). Questions are instead marked by rising intonation and negative commands by the insertion of *no* at the beginning of the sentence.
- Plurality is marked more redundantly in Spanish than in English. For instance, in the sentence "Han llegado los dos niños colombianos"/"The two Colombian boys have arrived," plurality is marked five times: on the auxiliary verb, the article, the quantifier, the noun, and the adjective. Such redundancy permits Spanish speakers to omit some of the markers without loss of information. Omission of plural markers is especially common in dialects that delete the postvocalic /s/ (Iglesias & Anderson, 1993).
- Negation is marked on all constituents of a negative sentence; for example, "Nunca veía a nadie en ninguna de las habitaciones" translates literally as "I never saw nobody in none of the rooms." *No* is used for all negation in the verb phrase, for example, "No puedo" ("I can't") or "No está aquí" ("He isn't here"). There is no equivalent to *not.*

Characteristics of Spanish-Influenced English. The basic framework for identifying and understanding characteristics of Spanish-influenced English is knowledge of the two languages and the differences between them. We should recall, however, that the interaction between the languages is influenced by dialectal variation within Spanish and English. Moreover, it is not clear that interference from Spanish is the major cause of errors in Hispanic American children's learning of English. Research on bilingual language learning suggests that grammatical forms are used in a language-specific manner (De Houwer, 1995). That is, children tend to maintain separation between the syntactic rules and morphological forms relevant to different languages they are acquiring.

Interference effects appear to be more potent in explaining the phonological characteristics of Spanish-influenced English. Table 9.6 provides examples of both grammatical and phonological interference errors that may be observed in Hispanic American children. The frequency and consistency of such errors is likely to vary depending on when and how the children begin to learn English as well as the degree of balance in their competence with the two languages.

African American Children

Many African American children learn a nonstandard dialect of American English. At one time, this dialect was commonly described as *Black English* or *Ebonics* (*Ebony Phonics*). However, these terms implied that the dialect was used by all African Americans, which is not the case. Consequently, a replacement term was the description *Black English Vernacular* and then, more recently, *African American English* (*AAE*) to emphasize that it is the dialect

TABLE 9.6 | Phonological and Grammatical Interference Errors Found in Spanish-Influenced English

Example	Errors	Explanation
She /tʃ i/ no can help	▪ Substitution of /tʃ/ "ch" for /ʃ/ "sh" ▪ Incorrect negative in the verb phrase	▪ /ʃ/ "sh" not used in Spanish; /tʃ/ "ch" is the closest form ▪ *no* is the only negative form in the verb phrase and always precedes the verb it modifies
I want /wan/ *the* /di/ *big*	▪ Reduction of cluster /nt/→ /n/ ▪ Substitution of /d/ for /ð/ ▪ Omission of indefinite pronoun *one*	▪ Spanish words do not end in /t/; cluster is reduced to conform with this rule ▪ /ð/ not used in word-initial position; /d/ is the closest form ▪ Article + adjective is the Spanish equivalent of the English phrase article + adjective + *one*
He wearing /werin/ *shirt* /tʃut/, *no?*	▪ Substitution of flap for /r/; substitution of /n/ for "ng"; substitution of "ch" for "sh" ▪ Omission of auxiliary verb *is* ▪ Omission of indefinite article *a* ▪ Use of *no* and rising intonation to form tag question	▪ Sounds do not exist in Spanish or are not allowed in certain phonetic contexts; closest forms are substituted ▪ Immature verb form (*not* an interference error) ▪ Indefinite articles not used following verb *wear* ▪ *No* + rising intonation is the Spanish tag form when seeking agreement from listener

of a particular speech community and not of an entire race. Sociolinguistic studies suggest that AAE is used to some extent by most African Americans but that the degree of usage varies by socioeconomic group. African Americans of lower-socioeconomic groups are more likely to use a higher percentage of AAE linguistic features, whereas those of upper- and middle-socioeconomic groups tend to use fewer features (Wolfram & Schilling-Estes, 1998). Although AAE is socially stratified, its use does not necessarily indicate a difference in the social background or education of the speaker. However, because the dialect can be difficult for SAE speakers to understand, even listeners who are professionals can mistakenly form impressions about intelligence from speech characteristics alone (Bleile, McGowan, & Bernthal, 1997).

Historical Issues. The origin of AAE has in the past been a disputed and controversial subject. Language is a major source of ethnic identity, and the origin of a language or dialect of a language can become an issue of ethnic pride as well as a topic of academic study. One early view of AAE was that it was merely a *restricted code*, that is, a variety of language used by lower social classes that is characterized by, among other things, reduced syntax and a reliance on context for the interpretation of meaning (Crystal, 1997). This opinion of AAE has been largely abandoned, though the issue of a restricted code among lower social classes continues to be argued.

Scholars agree that AAE had its origins among the slave communities of the American South and then spread to northern urban centers as African Americans migrated to those regions. There has been disagreement, however, about how the dialect first became established among the slaves. For example, some of the linguistic features of AAE are also found in British dialects that were spoken in the early periods of southern American history. The best-supported and most widely accepted view is that AAE began in Africa as a pidgin, or very limited trade language, used to facilitate commerce between Europeans and Africans. When a slave trade developed during the 1600s, this pidgin language came with the Africans to southeastern America. There it gradually merged with English to form a language of its own, known as a *creole* language, which has a systematic and elaborated grammar and vocabulary (Rickford, 1998). This creole language gradually evolved into what we recognize today as AAE. What is apparent from historical study is that AAE is a systematic and rule-governed variety of English that has evolved through processes that are well known to linguists. It should be viewed, therefore, as an independent linguistic system that is related to SAE but that has many of its own formal and functional characteristics.

Characteristics of AAE. AAE may be contrasted with SAE at each level of linguistic structure: pragmatics, semantics, phonology, and grammar. However, caution is warranted in making broad generalizations about these contrasts to most African American individuals. In an interview for a publication of the American Speech-Language-Hearing Association (ASHA), *The ASHA Leader* (Saad & Polovoy, 2009), Ida Stockman, recognized as a leader in SLP and issues related to CLD, reminded us that past perspectives of African Americans as making up a homogeneous group have meant that "we know little about how their dialect use varied with social class, gender, geographical location and other factors" (p. 24). She added that "normalcy is not absolute but relative" (p. 24). While caution about making broad generalizations is warranted, awareness of possible contrasts is important to working effectively with children who might use features of AAE. As an example, the interaction of AAE speakers may appear to a speaker of SAE to be highly assertive and perhaps even excessively demonstrative. Loud talking, heated public arguments, and frequent interruptions of one's conversational partners are considered acceptable pragmatic behaviors in AAE. On the other hand, certain behaviors that SAE speakers may consider acceptable or only mildly rude are intolerable to AAE speakers—for example, asking personal questions of a new acquaintance or trying to break in on a conversation. Thus, neither dialect should be considered more polite than the other.

AAE has been a fertile ground for the development of slang, especially among inner-city populations. This is hardly surprising because slang's most consistent function is to mark social or linguistic identity (Crystal, 1997). Some of the slang generated by AAE, such as the adjective *cool*, the verb *diss*, or the noun *props*, have crossed over and become part of SAE. Other words and idiomatic phrases have remained unique to AAE and are not understandable to individuals who do not know the dialect (Smitherman, 2000).

Some of the major phonological features of AAE affecting vowels and consonants are summarized in Table 9.7. Other phonological differences exist in the prosody of AAE, such as

TABLE 9.7 | Phonological Features of AAE

Phonological Variation	Example
Deletion of nasal at the end of a word and nasalization of the preceding vowel	comb→ co/ko/ (with vowel nasalized) man→ ma/mæ/ (with vowel nasalized)
Deletion of semivowels /r/ and /l/	store→ sto/sto/ fool→ foo/fu/ help→ hep/hɛp/
Devoicing and weakening of final stops	hat→ ha/hæ/ mad→ mat/mæt/ or ma/mæ/ big→ bid/bɪd/ or bi/bɪ/
Simplification of consonant clusters at the end of a word	last→ lass/læs/ soft→ sof/sɔf/
Substitution of f/θ in the middle and at the end of a word; substitution of /v/ð/ in the middle of a word	tooth→ toof/tuf/ brother→ brover/brʌvə/
Substitution of stop for interdental fricative at the beginning of a word	that→ dat/dæt/ thin→ tın/tın/

Sources: Craig, Thompson, Washington, and Potter (2003); Day-Vines et al. (2009); Pollock (2001).

TABLE 9.8 | Grammatical Features of AAE

Grammatical Variation	Example
Deletion of possessive marker with adjacent nouns	That Bobby bike (= Bobby's bike)
Deletion of plural marker when a numerical quantifier is used	I got two card
Different formation of indirect questions	I asked him did he know her name
No final *-s* in the third-person singular present tense	That dog bark all the time
Use of double negatives involving the auxiliary verb at the beginning of a sentence	Can't nobody fix that thing
Use of *be* to mark habitual action	I be goin' to school every day
Use of the copula is not obligatory	He mad
	My brother real big

Sources: Day-Vines et al. (2009); Nelson and Hyter (1990); Washington (2015); Wolfram and Schilling-Estes (1998).

greater vowel prolongation and varied intonation contours (Hyter, 1998). As indicated earlier, these features are characteristic of the dialect as a whole but are found to varying degrees in individual speakers. Many features common to AAE phonology, such as weak-syllable deletion and final cluster reduction, also occur in other English vernaculars, spoken by other ethnic groups (Pollock, 2001). There is also overlap between AAE and the phonological features common to young children, regardless of whether they are learning a standard or nonstandard dialect of English. It appears, therefore, that the phonological systems of AAE and SAE speakers do not become fully differentiated until later in childhood.

Table 9.8 shows some of the principal features of AAE grammar. Some grammatical markers that are obligatory in SAE are deleted in AAE in contexts where they are redundant. For example, the possessive noun marker will be absent in the sentence "That be Rhonda purse" but present in the sentence "That be Rhonda's." Interactions can occur between phonological and grammatical features of AAE (Stockman, 1996a). For example, the singular form of *desk* would be pronounced in AAE as /dɛs/. To form the plural and yet still avoid a consonant cluster, AAE speakers will produce /dɛsəz/ unless the word follows a numerical quantifier. In that case, the plural marker will be omitted: "My school got a hundred desk /dɛs/." Thus, the dialect's variations from SAE are both consistent and logical. The variations also avoid ambiguity in meaning, for example, omission of a plural marker on a noun if plurality is signaled elsewhere in an utterance, such as with a numerical marker but use of the marker if there is no other indication of plurality in an utterance (Washington, 2015).

A child's use of a dialect such as AAE, in the absence of impaired ability to learn language, is *not* a language disorder or impairment. However, we know from previous chapters that children's spoken language abilities have strong influences on how well children read. There is recent evidence that indicates the degree to which children use AAE features in their spoken language correlates inversely with their achievement, such that the greater occurrence of AAE features is associated with lower literacy achievement (Charity, Scarborough, & Griffin, 2004; Connor & Craig, 2006; Craig & Washington, 2004; Craig, Zhang, Hensel, & Quinn, 2009). We will see later in this chapter that this information has potential implications for intervention considerations.

Asian/Pacific Islander American Children

Asian/Pacific Islander (API) Americans are the most culturally and linguistically diverse of the major ethnic groups in the United States. There is no agreement on which nationalities should be included in the category of *Asian/Pacific Islander*, as it is not clear whether this

TABLE 9.9 | Examples of Languages Widely Spoken among Asian Immigrant Populations and Their Contrasting Phonological Features

Language(s)	Where Spoken	Contrasting Phonological Feature(s)
Japanese	Japan	No word-final consonants, only five vowels, contrastive vowel length
Korean	North and South Korea, parts of China, Japan, and Russia	Contrastive vowel length
Mon-Khmer family		
Khmer	Kampuchea (Cambodia)	Large repertoire of consonant clusters
Vietnamese	Kampuchea (Cambodia), Laos, Vietnam	Tone language, no consonant clusters, essentially monosyllabic, only six final consonants
Sino-Tibetan family		
Chinese (Cantonese and Mandarin)	China	Tone language, no consonant clusters, essentially monosyllabic, few final consonants
Hmong	Northern Laos, Thailand, Vietnam	Tone language, only word-initial consonant clusters, only one final consonant
Tai family		
Lao (Laotian)	Laos, Thailand	Tone language, essentially monosyllabic

Sources: Hirata, Whitehurst, and Cullings (2007); Hwa-Froelich, Hodson, and Edwards (2002); Mattock and Burnham (2006); Mugitani et al. (2009).

term refers to a racial subtype, a geographic area, or a linguistic grouping. For our purposes, it will refer to a particular group of languages.

Varieties of Asian/Pacific Islander Languages. The classification of languages raises some problems for which there are no clear solutions. Languages are usually compared in terms of their structural characteristics (grammar, vocabulary, and phonology) and historical origins. However, the weighting given to different structural levels is purely arbitrary. Thus, two languages that are grammatically distinct might be placed in different families, even though they share many phonological features. Historical information can assist in resolving some structural issues, but there are problems even here. Two languages that are historically distinct may be used by ethnic groups that, through migration and resettlement, come to live in the same area. For example, Pernagan is a mixture of Malay and Chinese and is spoken in Singapore and Malaysia. Over time, the two languages that were once distinct will begin to influence and borrow from one another.

Asian languages that are widely spoken by immigrants to the United States are listed in Table 9.9, along with some of the phonological features of those languages that contrast with English. As can be seen, the phonological structure of API languages is markedly different from that of English. They tend to have a simpler segmental structure, with fewer vowels and consonants and with word shapes that are largely monosyllabic and contain few consonant clusters. However, the suprasegmental structure of Asian languages, such as Chinese, Thai, Vietnamese, and Khmer, which are tonal languages, is generally richer than that of English, with variation in tone and vowel length used to signal differences in word meaning. In fact, intonation patterns are often identified as among the major contributors to linguistic differences between some Asian languages and English.

Pacific Islanders use various languages, mostly from the Austronesian language family, including Hawaiian, Maori, Nauruan, Marshallese, Tahitian, Tongan, Samoan, Tuvaluan, Gilbertese, Charmorro, and numerous others. Since the Colonial period, Pacific Islanders have been using English, French, Japanese, Chinese, Tagalog, Portuguese, and other languages. They also use creole languages that are heavily influenced by European languages. Bislama, for example, is the English-based creole of Vanuatu, and Tok Pisin is the lingua franca of New Guinea. The island of Papua New Guinea has more than 500 native languages, most of which are not known to be related to any other languages spoken outside of New

TABLE 9.10 | Phonological and Grammatical Interference Errors Found in the English of Native Chinese and Vietnamese Speakers

Example	Errors
We go you house /haʊ/ yesterday /jɛtu'de/ (= We went to your house yesterday)	■ Omission of word-final /s/ (*house*) ■ Reduction of cluster /st/→ /t/ (*yesterday*) ■ Incorrect syllable stress (*yesterday*) ■ Use of unmarked verb form (*go*) for irregular past-tense form (*went*) ■ Substitution of pronominal forms (*you/your*) ■ Omission of preposition *to*
Him no buy book /bʊ/? (= Didn't he buy the book?)	■ Omission of word-final /k/ (*book*) ■ Omission of article *the* ■ Simplified interrogative: auxiliary verb *did* omitted; question marked only by rising intonation ■ Use of unmarked verb form (*buy*) for expanded verb phrase (*did buy*) ■ Substitution of pronominal forms (*him/he*) ■ Simplified negation: marked only by use of *no*
That /dæ/ man two dollar /daral/ me (= That man gave me two dollars or That man gave two dollars to me)	■ Omission of word-final /t/ (*that*) ■ Substitution of /ð/→ /d/ (*that*) ■ Substitution of liquid consonants /r/ and /l/ (*dollar*) ■ Omission of plural marker when preceded by numerical quantifier (*two dollar*) ■ Reversed ordering of direct and indirect objects (*two dollar me*) or omission of preposition *to*

Sources: Cheng (1987a, 1987b); Hwa-Froelich et al. (2002); Jia and Fuse (2007); Trueba, Cheng, and Ima (1993).

Guinea. This makes them language isolates, which are languages with no known relatives or which belong to very small language families.

Characteristics of Asian-Influenced English. The English spoken by Asian American children may show the effect of interference from their native tongue. The extent of this interference depends on the bilingual profile presented by each child. Recall that Table 9.3 shows a range of profiles that may be demonstrated by different children learning two languages. The precise nature of the interference will depend on the cultural, social, education, migration, and linguistic experiences of each child. For example, the language and behavior of a Hmong child may show little resemblance to that of a Korean child. Table 9.10 summarizes some of the phonological and grammatical interference errors that are likely to occur in native speakers of Chinese or Vietnamese. Similar errors may be found among speakers of other Asian languages.

Besides their differences in language form, Asian American children may vary in their pragmatic behavior. Because Asian cultural mores generally discourage children from interrupting or asserting themselves with adults, they may appear passive when observed alongside other American children. They may seem to avoid eye contact in dyadic conversation and yet stare openly in other situations (Cheng, 1998). While pragmatic differences of this kind are subtle and may not interfere at all with peer interaction, they can interfere with assessment efforts and might be wrongly taken as an indication of limited language competence. In other situations, pragmatic differences, or even language/speech characteristics, may be erroneously attributed to cultural and/or linguistic differences when, in fact, a communication disorder exists. Asian culture in general is collectivist rather than individualistic (Cheng, 2007a). This means that a child is part of a very large family or clan and that a child's problem is not just his or her problem but the problem of the whole family. Cheng (2007a) has presented an excellent case study detailing the tragedy of the Virginia Tech massacre committed by a Korean American boy. He had a severe communicative disorder (selective mutism) and personality disorder (emotional disability), but his condition was not properly managed, leading to the tragedy that shook the world.

Native American Children

Roughly half a million American Indian and Alaska Native students attend elementary and secondary schools in the United States. About 90 percent of these students attend public schools, while 10 percent attend schools operated or funded by the Bureau of Indian Affairs and tribes. Although Native American students represent less than 1 percent of the school-age population, they make up 1.3 percent of the special education population (U.S. Department of Education, 2001). Native American students in special education are most often identified as having a specific learning disability, intellectual disability, emotional disturbance, or a speech–language impairment.

Language Preservation. There are only a few Native American languages that are being spoken today. Because most of the indigenous languages in the United States have disappeared, a unique consideration in discussing the language skills of Native American children is the growing efforts to preserve tribal languages. The issues surrounding these efforts are a complex mixture of history, linguistics, culture, and politics. Among the more pertinent considerations are these:

- Only a small proportion of limited-English-proficient students in the United States are Native American, for example, 2.5 percent in 1993 (Fleischman & Hopstock, 1993). This means that the vast majority of Native American children learn English as their first language. In fact, many of them only know English. In San Diego County, almost all Kumeyeey Native Americans have lost their ancestral language (C. Brown, personal communication, 2009).
- The impetus to maintain tribal languages is to prevent the demise of culture, though there is disagreement on this point within the Native American community.
- Few curriculum materials exist for the teaching of Native American languages. There is a paucity of materials regarding the linguistic and cultural history of the Native Americans.
- Although efforts to promote the preservation of history are being encouraged, some Native American students are under peer pressure not to learn or use their tribal language.
- Dialectic differences and the absence of an acceptable orthography (spelling of the language) impede language maintenance in some communities.
- Native American students living in cities may find access to tribal language instruction hindered by the fact that many different tribes and languages are represented in their schools and the community (Peacock & Day, 1999).

Cultural-Linguistic Differences. The assessment of language skills in Native American children is complicated by differences in parenting practices and overall cultural expectations for language use (Harris, 1985; Robinson-Zañartu, 1996; Westby, 2009). Because of these differences, children from Native American homes may appear delayed in language and other developmental traits compared to children from the cultural mainstream. Robinson-Zañartu (1996) alerts us to the possibility that

> direct and timed question and answer sequences common in psychometric testing and in classroom discourse are experienced as culturally inappropriate in many Native American groups. Such questioning may elicit silence, an "I don't know" response, or a reply that may seem unrelated. (p. 376)

Children may also struggle with the task of dealing with the materials used in many norm-referenced, standardized tests, such as pictures and booklets, particularly if their background is a more traditional one characterized by learning without books (Robinson-Zañartu, 1996). Cultural influences reflecting story traditions in Native American societies may also be seen in many of the narratives produced by these children, influences that potentially lead to content and structures of narratives that differ from those of mainstream narratives (John-Steiner & Panofsky, 1992; Kay-Raining Bird & Vetter, 1994; Westby & Roman, 1995). In particular, narratives may not progress in the linear, cause–effect fashion expected in most classrooms. Kaplan (1966) described the differences in cultural thought patterns,

TABLE 9.11 | Linguistic Features of English Spoken by Native Americans

Variation	Example
Phonology	
Vowel shifting	Among Navajo English speakers, exchange of /ɪ/ and /ɛ/, /i/ and /ɪ/, /e/ and /ɛ/
Morphology	
Frequent deletion of plural and possessive marker	I read Diane['s] book Many of my relative[s] live in Shiprock
Use of base form or overregularized form for past-tense verbs	I hear him sing yesterday I eated some
Syntax	
End-of-utterance dependent clauses	They ride bikes is what I see them do From the family is where we learn to be good
Deletion of articles and demonstratives	They find [a] bone in [that] deep yard He asked [the] shopkeeper for [that] sheep
Deletion of *be*, *have*, and *get* as auxiliary or copular verbs	She [is] Red Corn people Then they would tell them what law he [has] broken

Sources: Leap (1993); Thurston (1998).

differences that can be uniquely reflected in the characteristics of content and structure of narratives of various cultures. For example, Kaplan stated that Europeans have a tendency to be linear and straightforward in their cultural thought patterns, whereas other cultures have circular thought patterns (e.g., Chinese). Native Americans also have a tendency to be more circular rather than linear in their storytelling strategies. He asserted that, in contrast, users of the Romance language family have a tendency to be tangential in thought patterns. It is also possible that some children will not have had practice in telling stories or communicating events in narrative form because only adults have the privilege of being designated storytellers. Results from parent questionnaires and norm-referenced language tests, as well as narrative assessment, must therefore be interpreted with great care and an awareness of cultural influences (Long, 1998; Long & Christensen, 1998).

Characteristics of English Spoken by Native Americans. Although most Native Americans learn English as their first language, the dialect that many of them speak differs from SAE in terms of its grammar, phonology, semantics, and rules of discourse. Table 9.11 lists some of the most commonly observed linguistic differences in what has been termed Indian English (Leap, 1993). Even among individuals who speak their ancestral language, Standard English, or both, Indian English fluency is a way of reinforcing one's cultural identity for many Native Americans, especially where it is the only Indian-related language tradition that has been maintained in a community. Under such circumstances, Indian English fluency becomes a highly valued social skill, and the nonstandard features of the dialect take on an even greater cultural significance (St. Charles & Costantino, 2000).

A MATTER OF POVERTY

To this point, we have examined the language development and language differences of racial/ethnic groups of American children from a purely cultural and linguistic perspective. In an ideal world, this would be the only viewpoint we would need to consider. It is apparent, however, that in a disproportionate number of cases, these groups of children are also children of poverty.

Poverty in the United States and Globally

According to the 2016 report from the National Center for Children in Poverty, in 2014 there were about 72 million children under age 18 in the United States. These children represented 23 percent of the population. However, when we look at the percentage of children who live in families with *lower socioeconomic status (SES)*, that is, low-income families with annual incomes of about $48,000.00 or below in 2014 for a two-child family of four, they represent about 32 percent of the entire population. Of all children, approximately 44 percent, or 32 million, are in families in the low-income range, with about half living in families at or below the poverty level (about $24,008 for a family of four with two children). These data do not, however, tell the whole story. Table 9.12 provides a breakdown of the proportions of children by age and by race/ethnicity for whom their families fell into the 2014 U.S. low-income level, and of those, the proportions of children whose families fell into the poverty level. Thus, we see that a slightly greater proportion of younger children are represented in the low-income groups. We also see that notably higher proportions of children from African American, Hispanic, and Native American families fall in the low-income level.

Poor young children in the United States may be at a disadvantage from birth. According to Hart and Risley (1995), children in higher SES families have heard 30 million more words than children from underprivileged (low-SES) families by the age of 3, and their follow-up data indicated that the 3-year-old measures of accomplishment predicted third-grade school achievement. These poor children are behind to start with and they fall further and further behind as they grow. These data are telling and also make the point for the importance of early intervention and education for children in poverty. However, when we consider poverty from a global perspective, we see a relatively graver picture.

TABLE 9.12 | 2014 Percentage and Number of Children by Age and Race/Ethnicity Groups in U.S. Low-Income Level Families and of Those in Families in the Poverty Level

	Low-Income Children		Children in Poverty	
Age Groups of Children	*% of Children in Age Group in Low-Income Families*	*Number of Children (in millions)*	*% of Low-Income Children in Age Group in Poverty Level*	*Number of Children (in millions)*
■ Under 3 years	47	5.3	24	2.7
■ 3 through 5 years	47	5.6	23	2.8
■ 6 through 11 years	45	10.8	22	5.4
■ 12 through 17 years	40	9.7	19	4.6
Racial/Ethnic Groups of Children	*% of Children in Racial/Ethnic Group in Low-Income Families*	*Number of Children (in millions)*	*% of Low-Income Children in Racial/Ethnic Group in Poverty Level*	*Number of Children (in millions)*
■ Asian	30	1.0	12	0.12
■ Black	65	6.3	38	2.4
■ Hispanic	62	10.9	32	3.5
■ Native American	62	0.3	35	0.11
■ White	31	11.4	13	1.5

Source: From National Center for Children in Poverty (2016).

Below is a list of facts about world poverty, several of which arise from the World Bank's definition of poverty:

Overview:
- Each year, more than 8 million people around the world die because they are too poor to stay alive.

Housing:
- In many parts of Africa, a majority of the people has no homes.

Levels of Poverty:
- One sixth of the world's population earns less than U.S. $400 a year.
- 2.8 billion people in the world live on less than U.S. $2 a day.
- Over 50 percent of the world's population lives on less than U.S. $2 per day.
- More than 1 billion people live in extreme poverty, defined as living on less than U.S. $1 a day.
- There are nearly 3 billion people living in extreme poverty around the world.

Hunger and Malnutrition:
- More than 1 billion children suffer from hunger.
- According to the United Nations (UN), every 3.6 seconds, a person in the world dies because of poverty and starvation.
- More than 800 million people go hungry each day.
- Annually, 6 million children die from malnutrition before their fifth birthday.

Gender and Age:
- Most of the individuals who die from starvation every 3.6 seconds are children under 5 years of age.
- Women work 67 percent of the world's working hours and produce 50 percent of the world's food.
- Women earn only 10 percent of the world's income and own less than 1 percent of the world's property.
- Women and children, who make up 70 percent of the population, are the poorest in the world.
- Women are often ignored by conventional banks and financial institutions because of their lack of assets.
- Thus, millions of women in developing countries struggle to meet the daily needs of their families, and their children go hungry and have no opportunity for education.

Education:
- Over 100 million primary-school-age children cannot afford to go to school.
- Limited schooling and lack of appropriate health education are some of the chronic issues that strongly correlate to high poverty rates with women.

Diseases:
- Over 11 million children die each year from preventable causes like malaria, diarrhea, and pneumonia.

Although the UN World Food Program attempts to alleviate poverty and hunger, many countries and regions that are stricken by poverty also experience correlating famines, diseases, and civil wars, which, as we might suspect from the information above, seriously impact women and children. For example, the child soldiers of Sierra Leone are not only poor but experience many traumas, including being drugged and forced to kill (Beah, 2007). In his memoir *A Long Way Gone*, Beah (2007) describes both his descent into the madness of a brutal civil war and his emergence from that horror into a second life in which he has used his literary gifts to call attention to the terrible practices. As another example, the millions of street children in Brazil suffer from abuse, drug addiction, and communicable diseases, including AIDS, and are beggars and prostitutes (Freire, 2004, 2006). Poverty for them is a way of life. The plight of the world's poor, for the most part, is misery, suffering, and hopelessness and is perpetuated across generations, leading to a culture of poverty. When we put poverty in a global context, we begin to realize the enormity of the situation.

Culture of Poverty

Although poverty in the United States may have different descriptors than those associated with global poverty, poverty, regardless of location, has correlates, which we have seen above. The combined effects create and perpetuate vulnerability and a culture of poverty. The effects of poverty on the general health and development of children are well known. In the United States, many poor schoolchildren go to school hungry and go home to an unsupervised environment. Going home to noise, fights, and street violence makes a young person unsafe and insecure. The lack of home support for literacy and other activities related to schooling makes the children more vulnerable to educational and social failure. Many drop out from school and join a gang, deal with drugs and other crimes, and eventually end up in jail. The lack of social and economic resources can lead to family violence and other crimes. Work (1991) writes,

> Children of poverty lack food, clothing, housing, medicine, and early learning assistance. These children face sickness, psychological stress, malnutrition, and underdevelopment. As poor children progress through the school system, they face school failure, pregnancy, substance abuse, and economic stress. Illiteracy in the poor is endemic and cyclic as poor children become poor parents of more poor children. (p. 61)

The culture of poverty is transmitted from one generation to the next.

Each of the problems identified in the preceding paragraph can increase the risk of disabling conditions, including language disorders. Poor mothers may not have received prenatal care during their pregnancies, and malnutrition and substance abuse can lead to premature delivery of babies with low birth weight. These babies have a substantially greater risk of incurring developmental problems, among them fetal alcohol syndrome, which is associated with conditions such as language-learning disabilities and intellectual disability. Even when poor children are born healthy, they can be raised in an environment that can be less stimulating and more dangerous than that of other children. As a result, they are likely to be delayed in certain areas of language learning compared to middle-class children. Poverty is also not disassociated with what might be familial transmission of specific language impairment (SLI), given the resultant literacy and consequent academic difficulties of SLI with the related vocational and economic limitations. This means that some children of poor parents may have an inherited language impairment because one or both of their parents have a language impairment. These children likely experience a language delay as a result of limited environmental and early literacy experiences and a language delay as a result of language impairment. These children also have difficulty acquiring new language skills easily in the context of environmental experiences because of their language impairment.

All professionals should differentiate between environmental conditions that result from cultural differences and those that are due to poverty. Nutritional choices, methods of discipline, and styles of verbal interaction all vary across cultural groups. Although differences in these behaviors may have relatively short-term effects on language learning or in another cultural group's expectations for language performance, they are not associated with a greater prevalence of language disorders. In contrast, the consequences of poverty (e.g., poor health care, poor nutrition, effects of drugs) can harm a child's nervous system, either at or even before birth or during the early formative years. Such damage can lead to long-term language deficits from which a child is unlikely to recover. Further, the number of displaced and stateless populations has grown over the last decade and these children have not had proper education, schooling, nutrition, and even shelter. Many have missed the opportunity to go to school and are illiterate.

ISSUES IN ASSESSMENT

It is estimated that 10 percent of the members of all racial/ethnic minority groups have disorders of speech, language, or hearing, the same percentage as the U.S. population as a whole (Deal-Williams, 2002). The unique issue in the case of linguistically-culturally diverse children is that their language can be evaluated and categorized in any of four different ways:

1. Typically developing and speaking SAE
2. Typically developing and speaking a nonstandard dialect or form influenced by another language
3. Atypically developing for language learning and speaking SAE
4. Atypically developing for language learning and speaking a nonstandard dialect or form influenced by another language

The key to a culturally fair differential assessment is to determine each child's dialectal status and not allow a language variation to interfere with the judgments made about language-learning ability. This requires an awareness of the structural and pragmatic differences found in the particular linguistic influences, a critical attitude toward assessment instruments, which may ignore the possibility of linguistic variation (Seymour, Roeper, de Villiers, & deVilliers, 2003), and a commitment to using dynamic assessment and other non-normed approaches.

Testing Bias

Norm-referenced testing is based on the premise of peer comparison. Stimuli are presented in an invariant manner to children of the same age so that their responses can be compared and each child's performance ranked. In order to determine a valid ranking, no child can be put at a disadvantage in responding to the test items. Thus, a child who is ill would not be tested, and special assistance must be provided if tests are to be used with children who have sensory or motor handicaps. It is sometimes more difficult to recognize the disadvantages faced by linguistically-culturally diverse children who undergo norm-referenced testing. There are obstacles to be overcome in nearly every aspect of the evaluation process (Sattler, 2001). Some of the most common are as follows:

1. *Cultural bias.* Many norm-referenced tests reflect white, middle-class backgrounds. This is typically seen in the choice of tasks and stimulus items. For example, it is routinely assumed that children will enjoy the activities of listening to stories, pointing to pictures, and answering requests for information. Such activities are common in middle-class households, and children from these homes have usually been reinforced extensively for taking part. But linguistically-culturally diverse children may lack these experiences. Hence, these children may arrive at a testing session unprepared and unmotivated for the kinds of activities that will be presented to them. For example, children from cultures with an oral tradition tend to focus on the storytellers and watch their facial expressions and gestures rather than focusing on the pages from a book.
2. *Examiner sensitivity bias.* Professionals who administer norm-referenced tests may not be familiar with the linguistic and cultural characteristics of the linguistically-culturally diverse children they are asked to evaluate. This condition opens up the possibility of several types of misinterpretation. Because of phonological influences of dialectal or second language and/or because of phonological/articulatory disorder, the speech of the linguistically-culturally diverse children may be only marginally intelligible to the examiner, who then must frequently ask for repetition or clarification. Such frequent requests can be interpreted by children as an indication that they are performing poorly, which may make them reluctant to participate in the assessment. Another source of misinterpretation may be the pragmatic behavior of a child. As we have seen, linguistically-culturally diverse children may differ in their pattern of eye contact and in their willingness to respond to requests for information. An examiner who is unaware of these

differences may construe these behaviors as nervousness, uncertainty, ignorance, defiance, or disorder. For example, children from Thailand are taught not to look authorities in the eyes, told to bow their head, and in greeting others are told to put their hands together in a cultural protocol called "wai," a behavior that must be followed.

3. *Examiner expectations bias.* The experiences of certain examiners may lead them to anticipate a particular pattern of behavior from linguistically-culturally diverse children. Although norm-referenced tests try to reduce variation in examiner procedures, some discretion is always allowed. For example, most tests do not specify how long an examiner must wait for a child to respond to an item. Most examiners rely on their intuition in deciding whether a child is still thinking or does not know an answer. This intuition is formed from previous experiences with children. If those experiences suggest that a child will perform poorly, then the examiner is less likely to believe that additional time will enable a correct response. The sensitivity of an examiner is a key to a successful assessment. When children look confused, it may be because they do not know what to do rather than not knowing the answers.
4. *Overinterpretation bias.* A danger attached to all norm-referenced assessments is that the examiner will draw broad conclusions from limited test data. For instance, it is inappropriate to conclude that a child's language comprehension is generally impaired when the only data to support this statement is a low score on a test of receptive vocabulary. With monolingual, middle-class children without issues of linguistic and cultural variation, such bias is avoided by administering more than one test and by combining information from norm-referenced and unnormed standardized assessment procedures. The same practice should be followed with linguistically-culturally diverse children. However, fewer tests are available that have been normed on these populations, and unnormed standardized assessment can be difficult without the assistance of someone knowledgeable about a child's linguistic and cultural background. The use of interpreters and informants can help to ensure that communication does not break down.
5. *Linguistic bias.* Some tests may contain English words or idioms that are unfamiliar to linguistically-culturally diverse children. This may reduce the number of items to which a child responds or may change the demands of a task. For example, a bilingual child may not know some of the English words for common household items, which are frequently used in tests because they are assumed to be familiar. As a specific example, Chinese children might recognize chopsticks and bowls but may not recognize a cup with a saucer. Language bias may also occur inadvertently in the idiomatic prompts and reinforcers used by the examiner, such as "Don't take your eyes off it" or "That's the way."

The problem of bias is not limited to tests or examiners. Linguistically-culturally diverse children are likely to vary their performance, depending on how they perceive a communicative situation. For example, African American children may not use AAE in settings that are perceived as formal. If children try to communicate in SAE and they do not know this dialect as well as AAE, the results of the assessment will be misleadingly low. On the other hand, children who are able to code switch effectively from AAE to SAE may leave the impression that they speak only the standard dialect.

The concern over test bias applies to all instruments used to evaluate children's developmental abilities. Federal education law (the Individuals with Disabilities Education Act) mandates that all students be evaluated using nondiscriminatory evaluations and multiple forms of assessment. The act also requires that students be assessed in their native language or other mode of communication. If tests are not available in the student's native language, interpreters should be used. For students identified as limited English proficient, tests should focus on assessing the impact of the child's disability on his or her educational performance rather than assessing the child's English language skills.

Norm-referenced intelligence tests have long been criticized for underestimating the competence of linguistically-culturally diverse children. To reduce the bias inherent in intelligence instruments, one proposal has been that they be administered to linguistically-culturally diverse children only in a translated form. Translation of test items is difficult, however, without affecting the validity and sensitivity of the test. An alternative approach is sometimes to develop norms for specific ethnic groups, as has been done, for example, for the Wechsler Intelligence Scale for Children—Third Edition administered to Navajo children (Tempest, 1998).

For many years, norm-referenced language tests and other assessment procedures have been analyzed for evidence of bias. Examples of findings from the literature over several decades are the following:

- From kindergarten to fourth grade, African American students obtained increasingly lower scores than white students on the Grammatic Closure subtest of the Illinois Test of Psycholinguistic Abilities (Kirk, McCarthy, & Kirk, 1968). This appears to be due to the appearance of more AAE grammatical features in older African American students (Arnold & Reed, 1976).
- African American children in Head Start programs in a rural area of Alabama scored significantly lower on the Preschool Language Assessment Instrument (Blank, Rose, & Berlin, 1978) than white children from the same programs (Haynes, Haak, Moran, Rice, & Johnson, 1995). On components of the same tool that tap higher level, decentralized, and metalinguistic tasks (Levels III and IV), African American children in Georgia again performed significantly lower than their white peers (Fagundes, Haynes, Haak, & Moran, 1998).
- On another preschool language test, the Preschool Language Scale—3 (Zimmerman, Steiner, & Pond, 1992), African American preschoolers from low-income families scored an average of one standard deviation below the expected mean for their age, primarily because of their poor performance on items containing language features not part of their dialect (Qi, Kaiser, Milan, Yzquierdo, & Hancock, 2003).
- Both white and African American children from a rural area of northeastern Georgia obtained scores on the Wepman Auditory Discrimination Test (Wepman, 1958) that were lower than those predicted by the test's norms (Hirshoren & Ambrose, 1976).
- African American children matched for age and grade level with white children obtained statistically lower scores on the Peabody Picture Vocabulary Test (Dunn, 1965; Kreschek & Nicolosi, 1973). On the Peabody Picture Vocabulary Test—III (Dunn & Dunn, 1997), approximately 40 percent of the low-income African American preschoolers enrolled in Head Start who participated in the research scored greater than one standard deviation below the mean (Champion, Hyter, McCabe, & Bland-Stewart, 2003). Maternal education and the socioeconomic status of the families of African American children can likely influence the children's performances on this vocabulary test, with children whose mothers have no high school diploma and those from lower-SES families scoring notably lower than those with mothers with college degrees and those from middle-SES families (Horton-Ikard & Ellis Weismer, 2007; Qi, Kaiser, Milan, Yzquierdo, & Hancock, 2006; Restrepo et al., 2006).
- According to Teuber and Furlong's (1985) study, the scores of bilingual Hispanic children were almost two standard deviations below the mean for monolingual children on both the Expressive One-Word Picture Vocabulary Test (Gardner, 1979, 1983) and the Peabody Picture Vocabulary Test—Revised (Dunn & Dunn, 1981).
- Hispanic American and African American preschool children were more successful at imitating sentences containing AAE features, while their white counterparts performed better with SAE stimuli (Stephens, 1976).
- The Test of Language Development (Newcomer & Hammill, 1977), when administered to young AAE-speaking children, yielded scores significantly lower than those reported in the norms (Wiener, Lewnau, & Erway, 1983) and on the Test of Language Development—P:2 (Newcomer & Hammill, 1991). African American children received significantly lower total scores on all of the five core subtests than white children, and a substantial proportion of specific test items were biased in that they were more difficult for the African American children (Hammer, Pennock-Roman, Rzasa, & Tomblin, 2002).
- A wide range of scores has been obtained when the Spanish version of the Test for Auditory Comprehension of Language (Carrow, 1973) has been administered to different

> groups of Hispanic American children (Linares-Orama & Sanders, 1977; Rueda & Perozzi, 1977; Wilcox & Aasby, 1988). This variation appears to be due to differences in the socioeconomic status and educational experiences of the different subject groups. Similarly, Spanish-speaking bilingual children with normal language skills performed notably below the norms on the Spanish Version of the Preschool Language Scale—3 (Zimmerman, Steiner, & Pond, 1993), further indicating potential bias even in tests designed to be appropriate for bilingual children (Restrepo & Silverman, 2001).

Another potential source of bias—but one not always thought of—involves applying age-based norms of tests to children from linguistically and culturally diverse backgrounds. There are times when the true ages of some of these children cannot be determined because of a lack of birth records or missing paperwork.

It is apparent, therefore, that many norm-referenced language tests are significantly biased against linguistically-culturally diverse children. However, Stockman, in her interview for *The ASHA Leader* (Saad & Polovoy, 2009), cautioned us that we have not known much about how such tests might potentially be used in helpful ways, along with other assessments, to better identify children from linguistically-culturally diverse backgrounds. Nevertheless, the issue of test bias is of enormous concern to professional organizations involved in debates over assessment practices. Such concern, along with other efforts to increase professional awareness of multiculturalism, has prompted publishers to revise existing tests and develop new instruments that better meet the needs of linguistically-culturally diverse children. Examples are the Diagnostic Evaluation of Language Variance (DELV)—Screening Test (DELV-Screening) (Seymour et al., 2003) and Diagnostic Evaluation of Language Variation—Norm-Referenced (DELV-Norm-Referenced) (Seymour, Roeper, deVilliers, & deVilliers, 2005), which are language tests described as attempting to neutralize the impact of a child's use of nonmainstream American English on results. While these efforts to revise tests and develop new ones are positive steps in addressing the issues of test bias and producing valuable and useful assessment instruments, it is not always a strategy as successful or valid as it might appear (Anderson, 1996; Restrepo, 1998; Restrepo & Silverman, 2001). As we will see later in this chapter, renorming and/or translation of language tests that were developed initially for English-only, SAE-speaking children without validating, and likely modifying content and renorming the test, are fraught with multiple psychometric dangers, and thus, making the tests invalid.

Baker's (2000) Bilingual Family Profile can be helpful to professionals in reducing potential sources of bias in their language assessment. The Profile consists of nine elements, listed below, and a comprehensive assessment should be able to provide information about the child for each of the nine elements. Together, the combined information can provide a relatively complete picture of a child's language strengths and weaknesses. Elements of the profile include the following:

1. Development
2. Sequence
3. Competence
4. Function
5. Linguistic concepts
6. Interaction
7. Attitude
8. Conflicts/motivations
9. Exogenous aspects

The first and foremost important element is the history of a child's language development. The second element to be considered is the sequence of language exposure—which language was introduced first and which language was introduced later or which languages were introduced at the same time. The third is the informant's overall impression of the language competence of the child. The fourth is about what functions each language serves. The fifth element deals with the concepts learned from each of the languages. For example, some children learn about their home and items related to their home in their home language and learn concepts about school in their school language. The sixth is the interactions—who are the interactants, and what is the quality of the interactions? A child who is cared for mostly by a nanny may have a very limited vocabulary if the nanny basically takes care of the child's daily needs but is not engaged in verbal stimulation. The seventh element is attitude. Some children are eager to learn languages, and others are not. Children with language disorders are often among those less interested in learning language, regardless of what the language might be. This is an important factor to consider in taking the history of the child in question. The eighth element to consider is the potential conflicts and motivation about language learning. Some parents insist on their children speaking English, but they, themselves, can barely use the English language. Others are motivated to learn English. The final element includes all other exogenous factors that may impact on the language-learning process. Professionals need to consider each of these in assessing linguistically-culturally diverse children.

We know that children's production of narratives can especially reflect cultural differences. It is essential, therefore, that professionals attempt to consider the ways in which storytelling activities are reflected in children's particular cultures so that these can be analyzed in ways that do not lead to biased interpretations and misidentify different narrative structures, content, or sequences as evidence of impairment. These differences might be quite appropriate and consistent with expectations in the children's home and cultures. It is possible, however, that differences identified as culturally based can become a bridge to helping children learn other ways of conveying narratives that are more consistent with the mainstream classroom in which they are needing to function (Westby & Roman, 1995).

Differential Diagnosis of Communicative Behaviors

Professionals who work with linguistically-culturally diverse children face the challenge of distinguishing between language differences and language disorders. The principles and requirements of this task were stated succinctly in a 1983 position paper and have remained relevant since:

> No dialectal variety of English is a disorder or a pathological form of speech or language. Each social dialect is adequate as a functional and effective variety of English. . . . It is indeed possible for dialect speakers to have linguistic disorders within the dialect. An essential step toward making accurate assessments of communicative disorders is to distinguish between those aspects of linguistic variation that represent the diversity of the English language from those that represent speech, language, and hearing disorders. The SLP must have certain competencies to distinguish between dialectal differences and communicative disorders. These competencies include knowledge of the particular dialect as a rule-governed linguistic system, knowledge of the phonological and grammatical features of the dialect, and knowledge of nondiscriminatory testing procedures. (ASHA Committee on the Status of Racial Minorities, 1983).

The process of language assessment for linguistically-culturally diverse children follows the usual steps of screening and assessment, with a few additional considerations. Figure 9.1 illustrates the progression of a language evaluation for such a child. Because not all minority children are bilingual or use a nonstandard dialect, step 1 is to screen the child with an instrument that is based on and standardized for SAE. A passing score on this screening would tend to establish that a child is not language impaired but rather language different. However, children who fail the initial screening in SAE should then be tested in their native or nonstandard dialect (Peña, Bedore, & Rappazzo, 2003). This can help determine whether the child has competence in the second language or nonstandard dialect. If a child passes a screening in the second language or nonstandard dialect, there is greater evidence to believe that the child is not language impaired but rather language different. As Brice (2002) states, "It is not possible for a child to have a language disorder only in one language" (p. 48). A linguistically diverse child will exhibit a language impairment in both languages. This is among the essential evidence that the assessment process is looking for if a diagnosis of language impairment is to be appropriately made.

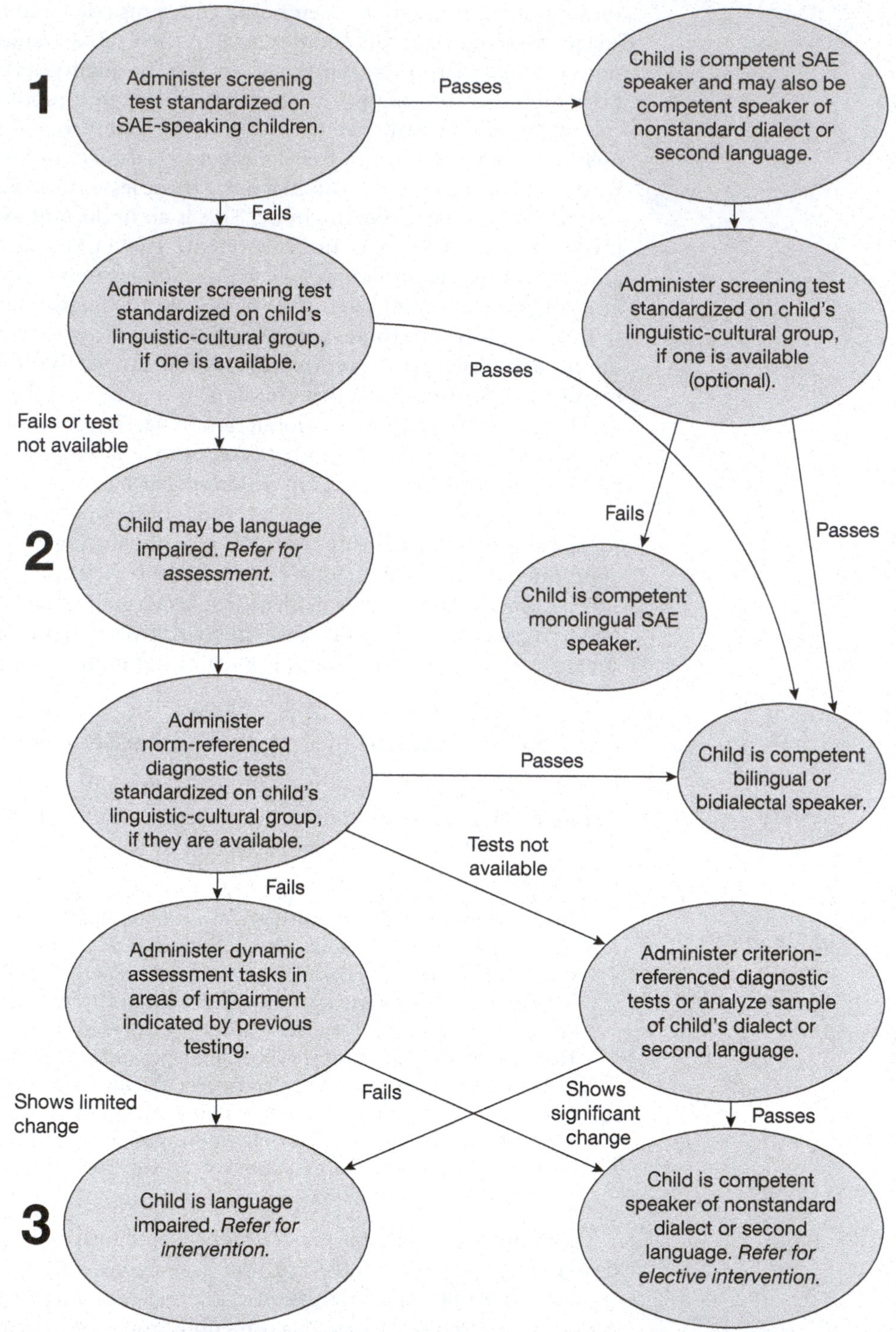

FIGURE 9.1 | Model of Differential Diagnosis for Linguistically-Culturally Diverse Children

Children who fail both language screenings arrive at step 2. These children should now be evaluated more fully to determine whether they are actually language impaired. Hemsley, Holm, and Dodd (2014) provide important advice for implementing culturally sensitive differential diagnosis for language differences and language disorder:

> Diagnosis requires the implementation of a range of alternative assessment techniques. No single methodology provides a definitive conclusion of difference versus disorder. A range of assessments considered together, however, provide a strong body of evidence outlining a child's language abilities in their unique cultural context. (p. 101)

If nonbiased, norm-referenced tests are available, they can be administered as one element in a range of assessment tasks. If a child receives passing scores on these tests, the result of the screenings would be discarded, and the child would be assessed as a competent speaker of a second language or nonstandard dialect. If appropriate norm-referenced instruments do not exist to suit a particular child, then criterion-referenced tests, often involving dynamic assessment tasks, or language sampling can be used to evaluate competence as other elements in the assessment process. Language samples can be obtained by recording conversation that occurs during play. During this interaction, however, care should be taken to avoid the kinds of interactions (e.g., interview) that are uncommon among members of certain racial/ethnic groups. Samples gathered in settings familiar to the children or while interacting with family members may increase the ecological validity of the samples (Gutiérrez-Clellen, Restrepo, Bedore, Peña, & Anderson, 2000; Hemsley et al., 2014). Collecting samples during parent–child interactions and/or peer-child interactions, in which the peer is not suspected of having a language impairment, provides the opportunity to compare a child's linguistic patterns to those of a competent language user (Hemsley et al., 2014; Terrell, Arensberg, & Rosa, 1992). This approach is known as a Parent (or Peer)-Child Comparative Analysis (PCCA). With all approaches, the samples that are gathered should be evaluated using developmental criteria that have been well referenced for the speech community to which a child belongs. For example, Black English Sentence Scoring (Nelson & Hyter, 1990), an adaptation of Developmental Sentence Scoring (DSS) (Lee, 1974), represents an attempt to honor the grammatical features of AAE as well as to compare young African American children to their linguistic peers. Toronto (1976) developed a variation of the DSS, the Developmental Assessment of Spanish Grammar, to examine the grammatical proficiency of Spanish-speaking children. As another example of an approach that attempts to reflect language features of non-SAE-speaking children, the Systematic Analysis of Language Transcripts (SALT) (Miller, Andriacchi, & Nockerts, 2015) provides procedures for collecting and analyzing samples for both Spanish-speaking and AAE-speaking children. Contrastive analysis is another procedure that can assist in differentiating which characteristics children exhibit in samples of their language represent patterns congruent with their first language or dialect and which are error patterns representing a language impairment (McGregor, Williams, Hearst, & Johnson, 1997). Characteristics representative of their primary language or dialect are likely due to a language difference, whereas error patterns that are inconsistent with their language or dialect are more likely the result of language impairment. However, contrastive analysis requires that the examiner be familiar with characteristics and features of the dialect or language of interest. In cases where the examiner is not bilingual or bidialectal, a PCCA analysis and/or collecting local norms derived from the children's linguistic environments can assist examiners in achieving reasonable degrees of familiarity with the language or dialect. Additional avenues for becoming familiar with other languages or dialects in order to conduct a contrastive analysis involve consulting literature that describes communicative and linguistic features of various languages and dialects, including the earlier sections of this chapter, professional interpreters, and representative members of the speech communities of the children who can act as cultural or linguistic brokers. Cultural and linguistic brokers are individuals in children's speech and/or cultural communities who can explain aspects of cultural experiences and/or inform about particular linguistic characteristics and communication norms (ASHA, n.d.).

Children who fail norm-referenced assessments using culturally and linguistically fair test instruments or who show problems in their language samples that have been evaluated with culturally and linguistically appropriate analysis approaches should then undergo dynamic assessment trials in those areas of language that appear deficient. If the child shows significant positive changes in their language behaviors during these trials, the poor test scores can be attributed to cultural differences rather than an underlying language impairment (Peña, Iglesias, & Lidz, 2001; Ukrainetz, Harpell, Walsh, & Coyle, 2000). Intervention in that case should focus on the elective goal of helping the child adjust to the mainstream culture and its methods of evaluation. However, if the child responds poorly to dynamic assessment—fails to attend or generalize new language learning—then intervention for language impairment should proceed (step 3), still with consideration of the child's multicultural needs.

The protocol just described and shown in Figure 9.1 is truly workable only if more nondiscriminatory norm-referenced assessment instruments become available. As a first step, some tests written in SAE and originally normed on mostly mainstream populations have been renormed on minority populations. Such an approach is inadequate, however, because it serves only to verify that a child is incompetent as a speaker of SAE. What is needed are measures that can establish children's competencies in their native languages or nonstandard dialects. To serve this purpose, the tests must be conceived and developed specifically to evaluate a minority population. For example, in the case of AAE speakers, test tasks and stimulus items should be developed and field tested with African American children to ensure that they are both motivating and familiar. The norming population for the test must be representative of AAE speakers nationwide, including accounting for socioeconomic differences that can affect the degree to which children's language includes features of AAE (Craig et al., 2009). In line with these requirements is Stockman's (1996b) Minimal Competency Core, which seeks to identify the linguistic components that differentiate typically developing and language-impaired children learning AAE. Investigations of the phonological and grammatical systems of AAE-speaking children have found that the features that best identify those with language impairments are ones shared between AAE and SAE (Bleile & Wallach, 1992; Seymour, Bland-Stewart, & Green, 1998). Thus, traditional measures of language performance, such as the number of different words, mean length of utterances, or complex syntactic constructions used in a language sample, can be used to identify children with language impairment when they speak a nonstandard dialect (Craig & Washington, 2000) or even speak another language in addition to learning English (Bedore, Peña, Gillam, & Hoa, 2010). The task of differentiation is made easier as normative data on the performance of minority populations become more widely available (Craig & Washington, 2002).

For children who speak languages other than English, the procedure of using traditional measures of language performance, such as the number of different words, mean length of utterances, or complex syntactic constructions used in a language sample, as noted above in reference to children who use a nonstandard dialect, is a key component of differential language assessment for these children. However, for children who are exposed to and are learning English in addition to one or more other languages, assessment must be conducted in each language in order to achieve adequate accuracy of differential classification, that is, language different, language impaired, language different and language impaired (Peña & Bedore, 2011). Therefore, such measures need to be derived from language samples collected in both languages.

As we noted previously, tests that were developed and normed for one language in one cultural context cannot be translated or modified by altering items (for example, using the Thai word for *fork* when asking a child exposed to Thai as the first language to point to the picture of a fork from a choice of four pictures, as in a receptive vocabulary test developed for SAE children) and maintain the validity and reliability of the tests. Frequencies with which words occur in languages and cultures differ, and therefore, children are differentially familiar with vocabulary words. (Relevant to our example, in Thailand the traditional and more frequently used utensil is a spoon, so we can expect that a child exposed to Thai as the first language would be less familiar with the item and the word *fork*, thus making it likely a more developmentally difficult word than in English.)

Currently, more tests and other assessment materials exist in Spanish than in any other foreign language. Table 9.13 presents a list of some of the child language tests available in Spanish. We can see that the list includes both language tests such as the Preschool Language Scales—Fifth Edition: Spanish Edition (Zimmerman, Steiner, & Pond, 2002) and parent report measures such as the MacArthur Inventarios del Desarrollo de Habilidades Comunicativas (Jackson-Maldonado et al., 2003). Although initially some of these instruments were developed in English and then translated into Spanish, a practice we now know is not psychometrically valid, more recent revisions of a number of them more accurately represent the Spanish language and its several dialects as well as experiences Hispanic American children might encounter as part of their cultural heritages. Nevertheless, it is important always to be alert to the possibility such versions of tests may or may not demonstrate good validity (Gutiérrez-Clellen et al., 2000; Restrepo & Silverman, 2001; Thal, Jackson-Maldonado,

TABLE 9.13 | Some Child Language Tests in Spanish

Test Name	Author(s)
Bilingual English Spanish Assessment (BESA)	Peña, Gutiérrez-Clellen, Iglesias, Goldstein, and Bedore (2014)
Bilingual English Spanish Oral Screener—Experimental Version (BESOS)	Peña, Bedore, Iglesias, Gutiérrez-Clellen, and Goldstein (2008)
Bracken Basic Concept Scale—Third Edition: Expressive (BBCS-3:E)—Spanish Adaptation	Bracken (2006a)
Bracken Basic Concept Scale—Third Edition: Receptive (BBCS-3:R)—Spanish Adaptation	Bracken (2006b)
Clinical Evaluation of Language Fundamentals—4 (Spanish) (CELF-4 Spanish)	Semel, Wiig, and Secord (2005)
Clinical Evaluation of Language Fundamentals (Preschool-2) (Spanish Edition) (CELF-Preschool-2 Spanish)	Wiig, Secord, and Semel (2009)
Expressive One-Word Picture Vocabulary Test—4: Spanish-Bilingual (EOWPVT-4:SBE)	Martin (2012a)
MacArthur Inventarios del Desarrollo de Habilidades Comunicativas	Jackson-Maldonado et al., (2003)
Preschool Language Scales—Fifth Edition: Spanish Edition (PLS-5 Spanish)	Zimmerman, Steiner, and Pond (2012a)
Preschool Language Scales Spanish Screening Test—Fifth Edition (PLSSST-5)	Zimmerman, Steiner, and Pond (2012b)
Receptive One-Word Picture Vocabulary Test—4: Spanish-Bilingual Edition (ROWPVT-4:SBE)	Martin (2012b)
Spanish Structured Photographic Expressive Language Test—3 (Spanish SPELT-3)	Langdon (2012)
Test of Early Language Development—3: Spanish (TELD-3:S)	Ramos, Ramos, Hresko, Reid, and Hammill (2007)
The Rossetti Infant-Toddler Scale	Rossetti (2006)
W-ABC Spanish Version	Wiig and Langdon (2006)

& Acosta, 2000). We need to keep in mind also that there are different dialects of Spanish and that what may be appropriate vocabulary and cultural assumptions for a Mexican American child may not be suitable for a child from El Salvador. Professionals need to evaluate these assessment instruments for adequate validity and reliability as thoroughly as they do for the other assessment instruments they use.

We saw previously that in all cases of assessment involving children who speak and have exposure to languages other than English, language sample analyses need to be conducted in each of a child's languages. This applies also to use of norm-referenced tests; children need to be tested in each of their languages. To do this, the examiner must possess "native or near-native proficiency" in the second language in addition to English proficiency (ASHA, 2016). However, this creates challenges for achieving valid assessment when there are discrepancies between the number of linguistically-culturally diverse children who require differential language assessment and the number of professionals who are qualified to conduct language assessments and are able to work in language forms other than SAE or who are from linguistically-culturally diverse backgrounds. SLPs are the professionals with the qualifications to conduct these assessments, but most of the SLPs in the United States are monolingual SAE speakers. As of the end of 2015, only 6.5 percent of the SLP members of

TABLE 9.14 | Cheng's (2006) RIOT Procedure

R Review	*I* Interview	*O* Observe	*T* Test
Review of all relevant data including the nine factors described by Baker (2000) listed earlier.	Interview all the people who are providers for the child, including parents, caretakers, other family members, and teachers.	Observe behaviors in various contexts with different interactants.	Test using dynamic assessment and other authentic test procedures.

ASHA identified themselves as being bilingual (excluding American Sign Language) (ASHA, 2016), and as of the end of 2014, only about 2.7 percent of the SLP membership was African American and about 3.6 percent was Hispanic American. Previously we introduced several options that might be used to help an examiner approach analyses of language samples if the examiner does not have bilingual or bidialectal skills. However, administration of norm-referenced tests raises the standard for the level of examiners' language proficiency to that of native or near-native levels. Interpreters and/or cultural or linguistic brokers may be necessary to assist in the assessment (ASHA, n.d.). If a parent or relative, community member, or even a professional interpreter serves this role, time must be allowed for adequate instruction and training for them regarding the purposes, procedures, and goals of the assessment. Working with interpreters, whether family members or professional interpreters, is far from straightforward and not an easily implemented alternative.

The RIOT process that Cheng (2006) has described provides a set of guidelines for professionals to use in assisting them to obtain an overall impression of a child's communicative performance. Table 9.14 explains this acronym—review, interview, observe, test—and provides a description of each element. The results from the RIOT procedures can form the basis for intervention and action plans appropriate to each child.

IMPLICATIONS FOR INTERVENTION

Language assessment of linguistically-culturally diverse children can have three different outcomes:

1. Intervention is not recommended for children who are competent users of SAE and who may also be competent users of another dialect or language.
2. *Therapeutic language intervention* is recommended for children who fail to show competence in *any* language or dialect.
3. *Elective language intervention* is recommended for children who are not competent users of SAE but who are competent in a nonstandard dialect or a language other than English.

The distinction between therapeutic and elective language intervention is based on the view that the traditional role of a language professional is to provide services to the communicatively disordered individuals, whereas children who do not use SAE may not be impaired in their ability to communicate; they merely communicate through another language form. Hence, following the traditional model, intervention would not be recommended for them. Nevertheless, professionals recognize that individuals who do not use SAE may be penalized educationally, socially, or vocationally. Recall we previously highlighted that there is evidence that the degree to which children use more AAE features in their spoken language correlates with poorer reading achievement (Charity et al., 2004; Connor & Craig, 2006; Craig et al., 2009). Many children or their parents may, therefore, request intervention to develop skills in the use of SAE. SLPs are often consulted regarding the issues of language differences and asked to assist in the teaching of English for school-age children and to assist reading specialists to help students with limited skills with SAE to code switch as a strategy to improve their literacy skills. SLPs have the expertise and skills to share best-practice models for language development with colleagues and serve as consultants in such cases. And, as Response to Intervention (RtI) models become more fully implemented in schools where the expertise and skills of SLPs are recognized in working with language and literacy of students who struggle with literacy and learning because of language delays in the absence of language impairment, we could anticipate greater SLP involvement in helping teachers and linguistically-culturally diverse children without language impairment.

Intervention for Language Differences and Language Disorders

Children recommended for therapeutic language intervention need to develop competence with some language form, whether it is Standard English, nonstandard English, or a language other than English. It is likely that many of the linguistically-culturally diverse children who are language impaired and learning English along with another language or a nonstandard dialect of English have a *low mixed language dominance*; that is, they combine elements of English and another language or dialect to form a mixture that is inadequate by the standards of both languages or dialects. Mixing of language elements is, by itself, not a sign of language disorder. Children with normal language-learning abilities whose language is influenced by a nonstandard dialect of English or another language may show signs of mixing. Language mixing is a normal part of the development for many children with normal language-learning abilities who are exposed to more than one language or dialect. Good models will help them distinguish between the two, and in general, with time and exposure, these children will be able to use the two separately in appropriate contexts. Among typically developing children, the acquisition of more than one language or dialect may slow rate of acquisition for the new language/dialect temporarily but not do so for extended periods. And, these children typically demonstrate competence in the other language or dialect or demonstrate the ability to learning elements of the other under conditions of dynamic assessment. However, this is typically not true for children with a language impairment. The different rules for phonology and grammar, the greater vocabulary load, and the need to master the subtleties of code switching all can place additional demands on the children with language impairment without necessarily improving the child's communicative effectiveness. The routine practice, therefore, is for professionals to begin by determining which language form will serve as the primary target of intervention.

There are several factors that must be considered in determining which language form will serve as the primary target of intervention:

- *Dominant language or dialect.* Although children receiving therapeutic intervention are not competent in any language form, they may show greater strength in one than another. For example, a 4-year-old Asian American child from Korea may respond to simple commands in both Korean and English but display a larger receptive vocabulary in English. The child may speak in both languages but produce only minor or formulaic utterances in Korean, in contrast to two- and three-word generative combinations in English. In both languages, then, the competence is less than would be expected of a typically developing child of this age, yet English appears to be the dominant language. The possibility should also be considered that a child will have "domain-specific" competencies in different languages, for example, better speaking ability in one language but better reading ability in another (American Educational Research Association, American Psychological Association, & National Council on Measurement and Education, 1999). Even though intervention may focus on one language, there is increasingly a case being made to maintain bilingual input to children with language impairment (Cheng, 2007a; Gutiérrez-Clellen, 1999; Kohnert, Windsor, & Ebert, 2009; Langdon & Cheng, 2009).
- *Availability of service provider.* If intervention is to be provided in a language form other than SAE, it must be conducted by a professional or by an interpreter who is fully proficient in that other language. In cases where the professionals are bilingual and speak the

home language of the students, bilingual language therapy or home language therapy can be used. However, as we saw previously, this may not be possible given the shortage of professionals with necessary qualifications. In many instances, therefore, professionals will need to rely on an interpreter or substantially improve their knowledge of a nonstandard dialect, such as AAE.

- *Parental preference.* In all language intervention, the support and assistance of a child's parents is essential. This will obviously be difficult if (1) the parents are opposed to the proposed language form selected for intervention, (2) they themselves are not proficient in that language form, and/or (3) they have different culturally based beliefs about adult–child communication patterns and/or education and health services for children and their families, and child-rearing practices. Some parents want their children to become SAE speakers even though they themselves may not be. Families may insist that their children learn SAE, as it is viewed as crucial to their economic improvement and cultural assimilation. Parent counseling may help to create an optimal language-learning environment at home and at school.
- *Speech community.* One of the most important insights that sociolinguistic study affords us is that language develops within a cultural context. We learn to speak and understand the variety of language used by those with whom we live and interact. For children, this means that peers and adult supervisors (parents, teachers, day care providers, relatives, and so on) will be the most important linguistic influences.

Once a language form is chosen as the target for intervention, goals should be formulated that will increase the linguistically-culturally diverse child's language competence. In the main, the process of goal selection should observe the same principles as with mainstream language-impaired children. Some multicultural materials are available that may enhance a child's progress by providing stimuli that are more personally relevant. The major differences in the intervention procedure will be to (1) identify instances when a child's performance in the target language form appears to be influenced by the other language or dialect, (2) use assistants as models when necessary, and (3) clearly identify what is an acceptable target behavior. An example of the first point is that Hispanic American children being taught SAE syntax may be slow to learn interrogative reversals because of interference from Spanish syntax. This does not affect the manner in which the form is introduced (operant learning, modeling, and so on), but it does lead to a different expectation for how quickly the children will progress with that form. A case could be made for initially avoiding certain target forms when large degrees of interference can be anticipated. As we have already seen, this means the intervention professional needs to be familiar or become familiar with the linguistic features of the other language or dialect. And, as we have already outlined, there are multiple avenues and resources available to these professionals.

If intervention is not able to ensure that correct models are presented, the use of an assistant who can present stimuli under the guidance of the professional may be required. The intervention task and the stimuli to be presented should be worked out in advance so that the interaction with the child is as natural and uninterrupted as possible. Similarly, professionals must identify, perhaps with the assistant's, parents', or linguistic/cultural broker's help, what are acceptable responses to certain tasks. Once these are determined, the professional and the supporting individuals may share the job of reinforcing the behaviors when they are produced by the child. The parents, assistants, and/or brokers can also help to select what are culturally as well as linguistically appropriate intervention objectives and even intervention materials.

Intervention for Language Differences

Elective language intervention can occur under the following circumstances:

- A child is a proficient speaker of a nonstandard dialect or language other than English.
- The child or his or her parents request intervention to facilitate the acquisition of SAE.

- Resources are available to support elective intervention for children with language differences as well as therapeutic intervention for children with language impairment.

The proficiency of these linguistically-culturally diverse children in a language form other than SAE means that they are competent language learners and should respond well to instruction. This conclusion, in turn, provides a rationale for working with the children in larger groups and using teacher aides and peer instructors to maximize resources. The role of the professional may vary from providing direct, individualized instruction to consulting with teachers, conducting in-service training, and collaborating in classroom activities.

With the increasing body of evidence that links degree of use of AAE features in speaking and degree of code switching between AAE and SAE with reading proficiency (Charity et al., 2004; Connor & Craig, 2006; Craig & Washington, 2004; Craig et al., 2009), we could anticipate that the argument for providing elective intervention for children who have sizable numbers of AAE features in their speech and are also struggling with literacy will strengthen. This argument would be consistent with RtI frameworks that include providing specialist services for children without diagnosed disabilities but with educational achievement challenges. An overarching goal of such intervention would be to assist these typically developing children to learn the features of SAE to become effective code switchers.

Despite this emerging evidence providing reasons for providing assistance for linguistically-culturally diverse children who might struggle with literacy acquisition, the practice of elective language intervention remains controversial and raises issues of ethnic identity, nationalism, economics, and professional training. To some extent, the issues are different for speakers of nonstandard dialects and speakers of languages other than English. In 1977, a lawsuit was brought in Ann Arbor, Michigan, by African American elementary schoolchildren because they were faring poorly as a result of the disadvantage they faced because they were required to speak and read SAE in school even though they were speakers of AAE (*Martin Luther King Jr. Elementary School Children v. Ann Arbor School District Board*, 1977). The interpretation of the problem was not the use of SAE in the classroom but the fact that teachers were insensitive to the African American children's problems with learning related to AAE dialectal use. The solution devised by the Ann Arbor School Board, under court order, was to organize in-service programs to increase teachers' awareness of AAE and improve their ability to teach SAE to the African American children.

The issue of ethnic sensitivity involves a different response in the case of children who speak little or no English. Politically, it has been more difficult to make the case that these children should receive special instruction to help them make the transition to the use of SAE. As of 2009, 29 states had declared by statute, resolution, or constitutional amendment that English was the official language of the state (Mujica, 2009). The effect of these laws has been mixed, and they have been challenged in court. However, they speak to the concern many citizens feel over the increasing linguistic diversity of the United States, in large part because of apprehension that programs to accommodate non-English-speaking children will take resources away from other aspects of public education.

There is disagreement over which group of professionals should be responsible for elective language intervention. Some within the field of SLP feel competent to serve as teachers and are supportive of the practice. The position of ASHA is that SLPs may, by virtue of their individual experiences and education, be qualified to provide English as a second language (ESL) instruction. Others argue that elective intervention, especially for non-English speakers, requires skills, such as those possessed by teachers with specific training and credentialing in ESL education, which are not possessed by SLPs. Without such skills, SLPs might better limit their role to collaboration with ESL instructors in providing assessment and/or intervention services in school settings (ASHA, 2001; Cheng, 2007a). However, as we noted previously, increasing implementation of RtI in schools may lead to greater involvement of SLPs in order to capitalize on their expertise on how children learn language and in facilitating children's language learning beyond their essential role in differential diagnosis of children with language impairment with language differences and children with language differences only.

At least three distinct purposes for elective language intervention can be identified. It may be that some but not all of these objectives are relevant to professionals in different settings:

1. *Acculturation.* Especially in conditions where linguistically-culturally diverse children are a small minority, the mastery of SAE may help the development of peer relationships and facilitate interactions with adults at school and in the community.
2. *Career opportunity.* Difficulty in obtaining work is a problem that many children will face in the future if they do not speak SAE. It is futile to prepare children in other areas if they will be denied opportunities because of their language differences.
3. *Literacy instruction.* This was the basis of the Ann Arbor litigation, and it remains a significant issue. The only form of English that is written—apart from creative works—is the standard dialect. For literacy success, therefore, a child must learn that dialect for the purposes of, at a minimum, code switching for the purposes of reading and writing achievement. We have already seen the emerging evidence with regard to the association between AAE use and reading difficulty. Experience with Hispanic American children suggests that their reading success correlates with their oral language proficiency (Gottardo, 2002; Quiroga, Lemos-Britton, Mostafapour, Abbott, & Berninger, 2002). However, it is also important to recognize that lack of English proficiency is not the sole cause of poor reading skills. Other factors that must be considered are cultural differences in family attitudes toward literacy, as well as low motivation and low educational aspirations that are the result of discrimination (Snow, Burns, & Griffin, 1998).

If the decision is made to support elective language intervention for linguistically-culturally diverse children, instructional procedures should be tailored to match their age, environment, and language needs. Young children who speak languages other than English are often mainstreamed successfully in classes of predominantly SAE-speaking peers. They may require some initial support in making their needs known, and some of them will be silent for an extended period before they begin speaking in English. In circumstances where bilingual children form a sizable percentage of a class, mainstreaming may need to be supplemented with special programs to introduce ESL, an acronym that refers to "English as a Second Language." The terms "English Language Learner" (ELL) and "English as a New Language" (ENL) are now appearing in the literature as replacements for the term ESL. A committee on ENL was established in 2009 (Cheng, 2010) to address issues encountered by ENL learners.

Children who use a nonstandard dialect should receive instruction targeted at contrasting structures in SAE. For example, speakers of AAE may benefit from SAE practice in the use of the copula, the formation of indirect questions, and the use of negation (*see* Table 9.8). Children can benefit from practice in code switching from nonstandard to standard dialectal forms within the same communication task. Emphasizing the relation of spoken AAE and SAE to written forms of SAE is an important component of intervention.

A child's age must be considered in relation to interference effects and to the amount of time available for instruction. In general, older nonnative speakers of English will have more difficulty with interference from their native languages. The same might be presumed to be true for speakers of nonstandard dialects. In both cases, however, a child's age may be offset by a high motivation to learn SAE. The linguistic needs of older children are more immediate, as they have fewer remaining years of school. In this case, professionals may opt for a more intense and selective approach to instruction, emphasizing those features of SAE that will most improve the intelligibility and broad public acceptability of an individual's communication.

Intervention for Linguistically-Culturally Diverse Children with Other Disabilities

As we have seen in many of the chapters in this book, the underlying deficits of intellectual disabilities, autism, specific language impairment, and other developmental disorders have particular negative effects on language acquisition mechanisms. Linguistically-culturally diverse children with these deficits are especially at risk. Furthermore, the association between language impairment and emotional or behavioral disorder is high in linguistically-culturally diverse children (Toppelberg, Medrano, Pena Morgens, & Nieto-Castanon, 2002). Decisions regarding language input to these children are especially important because they are generally more dependent on that input and their pragmatic deficits make them less likely to engage speakers in conversation on their own. As we noted earlier, a more current perspective is to continue bilingual input to children with language impairment (Cheng, 2007b; Gutiérrez-Clellen, 1999; Langdon & Cheng, 2009). Given the number of linguistic and social variables at issue, however, it is difficult to justify a single approach. Instead, professionals should follow a set of guidelines such as these (Kohnert, Kennedy, Glaze, Kan, & Carney, 2003; Kohnert et al., 2009; Toppelberg, Snow, & Tager-Flusberg, 1999):

1. Determine the critical communicative needs of the child and the language(s) with which the child absolutely must be familiar.
2. Determine the child's relative ability in the first and second languages, the willingness and ability of family members and school personnel to function in the various possible languages, and the child's attitude toward and aptitude for language in general and learning a second language in particular.
3. Discuss with the family the risks, benefits, and availability of a particular language given the child's abilities and needs. The value of maintaining the home language (for emotional and behavioral regulation and for family and cultural relatedness) is paramount.
4. Provide an optimal language-learning experience and environment, that is, the OLLEE (Cheng, 2009) introduced earlier in this chapter.

EMERGING ISSUES

Cheng (2010), in the special issue of *Topics in Language Disorders*, focused on *Education for Speech and Language Pathologists: Emerging Issues*, discussed a number of emerging issues surrounding the delivery of speech-language services at a global level and specific topics dealing with services needed in underserved areas. Dialogues around topics related to underserved and unserved populations have also emerged. Two of these topics are highlighted here.

Slavery

Modern day slavery is a topic that has not been largely explored in our literature of underserved/unserved populations. It is difficult to imagine that in the 21st century there are still millions of slaves. According to the Walk Free Foundation (2016), there were 45.8 million people in 2016 who were modern day slaves because of circumstances such as human trafficking, forced labor, debt bondage, forced or servile marriage, or commercial sexual exploitation. The top five countries for high prevalence for modern slavery as a proportion of population are: North Korea, Uzbekistan, Cambodia, India, and Qatar, and 11 more tie for sixth as a proportion of population: Pakistan, Democratic Republic of the Congo, Sudan, Iraq, Afghanistan, Yemen, Syria, South Sudan, Somalia, Libya, and Central African Republic (Global Slavery Index, 2016). Low prevalence countries, all tied for lowest proportion by population, are: the Netherlands, Brazil, United States, Germany, France, United Kingdom, Spain, Canada, Australia, Belgium, Sweden, Austria, Switzerland, Denmark, Norway, Ireland, New Zealand, and Luxembourg (Global Slavery Index, 2016).

Refugees and Stateless/Displaced Populations

Geographically, the problems of displaced people are pressing in Southeast and Central Asia, Central and Eastern Europe, and many countries in Africa. Estonia, Nepal, and Thailand also have large numbers of displaced populations. And recent events in countries such as Libya, Syria, Pakistan, Iraq, Egypt, and the Ukraine, have led to the fleeing of millions of people. For example, there are many unaccompanied minors in Jordan, often from Syria and without guardians. Beyond these areas there are thousands of other children and families in the world today who are displaced and stateless. The UN believes there could be as many as 10 to 12 million stateless people around the world (UN High Commissioner for Refugees, 2012). Many have witnessed such atrocities that they suffer from post-traumatic stress disorder (PTSD). Children who have grown up in refugee camps will have had very different experiences from those of children who grow up in a slum in big cities or in other poverty circumstances, such as rural or isolated areas. Obviously, these thousands upon thousands of displaced people have had no SLP services. Even their basic needs cannot be met. As families become relocated to more stable areas, children who have grown up in refugee camps experience dramatically different environments and face huge adjustments.

These issues likely foreshadow a number of those that will impact future intervention directions for linguistically-culturally diverse children.

SUMMARY

In this chapter we have seen that

- Changes in the population of the United States are resulting in increased immigration and multiculturalism, that is, variation in race, ethnicity, language, history, and culture.
- Language variation exists on many levels: in different nations, in different regions of the same nation, among different ethnic and sociocultural groups, in different social situations, and among different individual speakers.
- Children learning more than one language can show varying degrees of competence with the different languages. Bilingual learning is affected by many factors. Patterns of acquisition appear to be different in children who learn the languages sequentially rather than simultaneously.
- A major influence on the English produced by Hispanic American bilingual/bicultural children is the Spanish language. Most of the phonological variation and some of the grammatical differences they show from SAE can be explained as interference from a dialect of Spanish.
- Some African American children learn a nonstandard dialect, known as African American English that evolved from the interaction of English and African languages mostly from the west coast of Africa. The dialect is systematic, with rule-governed features of phonology, grammar, semantics, and pragmatics.
- The English of Asian/Pacific Islander American children may be influenced by the phonological and grammatical features of their native languages and dialects as well as suprasegmental characteristics. Some general contrasts exist between English and several Asian languages. However, there is considerable variation in the linguistic and cultural behaviors of Asian/Pacific Islander American children.
- The majority of Native American children learn English as their first language, with many learning a nonstandard dialect. Many of the Native American languages are dying out. Differences between Native American and the mainstream white culture increase the threat of bias in standard language assessment.
- A high percentage of linguistically-culturally diverse children live in conditions of poverty. This may be responsible for a higher prevalence of certain language disorders in this population.
- Professionals who assess linguistically-culturally diverse children must distinguish between language differences and language disorders, either or both of which can occur in an individual.
- Many current tests of language contain significant sources of bias when they are used with linguistically-culturally diverse children. They should be administered with caution, if used at all; more optimally, they should be replaced by methods that are authentic and relevant to the cultural and social background of such children.

- Therapeutic language intervention is for children who do not show proficiency in any language or dialect. Several factors must be considered by professionals in selecting the language or dialect for use in instruction. Assistance in interpreting a child's language or culture may be necessary, but working with interpreters requires training and is not a perfect solution.
- Elective language intervention is for children who are competent in a nonstandard dialect or another language but not in SAE. It may not be supported by all professionals or political factions. The form of intervention will vary, depending on the identified purposes of instruction, the number and ages of the children to be seen, and the resources that are provided.

The communication needs of linguistically-culturally diverse children have been highlighted by demographic changes, linguistic research, and legal action. Professionals need to learn about the needs of these populations. New paradigms, which require many changes in traditional methods of assessment and intervention, must be created and adopted in order to serve these children. It is a work in progress.

10

Children with Acquired Language Disorders

Cynthia R. O'Donoghue • Sarah E. Hegyi

LEARNING OBJECTIVES

After reading this chapter, you should be able to

- Provide an overview of acquired aphasia in children
- Describe language development and language recovery of children with acquired aphasia
- Describe the language characteristics of children with acquired aphasia
- Describe the academic achievement of children with acquired aphasia
- Identify the differences between developmental and acquired language disorders in children
- Discuss implications for assessment and intervention

The language skills of talking, listening, reading, and writing are readily developed by most children through their life experiences and formal education. When language learning is abruptly interrupted by devastating neurological events such as brain injury or stroke, these children are at risk for lifelong deficits across all domains of language. Fortunately, nature heals and compensates for much of the damage that occurs. However, recovery is typically neither immediate nor complete, and the resulting changes that children face create enormous challenges for them and their families (Hawley, Ward, Magnay, & Long, 2003). Professionals must be competent to evaluate and explain these changes as well as to provide intervention that complements the natural recovery process.

AN OVERVIEW OF ACQUIRED APHASIA IN CHILDREN

Definition

Historically, the term *aphasia* has been used to describe two different conditions in children. Chapter 3 explained that the terms *developmental* or *congenital* aphasia have sometimes been used to describe children who show language impairment without sensory dysfunction, intellectual disability, or other neurological damage. In more recent clinical and research literature, these terms have been replaced by *developmental language disorder* or *specific language impairment.* In contrast, the term *childhood aphasia* or, preferably, *acquired aphasia* refers to children who have a language disorder secondary to an accident or a disease that alters neurological functioning. Children with acquired aphasia will have begun to develop language normally but then lose all or part of their communicative abilities as a result of neurological damage they sustain.

Types of Acquired Brain Injury

Acquired brain injuries (ABI) occur in localized and diffuse forms. Localized or focal lesions are confined to discrete areas of the brain and typically result from penetrating injuries (e.g., gunshot wounds), cerebrovascular lesions (e.g., strokes or aneurysms), or tumors. Diffuse lesions are vast and encompass many brain regions and usually result from traumatic head injuries, poisoning, or infections. When brain injury occurs, nerve cells become necrotic (i.e., die) because of the following:

1. Lack of oxygen carried by blood
2. Mechanical shearing of neuronal axons
3. Degradation or disruption of their connections with other nerve cells
4. Electrical overstimulation

Nerve cell death caused by overstimulation has been discovered relatively recently and appears to be amenable to early drug treatment (Almli & Finger, 1992; Felberg, Burgin, & Grotta, 2000). Thus, in the future, it may be possible to reduce the amount of permanent damage caused by certain kinds of brain injuries.

Traumatic Brain Injury. Every year, American children 14 years and younger sustain traumatic brain injuries (TBI) that result in an estimated 2,147 deaths, 35,000 hospitalizations, and 473,000 emergency department visits (Faul, Xu, Wald, & Coronado, 2010). Since 2006, the number of brain injuries resulting in death has decreased. The decrease in death and mortality has led to an increase in the number of individuals surviving with brain injury. The National Head Injury Foundation (1985) defines TBI as

> an insult to the brain, not of a degenerative or congenital nature but caused by an external physical force, that may produce a diminished or altered state of consciousness, which results in impairment of cognitive abilities or physical functioning. It can also result in the disturbance of behavioral or emotional functioning. These impairments may be either temporary or permanent and cause partial or total functional disability or psychosocial maladjustment. (p. 3)

TBI should not be confused with minimal brain dysfunction, an older term for children with behavioral evidence of neurological dysfunction but no history of injury (*see* Chapters 3 and 4). Professionals often use the terms *head injury* and *traumatic brain injury* interchangeably.

TBI results from several causes, and these etiologies vary somewhat by age groupings. Infants and toddlers are generally hurt through falls or abuse. Older preschoolers suffer falls, while young school-age children suffer injuries through sports and accidents involving them as pedestrians, bike or skateboard riders, or passengers. Adolescents sustain most accidents primarily as the result of motor vehicle accidents or assault-related incidents (Faul et al., 2010). Beginning in the preschool years, boys become 2 to 4 times more likely than girls to suffer a TBI. In fact, TBI rates are higher for males compared to females across almost every age group (Faul et al., 2010). Children and adolescents with TBI are a much higher incidence population than is generally realized, and very young children have the highest rate of TBI-related emergency department visits, followed by adolescents, according to data from the Centers for Disease Control and Prevention (Faul et al., 2010). Estimates are that approximately 4 percent of all children in kindergarten through grade 12 have experienced some type of head trauma (Faul et al., 2010). Among children enrolled in special education, this figure jumps to somewhere between 8 and 20 percent (Savage, 1991). Automobile accidents causing head injury in children are more likely to be at low speeds. The rotational acceleration to which their brains are subjected is, therefore, likely to be less than that of adolescents and adults whose accidents are more likely to be high-speed crashes. Damage to children may, therefore, be confined to the cortex of the brain, whereas in adolescents and adults it can extend into the deeper white matter. In addition, children are less likely to develop contusions, hematomas, and white matter damage (because their brains have little myelination). Unfortunately, however, when children's trauma is caused by abuse, there is frequently a delay in receiving medical attention (Duhaime, Christian, Rorke, & Zimmerman, 1998). Overall, it is estimated that falls are the leading cause of TBI (38 percent), followed by struck by/against events (20 percent), traffic accidents (16 percent), and assaults (11 percent) (Faul et al., 2010).

Classification of brain injury severity is determined using the *Glasgow Coma Scale* (GCS) (Teasdale & Jennett, 1974). The GCS measures best performance for three categories of an individual's functional response performance following an incident. The three categories are: eye opening, motor responses, and verbal responses. For each category, points are assigned based on the quality of the person's responses, with higher points for better responses. For the eye-opening category: points range from 4 for individuals opening their eyes on their own, 3 for opening eyes when requested, 2 for opening when pinched, and 1 if not able to open eyes. There is a range of 6 points in the motor response category: 6 for following simple commands, 5 for pushing an examiner's hand away if pinched, 4 for pulling a body part away from an examiner if pinched, 3 for flexing in response to pain, 2 for the body becoming rigid in response to pain, and 1 if no motor response is present. In terms of the verbal response category, 5 points are given for carrying on a conversation and providing answers to orientation questions such as name and date, 4 if verbalizations suggest confusion or disorientation, 3 if responses are intelligible but nonsensical, 2 for unintelligible vocalizations, and 1 if there are no vocalizations or verbalizations. Scores from the three categories are summed, and then a severity rating is assigned:

13–15	mild brain injury
9–12	moderate brain injury
3–8	severe brain injury

Correlation between GCS score and later cerebral atrophy (i.e., lost brain tissue) supports the GCS as a valid prognostic tool of recovery and outcome in children (Ghosh et al., 2009). Although initial GCS scores are generally predictive of which children will die or have a poor outcome from an accident, the ratings do not necessarily correlate with the functional level that surviving children will experience in motor performance, education, and socialization (Haley, Cioffi, Lewin, & Barqza, 1990; Savage, 1991). Even though the GCS was originally developed a number of years ago for use with adults, it remains the most commonly used scoring tool for children. However, it is less appropriate for very young children whose motor and verbal skills are not yet fully developed, and for this reason alternative scales have been developed (Durham et al., 2000; Simpson, Cockington, Hanieh, Raftos, & Reilly, 1991). The Modified GCS for Infants and Children uses a 15-point rating scale with lower composite scores (i.e., 3–8) indicating a more severe injury (Koch, Narayan, & Timmons, 2007; Reilly, Simpson, Sprod, & Thomas, 1988). The Modified GCS appears to be a better predictor of functional outcome if coupled with other measures, such as the Abbreviated Injury Score and the Injury Severity Score (Foreman et al., 2007; Heather et al., 2013).

The National Center for Injury Prevention and Control (NCIPC) (2003) reports that of the traumatic brain injuries that occur in the United States in any given year, 75 percent of these are mild brain injuries. Mild traumatic brain injury (MTBI) is also referred to as concussion, minor head injury, and postconcussive syndrome (Hux, 2011). According to the NCIPC:

> A case of MTBI is an occurrence of injury to the head resulting from blunt trauma or acceleration or deceleration forces with one or more of the following conditions:
>
> - Any period of observed or self-reported:
>   - Transient confusion, disorientation, or impaired consciousness
>   - Dysfunction of memory around the time of injury
>   - Loss of consciousness lasting less than 30 minutes
> - Observed signs of neurological or neuropsychological dysfunction such as:
>   - Seizures acutely following injury to the head
>   - Among infants and very young children: irritability, lethargy, or vomiting following head injury
>   - Symptoms among older children and adults such as headache, dizziness, irritability, fatigue or poor concentration can be used to support the diagnosis of MTBI, but cannot be used to make the diagnosis in the absence of loss of consciousness or altered consciousness (p. 2)

In children with MTBI, persistent symptoms generally resolve within 2 to 3 months after injury (Carroll et al., 2004). Sports injuries are the leading cause of MTBI in children under 20 (CDC, 2011). For high school males, MTBI occurs most frequently in football and soccer (Giza et al., 2013). Soccer and basketball are the most common source of mild head injury for female athletes (Giza et al., 2013). The interaction between postconcussive symptoms and prognosis is not fully understood, and more research is needed to help professionals better address the needs of children with MTBI.

Children who have had an MTBI are 3 to 6 times more likely to sustain a second head injury (Mason, 2013). If the second MTBI occurs before the symptoms of the first head injury fully resolve, the repeated injury may result in what is referred to as *Second impact syndrome*. Second impact syndrome may lead to severe cerebral swelling, herniation, and death (Bey & Ostick, 2009). Extending the time allotted to recover from an MTBI before returning to play is currently considered the best way to prevent Second impact syndrome (Hux, 2011). Research will help to set more clearly defined guidelines for determining when young athletes can safely return to play following a head injury.

Strokes and Tumors. Strokes, the most common cause of aphasia in adults, are relatively uncommon in children. In 2000, the death rate for cerebrovascular disease in the United States was 0.5 per 100,000 (for children under 15 years of age). A California-wide hospital discharge database (from 1991 to 2000) found an annual stroke incidence rate of 2.3 per 100,000 children aged 1 month to 19 years of age (Fullerton, Wu, Zhao, & Johnston, 2003). The comparable figure for adults age 65 and older was 422. Similarly, the death rate for cancerous tumors of all kinds was 4.6 per 100,000 for children ages 0 to 19, while for adults it was 1,127 (Minino & Smith, 2001; Roger et al., 2011). Although the incidence of traumatic injuries, vascular lesions, and tumors is less frequently occurring in children than adults, when they do occur and produce unilateral damage to the left hemisphere, they result in aphasia-like symptoms that are comparable to those seen in adults.

More than a third of childhood strokes occur during the first 2 years of life. The usual causes are vascular malformation, cardiac disease, vascular occlusion, sickle cell disease, or hemorrhage. Blockage of a cerebral artery may result from trauma, infection, or cellular changes or for no discernible reason. In sickle cell anemia, deformed red cells cause vascular obstruction, leading to a crisis in which coma and seizures occur. Cerebral hemorrhage is often produced by the rupture of malformed blood vessels. Sadly, children with this condition are at risk for recurrence throughout their lives.

Associated Problems

Children with acquired aphasia generally manifest associated problems as a result of their brain injuries. These concomitant difficulties vary widely across children. Findings for these coexisting problems are shown in Table 10.1. The impairments associated with acquired

TABLE 10.1 | Associated Physical, Cognitive, Perceptual Motor, Behavioral, and Social Problems in Children with Acquired Aphasia

Functions	Etiology	
	TBI	*Vascular Lesion*
Gross and fine motor	Moderate TBI: spasticity, ataxia, delayed motor milestones Mild TBI: fine motor and visuomotor deficits, reduction in age-appropriate play and physical activity	Hemiparesis on side opposite to brain injury
Cognitive	Problems with long- and short-term memory, conceptual skills, problem solving Reduced speed of information processing Reduced attending skills	Lower scores on norm-referenced intelligence tests with performance scores higher than verbal scores
Perceptual motor	Visual neglect, visual field cuts Motor apraxia, reduced motor speed, poor motor sequencing	Visual neglect, motor apraxia Visual discrimination problems in cases of crossed aphasia (right-hemisphere lesion)
Behavioral	Impulsivity, poor judgment, disinhibition, dependency, anger outbursts, denial, depression, emotional lability, apathy, lethargy, poor motivation	Inattention, distractibility
Social	Does not learn from peers, does not generalize from social situations Behaves like a much younger child, withdraws Becomes distracted in noisy surroundings and becomes lost even in familiar surroundings	May have periods of social withdrawal (elective mutism reported in one case)

Sources: Brain Injury Association of Virginia (2013); Catroppa and Anderson (2003); DePompei and Blosser (1987); Haley et al. (1990); Raybarman (2002); Ylvisaker (1989).

aphasia can have a significant impact on the procedures used for evaluating and treating the language disorder. For example, perceptual and motor difficulties may make it necessary to adapt test materials and procedures. Behavioral disturbances may interfere with attempts to include a child in group instruction or recreation.

LANGUAGE DEVELOPMENT AND LANGUAGE RECOVERY

It is evident that similar types of brain injuries affect both children and adults. However, these brain injuries influence language differently for the two age groups. A common thought is that brain-injured children differ in at least three respects (Dennis, 2000):

1. They have a lower risk of aphasia.
2. They present with different language symptoms.
3. They recover faster and more fully than adults.

This thinking has been tempered as research has progressed. A key issue has been the validity of the progressive laterality or equipotentiality hypothesis, which maintains that cerebral dominance is not present at birth but develops slowly over the course of childhood (Lenneberg, 1967). Cross-modal plasticity is greater in younger brains even though the adult brain is also able to reorganize (Johansson, 2004). If it is true that language has not yet fully lateralized in preadolescents, then it is understandable that damage to the dominant hemisphere (usually the left one) would not produce aphasia or would produce milder symptoms. Moreover, the absence of cerebral dominance suggests that higher-level functions, including language, are less localized in a child's brain. This means that uninjured parts of the brain might be able to assume the functions previously handled by injured regions because of neurological plasticity, a concept introduced in Chapter 1. Some of the research suggests a great deal of neuronal plasticity in young children's brains (Dapretto, Woods, & Bookheimer, 2000; Mills, Coffey-Corina, & Neville, 1993). However, not all the evidence supports the notion of progressive laterality. Certain anatomical and electrophysiological studies indicate that some features of lateralization, such as dichotic ear preference, are present very early in life. Studies of children's recovery from unilateral damage to the left hemisphere of the brain are also difficult to interpret because of differences in methods of investigation. Taken as a whole, however, the evidence to date does not support the notion that a child's chances of recovery decline consistently (monotonically) with age. Additionally, age-based functional plasticity is confounded by the fact that different recovery patterns exist for various causes (e.g., stroke versus TBI) regardless of age (Dennis, 2000). Further studies are needed to determine exactly how plasticity varies with age and impacts the chances for recovery from brain injury (Bates & Roe, 2001). It is possible that language representation in children is like that of adults, but this similarity is masked by the greater neural interconnections that characterize the young brain (de Bode & Curtiss, 2001).

The language symptoms of children with aphasia have traditionally been thought to be different from those of adults. Aphasia in adults is broadly categorized into two groups: *nonfluent*, in which speech is halting, speech comprehension is relatively good, and the site of injury is in the frontal lobe of the brain, and *fluent*, in which speech contains errors but is produced without effort, speech comprehension is poor, and the site of injury is in the parietal and temporal lobes. Most cases of acquired aphasia in children have been traditionally described as presenting as nonfluent regardless of the location of the brain injury (Satz & Bullard-Bates, 1981). As more studies have been conducted, however, it appears that, as with adults, children with aphasia demonstrate either nonfluent or fluent types (van Dongen, Paquier, Creten, van Borsel, & Catsman-Berrevoets, 2001), although descriptions of the nonfluent form still predominate in the literature. In other respects, children also appear to show disturbances across language modalities. These disordered areas include, like adults, auditory comprehension, writing, reading, naming, and working memory (Aram, 1988; Jordan & Ashton, 1996; Levin et al., 2004; Mandalis, Kinsella, Ong, & Anderson, 2007).

Although the symptoms of children with aphasia are similar to those of adults, the prognosis for the two groups is considerably different. When all cases of acquired aphasia are taken together, the great majority of children—estimated at about 75 percent—shows a dramatic recovery of language that is unrelated to their recovery of motor function (Aram, 1988; Eisele & Aram, 1995; Satz & Bullard-Bates, 1981). The rate of recovery is considerably lower for children who suffer from seizures (Bates & Roe, 2001). Seizures negatively impact brain plasticity as evidenced by lower performance scores on intellectual and language measures (i.e., two longitudinal studies of children with unilateral ischemic perinatal stroke) (Ballantyne, Spilkin, Hesselink, & Trauner, 2008). Of children who suffer a TBI, 12 to 35 percent have seizures postinjury (Statler, Swank, Abildskov, Bigler, & White, 2008). Recovery is rarely complete. One fourth or more of children with brain injuries show residual aphasia more than a year postonset, and even in cases where they appear to be clinically recovered from the aphasia, they continue to show deficits on tests of intelligence and academic achievement (Jordan & Murdoch, 1994). The formidable functional recovery of some children with aphasia raises two questions:

1. Why do other children not recover as well?
2. Why do children recover so much better than adults?

Recovery in adults with aphasia has been related to factors such as age, etiology, aphasia type, and injury severity. These factors are presumed also to affect recovery in children. For adults who suffer strokes, younger age is regarded as a positive prognostic factor (Sarno, 1998). Among children who suffer traumatic brain injuries, age interacts with factors such as anatomical development, type of injury, and state of language development to determine the prognosis (Anderson et al., 1997). Important prognostic factors for young children (i.e., aged 2 to 7 years) include socioeconomic status, injury severity, preinjury adaptive abilities, and age (Anderson, Morse, Catroppa, Haritou, & Rosenfeld, 2004). More recent studies are investigating biochemical markers as possible prognostic indicators (Kochanek et al., 2008).

Other potential factors such as preinjury communication skills, age at injury, and vocabulary may serve as predictors of language and literacy skills post-TBI in children (Catroppa & Anderson, 2004). Toddlers and young children generally appear to recover best because (1) their brains withstand injury better than those of infants, (2) they have established certain spoken language skills and sometimes written language skills prior to injury, and (3) they have neuroplasticity adequate for functional reorganization of the brain to occur. However, after age 5, children's patterns of recovery from TBI become increasingly like those of adults (Chapman, Levin, Wanek, Weyrauch, & Kufera, 1998). A prospective longitudinal study of children ages 5 to 15 with mild to severe TBI found more severe cases to have deficits in certain academic skills for a longer time postinjury compared to mild cases. Further, children with a younger age of onset have been found to have smaller increases in academic achievement (Ewing-Cobbs et al., 2004). Studies have demonstrated that children under 2 who sustain severe injuries have the poorest functional outcomes overall (Anderson, Catroppa, Morse, Haritou, & Rosenfeld, 2005).

The type and location of a brain injury may also affect a child's recovery, though evidence is conflicting. For example, specific lesion characteristics did not play a significant prognostic role in one prospective longitudinal study of young children who suffered TBI (Anderson et al., 2004). In the smaller number of instances where brain-injured children present with the symptoms of fluent aphasia immediately after the injury, the prognosis for recovery is generally worse (Martins & Ferro, 1992). Also affecting the prognosis for recovery is the cause of brain injury. The pattern most often observed is that recovery is best with localized traumatic injuries, not as good with vascular lesions, and poorest with infectious etiologies (Dennis, 1992; Martins & Ferro, 1992).

LANGUAGE CHARACTERISTICS OF CHILDREN WITH ACQUIRED APHASIA

There is no single way to characterize the language characteristics of acquired aphasia in children. This is because of the variability of injury severity coupled with the child's language development at the time of injury. Aphasiologists characterize the first 3 to 12 months following brain injury as a period of "spontaneous recovery" during which the nervous system is most able to recover a number of functions even without any type of intervention (Helm-Estabrooks & Albert, 2004; Sarno, 1998). Although language impairment is most pronounced during the acute period, children who have sustained a brain injury typically have residual language difficulties. These difficulties affect interpersonal communication but are most detrimental to academic performance, mostly because of the dependence of academic performance on the robustness of language ability. The following sections delineate the common language characteristics during the acute, or early, recovery period and afterward. Distinctions between the behaviors of children with TBI and vascular injury are discussed.

Early Recovery and Language Impairment

Comprehension. A wide range of comprehension impairments is possible during the initial recovery period. In general, the severity of the comprehension disorder corresponds to the severity of the injury. For example, a child with a severe TBI usually shows more difficulty at first than a child with a MTBI. Complexity of what is to be comprehended is also a factor. A study of 57 children and adolescents with mild to moderate/severe brain injury found that more than 18 percent had poor auditory comprehension of syntactically complex sentences but that only 2 percent had trouble understanding single words (Ewing-Cobbs, Fletcher, Landry, & Levin, 1985). While children with severe TBI have been shown to understand the literal aspects of a story when compared to the control group, they have trouble making inferences to help them understand what was read. Oral and written comprehension is also often significantly affected by working memory strain and inferential processing deficits (Ewing-Cobbs & Barnes, 2002).

Children with vascular lesions also show individual variability in their comprehension problems. Dennis (1980) described a 9-year-old girl who, immediately following a left-sided stroke, was impaired in her auditory comprehension of words and simple commands.

Her silent reading comprehension of the same content was better but suffered interference if she read aloud. In another investigation, two of eight children with left-sided nontraumatic brain injuries exhibited problems of auditory comprehension (Hécaen, 1976).

Word Retrieval. Difficulties with word retrieval or anomia are pervasive in children with acquired aphasia. Anomia presents as an inability to name or a misnaming of pictures and objects (e.g., couch for chair) or as excessive hesitation and nonspecific word use in spontaneous speech. In one study, a relatively small percentage (9 percent) of children and adolescents with mild to moderate/severe head injuries were impaired in confrontation naming; a larger number (more than 18 percent) had trouble retrieving words in a specific category (Ewing-Cobbs et al., 1985). In their spontaneous speech, children and adolescents with TBI produce significantly fewer words and fewer word types (e.g., nouns, verbs, and so on) than control subjects. Significant improvement in vocabulary usage occurs for most children during the first year following injury, although some anomic behaviors may persist (Campbell & Dollaghan, 1990). In general, some word-finding difficulty can be expected in children with head injury regardless of the severity of the injury or age of the child (Dennis, 1992; Jordan, Murdoch, Hudson-Tennent, & Boon, 1996).

Few studies have documented lexical difficulties in children with left-sided vascular lesions. The 9-year-old girl described previously (Dennis, 1980) had a number of word-finding impairments 2 weeks after her stroke, including semantic paraphasias (*bottle* for *cup*) and random misnamings. Perseverative or repetitive responses were common. Her ability to write names was better than her ability to speak them. Lexical problems have been reported in other children with nontraumatic brain injuries, though these may appear more on word association rather than naming tasks (Jordan, Murdoch, et al., 1996).

Syntax. Children and adolescents evaluated shortly after the onset of brain injury show significant differences on many global measures of spontaneous speech: a smaller number of utterances produced, a shorter mean length of utterance, a smaller percentage of complex utterances, and a larger percentage of utterances with mazes and disruptions (i.e., filled pauses, false starts, revisions, and so on) (Campbell & Dollaghan, 1990). Performance is also impaired on various structured communication tasks such as object description, sentence repetition, and formulation of sentences containing target words. Writing tends to be even more impaired than speaking.

Case studies of children who suffer strokes suggest a similar pattern of syntactic deficits. A child who suffered a massive left-sided stroke was impaired, 2 weeks postonset, in describing the use of common objects, repeating sentences, and formulating sentences with target words. These difficulties were still present at 3 months postonset (Dennis, 1980). Another child, a 5-year-old who exhibited a crossed aphasia (i.e., resulting from a right-hemisphere lesion), was initially mute. Over the next 3 months, syntax progressed to single words, then two- and three-word combinations with lengthy delays between words, then short phrases, and, finally, short sentences (Burd, Gascon, Swenson, & Hankey, 1990). A case study of a child, age 3 years, 4 months, who suffered a stroke in the left Sylvian area resulting in global aphasia, showed deficits in mean length of utterance and morphological markers at 6 months postinjury (Chilosi et al., 2008).

Speech Production. Many children with acquired aphasia demonstrate speech intelligibility problems. Brain damage affecting motor-planning regions of the brain or cranial nerve pathways alters sound productions. Manifestations include sound substitutions, omissions, distortions, or "slurred" speech that suggest the presence of an apraxia and/or dysarthria. During the first year post-TBI, many children show improved articulation skills. In fact, articulation can be the earliest and strongest of gains in expressive language (Campbell & Dollaghan, 1990), although one controlled study found markedly slowed articulatory rate persisting more than 1 year post-TBI (Campbell & Dollaghan, 1995). Similar articulation problems are also observed in children with left-sided nontraumatic brain injuries (Dennis, 1980; Hécaen, 1976). For example, children with cerebellar tumors may present with imprecise consonants, decreased speech intelligibility, and slow rate (Cornwell, Murdoch, Ward, & Kellie, 2003; van Mourik, Catsman-Berrevoets, Yousef-Bak, Paquier, & van Dongen, 1998).

Later Recovery and Residual Language Impairment

Though children with aphasia generally recover language functions more fully than adults, recent findings also indicate that children experience some persistent language impairments. This appears to be true regardless of the etiology of the aphasia. Following TBI, the persistent difficulties are often subtle higher-level language skills. For example, in spontaneous conversation or in narrative accounts, residual problems in word retrieval, recall and organization of information, syntactic formulation, and use of cohesion devices that help the listener follow the events and characters of a story are lacking (Brookshire, Chapman, Song, & Levin, 2000; Chapman et al., 1998; Dollaghan & Campbell, 1992). Residual impairments may include poor syntax, nonfluent speech, and word retrieval deficits (Chilosi et al., 2008). Verbal explanations may be disorganized, confusing, and ineffective because of unnecessary repetition or the inclusion of irrelevant details (McDonald, 1993). In reading or listening, children with brain injury may understand facts that are stated directly but fail to comprehend information that must be inferred (Barnes & Dennis, 2001; Dennis & Barnes, 2001). The superficial emotions of characters in a story may be understood but not the more deceptive emotions that motivate certain behaviors (Dennis, Barnes, Wilkinson, & Humphreys, 1998). In language tasks involving nonliteral meanings, such as understanding humor or sarcasm, children with acquired aphasia are more prone to misunderstandings than their peers (Dennis, Purvis, Barnes, Wilkinson, & Winner, 2001; Jordan, Cremona-Meteyard, & King, 1996). Higher-level language abilities are among the most debilitating communication problems these children experience because of the potential compromise to their academic and social success. These are also the more discrete language functions that are prone to oversight when testing. Professionals need to be alert to the high probability of these difficulties.

Children's recoveries from vascular lesions show similar patterns. There appears to be a strong initial recovery of language functions, but despite their early progress, most children experience some level of long-term impairment. For example, an evaluation of 11 children and adolescents with nontraumatic brain injuries more than a year postonset found that they were able to communicate verbally and engage in conversation but still exhibited residual language and academic difficulties (Cooper & Flowers, 1987). The spontaneous spoken language of these children is less elaborated syntactically and contains more errors in the complex sentences that are produced (Aram, Ekelman, & Whitaker, 1986). Naming is slower than in normal subjects, but the pattern of errors produced is generally similar to that of normal children and does not resemble the anomia of adults with aphasia (Aram, Ekelman, & Whitaker, 1987). Unfortunately, time alone does not heal these problems. Longitudinal studies of young adults who experienced strokes in childhood show a broad range of language impairments, with resultant compromise on not only their academic performance but also their vocational and social lives (Watamori, Sasanuma, & Ueda, 1990). It is reasonable to expect that children with acquired aphasia will exhibit some degree of language difficulty following their brain damage and probably well into adulthood.

ACADEMIC ACHIEVEMENT

Despite the previous statement, there can be a tendency to view many children with acquired aphasia as "fully recovered" given the amount of recovery that is often achieved. However, it is apparent that the more subtle deficits of brain damage and its detrimental impact on language functioning influence a child's performance, particularly at school. Even intelligence testing is often insensitive to these subtle deficits and consequently hinders prediction of academic success (Ewing-Cobbs, Levin, & Fletcher, 1998).

Classroom performance is affected in many different ways. In an early study, Cooper and Flowers (1987) followed up 15 children with acquired aphasia between 1 and 10 years postonset and tested their language and academic performances. The several tests of language included tasks that tapped, for example, comprehension abilities (i.e., comprehension of single words, sentences, and connected language) and those that examined expressive skills (e.g., sentence complexity, vocabulary recall and semantic association, picture labeling). Performances of the children with acquired aphasia indicated deficits in all of the language areas examined. Four of 15 children (approximately 25 percent of them) obtained test scores two or more standard deviations below the mean of the relevant peer age groups on two tasks—comprehension of connected spoken language and vocabulary recall and semantic association. Performances were poorer in the other areas, ranging from approximately one-half of the children obtaining test scores two or more standard deviations below the mean for comprehension of sentences to nine of the 15 children (60 percent of them) obtaining test scores two or more standard deviations below the mean for comprehension of single words and expressive sentence complexity. For the four areas of academic performance that were tested (i.e., reading recognition, reading comprehension, spelling, arithmetic), the children also demonstrated difficulties with all of the areas. The children's best performances were in the area of reading recognition, with three of the 15 children (20 percent of the children) receiving scores one or more standard deviations below the mean. One third of the children (5/15) and eight of 15 (53 percent) obtained scores one or more standard deviations below the mean for reading comprehension and spelling, respectively. Their worst performance was in the area of arithmetic; 86 percent of the children obtained scores at or below one standard deviation. Ewing-Cobbs et al. (2006) obtained similar results. They studied the longitudinal academic achievements of 23 children who suffered a moderate to severe TBI before 6 years of age and found the following results:

> Both IQ and academic achievement test scores were significantly related to the number of intracranial lesions and the lowest post-resuscitation Glasgow Coma Scale score but not to age at the time of injury. Nearly 50% of the TBI group failed a school grade and/or required placement in self-contained special education classrooms; the odds of unfavorable academic performance were 18 times higher for the TBI group than the comparison group. (p. 287)

Although most children with acquired aphasia continue in regular school, the research clearly indicates that academic and language difficulties are likely.

Writing skills appear especially susceptible to impairment as a result of brain injury. These skills seem more affected in younger children with head injury than in adolescents. This is possibly due to the effect of the injury on acquiring new skills or to the greater writing experience of adolescents, which makes their writing more resistant to disruption (Ewing-Cobbs et al., 1985). Regardless of age, the prognosis for recovery of writing skills is worse for individuals who sustain more severe head injuries (Yorkston, Jaffe, Liao, & Polissar, 1999). Severe TBI cases showed continuing deficits compared to mild and moderate TBI cases on academic scores (Ewing-Cobbs et al., 2004). Discourse ability is more impaired in children with severe TBI than in children with mild to moderate TBI (Chapman et al., 2001).

Much of the research that has documented academic difficulties among children with acquired aphasia has relied on norm-referenced language or achievement tests to measure their abilities. These tests do not expose the full extent of the problems these children experience in the classroom (Ewing-Cobbs, Brookshire, Scott, & Fletcher, 1998). A survey of the teachers of severely head-injured students indicated an even wider range of academic difficulties, especially with more complex tasks requiring processing and integration of information (Ylvisaker, 1989). The teachers' ratings of these students' academic performances indicated that 25 percent had problems with reading vocabulary, even more students had difficulties with reading rate and higher levels of reading comprehension, and almost all of them had problems with reading passages of substantial length. For expressive language, teachers' reports indicated that 14 percent had problems conveying relatively simple ideas but 75 percent had notable difficulties expressing complex ideas, both in their spoken and written language. In areas related to processing, 77 percent were reported to show deficits in long-term recall of verbal material, possibly associated with their language comprehension issues that their teachers reported, and 60 percent were identified by teachers as being distracted by both visual and auditory stimuli in the classroom. Clearly, the problems these children can face in school are extensive. As a result of their acquired language and language-related difficiulties, these problems affect almost all academic areas.

The academic problems created by brain damage are not limited to deficits in specific skills. It is common to find disturbances of metacognitive and metalinguistic functions. Problems identified include the following (Janusz, Kirkwood, Yeates, & Taylor, 2002; Taylor et al., 2002; Ylvisaker & Szekeres, 1989):

1. *Limited self-awareness* of communication problems, leading to a reluctance or unwillingness to work on them
2. *Poor planning* of language responses, resulting in disorganized, haphazard narratives
3. *Difficulty in initiating* conversation
4. *Problems in inhibiting* inappropriate remarks
5. *Failure to self-monitor* situations and conversations, resulting in inappropriate behavior or poor comprehension
6. *General self-evaluations* ("it's okay" or "it's all wrong") that do not lead to constructive responses
7. *Lack of flexibility* in considering various solutions to problems
8. *Impairment of higher-level discourse skills*, such as summarizing, outlining, or identifying main ideas

Thus far, metacognitive/metalinguistic problems have been described in the literature in any degree of detail only for children with head injury. Children with vascular lesions also have difficulties with narrative organization, self-awareness of their impairments, and timely initiation of speech. Future studies to advance the understanding of metacognitive/metalinguistic deficits in acquired aphasia are necessary.

DIFFERENCES BETWEEN DEVELOPMENTAL AND ACQUIRED LANGUAGE DISORDERS IN CHILDREN

Throughout this chapter, we have seen that children with acquired aphasia are a unique population because they have developed and then lost some competence with language. The evidence of rapid recovery of skills suggests that children may not actually relearn language following a brain injury. They appear to reaccess some of the abilities that existed premorbidly, to compensate for some of the abilities that are lost, and to resume acquiring new skills.

Compared to children with developmental language disorders, children with acquired aphasia differ in attitude, in profile of abilities, and in pattern of improvement. Among the characteristics commonly noted in children with head injury are the following (Catroppa & Anderson, 1999, 2003; DePompei & Blosser, 1987; Tucker & Colson, 1992; Ylvisaker & Gioia, 1998):

- They have previous successful experiences in social and academic settings.
- Before their injury, they had a self-concept of being normal.
- They have many discrepancies in ability levels.
- They show inconsistent patterns of performance.
- During recovery, they are likely to show great variability and fluctuation.
- They have greater problems in generalizing, structuring, and integrating new information.

The differences in the experiences of these children and in our expectations for their rate of progress leads us to organize intervention programs that cater to their individualized needs and yet still recognize their commonality with other children. Intervention for children with acquired aphasia cannot rely solely on the strategies that are used for developmental language disorders. Many professionals have reported that they feel unprepared to serve students with TBI. Although increased training opportunities in this domain have enhanced the overall quality of service, there remain significant gaps in knowledge and uncertainties about professional competence (Hux, Walker, & Sanger, 1996). There remains a lack of diagnostic tools sensitive to cognitive deficits in mild cases of TBI, insufficient training of speech–language pathologists in regard to counseling families of children with MTBI, and inadequate referral and follow-up protocols for the increasing population of MTBI cases (Duff, Proctor, & Haley, 2002). To assist professionals, an interdisciplinary group of Australian researchers developed a database that evaluates the available evidence about practices, including language interventions for people with acquired brain injury who are 5 years of age and older (Tate & Douglas, 2002). The database, known as PsycBITE™, is available free of charge at http://www.psycBITE.com.

IMPLICATIONS FOR ASSESSMENT AND INTERVENTION

Assessment

Since the incidence of acquired aphasia in children is significantly lower than either the incidence of developmental language disorders or the incidence of aphasia in adults, few tests have been designed to evaluate childhood aphasia. It is possible to administer norm-referenced tests that are used to identify developmental language disorders. These will at least establish how children with acquired aphasia compare to their typically developing peers. However, these tests cannot be used to answer questions about rate or pattern of recovery. When testing the language of children with acquired aphasia, it is crucial to differentiate issues of language (e.g., language comprehension deficits) from issues of testing measures (e.g., sustained attention and speed of information processing) (Turkstra & Holland, 1998). Unfortunately, some diagnostic tools lack sensitivity to subtle cognitive communication deficits (Duff et al., 2002).

It is tempting to administer a battery of tests to compare a child's performance across different modalities (e.g., speaking, listening, reading, and writing). However, in most instances these tests are normed on different populations, and any conclusions about patterns of delay are limited (Swisher, 1985). Even tests such as the *Clinical Evaluation of Language Fundamentals—Fifth Edition* (*CELF-5*) (Semel, Wiig, & Secord, 2013), which assesses both receptive and expressive language abilities, must be used with caution. Tests like various versions of the *CELF* are intended to identify linguistic delay but do not necessarily identify problems of verbal memory, learning, and fluency that can significantly affect a student's academic performance (Turkstra, 1999).

Some of the available tests are adaptations of instruments originally devised for use with adults. The child adaptation of the *Neurosensory Center Comprehensive Examination for Aphasia* (Gaddes & Crockett, 1975) provides norms for children from 6 to 13 years of age. The *Porch Index of Communicative Ability in Children* (Porch, 1979) has norms from 3 to 12 years. These tests cannot be interpreted in the same fashion as their adult counterparts, and questions remain about whether the aphasia models they are based on can be validly applied to children. Further, the mere time since their development makes their current value questionable.

A preferable means for assessment comes from the development of tests that are normed on children and adolescents with acquired aphasia. One such instrument, the *Pediatric Test of Traumatic Brain Injury*, is designed for use with school-age children and adolescents in acute care and rehabilitation settings (Hotz, Helm-Estabrooks, & Nelson, 2001). It allows for the evaluation of cognitive and linguistic skills immediately following injury and during the period of recovery. Eventually, this information will enable researchers to develop psychometric profiles for recovery based on a child's age and type and severity of injury. Other instruments will assist in the detection of subtle deficits in pragmatic skills, such as the ability to negotiate, hint, describe a simple procedure, or understand sarcasm (McDonald & Turkstra, 1998; Turkstra, Politis, & Forsyth, 2015).

The assessment process for children with acquired aphasia needs to be multidisciplinary. Among the professionals who may be involved are a classroom teacher, nurse, occupational therapist, pediatrician, physical therapist, psychologist, recreational therapist, and speech–language pathologist. Parents must be involved. To synthesize information from a variety of sources (tests, interviews, and observations) and facilitate team decision making, a common rating scale may be used to track a child's progress (Bagnato et al., 1988). Examples of frequently used instruments to measure and track outcomes include the *Functional Independence Measure* and the *Level of Cognitive Functioning Scale*. The *Functional Independence Measure for Children* (WeeFIM) is designed specifically to determine and track the level of disability in children across a variety of conditions including brain injury (Msall et al., 1994). The WeeFIM is an accurate, reliable, and valid measure of functional abilities at home and in school settings (Msall et al., 1994; Ottenbacher et al., 2008; Ziviani et al., 2001). These tools, and numerous others, are available online and free of charge from the Center for Outcome Measurement in Brain Injury (COMBI) at http://www.tbims.org/combi (Sander, 2002; Wright, 2000).

Social and Legislative Influences

Children with acquired aphasia secondary to TBI or vascular episodes are now included in the federal laws on education for children with disabilities and, thus, are eligible for services from public school systems. However, the cost of such services is challenging for many schools. Consequently, it is suspected that children with mild and moderate language problems are underserved.

Interestingly, these laws do not define what "education" is, with the result that education and rehabilitation professionals may disagree on what are appropriate services for a child. A plan for therapy that is recommended by medically based personnel may be rejected or reduced by public schools on the grounds that it is not relevant to the child's educational success (Savage, DePompei, Tyler, & Lash, 2005).

Augmentative and Alternative Communication

Later in this text is a discussion of augmentative and alternative communication (AAC) and the relevance to children with acquired aphasia. In early stages of recovery following acquired brain injury, AAC may be necessary for the children to communicate. AAC may also be part of their intervention, as discussed in Chapter 12.

Behavior Disorders

Professionals working with children with acquired language disorders need to be prepared for the possibility of behavior problems (Yeates & Taylor, 2006). These include aggressive, impulsive, disinhibited, or antisocial behaviors. Additional behaviors can include lack of drive, poor motivation, or depression. The behavioral profile results from an interaction among the effects of the brain injury, the adjustment made to the new situation created by the accident (e.g., new living quarters, parent–child relationships, school, and peer group), and the behavioral predisposition of the individual (e.g., tendencies toward aggressiveness, depression). In some cases, these behaviors may have been associated with the reasons for their injury in the first place. All these factors must be considered when developing a successful behavior intervention plan. The Brain Injury Association of Virginia (BIAV, 2013) has provided professionals with suggestions to help children who demonstrate problematic behaviors. These include providing the children with direct feedback, predictable routines, and periods of rest and implementing environmental modifications to best manage the behavior of students with TBI. For some students, postinjury behavioral problems are driven by neurological damage and will require adjunctive drug therapy.

Intelligibility

Children with acquired aphasia who also present with speech production problems require intervention so that language recovery is not hindered by poor intelligibility. Improved intelligibility allows children to display linguistic abilities without frustration. Further, gains in intelligibility enhance other intervention strategies that require judgments about the correctness of children's attempts at target forms. It is important to remember that acquired aphasia, dysarthria, and apraxia of speech are not mutually exclusive problems. Articulatory impairments are usually amendable to phonetic placement approaches or drills designed to increase gradually the length and complexity of phonetic units that a child can produce.

Developmental versus Remedial Logic

Depending on the age at which a child acquires aphasia, professionals may apply different models of recovery. Preschool children are likely to be learning fundamental syntactic and phonological skills at the time of their injury (Eisele & Aram, 1995). Consequently, a developmental model likely remains appropriate and may be used to select goals and teaching strategies for these children (Ylvisaker & Holland, 1984). With older children and adolescents, a model based on observed patterns of physiological recovery may be more useful. Table 10.2

TABLE 10.2 | Characteristics of Recovery Stages of Older Children and Adolescents and Intervention Implications

	Recovery Stages		
	Early	*Middle*	*Late*
Child/Adolescent Characteristics	■ Responsive to stimulation ■ Easily overstimulated ■ Inconsistent memory, especially for recent events ■ Inconsistency in language comprehension ■ Simple gestures used for communication ■ Difficulties with executive functioning, e.g., planning and organizing activities and behaviors ■ Possible unintelligible speech, echolalia, perseveration, and/or disfluent with considerable mazes ■ Social communication and interaction difficulties	■ Alert and more oriented but still confused about schedules and own condition ■ Limited attention span and concentration ■ Information processing and language comprehension limited to small amounts and simple concepts and words ■ Speaks but may require prompting ■ Loses train of thought while talking and has difficulty with word retrieval ■ Executive functioning problems ■ Difficulties sequencing activities ■ Problems with conversational pragmatics in conversations and cohesion in narratives ■ Social communication and interaction difficulties	■ Oriented as long as a routine is followed ■ Difficulty in shifting from one task to another ■ Able to learn new skills and information, though slowly and with effort ■ Difficulty with comprehension of nonliteral language (metaphors, verbal humor) ■ Disorganization evident at all levels of language discourse ■ Difficulty focusing on main points or staying on topic ■ Few syntactic errors ■ Word-finding problems and difficulty with new word learning ■ Continuing issues with executive functioning
Intervention Implications	■ Control amount and type of stimulation child receives ■ Counsel and educate family members ■ Determine and provide stimuli to which child is most appropriately responsive ■ Reassess frequently for evidence of change ■ Modify environment to suit needs of child ■ Provide familiar pictures, objects, music, and so on ■ Verbally orient child to time and place ■ Encourage communicative interaction	■ Begin practice of cognitive and communicative functions ■ Structure child's day ■ Provide ongoing orientation by means of schedules and logbooks ■ Schedule intervention in group (for social communication opportunities) and individual sessions (to reduce distractions) ■ Work on attending behavior, memory function, and information processing by gradually increasing length and complexity of tasks ■ Employ graphic organizers and visual reminders ■ Ensure high success rate (errorless learning), vary activities, and use video to maintain child's motivation ■ Focus on improving comprehension of longer and more complex stimuli	■ Teach compensatory strategies ■ Introduce AAC devices, if appropriate ■ Practice deductive reasoning and problem solving (e.g., "20 questions") ■ Vary activities and discussions to encourage cognitive flexibility (e.g., change rules of a game slightly) ■ Practice self-monitoring ■ Practice requesting clarification of information that is not understood ■ Compensate for poor memory with associative strategies and memo books ■ Practice analyzing information for main ideas ■ Work on cohesion of ideas in spoken and written discourse ■ Practice social interaction skills ■ Introduce analysis of figurative language expressions

Sources: Braga, Da Paz Júnior, and Ylvisaker (2005); Catroppa, Anderson, Morse, Haritou, and Rosenfeld (2008); Kirkwood et al. (2008); Ross, Dorris, and McMillan (2011); Sullivan and Riccio (2010); Ylvisaker and Feeney (2007); Ylvisaker and Holland (1984); Ylvisaker et al. (2005).

suggests intervention implications and strategies for older children and adolescents associated with early, middle, and late stages of recovery following brain injury. Unfortunately, the evidence base for particular intervention approaches or strategies for addressing language and communication deficits is relatively limited (Laatsch et al., 2007; Ylvisaker, Turkstra, & Coelho, 2005). Therefore, the words of Kirkwood et al. (2008, p. 773) provide a useful perspective for considering the intervention implications and strategies presented in Table 10.2 as "recommendations . . . offered not as evidenced based standards or guidelines but as scientifically informed propositions to assist in clinical planning and identifying potentially fruitful areas for future research."

Facilitating versus Compensatory Intervention

Children with acquired aphasia are still learning language when their brain injury occurs. Although adolescents have acquired more language abilities, brain injury in the teenage years not only disrupts existing communication skills but also affects further learning. Unlike their younger counterparts who sustain brain injury, these adolescents have less neurological plasticity to accelerate their recovery. However, whether intervention for children or adolescents, the goals aim to restore what was lost and to facilitate the new learning that was interrupted. Haley et al. (1990) describe this with four objectives:

1. Restoration of function
2. Compensation for function
3. Adaptation of the environment to facilitate function
4. Normal acquisition of developmental skills

In the late stages of recovery, the role served by the professional is to assist children and adolescents in compensating for skills that are lost or to help in adapting to the environment. Many techniques and strategies can be applied in this process, some of which are listed in Table 10.3.

Returning to School

Special education services for intellectual disabilities, learning disabilities, or emotional disturbances are likely inappropriate for children with acquired aphasia. On the other hand, full-time reentry into a regular/general education classroom may be overwhelming for a child who has been in a hospital environment for several months (Blosser & DePompei, 1994; DePompei & Blosser, 1987; Savage & Wolcott, 1994; Ylvisaker et al., 1991). The rapid rate of recovery for many children with brain injuries means that their individualized educational plans must be reviewed and modified more frequently than those of other children (Savage, 1991; Ylvisaker et al., 1991).

To function effectively in school, children must be able to cope with demands for attention, concentration, and socialization. Cohen, Joyce, Rhoades, and Welks (1985) suggest several requisite skills for a positive reentry to school:

- Attend to a task for 10 to 15 minutes
- Tolerate 20 to 30 minutes of general classroom stimulation, such as movement, noises, and visual distractions
- Function within a group of two or more students
- Engage in meaningful communication through speech, gesture, or alternative/augmentative communication device
- Follow simple directions
- Show potential for learning

Successful return to school requires cooperation of professionals at the hospital and school, family members, and individuals in the community (Taylor et al., 2002). Many areas require planning and follow-up (Hawley, Ward, Magnay, & Mychalkiw, 2004; Jantz & Coulter, 2007; New Zealand Guidelines Group, 1998; Ylvisaker et al., 1991):

TABLE 10.3 | Compensatory Teaching Strategies

Socialization and emotional support	■ Plan small-group activities with unimpaired children to facilitate interaction skills. ■ Schedule time for rest and emotional release. Encourage child to discuss problems as they come up.
Instruction	■ Give instructions both verbally and in writing. Repeat or paraphrase them as necessary. If understanding is critical, ask the student to repeat information or respond to a few questions about the instructions. ■ Encourage student to self-monitor comprehension and to request repetition or rephrasing of instructions. ■ Develop a verbal (e.g., calling student's name) or nonverbal system (e.g., posting a symbol or picture) for cuing the student to attend, respond, or change some aspect of behavior. ■ Allow additional time for processing of instructions, responding to questions, and completing assignments. ■ Provide child with a "buddy" to assist in following classroom directions, completing assignments, and traveling within the school.
Assistive devices	■ Allow and encourage the use of calculators, tape recorders, and computers. ■ Have the student maintain a schedule and logbook in which all classes, appointments, assignments and due dates, and room locations are tracked. Include pictures of persons who are not readily identified. ■ Provide maps for finding locations within the school.
Modification of materials	■ As far as possible, structure the physical environment to reduce distractions and allow freedom of movement. ■ Use enlarged print in reading materials and supplement texts with pictures and other resources (vocabulary lists and outlines of key points) to facilitate comprehension. ■ Cover parts of the page during reading and look at exposed area systematically; use finger or index card to help in scanning. ■ Modify assignments and tests according to the student's abilities by reducing the amount of reading or number of problems.

Sources: Blosser and DePompei (1994); DePompei et al. (2008); New Zealand Guidelines Group (1998); Ylvisaker, Hartwick, and Stevens (1991).

1. The parents must be prepared for their role as advocates for their child's education. They must receive information about medical and social aspects of brain injury, entitlement to special education under federal laws, and cost sharing between schools and insurance companies.
2. Children with brain injuries must maintain peer relationships that are as close to normal as possible. Friends and classmates should be informed about the child's condition and how it affects and does not affect participation in various games and activities. Children who are willing can be involved in explaining their injuries to their peers.
3. Children should be prepared for the demands of school before they return. Environmental conditions, such as noisy classrooms and crowded hallways, can be simulated in the hospital, and children can be encouraged to visit their schools before they return full time. Special instructional materials (e.g., large-print books and modified worksheets) and procedures should be tested and evaluated before they are used on a regular basis.
4. Teachers and other school staff should be educated about the child's condition, needs, and abilities. One individual should be appointed as case manager to coordinate services provided by the school.
5. The need for vocational rehabilitation should be considered from an early age. Efforts should be made to provide work experiences to children with brain injuries so that they develop normal expectations for and attitudes about employment.
6. Children who are discharged from the hospital during the summer months will require special planning to see them through the period until school begins.

7. Physical, health, or cognitive problems may prevent some children from attending school. In this case, they are entitled to homebound services from the school system, which require special coordination efforts.

The BIAV has developed an extensive guide for educators to better serve students with TBI. The guide details the educational implications of TBI in each core subject and provides educators with strategies to manage persistent symptoms (BIAV, 2013). Key elements of the guide include:

- Cognitive: Difficulty with attention, response time, organization, generalization, abstraction, and judgment.
  - Persistent cognitive symptoms may cause the student difficulty when learning new information.
- Behavioral: Difficulty with self-control, insight, initiation, compliance, and following rules. Decreased mood regulation, threshold for stimulation, and frustration tolerance.
  - Dysfunction in sensory processing can cause withdrawal behavior if a student is overstimulated and overwhelmed at school, and impulsive behavior in students who are understimulated.
  - Cognitive difficulties can cause behavioral problems when students do not attend to or comprehend directions, expectations, and new material.
- Physical: Vision and hearing loss, loss of or reduced motor and sensory abilities, seizures, headache, and fatigue.
  - Preferential seating, small-group instruction, increased response time, minimal distractions, assigned peer note takers, and shortened school days are strategies that can be used to reduce the impact of physical TBI symptoms on education.

As an example of one state's approach to educating students with TBI, the Virginia Department of Education promotes a train-the-trainer approach to evaluate and monitor students who have sustained a traumatic brain injury. Each school district sends a team of educators to be trained by recognized experts on the physical, neurological, and cognitive effects of brain injury and the subsequent implications for learning. Educational teams are typically comprised of teachers, school psychologists, speech–language pathologists, athletic trainers, physical therapists, and occupational therapists. The panel of experts includes physiatrists, neuropsychologists, neurologists, rehabilitation specialists, and social workers. During the training, each team establishes a district-wide approach to developing the Individualized Education Plan for students with TBI and their families (BIAV, 2013).

Plainly, the transition back to school is a challenge to friends, parents, school personnel, and, most of all, the child. Professionals should be ready to help organize and assist in this crucial process.

SUMMARY

In this chapter we have seen that

- Acquired aphasia is a condition in which a child begins to develop language and then loses all or part of that ability following an acquired brain injury.
- The major causes of acquired aphasia in children are traumatic head injury and vascular disorders.
- Besides causing aphasia, acquired brain injuries can produce impairments of gross and fine motor skills, cognition, perception, and social behavior.
- Many children spontaneously recover a substantial portion of their premorbid communicative abilities.
- During the early period immediately following injury, children with acquired aphasia often show a dramatic loss of language abilities. In the most severe cases, they may be mute and completely unresponsive to speech stimuli.
- Most children recover much of their ability to comprehend and produce language during the first year following their injury. Thereafter, they are often plagued with residual

communicative difficulties, often high-level language skills and/or pragmatic abilities that can seriously affect academic and social performance.

- Assessment and intervention for children with acquired aphasia is a multidisciplinary endeavor. It must be planned with consideration of each child's intelligibility, behavior problems, preferred modality, and changing needs over the course of recovery.
- The aims of intervention are to assist in the restoration of language functions and acquisition of skills for which development was interrupted and to help children compensate for other functions that remain impaired.
- The transition back to school is a complex undertaking that requires considerable cooperation, organization, and sensitivity to the host of physical, educational, and social problems a child will encounter.

Children with acquired aphasia pose special challenges to professionals working with language disorders. Over the course of recovery, these children gradually exchange medical problems for social and educational ones. In most instances, professionals working in hospital settings hand over the intervention to school personnel. There is opportunity for confusion as these changes in service occur. The problem is best avoided by increasing everyone's awareness and understanding of these children's capabilities, disabilities, and needs.

11

Language and Other Special Populations of Children

Mona R. Griffer • Vijayachandra Ramachandra

LEARNING OBJECTIVES

After reading this chapter, you should be able to

- Discuss the language of children who are gifted
- Discuss the language of children with visual impairment
- Discuss the language of children with neuromotor impairment
- Discuss the language of children with cleft palate
- Discuss language difficulties of some children who stutter

This chapter takes a brief look at five populations of children whose language can be affected by their special conditions. In the first part of the chapter, we discuss the language in two different special populations: the gifted and the blind. From reading this part of the chapter, we will understand that language ability plays an important role in the children's development. In the latter part of the chapter, we review language abilities of children with neuromotor impairments, cleft palate, and stuttering.

LANGUAGE AND GIFTED CHILDREN

There are at least four reasons for understanding and describing the language of gifted children. First, gifted children, like children with language impairments, are different and fall outside the typical pattern of language and cognitive development. The psychometric procedures for identifying both groups of children are quite similar, and *gifted education* is commonly viewed either as a branch of *special education* or as a parallel division of education. Second, children who are gifted or talented are sometimes disruptive in the classroom because they are not sufficiently challenged by the style and pace of the curriculum (Cline & Hegeman, 2005; Cline & Schwartz, 1999; Webb, 1993). Third, these children may have emotion-related issues, and the emotional side of gifted children is not always well understood, even by their parents. An investigation by Solow (1995) indicated that parents who did understand their gifted children's cognitive and emotional aspects were in a better position to respond appropriately to their behaviors, but most of the parents in the study understood the intellectual aspects of their children's giftedness better than the emotional and social aspects. In other instances, teachers may fail to recognize the special needs of gifted children because of negative biases that they can have toward these children. A large analysis of 377 teachers from Australia, England, and Scotland who were undergoing training in gifted education revealed that teachers subconsciously associated giftedness with negative attitudes, such as "disrespectful of others," "insensitive to others," and "social isolates" (Geake & Gross, 2008). More recently, an analysis of British newspaper stories on gifted children revealed that children who were identified as gifted in academics were viewed more negatively than children who were exceptional in music or sports (O'Connor, 2012). Gifted children may also have a different perception about their social self-concept. A survey of 1,526 adolescents who had participated in gifted programs showed that being gifted did not have a negative impact on their ability to form and maintain social relationships with their peers but they rated their academic self-concept higher than their social self-concept (Lee, Olszewski-Kubilius, & Thomson, 2012).

The fourth reason, and the one most significant for our discussion, is that the population of gifted children overlaps with three other groups: linguistically-culturally diverse children, children with physical or sensory impairments, and children with learning disabilities. One of the issues noted by experts in gifted education as most important to that field is how best to identify and serve gifted children who come from a culturally different background, are economically disadvantaged, or have disabilities that limit the expression of their abilities (Ford, 1996, 1997; Winebrenner, 2003). A new category of learners, known as twice-exceptional students, have superior abilities in one or more areas but demonstrate weaknesses in others, such as the sensory, emotional, and physical areas. Professionals—in particular, counselors—who can understand the needs of such children and provide recommendations to parents and teachers about providing services to these children play important roles in their rehabilitation (Assouline, Nicpon, & Huber, 2006).

An Overview of Giftedness

Definition. In popular thinking, there seems to be little argument that some individuals are more able than others. Our language has a number of words—*gifted*, *genius*, and *talented* among them—to distinguish those with exceptional abilities. Despite the labels used to refer to a child with exceptional abilities and the continuing debate in psychology about environmental versus genetic factors of giftedness, one thing is clear: there is no single definition of *giftedness*. The difficulty in defining this term is much like the problem of defining *disordered* or *impaired*. Children may be viewed as disordered if they display characteristics that will hinder them from achieving socially valued goals such as getting along with peers, gaining an education, or finding a job. Similarly, children may be considered gifted if they show superior abilities in domains that society values: speech and language, writing, music, athletics, art, and others. In 1993, the U.S. Department of Educational Research and Improvement (U.S. Department of Education, 1993) provided the following definition of giftedness:

> Children and youth with outstanding talent perform or show the potential for performing at remarkably high levels of accomplishment when compared with others of their age, experience, or environment. These children and youth exhibit high performance capability in intellectual, creative, and/or artistic areas, possess an unusual leadership capacity, or excel in specific academic fields. They require services or activities not ordinarily provided by the schools. Outstanding talents are present in children and youth from all cultural groups, across all economic strata, and in all areas of human endeavor. (p. 26)

This definition is deliberately broad and calls attention to the special educational needs of these children. Another definition of giftedness, based on opinions contributed by a panel of experts in the field, is shown in Table 11.1. This definition is more detailed and reflects the evolution of thinking among educators from the 1970s to the 21st century.

In principle, children may display giftedness in several different ways. They may score very highly on general tests of intelligence, suggesting that they are developmentally advanced in a number of areas. Or they may achieve high scores on tests of aptitude in only one or two domains, such as visuospatial abilities or mathematics. Another possibility is that

TABLE 11.1 | A Consensus Definition of Giftedness by Experts in Gifted Education

1. Giftedness is the potential for exceptional development of specific abilities as well as the demonstration of performance at the upper end of a talent continuum; it is not limited by age, gender, race, socioeconomic status, or ethnicity.
2. A gifted child is one who is developmentally advanced in one or more areas; he or she has potential or demonstrated ability in general intellectual ability, specific academic aptitude, leadership, creative productive thinking, or the visual and performing arts; because of this potential or demonstrated ability, the child requires differentiated education services in order to function at the level appropriate to his or her potential.
3. A gifted adult is one who shows unusual skill, ability, or talent in one or more areas of intellect, leadership, or the visual or performing arts; he or she makes independent and creative contributions to a field.

Sources: Cramer (1991); Ross (1993); VanTassel-Baska (1992).

they will not distinguish themselves on any formal test but will manifest their special abilities through their behavior in natural surroundings. Table 11.2 lists some of the behavioral characteristics of gifted children that can be observed informally. As with their performance on norm-referenced tests, gifted children may display exceptional behaviors in all or just a few of the categories shown. Of particular relevance to this chapter is the number of references in the table to language and language-related skills.

Identification. There is a heavy reliance on IQ scores for the identification of gifted students. Giftedness is not the same as high IQ scores. This may be the reason why children from certain ethnic minorities and low socioeconomic backgrounds may be underrepresented in gifted programs. Also the cutoff scores for determining eligibility to gifted programs may lead to illogical decisions like admitting someone with an IQ of 130 and excluding someone with an IQ of 129. The assessment of gifted children should be multifaceted and we should not overly depend on IQ scores. The notion that "once gifted, always gifted" is not true. Reevaluations are necessary at different stages of their development. Some children may be gifted at one stage but may lose that ability when they grow, and on the other hand, some children who are not identified as gifted may develop gifts/talents at a later stage in their lives. It is necessary to monitor the progress of gifted children at different stages of their academic life. School psychologists should play a role in identifying giftedness in children who are of different color, socioeconomic background, English as a second language (ESL), and rural communities (McClain & Pfeiffer, 2012; Pfeiffer, 2012).

Prevalence. Because of variation in definitions and eligibility criteria, prevalence estimates for giftedness can range from 2 percent to almost 90 percent (Fenstermacher, 1982; Gagne, 1998). Very high estimates are nearly always based on definitions that focus on children's potential for achievement, not their actual achievement. Some educators, especially in the United States, are reluctant to recognize a category of gifted children because it smacks of elitism and therefore runs contrary to inclusive, egalitarian principles (Mills & Durden, 1992; Runco, 1997). Individuals who share this view prefer to highlight the latent abilities that all children have if provided stimulation and educational opportunity. This opinion is supported by psychological research indicating that most children's abilities can be accelerated beyond what is currently considered average by means of well-designed programs of instruction and encouragement (Howe, 1990). In the following discussion, we use *gifted* in its more narrow sense of children who appear to excel without special instruction.

Language Characteristics of Gifted Children

One of the most common and striking features of gifted children is their accelerated language development. Other than its fast rate of development, there is no evidence that the language learning of gifted children differs from that of typically developing children. Thus,

TABLE 11.2 | Behavioral Characteristics of Gifted Children

Category	Behavior
Communication	Has unusually advanced vocabulary for age or grade level; uses terms in a meaningful way; has verbal behavior characterized by richness of expression, elaboration, and fluency
	Strong transmission and reception of signals or meanings through a system of symbols (codes, gestures, language, and numbers)
	Demonstrates a flair for dramatic or oral presentations
Learning	Has quick mastery and recall of facts
	Quickly grasps new concepts and makes connections; senses deeper meanings
	Highly conscious, directed, controlled, goal-oriented thought
	Has rapid insight into cause–effect relationships; tries to discover the how and why of things; asks many thought-provoking questions (as distinct from information or factual questions)
	Logical approaches to figuring out solutions; effective (often inventive) strategies for recognizing and solving problems
	Determines alternatives to reach a desired goal
	Learns from experience and seldom repeats mistakes
	Transfers learning easily from one situation to another
	Exceptional ability to memorize, retain, and retrieve information; has large storehouse of information on school or nonschool topics
Motivation	Evidences strong desire to learn, satisfy a need, or attain a goal
	Becomes absorbed and involved in certain topics or problems; is persistent in seeking task completion; displays long attention span
	Strives toward perfection; is self-critical; is not easily satisfied with work
	Often is self-assertive (sometimes even aggressive); stubborn in beliefs
Creativity/ sensitivity	Displays a great deal of curiosity about many things; constantly asks questions about anything and everything; has strong insight; explores, experiments
	Displays much intellectual playfulness; fantasizes; imagines ("I wonder what would happen if . . ."); produces many ideas; is highly original
	Shows ability to form mental images of objects, qualities, situations, or relationships that are not immediately apparent to the senses
	Is unusually aware of impulses and more open to the irrational (freer expression of feminine interest for boys and greater-than-usual independence for girls); shows emotional sensitivity
	May have intense (sometimes unusual) interests; activities and objects may have special worth or significance and are given special attention
Leadership	Carries responsibility well; can be counted on to fulfill promises and usually does it well
	Is self-confident with peers as well as adults; seems comfortable when asked to show work to the class
	Adapts readily to new situations; is flexible in thought and action and does not seem disturbed when the normal routine is changed
Humor	Conveys and picks up on humor well
	Shows ability to synthesize key ideas or problems in a humorous way; exceptional sense of timing in words and gestures

Sources: Alexander and Muia (1982); Frasier et al. (1995).

it is likely that a developmental model can be used to describe their language skills. Gifted preschool children may produce and understand language at a level that would be expected of elementary school children, and gifted children between 5 and 10 years of age may show language skills that resemble those of middle and high school children. We need to remember, however, that although a common characteristic of gifted children, superior language abilities are not a requirement for giftedness.

Oral Language. Gifted children are often said to be precocious talkers. One frequently cited milestone is the age at which first words are spoken. For example, studies of gifted children have reported that the average age of first words is 9 months, and some children begin to talk as early as 6 months of age (Price, 1976; Rogers & Silverman, 1997). More reliable indicators of advanced verbal development are the rate at which a child progresses from single words to word combinations and the rate at which vocabulary is acquired during the single-word period. Recall that typically developing children make the transition from single words to syntax over a period of about 6 to 12 months. Gifted children may exceed both of these expectations by moving rapidly beyond single words into syntax and/or by acquiring an exceptionally large vocabulary before they begin to combine words. Gifted children are also frequently advanced in their knowledge of abstract vocabulary and of word relationships. This is shown in their spontaneous use of higher-order words, their ability to paraphrase, and their ability to define words, a task included in the verbal portion of many intelligence tests. In relation to precocious vocabulary development, advanced syntactic abilities may not be as dazzling but are further indications of oral language proficiency. Hoh (2005) followed a gifted child who was also bilingual from birth to 7 years and reported that the child had an accelerated development with all aspects of language, including syntax, morphology, phonology, and semantics and figurative language (humor, metaphor, ambiguity, and social competence). However, with regard to pragmatic language development, there is little research directly comparing the pragmatic language skills of gifted and typically developing children. Following the general principle that gifted children show normal but accelerated development, we might anticipate that they would be superior in their skills of referential communication, conversational repair, and topic management, but this hypothesis needs empirical investigation.

Reading and Writing. It is assumed most of the time that gifted children read well and that direct teaching of reading to these children may not be needed, and this can be the case. However, opinion is divided on the significance of early reading ability in giftedness. Some assert that early reading is characteristic of gifted children, but in a survey of parents of preschoolers believed to be gifted, only 16 percent mentioned an early interest in books and reading. Even when early reading was reported, it was not predictive of whether the child was actually gifted (Louis & Lewis, 1992). This is consistent with some research suggesting that early reading is not strongly related to intellectual ability, does not always predict later levels of reading achievement, and is probably attributable in part to child-rearing practices (Jackson, 1988; Jackson & Kearney, 1995), such as the availability of reading materials in the home and the value placed by families on education. Precocious readers, who constitute only 1 percent of children who enter preschool, kindergarten, and first grade, show interindividual differences, and there is no single basic reading measure that is predictive of future success in reading. Olson, Evans, and Keckler (2006) suggest that future research on precocious readers should focus more on application of what is known about these children rather than simply describing their characteristics.

There is better agreement that, once they begin to read, many gifted children show an exceptional enthusiasm for books and quickly become extremely able readers. However, gifted children may sometimes need support from others to help them choose the right kind of books that can enhance their knowledge and deal with their emotional issues (Cramond, 2004).

Flexible and effective use of reading strategies and the ability of a child to monitor and make modifications in his or her reading strategies are what separate a good from a poor reader (Jackson, Donaldson, & Cleland, 1988). With regard to reading strategies, a study of students in grades 8, 10, and 12 indicated that gifted students did not differ from the average readers in terms of the various types of strategies they used. However, the gifted students employed more frequent use of the more effective strategies, such as rereading, inferring, predicting, and relating to content area, whereas the average readers were more often concerned about word pronunciation and made more inaccurate summaries of what they were reading (Fehrenbach, 1991, 1994). The more effective strategies used by gifted children enable them to read with greater comprehension than their peers. This provides them with a tremendous advantage in all academic areas, especially as they advance in school, and reading becomes a principal method for acquiring new information.

In comparison to their oral expression and reading skills, the writing ability of many gifted children is less impressive, although the content of what they write is frequently above average (Yates, Berninger, & Abbott, 1995). The form of their writing often resembles that of their typically developing peers. They may write in simple sentences and use a limited vocabulary (Mindell & Stracher, 1980). The discrepancy between writing and other language skills is usually explained in terms of motivation. Good writing requires a command of form—punctuation, spelling, and organization—that is unnecessary for other language behaviors. Writing is also a motor skill that must be learned and integrated with the pace at which thinking occurs. Many gifted children appear to be put off by the work that is demanded for writing and by the way it slows self-expression (Freeman, 1979; McCluckey & Walker, 1986). Consequently, they may not practice their writing sufficiently to develop a level of skill equal to their other language abilities. Use of word-processing computer programs is one possible alternative for these children.

Language in Disadvantaged or Disabled Gifted Children

One issue in gifted education is that of special populations of gifted children (Cramer, 1991). Three groups of these children that have been identified:

1. Children from economically disadvantaged backgrounds, the majority of whom are members of racial/ethnic minorities
2. Children with motor or sensory disabilities
3. Children who are underachieving because of learning disabilities superimposed on a high level of intelligence

There has been little study of these groups, and they have proven difficult to identify and serve.

Disadvantaged children who are also gifted are frequently not recognized. Perhaps because they anticipate and actively look for signs of giftedness in their children, mainstream parents are far more likely to seek specialized evaluation and educational services for preschoolers (Louis & Lewis, 1992). The parents of disadvantaged children may not recognize giftedness, or they may lack the means or motivation to pursue special services. Cultural and linguistic factors also appear to play a role, as children from Asian American families tend to be overrepresented in giftedness programs relative to their population numbers and children from African American, Hispanic, and Native American families tend to be underrepresented (Cohen, 1990). Vanderslice (1998) discussed some of the reasons for underidentification of Hispanic gifted children in schools. She suggested that most of the reading tests used to identify gifted children are in English, and gifted Hispanic children may be at a disadvantage when tested in English if it is not their primary language. Even Hispanic gifted children who have good English vocabularies may tend to obtain low reading scores in English. Because performances on many intelligence tests are dependent on previous exposure and experience, these measures are inadequate for identifying the intellectual abilities of these children.

A different category of children with discrepant abilities is those described as underachievers. These children function at levels that are roughly age appropriate, but they are hindered by learning disabilities or adverse social or emotional conditions that prevent them from realizing their potential (Brody & Mills, 1997). Formally, these children are identified by the inconsistency between their scores on IQ or achievement tests and their actual classroom performance (National Joint Committee on Learning Disabilities, 1998). Informally, these children often call attention to themselves because of personality and behavioral disturbances. Researchers have found that gifted children who do not achieve often lack self-confidence, have lower self-concepts, may have difficulty forming social relationships, and/or exhibit aggression (Mendaglio, 1993; Olenchak, 1994; Schiff, Kaufman, & Kaufman, 1981). Those gifted underachievers who have learning disabilities are often verbally superior in contrast to most children with learning disabilities (but not gifted) who are usually linguistically deficient and perform better on nonverbal tasks. One study (Waldron & Saphire, 1990) compared performances of gifted children with learning disabilities and those without learning disabilities on the Wechsler Intelligence Scale for Children—Revised (WISC-R) and revealed that the gifted children with learning disabilities had relatively better "verbal conceptualization" skills and "reasoning" but poorer "rote short-term memory." The superior verbal conceptualization skills that these children possess may conceal the academic difficulties that they face in school. One of the important findings that emerged from this study was that the gifted children with learning disabilities obtained significantly lower scores on what the researchers referred to as the "organic brain syndrome" factor, which included digit span, coding, and block design tasks. This factor may be important in differentially diagnosing gifted children with learning disabilities from those without learning disabilities and should be used for future investigations and clinical assessments (Waldron & Saphire, 1990).

Implications for Intervention

Professionals who serve children with language disorders have a different role to play with various groups of gifted children. With advantaged children who are verbally gifted, professionals in most educational settings defer to a teacher who has been charged with developing a gifted education program.

A program for the gifted will vary from one school to another but likely will consist of some combination of *acceleration* and *enrichment* approaches, which attempt to provide a curriculum that matches gifted children's abilities, and *grouping* approaches, which separate gifted children from other students during certain instructional periods so that they can work at a faster pace (VanTassel-Baska, 1992). Computers are also important tools in teaching children who are gifted. Some children who are gifted may be better visual learners, but others may be better auditory or tactile learners. Computers have the ability to present study materials in multiple modalities that are conducive for learning (Parette, Hourcade, & Ginny, 2000).

With disadvantaged gifted students, professionals have more responsibility in evaluating their abilities and interpreting issues of language difference to other educators. Gifted children with linguistically-culturally diverse backgrounds require attention to matters of nonbiased assessment and nonstandard dialect, as discussed in Chapter 9. They also may need help in understanding and adjusting to their own giftedness. As we observed earlier, these children are much less likely to be identified by their families. Therefore, it is important for professionals working with this population to devise culturally and linguistically sensitive assessment procedures that are appropriate for identification of these children. Giftedness of children with culturally and/or linguistically diverse backgrounds may emerge if they are provided with supportive and facilitative opportunities (Gentry, 2009), such as programs in which they direct and design their own learning strategies (Uresti, Goertz, & Bernal, 2002).

Gifted children who have physical, sensory, or learning disabilities are referred for intervention often more for what they cannot do than for what they can do. These children demonstrate both inter- and intraindividual differences in cognitive and emotional abilities so that the intervention strategies for the children should be tailor-made and based on their profiles of strengths and weaknesses. For example, in their study including three children with superior IQ scores but poor decoding skills, Crawford and Snart (1994) found that of the three children, only one benefited from a cognitive remediation therapy program that focused on successive processing. This indicates a need for individualized intervention for gifted children. An instructional program for gifted children with learning disabilities developed by one public school system emphasizes development of the children's strengths and improvement of their weaknesses rather than focusing on remediation (Weinfeld, Barnes-Robinson, Jeweler, & Shevitz, 2002). The gifted children in this program interact with the general education students on a regular basis for arts, physical education, and lunch; are respected for who they are; and are provided with technological support to maximize their potentials.

LANGUAGE AND CHILDREN WITH VISUAL IMPAIRMENT

Judged by their progress through major language milestones, few children with only visual impairment will meet the criteria for a language disorder. Because of their sensory deficit, however, these children acquire language differently from sighted children, which often leads to a request for professional evaluation and consultation. In addition, until complete developmental and sensory evaluations can be performed, there will be a concern that a child with visual impairment may also have hearing impairment, learning disabilities, or intellectual disabilities. In that event, the prognosis for normal development of language is considerably poorer. All children with intellectual disabilities will have difficulty with language; visual impairment adds to that problem and raises a serious obstacle to intervention efforts.

An Overview of Visual Impairment

According to the World Health Organization (2014) there are about 19 million children in the world living with visual impairment and about 1.4 million of them are blind. Several terms are used by professionals in medicine, education, and rehabilitation to describe loss of vision. *Blindness* has no fixed definition. It is possible to measure vision in different ways. The standard optometric test is a measure of visual acuity for objects at a distance. However, many individuals with visual impairment cannot see at a distance but do possess some near vision. Furthermore, vision does not operate independently of other sensory and cognitive systems. It is possible to have some functional vision if the nervous system is able to augment a very weak visual signal with information gained from other sensory channels and from previous experiences.

The American Foundation for the Blind recommends that the term *blind* be used to refer to individuals with no usable sight. Persons with usable vision, no matter how little, should be described as *visually impaired*, *partially sighted*, or *low vision*. Within the category of blindness, distinctions are made between individuals who do and do not have light perception and between those who can and cannot detect movement, as when a hand is waved in front of the face. Blindness may be congenital, with onset at birth or shortly after, or adventitious, occurring later in life. Children who become blind after 5 years of age retain visual memories and are able to visualize as an adjunct to thinking (Sardegna & Otis, 1991). Among children with visual impairment and no other deficits, language development is seriously affected only in children with congenital blindness who have no pattern recognition (Freeman & Blockberger, 1987). In the remainder of this section, we limit discussion to children who are congenitally blind. Children with lesser degrees of visual impairment can be expected to show greater parallels with the language development of sighted children. Children with visual impairment along with intellectual disabilities or physical disabilities will have wide-ranging language impairments.

Congenital blindness results from diseases or conditions that are either inherited or occur in utero. Damage may affect either nonneural (lens, cornea, and/or iris) or neural (retina and/or optic nerve) portions of the visual system. Certain conditions, such as retinitis pigmentosa, are degenerative so that vision will become worse as a child grows older. Recent improvements in obstetric and neonatal care now allow many extremely premature infants to survive. These infants, however, have a high incidence of impaired vision (Powls, Botting, Cooke, Stephenson, & Marlow, 1997). Data from a U.S. urban survey found that slightly less than 1 in 1,000 children between ages 3 and 10 had a vision impairment, mostly of prenatal origin (Mervis, Yeargin-Allsopp, Winter, & Boyle, 2000). For the 2006–2007 school year, the

U.S. Department of Education (2007) reported that an estimated 33,000 visually impaired or blind students (in the absence of other impairments) were identified as receiving some form of special education in the United States.

Language Characteristics of Blind Children

In general, what is observed in the language development of blind children is neither delayed nor deviant but rather an alternative route to language acquisition that utilizes sensory and motor resources in ways different from sighted children (Perez-Pereira & Conti-Ramsden, 1999). Despite a few differences and delay in vocabulary and syntax of blind children during the early years, most of these children catch up with their sighted peers at around school age by adopting this alternative route to acquire language (Landau & Gleitman, 1985).

Mothers of visually impaired children have been found to talk more and use more directives—such as "Look at it with your nose to see what it smells like" or "First pick it up with your hand and then do not drop it until it is inside the container" or "Put this hand out and search for it—look for it with this hand" (Conti-Ramsden & Perez-Pereira, 1999; Perez-Pereira & Conti-Ramsden, 2001)—than generally observed in interactions between mothers and their sighted children and may use touch and body contact to maintain a link with the child. Like mothers of sighted children, mothers of children who are blind engage in joint action routines with their children, such as games involving repetition and anticipation comparable to peekaboo. The mothers may, however, rely less on facial expressions, eye gaze, and other typical gestures to maintain contact with their children during these activities. Instead, they may use other nonvisual communicative signals, such as body pointing (Loots, Devisé, & Sermijn, 2003), tickling, and stroking. The infant's vocalizations are actively encouraged during these routines. The routines, though they also occur in sighted children, are especially important to the development of blind children because they serve as both an emotional link to the caretaker and a key sensory experience (Chen, 1996). There is, however, a concern that such routines can be encouraged to the point that idiosyncratic routines may develop. Visually impaired children do communicate using gestures during the early stages of language development just like the sighted children, indicating that gestures can develop in children even in the absence of vision. However, the frequency of gesture use may be limited in visually impaired children given their reliance on other modalities for communication (Iverson, 2000).

Children who are blind become more developmentally heterogeneous as they grow older. Many factors have an impact on their language development, including the degree of visual loss, the presence of other impairments, and the response of caretakers to their impairment. Nevertheless, certain behaviors occur with sufficient frequency in these children to be considered generally characteristic.

Syntax. The syntactic development of blind children differs little from that of sighted children. They are slightly delayed in beginning to use word combinations, but by age 3, their mean length of utterance is comparable to that of their typically developing peers (Landau & Gleitman, 1985; Perez-Pereira & Conti-Ramsden, 1999). Utterance length may be less representative of syntactic competence than it is in typically developing children because of blind children's tendency to echo phrases they hear before they have productive control of the syntax of those phrases.

Semantics. As vocabulary is learned, the contexts and functions of words tend to be restricted. Words first learned in the context of routine activities, such as eating or bathing, may not be used outside those contexts until a child is much older. Typically developing children commonly overextend the meanings of early words, for example, using *juice* to refer to all potable liquids. Many of these overextensions are based on visual similarities among objects. As might be expected, blind children rarely overextend the meanings of words they acquire (Andersen, Dunlea, & Kekelis, 1984).

A number of early-developing concepts are closely linked to visual experiences. Thus, children who are blind may be slow to understand or use words such as *dirty*, *clean*, *open*, *shut, in, out, up,* and *down*. This delay appears to be due exclusively to the lack of sensory experience. Concepts and words that can be learned through other sense information, such as *sticky, sweet, hot, cold,* and *big,* are readily learned (Sardegna & Otis, 1991).

Echolalia. A characteristic of blind children's communication that draws frequent comment is their use of imitation. As in children with autism, this behavior is described as *echolalia* when it appears to occur in an automatic and unthinking way. A high proportion of blind children's utterances may be echoic. In one study of a 3-year-old girl, the percentage of echoed utterances in spontaneous speech was 20.7 percent with her mother and 35.7 percent with an adult she knew slightly (Kitzinger, 1984).

Echoed utterances may appear more unusual than they really are. Lacking sight, blind children must find substitutes for many communicative behaviors that are typically accomplished with nonverbal visual signals. For example, repetition frequently serves the function of acknowledgment, which sighted children perform nonverbally by looking, nodding the head, changing facial expression, and so on. Sighted children are known to produce monologues that serve the purposes of verbal rehearsal, dramatic play, and direction of their own actions. Yet this speech is typically accompanied by movement, especially with the hands, that gives the words a context.

Pragmatics. Blindness has some inevitable consequences for the way in which children use language. For example, although young blind children generally display a similar profile of communicative functions, they use language less often to name or request objects that are remote and cannot be touched. They produce fewer utterances describing the perceptions of others (that they cannot see) and more about ongoing or intended action (Perez-Pereira & Conti-Ramsden, 1999). Unusual nonverbal mannerisms may develop in blind children because they cannot observe certain behaviors during conversation. For obvious reasons, they have more difficulty in adjusting their vocal loudness to suit the distance of the listener. Therefore, they tend to speak at a constant, loud level (Freeman & Blockberger, 1987). Blind children tend to nod their heads less often but to smile more often. They may have eyebrow movements that appear inappropriate because they are not used to indicating interest or give emphasis to what is being spoken (Parke, Shallcross, & Anderson, 1980), and they may use more facial muscle movements than sighted children (Galati, 1997). A recent study showed that children with congenital visual impairment have difficulties in social communication despite having strong structural language abilities. The pragmatic skills of these children are similar to the pattern seen in sighted children on the autism spectrum. Some researchers have argued that the poor pragmatic skills in these children could be attributed to the delay in development of theory of mind in blind children (James & Stojanovik, 2007; Tadic, Pring, & Dale, 2010).

Phonology and Reading. As discussed elsewhere in this text, reading disorders are viewed today from a developmental language perspective, emphasizing the relationship between reading and other language skills, especially in the domain of phonology. Sighted children must develop phonological awareness that allows them to decode the relationship between speech sounds and printed letters. Blind children must develop this same awareness, as Braille is also based on the alphabetic principle. Research indicates that blind children who do not read at age level are delayed in their ability to understand and apply the sound structure of spoken language (Gillon & Young, 2002). In an investigation by Barlow-Brown and Connelly (2002), the blind children with no knowledge of written letters and words had limited phonological awareness, but the blind children (trained in Braille) who had knowledge of written letters alone had increased phonological awareness. However, the blind children who were proficient Braille readers and who had developed knowledge of both written letters and words had significantly greater phonological sensitivity.

Implications for Intervention

Unlike many other groups of children with language disorders, there is some question whether language intervention is necessary for blind children. Most professionals agree,

TABLE 11.3 | Suggestions for Interacting with Blind Children

Talk in a normal voice.
Provide verbal signals to substitute for nonverbal cues. For example, narrate what you are doing when you introduce or change materials.
Make sure that drawers, cabinet doors, and other obstacles are either fully open or shut.
Feel comfortable using "sighted" words such as *see*, *look*, or *pretty*. Blind children will interpret these appropriately in relationship to their abilities.
Tell the child when you are going to move to another part of the room.
Don't be surprised if the child reacts negatively to being suddenly held or picked up. This is not a rejection of affection but a response to being interrupted unexpectedly.
State your name when you approach the child, unless you are well known. Don't expect that the child will recognize your voice.
Don't use toy miniatures unless the child has previous experience with them.
Remember that most representational toys rely on visual analogy with the real objects.
Facilitate interaction between the child and one peer and then gradually increase the number of children in a play situation.

Sources: Rettig (1994); Sardegna and Otis (1991); van Kleeck and Richardson (1988).

however, that intervention is needed to monitor and interpret the child's language acquisition because it can be expected to follow a different developmental path.

Blind children comprise a small population, and it can therefore be difficult to develop a large experiential base for working with them and their families. Despite their training, many professionals may tend to overcompensate for the visual impairment rather than relying on a style of interaction that is generally effective with children. On the other hand, some necessary modifications are easily forgotten because visual ability is so easily assumed. Table 11.3 lists some suggestions that may facilitate interactions with blind children.

On the whole, progress in language acquisition cannot always be judged accurately by comparing blind children to the milestones observed in typically developing children. Some early communicative behaviors are delayed because they must be mediated through touch or hearing, which are less efficient sources of information. As a general guideline, professionals should always ask themselves whether a child's behavior is reasonable and even understandable in view of the sensory deficit.

LANGUAGE AND CHILDREN WITH NEUROMOTOR IMPAIRMENT

Unlike many of the other populations of children discussed in this text, children with neuromotor impairments do not present unique symptoms of language disorder. This does not mean that they are free of language difficulties. Their language problems, though, are not the direct result of the neuromotor disorders that interfere with posture and movement. Instead, these children are impaired communicators because of conditions that frequently coexist with neuromuscular disorders: intellectual disabilities, hearing impairment, visual impairment, and seizure disorders. And, as with any children, children with neuromotor impairments can have specific language impairment (SLI) but, as stated above, this is not the direct result of their neuromotor disorders. They may also suffer from general delays because motoric disabilities interfere with their abilities to explore the environment and to speak, gesture, and engage in social interaction.

Children with Cerebral Palsy

The most common neuromotor disorder in children is cerebral palsy. It is a neurodevelopmental disorder that begins in early childhood and persists into adulthood (Bottcher, Flachs, & Uldall, 2010). This condition has no single cause and includes many different types and distributions of muscular impairment. The common elements in cerebral palsy are as follows:

- It is caused by an injury to the brain.
- It appears very early in life and persists into adulthood.
- The damage to the brain does not become worse over time, though an individual's capability for functional movement may deteriorate.

Etiology and Types of Cerebral Palsy. The causes of cerebral palsy are classified by when they occur: during the pregnancy (prenatal), during birth (perinatal), or during the first few years of life (postnatal). Prenatal events, such as infection, physical injury, or substance abuse, may cause injury to the fetus or disrupt the normal development of the nervous system. During delivery, the major risks are lack of oxygen (anoxia), infection, and cerebral hemorrhage. Postnatal causes include cerebrovascular accidents, brain infection, and trauma. We see that there is overlap between the etiological categories of postnatal cerebral palsy and acquired childhood aphasia. The latter is discussed in Chapter 10.

About 8,000 babies and infants are diagnosed with cerebral palsy each year. In addition, some 1,200 to 1,500 preschool-age children are recognized each year to have the condition (United Cerebral Palsy, 2002). Studies have indicated two opposite trends in the frequency of the disorder. The number of perinatal cases appears to be declining, probably as the result of improvements in obstetric care and fetal monitoring equipment used during delivery. On the other hand, improvements in neonatal medicine have increased the survival of low-birth-weight (premature) babies, who have an elevated risk of cerebral palsy (Pharoah, Cooke, Johnson, King, & Mutch, 1998; Skidmore, Rivers, & Hack, 1990). A survey conducted in 2006 by the Autism and Developmental Disabilities Monitoring Network to identify the prevalence of cerebral palsy among 8-year-olds in Georgia, Alabama, and Wisconsin found an average prevalence rate of 3.3 cases per 1,000, with rates ranging from 2.9 in Wisconsin to 3.8 in Georgia. Spastic cerebral palsy was the most common type (81 percent). The survey also showed that 8 percent of children with cerebral palsy had autism spectrum disorders, and 35 percent had epilepsy (Kirby et al., 2011). A meta-analysis that examined the relationship between cerebral palsy and gestational age revealed that the prevalence of cerebral palsy decreased with gestational age from 27 weeks to term (Himpens, Van den Broeck, Oostra, Calders, & Vanhaesebrouck, 2008). It was also found that spastic cerebral palsy was more prevalent in preterm infants, whereas nonspastic and unilateral cerebral palsy types were seen more often in full-term infants. Bilateral cerebral palsy was, however, equally prevalent among both preterm and full-term infants. It is important to note that prematurity and low birth weights are the most important risk factors associated with cerebral palsy (Sankar & Mundkur, 2005).

Associated Problems. Rarely are the problems of children with cerebral palsy limited to their neuromotor difficulties. Table 11.4 summarizes information on some of the most commonly associated problems. In children with multiple disabilities, it is exceedingly difficult to judge the contribution of each impairment to the whole. For example, we might expect children with cerebral palsy to be slightly delayed in their cognitive development because of the limitations imposed on their physical exploration of the environment. If these children are also visually impaired, their ability to learn through observation will be compromised, leading to much greater restrictions on cognitive growth. And if these children are further affected by seizures, the pace of learning can slow markedly or even regress if the seizures are severe enough to produce brain damage.

Language Characteristics of Children with Cerebral Palsy. There is no pattern of communication deficits that is consistently identified with cerebral palsy. Every child with this condition has a profile of language skills that is derived from the severity of the neuromotor disorder, the number of associated problems, and the manner in which all of these impairments interact. Generally, the extent of motor impairment along with intellectual level determines the language and motor speech problems in children with cerebral palsy. Children with motor

TABLE 11.4 | Associated Problems in Children with Cerebral Palsy

Intellectual disability	Many but not all are estimated to have intellectual disabilities. Testing is difficult or impossible with some children because of their inability to produce reliable verbal or other motor responses.
Orthopedic problems	Nearly all children have some orthopedic problem stemming from an imbalance in muscle forces. Physical therapy is prescribed to facilitate the development of motor reflexes and reduce the imbalances. Bracing is used to stabilize limbs, permitting greater mobility, and to counteract muscular pressure that leads to bone deformities. If these therapies are ineffective, surgery may be recommended to restore muscle balance or stabilize certain joints.
Feeding problems	Feeding problems result from abnormal development of oral reflexes and damage to the cranial nerves that supply the muscles of the face and mouth. Dental problems may also develop. Children will have difficulty with all phases of eating: sucking, chewing, and swallowing. Problems can be reduced through customized feeding programs that include precise positioning, relaxation and desensitization exercises, and special procedures for introducing food into the mouth (Gisel, Birnbaum, & Schwartz, 1998).
Hearing loss	Estimates of hearing loss vary, but prevalence can be sufficiently high, approximately 50%, to warrant vigilance. Both conductive and sensorineural losses are found, though severe sensorineural cases appear in less than 1% of children (Pharoah et al., 1998).
Seizures	Seizures occur commonly, especially in children of the spastic type. Anticonvulsant medications are often prescribed to control seizure activity. Some medications can adversely affect attention.
Visual impairment	Severe visual disability has been found in around 9% of children (Pharoah et al., 1998). Visual problems can result in an expressionless appearance and are associated with poor head control. Perception of color will be better than perception of shape. Spatial perception is frequently poor, causing difficulty in reaching for objects (Jan, Groenveld, Sykanda, & Hoyt, 1987).

impairment and normal/near-normal intelligence suffer from motor speech problems alone. In comparison, children who have an intellectual impairment along with motor impairments show problems in both language and motor speech (Pirila, van der Meer, Pentikainen, Ruusu-Niem, & Korpela, 2007). A study conducted recently in Iceland on 5-year-old children with cerebral palsy showed that 72 percent of them spoke in sentences and phrases consisting of at least three words, and 16 percent of the children were nonverbal. The subtype of cerebral palsy, the degree of gross motor impairment, and level of intellectual functioning were associated with the speech and language level of these children. Interestingly, more than half of the children with cerebral palsy had normal verbal cognition (Sigurdardottir & Vik, 2011).

Several other chapters in this text contain discussions of language characteristics that are potentially relevant to children with cerebral palsy. The characteristics of children with intellectual disabilities are described in Chapter 6, children with learning disabilities in Chapter 4, children with hearing impairment in Chapter 8, children with acquired aphasia in Chapter 10, and children with visual impairment in this chapter. If a child with cerebral palsy comes from a linguistically-culturally diverse background, then Chapter 9 is also pertinent.

A key to predicting the language deficits and potential of children with cerebral palsy is to assess their ability to compensate. Table 11.5 shows a simple outline of five resources for language learning and suggests how a child can compensate for the loss of each. For example, children with neuromotor disorders are denied normal opportunities for physical exploration of the environment. In typically developing children, this exploration increases their knowledge of the world and leads to preverbal communicative interactions. Children with cerebral palsy need to compensate through vicarious experience, which is most effective if they possess normal hearing, sight, and intelligence.

The primary speech impairment in cerebral palsy is dysarthria, produced by neuromuscular damage affecting the systems for respiration, phonation, and articulation. The likelihood of dysarthria increases with the amount of upper-limb involvement. Thus, it is

TABLE 11.5 | Compensation for Loss of Language Learning Resources

Resource	Compensation
Physical exploration	Hearing, sight, intelligence
Hearing	Sight, physical exploration, intelligence
Sight	Hearing, physical exploration, intelligence
Intelligence	Social interaction
Social interaction	Intelligence

uncommon in children with hemiplegia (motor impairment on one side of the body) or paraplegia (motor impairment of the lower part of the body) and most frequent and severe for children with quadriplegia (motor impairment of all limbs). The major symptoms of dysarthria found in children with different types of cerebral palsy are shown in Table 11.6. There may also be articulatory symptoms, such as difficulty with speech initiation or inconsistent error patterns, that are better attributed to an apraxia of speech (a neurological disorder that affects the ability to plan speech movements). A study (Nordberg, Miniscalco, Lohmander, & Himmelmann, 2013) conducted in Sweden found that 53 percent of children with cerebral palsy (out of the 129 children who participated) had some form of speech difficulty. Twenty-one percent of them had speech disorders and the remaining 32 percent were nonverbal. However, the researchers of this study noted that the type of cerebral palsy, degree of gross motor impairment, and area of lesion in the brain were important factors that determine the amount and type of speech difficulties. Speech impairment was not seen in a majority of the children with unilateral spastic cerebral palsy but a majority of the children with a dyskinetic type of cerebral palsy were nonverbal. Therefore, in most cases, bilateral lesions may be necessary to cause a significant speech deficit. The degree of speech impairment was directly related

TABLE 11.6 | Symptoms of Developmental Dysarthria in Children with Cerebral Palsy

Subsystem	Nonspeech Problems	Speech Problems
Respiration	Reversed breathing (simultaneous muscle movements for inhalation and exhalation)	Short phrasing (small number of words spoken per breath)
	Rapid, shallow breathing	Frequent inspiration
	Involuntary movement of respiratory muscles	Decreased rate of speech
Phonation	Vocal folds do not come together fully	Breathy voice
	Involuntary spasms of vocal folds	
	Increased or decreased tension of vocal folds, depending on type of cerebral palsy	
Resonance	Inadequate velopharyngeal closure	Hypernasality
Articulation	Weakness in articulatory muscles	Midvowels are most accurate, front and back vowels more difficult
	Reduced range of motion	Consonant manner errors predominate, especially with fricatives and affricates
	Variation in muscle tone	Final-consonant sounds are more difficult
	Abnormal jaw and tongue reflexes	Individuals with athetosis present more severe problems than those with spasticity

to the severity of motor impairment. Although a variety of lesions in the brain were found in children with cerebral palsy, cerebellar lesions were found only in the speech-disordered group. Interestingly, the timing of the brain damage may also be critical. Damage that occurs late into gestation may result in a nonverbal type of cerebral palsy but periventricular white matter lesions during the second or third trimesters were seen in cerebral palsy children without speech disorders (Nordberg et al., 2013). Regardless of the diagnosis, the effect on language acquisition will be to reduce the child's ability for self-expression. Communication may still be possible but never at the speed or level of sophistication of the child's typically developing peers.

Implications for Intervention. Because children with cerebral palsy are likely to have multiple disabilities that require intervention, several professionals need to work together. The goals of language intervention can vary considerably, depending on the type, distribution, and severity of each child's neuromotor impairment and the number of associated problems. For instance, a child with mild hemiplegia and moderate hearing loss might require amplification and short-term articulation therapy. But a child with severe quadriplegia and intellectual disabilities would most likely be a candidate for augmentative and alternative communication (AAC). In all cases, language intervention has three purposes:

1. To compensate for impaired motor and sensory functions
2. To facilitate the development of motor speech skills and cognitive–linguistic abilities
3. To modify the environment so that the child is able to communicate more independently

Because cerebral palsy is usually detected at birth or soon afterward, early intervention is possible and desirable, especially for efforts at compensation and facilitation. A study by Hustad, Allison, McFadd, and Riehle (2013) showed that 85 percent of children with cerebral palsy as young as 2 years had clinical speech and language delays. Therefore, speech therapy should be started before the age of 2 years in these children. Environmental adaptations that move a child in the direction of independence naturally become more important in later years.

Compensation for sensory impairments must begin with auditory and visual assessment. Depending on the extent of any losses that are discovered, three avenues of intervention are available: (1) amplification of input by means such as hearing aids and glasses; (2) training to improve specific subskills, such as visual tracking, scanning, use of peripheral vision, sound localization, and sound discrimination; and (3) use of alternative input sources, such as vibrotactile units that convert sound into vibrations felt on the skin (Marchant, 1992).

Motor speech skills can be facilitated in the context of feeding. Special exercises and feeding techniques have been developed to reduce the interference of oral reflexes during biting, chewing, and swallowing (Morris & Klein, 1987). These procedures are implemented during infancy, before a child would be expected to talk, in order to provide a better foundation of oral motor skills. Once the child's motor and sensory abilities have been attended to, language and cognitive development are promoted through a home program of stimulation and social interaction. It is important to choose activities and materials that are familiar to the child and relevant to his or her needs, interests, and experience (Chen & Whittington, 2006). The task of the professional is often to help interpret the child's communicative behaviors, which may be ambiguous at first glance, and to offer steadfast encouragement to the parents, who must continue to provide stimulation even when there may be little response in return.

A chief adaptation that can be made to help the communication of children with cerebral palsy is to introduce AAC. Further discussion of children with cerebral palsy and AAC is found in the next chapter. Considerations of AAC as an intervention generally are also discussed in that chapter.

Children with cerebral palsy require intervention in almost all aspects of their lives. Because the intervention is so pervasive, it imposes a particular burden on the family of the child. Professionals should be especially sensitive to parents' need to be the child's primary caretakers. Research suggests that parental distress as caretakers of children with cerebral palsy is related to their perception of unequal role distribution and lack of family support with day-to-day family tasks (Wiegner & Donders, 2000). Increasingly, professionals favor a family-centered approach to assessment and intervention because of its greater ecological validity (Morris & Klein, 1987; Wilcox, 1989). Finally, the role of nonaffected siblings of a child with cerebral palsy cannot be forgotten. Given the demands made on the time and resources of the parents by the disabled child, siblings can easily develop feelings of resentment and jealousy. Increasing the nonaffected sibling's knowledge about cerebral palsy and its effects can help improve that child's behavior (Williams et al., 2002).

Communication of Other Children with Neuromotor Impairment

Although cerebral palsy is the most common form of neuromotor impairment, it is not the only one. Other neurological diseases and injuries can impair a child's ability to communicate. A brief summary of some of those conditions is presented here.

Muscular Dystrophy. In contrast to cerebral palsy, muscular dystrophy is a progressive disorder that produces weakness and wasting of muscles (Cutler, 1992). The earliest signs of the condition are problems of balance and motor coordination. Over time, the arms, legs, and face are affected so that eventually children are unable to walk or talk. There are more than 20 types of muscular dystrophy, most of which are genetically determined metabolic disorders that result in poor oxygenation and nutrition of muscle tissue. Duchenne muscular dystrophy, the most common type affecting children, has its onset in early childhood. Boys are affected almost exclusively, and most children are wheelchair bound by age 10. Children frequently die within 10 to 15 years after the first symptoms are observed, usually as the result of respiratory or acute infections (Muscular Dystrophy Campaign, 2002).

Most studies of children with Duchenne muscular dystrophy indicate that they generally have lowered intellectual functioning, but the findings are inconsistent (Cotton, Voudouris, & Greenwood, 2001). One study (Cyrulnik et al., 2008) suggested that these children have a general cognitive processing problem, which includes attention, memory, and visuospatial skills, and language comprehension and production problems. Deficits in verbal abilities have been attributed to the children's problems in verbal short-term memory span rather than problems with executive functions or physical or behavioral disabilities associated with this condition (Hinton, De Vivo, Fee, Goldstein, & Stern, 2004; Hinton, Fee, Goldstein, & De Vivo, 2007). Speech production abilities are related to the progress of the disorder. As muscular degeneration occurs, it affects respiratory, phonatory, and articulatory systems, producing a gradually worsening dysarthria. Intervention is usually targeted at each child's specific language difficulties and at achieving the best possible compensation for the motor speech disorder. AAC may be used when intelligible speech becomes impossible.

Spina Bifida. Spina bifida refers to a range of defects caused by a cleft in the spinal column. It is the most common central nervous system malformation. The spinal cord, the protective sheath around it, or the vertebrae of the spine can be affected. The defects usually occur in the lower portions of the spinal column. Milder forms of spina bifida do not affect the spinal cord itself and can, if necessary, be corrected by surgery. The most severe form of the disorder, spina bifida myelomeningocele, is caused by a large opening in the vertebral column through which the spinal cord and nerve roots protrude. Surgery, performed to repair the open defects, typically results in the loss of sensation and voluntary movement below the level of the vertebral anomaly. Most children with spina bifida myelomeningocele also have hydrocephalus and are therefore at risk for intellectual disabilities.

Speech and language disturbances in children with spina bifida result primarily from any associated intellectual disabilities (Byrne, Abbeduto, & Brooks, 1990; Tew, 1991). Young children with spina bifida tend to perform poorly on cognitive, motor, and language tasks, but their performance on cognitive and language tasks may be poorer relative to their motor skills (Lomax-Bream et al., 2007). Although these children may not regularly show problems in syntax and lexicon, relative to their cognitive levels, they have more deficits in real-time language processing tasks, such as pragmatics and meaning generation (Fletcher, Barnes, & Dennis, 2002). As with children with cerebral palsy, the motor impairment severely reduces the opportunities for physical exploration and may therefore contribute to cognitive delays. High-quality parenting is an important factor in spina bifida because it leads to faster development of motor, language, and cognitive skills (Lomax-Bream et al., 2007).

Spinal Cord Injury. The most common cause of spinal cord injury is trauma from motor vehicle and sports accidents. Typically, the injury results in fracture and dislocation of the cervical vertebra. The spinal cord is compressed, and the blood supply may be reduced by damage to the anterior spinal artery. Sudden quadriplegia can occur if the head is severely flexed or extended. Recovery can be improved by steroid treatment if it is administered shortly after the accident (Cutler, 1992). There are typically no direct effects on speech and language from a spinal cord injury. If a child sustains head trauma in the same accident, then acquired aphasia may result, as discussed in Chapter 10.

LANGUAGE AND CHILDREN WITH CLEFT PALATE

There is no question that children with cleft palate have unique problems in mastering phonetic skills. The patterns of articulation and resonance that are characteristic of these children are strongly related to the severity of their clefts and the adequacy of the result achieved by corrective surgery. This relationship is captured in the commonly used phrase, *cleft palate speech*, which indicates that the quality of speech is determined in most respects by the nature of the structural deficit. The question raised here is whether language impairments are also part of the communication problems some of these children experience.

An Overview of Cleft Palate

Cleft lip, cleft palate, and related disorders are congenital malformations of the midface and oral cavity. A variety of forms occur, ranging from a small notch of the lip to a total cleavage affecting the lip, bony palate, soft palate, and other facial structures. Genetic factors are the most important influence on the development of clefts, but certain drugs and environmental pollutants have also been implicated. In certain cases, clefting occurs as part of a larger syndrome that can include intellectual disabilities and other disabilities as concomitant problems. Perhaps the best recognized of these syndromes is velocardiofacial syndrome (VCFS). VCFS was described in the 1960s by Kirkpatrick and DiGeorge (known as DiGeorge syndrome) and later in the 1970s by Shprintzen and colleagues (known as Shprintzen syndrome) before being referred to as VCFS. As the name implies, it is characterized by cardiac as well as cleft and facial abnormalities. VCFS results from a microdeletion in the long arm of chromosome 22. In addition to the "velo," "cardio," and "facial" anomalies, children and adolescents with this genetic condition may suffer from particular cognitive and/or psychiatric conditions, such as attention-deficit/hyperactivity disorders, oppositional defiant disorder, specific and social phobias, generalized anxiety disorder, separation anxiety disorder, obsessive-compulsive disorder, and autism spectrum disorder (Carneol, Marks, & Weik, 1999; Gothelf, 2007; Gothelf, Schaer, & Eliez, 2008; Kummer, 2014; Scherer, D'Antonio, & Kalbfleisch, 1999). From information elsewhere in this text, we know that several of these are also associated with problems with language functioning.

Incidence figures for cleft palates vary, depending on the range of clefting that is included. The March of Dimes Birth Defects Foundation (2002) estimates that 1 child in every 1,000 is born with cleft lip, cleft palate, or both. The frequency of clefting is lowest for African Americans and grows progressively higher for white Americans, Asian Americans, and certain groups of Native Americans (Croen, Shaw, Wasserman, & Tolarova, 1998). Racial/ethnic differences may be caused by genetic variation across groups or by cultural practices, including diet and other habits, that affect environmental exposures during pregnancy (California Birth Defects Monitoring Program, 2002). The occurrence of combined cleft lip and palate is nearly twice as great for males, but females have a higher incidence of isolated cleft palate (Robert, Kallen, & Harris, 1996).

One of the major complications of palatal clefting for language ability is the elevated risk it brings for middle-ear disease and conductive hearing loss. This problem exists for most children both before and after surgical repair of the palatal opening. It is caused by a combination of impaired eustachian tube functioning and upper-respiratory infection and inflammation (Paradise, Elster, & Lingshi, 1994). Vigilance in diagnosing and treating middle-ear disease in children with clefts appears to bring the frequency of conductive hearing loss in line with that of typically developing children (Broen, Doyle, Moller, & Prouty, 1991).

Language Characteristics of Children with Cleft Palate

From one perspective, in the absence of particular syndromes such as VCFS, the effect of cleft palate on language development can be conceived of as a set of interacting risk factors. Individually, the impact of these factors is probably quite limited. Collectively, however, these appear capable of disrupting the normal processes of language acquisition. These factors are listed in Table 11.7.

TABLE 11.7 | Variables Potentially Disrupting Language Acquisition in Children with Cleft Palate

Variable	Explanatory Points
Intellectual disability	Risk of intellectual disability is high only among children who have clefts as part of a syndrome that includes other anomalies, such as velocardiofacial syndrome (Gerdes et al., 1999).
Hearing loss	Risk of developing middle-ear disease is likely to lead to fluctuating conductive hearing loss.
	In one study, children followed from 9 to 24 months had depressed hearing on 16% of the days (Broen et al., 1991).
	Frequency of hearing loss is probably higher for children who are not monitored so closely.
Surgery and recuperation	Surgery for cleft lip is usually performed at about 10 weeks of age; repair of the palate is commonly postponed until later but in most cases is completed before 12 months.
	Postsurgically, children are somewhat limited in their activities in order to protect the wound and prevent infection.
	Effects of these experiences on language development are not well known and seem likely to vary among children.
	Nevertheless, these appear to alter, at least temporarily, the normal patterns of parent–child interaction and motor exploration.
	During the first 2 years of life, children with clefts show relative delays in cognitive and psychomotor development (Speltz et al., 2000).
	These developmental delays may slow progress in certain aspects of language acquisition.
Disruption in speech production	Palatal surgery is performed most often during the period when children are babbling or beginning to use their first words.
	Studies of the prelinguistic vocalizations of babies with cleft palate show that they produce fewer oral sounds in general and fewer plosives in particular and more nasal and glottal sounds (Devers & Broen, 1991; Grunwell & Russell, 1987; O'Gara & Logemann, 1988; Willadsen & Enemark, 2000).
	Following the surgery, which facilitates oral sound production, there is probably a reorganization of the motor schemes for producing speech (Broen et al., 1991). This may cause a delay in the acquisition and use of meaningful vocabulary
Unintelligible speech	Nearly all children with cleft palate will have reduced speech intelligibility, especially until the cleft has been surgically corrected and they have had time to adjust to the changes in the speech mechanism.
	Poor intelligibility can hinder parents and other conversational partners from responding appropriately to children's speech attempts.
	The number of successful communicative interactions is diminished, and language learning may be curbed.

Many studies on the language development of children with cleft palate over 50 years indicate that these children do display delays in language acquisition (Ceponiene et al., 2000; Richman & Eliason, 1993; Scherer & D'Antonio, 1997). In early childhood, both language comprehension and production are affected. After the preschool years, the problems tend to become expressive. Vocabulary learning may be one of the more consistent areas of deficit. Vocabulary measures taken at 15, 18, and 21 months showed that toddlers with cleft palate were delayed by 3 months in lexical acquisition when compared to their non-cleft peers (Broen et al., 1991). A study by Chapman et al. (2008) showed that only 5 out of the 40 toddlers with cleft who participated in a longitudinal study of palatal surgery, timing, and speech outcome could be labeled as "delayed" in lexical acquisition and some of them continued to make progress during the span of the study. This indicates that not all children with cleft palate show delay in acquisition of words (Hardin-Jones & Chapman, 2011).

Compared to their typically developing peers, children with cleft palate have a tendency to produce words beginning with sonorants and have difficulty producing words that begin with obstruents. It has also been found that the early appearance of true stop consonants, either before or after early palatal surgery, is associated with better speech production and lexical development roughly 9 months later (Chapman, Hardin-Jones, & Halter, 2003). However, a study by Chapman (2004) showed that speech measures taken at presurgery and early postsurgery were generally poorly correlated with speech and language skills at 39 months. Therefore, although a child with good presurgery/early postsurgery speech scores may perform well in speech and language measures a few months later, the same child may not be able to maintain acquisition of skills across time. Cumulative records of the vocabulary used during the second year of life have also shown that children with clefts consistently lag behind in lexical acquisition (Broen et al., 1991). However, as children grow older, the gap in language abilities between those with and without clefts may gradually close. The problems that remain often appear related to interpersonal factors, such as concerns about appearance and peer acceptance.

Children with cleft palates and lips can have problems with their conversational abilities. They have been described as producing fewer assertive utterances and not responding very well to their caregivers. The conversational assertiveness of these children has been found to positively correlate with their speech production skills. The passive communication style of children with cleft palate may be related to their shy personality or their reluctance to interact with others due to poor speech intelligibility. Work on the children's pragmatic aspects of their language is, therefore, important as part of their intervention program (Frederickson, Chapman, & Hardin-Jones, 2006; Hardin-Jones, Chapman, & Schulte, 2003).

Given the evidence for the existence of language problems in children with palatal clefts, it is important to determine some prelinguistic indicators of future language problems in children with cleft palates and lips. Frequency of babbling and mean level of babbling taken at 6 months are good indicators of number of consonants produced and vocabulary development at 30 months for children with cleft palates (Scherer, Williams, & Proctor-Williams, 2008). Symbolic play may be another important indicator of later language development. The symbolic play measured at 18 months for the children in the isolated cleft palate group was a good indicator of later language development measured in terms of vocabulary at 30 months and mean length of utterance at 24 and 30 months. In contrast, for the children with combined cleft lip and palates, there were only a few significant correlations between symbolic play at 18 months and later language development (Snyder & Scherer, 2004). These findings indicate the importance of symbolic play assessments in young children with palatal clefts, especially those with isolated cleft palates.

Learning Disabilities/Language Impairment in Children with Cleft Lips and Palates

Besides early delays in vocabulary and morphosyntax (Broen et al., 1991; McWilliams, Morris, & Shelton, 1990), when children with clefts enter school, a greater proportion of the children could be expected to have been identified with learning disabilities, including reading problems (Broder, Richman, & Matheson, 1998; Richman & Eliason, 1993; Richman, Eliason, & Lindgren, 1988). Some suggest that about half of individuals with clefts have language and learning disabilities (Ceponiene et al., 2000). Older children with cleft palate who have learning disabilities have been found to differ from those with no learning disabilities in expressive language and rapid naming but do not differ on measures of phonemic awareness (Richman & Ryan, 2003). Because of their problems in rapid naming, which can potentially impact sight word reading ability, reading remediation for these children that capitalizes on their relative strengths in phonemic awareness may be an effective strategy to help their reading achievement.

There is also evidence that language and learning disabilities are more prevalent among children with certain types of clefts, in particular children who have clefts of the palate only rather than clefts of both the lip and palate (Broder et al., 1998; Scherer & D'Antonio, 1997).

The reasons are not fully known why some children with clefts might have language disorders not directly attributable to their craniofacial anomalies and early efforts to cope with and treat their medical needs and related speech and hearing problems. The reasons that caused the children's clefting in the first place are certainly suspect, including the possibility of subtle syndromes not yet identified. One line of research has begun to look at the brain morphology of individuals with clefts. Nopoulos et al. (2000) found that the frontal lobes of men with orofacial clefts were larger and the temporal and occipital lobes were significantly smaller than those of the control subjects. Another line of research has investigated the ability of the brains of infants with clefts to detect changes in and retain auditory stimuli (Ceponiene et al., 1999, 2000). Results have indicated that neonates with clefts only, as opposed to other forms of clefting, may be born with differences in auditory cortex functioning that might be associated with language acquisition and later learning problems and that the early differences in auditory perceptual functioning may persist into later infancy.

To the extent that children with clefts are at risk for language problems not directly associated with their speech and other medical problems, professionals need to be careful not to attribute signs of early language delays to the wrong reasons. They also need to be prepared to provide early language as well as early speech intervention. If these children are in school and learning difficulties emerge, professionals need to be suspicious that these, too, may have a language basis and be an intrinsic part of the children's cleft palate condition.

LANGUAGE IN CHILDREN WHO STUTTER

An Overview of Language Problems in Children Who Stutter

The findings that have emerged from studies that have investigated the language skills in children who stutter have been contradictory. Some studies show that children who stutter have problems in expressive language skills (Byrd & Cooper, 1989; Silverman & Bernstein Ratner, 2002). In contrast, there is other evidence suggesting that preschool children with both persistent and recovered stuttering have expressive language skills that exceed their developmental expectations (Watkins, Yairi, & Ambrose, 1999). There are also a few studies that indicate that children with stuttering do not significantly differ from those without stuttering in areas of language (e.g., Howell, Davis, & Au-Yeung, 2003). A study by Bajaj (2007) found that children with stuttering did not significantly differ from typically fluent children even in language performance tasks such as oral narratives.

A survey by Arndt and Healey (2001) of children served by 241 speech–language pathologists revealed that out of 467 children between the ages of 3 and 20 years who stuttered, 262 (56 percent) had only stuttering and 205 (44 percent) had associated communication disorders. Among those with additional communication problems, 66 (32 percent) had phonological problems alone, 72 (35 percent) had language problems alone, and 67 (33 percent) had both phonological and language problems. In another study, Blood and

Seider (1981), who surveyed 358 speech–language pathologists, found that of the 1,060 children with stuttering who were age 14 years or younger, 335 (32 percent) had stuttering alone and 725 (68 percent) had other communication problems in addition to stuttering. Of the 725 children with additional communication problems, 170 (23 percent) had phonological disorders; 104 (14 percent) had language disorders; only 42 (6 percent) had both phonological and language problems; and 316 (44 percent) had other communication problems, such as voice problems or hearing loss, or other concomitant problems, such as cerebral palsy. In explaining such findings, it is possible that children with both stuttering and additional communication problems may be more likely than children with stuttering alone to receive help from speech–language pathologists. Therefore, by surveying practicing speech–language pathologists, we may be overestimating the prevalence of additional communication problems in children who stutter. In order to obtain a more representative sample, we need to conduct a broader epidemiological study (Nippold, 2004). Nevertheless, by combining the findings of the studies that have been conducted to date, we can conclude that children who stutter constitute a heterogeneous group that likely consists of different subgroups and that a proportion of children with stuttering can exhibit language problems as well as their stuttering. These language problems may vary across the life span of a person with stuttering (Watkins & Yairi, 1997).

A meta-analysis of the language abilities of children who stutter and those who do not revealed some differences between the two groups (Ntourou, Conture, & Lipsey, 2011). Receptive and expressive vocabulary seems to be more affected in children who stutter. This could be attributed to underlying poor attention and/or a deficit in phonological working memory. Children who stutter also have a lower mean length of utterance (MLU) when compared to their non-stuttering peers. This may not be indicative of an underlying grammatical deficit. This could perhaps suggest that children who stutter avoid production of longer utterances to enhance their fluency. They may also be emotionally reactive and reluctant to speak in new situations (Ntourou et al., 2011).

Implications for Intervention

Given a possible relationship between language and stuttering, it is reasonable to hypothesize that language deficits may cause some cases of stuttering or that, for some, language and stuttering are served by the same set of neurological processes. Therefore, we could think that a treatment program that focuses on language may bring about positive changes in both fluency and language in children who stutter and have concomitant language deficits. Most of the treatment studies in this area involved training different linguistic contexts and complexities (from simple to complex), and the findings have been promising. Unfortunately, however, language training was not the only procedure employed in these investigations so we cannot conclude that just language training led to improvements in fluency (Culp, 1984; Riley & Riley, 1984). An investigation by Butcher, McFadden, Quinn, and Ryan (2003) was the first experimental study to examine the effects of language training alone (vocabulary, irregular verbs, and pragmatic use of conversational speech acts) on stuttering in 3-year-old children. The results indicated that language training alone led to improvements in either language or fluency but not both. On the other hand, a response contingency intervention in which the children were asked to stop and speak fluently after each stuttered utterance led to significant improvements only in fluency. Therefore, language intervention alone may not improve stuttering, suggesting that intervention for both language and fluency may be necessary in order to see gains in both areas for a child who has concomitant language problems and stuttering.

There is ample evidence indicating that in both stuttering and typically fluent children, the frequency of dysfluencies increases with increase in length and grammatical complexity of utterances. Therefore, when working with children who stutter, it is important to control for language complexity demands by starting with grammatically simpler targets where frequency of stuttering is relatively less and gradually proceed to grammatically more complex targets (Bernstein Ratner, 1995; Colburn & Mysak, 1982a, 1982b; Hall, Yamashita, & Aram, 1993).

SUMMARY

In this chapter we have seen that

- Giftedness has no sanctioned definition. Experts generally describe it as either the potential or the actual demonstration of exceptional abilities.
- Many but not all gifted children have exceptional verbal abilities. Those who do have exceptional abilities follow typical developmental paths but at an accelerated rate.
- Three special populations of gifted children are those from disadvantaged backgrounds, those with physical or sensory disabilities, and those with concomitant learning disabilities.
- Intervention with disabled gifted children is designed to help them compensate for their impairments. The superior intelligence of these children may facilitate the use of technology and cognitive teaching strategies.
- The major variables in visual impairment are degree of loss and age of onset. Children with no useful sight from birth are described as congenitally blind and show a different pattern of language development.
- The early language development of blind children is affected by the unavailability of vision to guide early mother–infant interactions.
- The major differences in blind children's language are semantic and pragmatic. Words are used more restrictively and may be acquired later if the underlying concept is visual. Language functions related to sight are also delayed. Unusual or inappropriate nonverbal behaviors may develop.
- Intervention with blind children should help to compensate for sensory loss, facilitate parent–child interaction, and reduce the frequency of inappropriate behaviors.
- Cerebral palsy is a set of nonprogressive neuromotor disorders caused by brain damage during fetal development or infancy.
- There is no standard profile of language disability in children with cerebral palsy. Problems result from the combined effect of neuromotor impairment, seizures, sensory loss, and intellectual disabilities.
- Language intervention in cases of nonprogressive neuromotor impairment aims to compensate for those motor and sensory functions that will remain impaired, to stimulate cognitive–linguistic abilities, and to modify the environment so that the child can function more independently within it.
- Neuromotor disorders other than cerebral palsy have different effects on speech and language abilities. Progressive disorders cause steady deterioration of function. Some disorders have little or no effect on communication.
- Children with cleft palate who do not have other disabilities exhibit some delays in language acquisition. Some of these may be outgrown, but other children may continue to have language problems and experience learning disabilities when they enter school. Continuing language problems may be associated with cleft types. Congenital auditory perceptual problems have recently been suspected.
- Hearing loss, time spent in surgery and recuperation, structural changes in the speech mechanism, and unintelligible speech are conspicuous factors affecting the language development of children with clefts but may not account for all language problems these children can have.
- All children with stuttering may not show problems in language, but some do. A small subgroup of children who do show deficits in language along with stuttering may benefit from both language and fluency intervention.

In this chapter, we have examined five groups of children who present with very different language characteristics. Their needs for language intervention may range from comprehensive services to no services at all. Professionals must be prepared to encounter a variety of associated problems and ability levels. They should be careful not to assume that certain competencies are present. Neither should they restrict their expectations of what these children can accomplish.

PART 3

Language Intervention

12

Language and Augmentative and Alternative Communication

Susan Balandin • Kate L. Anderson

LEARNING OBJECTIVES

After reading this chapter, you should be able to

- Describe what augmentative and alternative communication (AAC) is and its different types
- Discuss the variety of children who benefit from use of AAC
- Explain the principles of AAC assessment
- Discuss the principles of AAC intervention, including the importance of ensuring children's language and literacy development

Some children described in previous chapters are likely candidates for *augmentative and alternative communication* (AAC). The use of AAC can support children's receptive and expressive language and/or facilitate their language development. Because the implementation of an AAC system is an intervention, we have chosen to locate this chapter at the beginning of this part of this text.

Families, clinicians, and educators may find themselves in the situation of considering AAC systems for a child with language impairment. Questions arise as to what this might mean for the child in terms of the types of systems available, which system is most appropriate for the child, what the implications might be for a child learning to talk, and the impact of AAC on literacy development and reading achievement.

The discipline of AAC began to take shape in the United States in the early 1980s. It was at this time that a group of clinicians created a journal dedicated to AAC, appropriately titled *Augmentative and Alternative Communication*, which encouraged development of college course work in the area and created a number of conferences and organizations, including the International Society for Augmentative and Alternative Communication. Prior to this, in the 1970s, Margaret Walker, Kathy Johnston, and Tony Cornforth had developed the Makaton vocabulary in the United Kingdom. The Makaton vocabulary is a sign vocabulary that was originally used across the world with people with cognitive disability (Walker, 1976). Over the years it has undergone many adaptations, and since 2010 it has been known as Key Word Sign (KWS). KWS is used by adults and children with little or no functional speech across the world and uses the signs of the host country. Today, the ongoing development of mobile technology, apps, and tablets has increased the availability, reduced the cost, and raised the profile of AAC so that it is more widely used than ever before. Thus, in the past 40 years, the discipline of AAC has become a rich, multidisciplinary field in which people who use AAC, families, computer engineers and software developers, speech–language pathologists, teachers, occupational therapists, and many other professionals contribute to the advancement of the field.

More recently, there has been a growing interest in the relationship between the use of alternative communicative modes and the language development of the children who use them (Drager, Light, & McNaughton, 2010; Murray & Goldbart, 2009). Research to date indicates that the use of AAC does not hinder spoken language development, and there is some evidence that it may encourage speech and language production (Binger, Berens, Kent-Walsh, & Taylor, 2008; Leech & Cress, 2011; Millar, Light, & Schlosser, 2006; Schlosser & Wendt, 2008). Importantly, AAC can provide a means of expression or aid comprehension for those with little or no functional speech. Furthermore, it facilitates the learning, social interactions, and inclusion of children with little or no speech.

This chapter provides an overview of the concepts of AAC, including the types of technology and communication modalities commonly employed by children with language impairments. It explores the identification of children who may benefit from AAC interventions and the principles of assessment and intervention of AAC systems. Finally, the chapter addresses the influence of AAC on language and literacy development and the use of AAC in the management of behavioral issues.

WHAT IS AAC?

An Overview and Definitions

AAC refers to an area of research, clinical, and educational practice. It involves the study of and, as necessary, provision of communication approaches that compensate for temporary or permanent communication impairments, activity limitations, and/or participation restrictions of individuals with severe disorders of speech production and/or comprehension, including spoken and written modes of communication (American Speech-Language-Hearing Association [ASHA], 2005). A comprehensive AAC system includes a set of procedures and processes (ASHA, 2002) to maximize functional and effective communication through use of aided (e.g., speech-generating devices [SGDs], picture communication symbols, line drawings, Bliss symbols, tangible objects) and/or unaided symbols (e.g., manual signs, gestures, finger spelling) (ASHA, 2002). As shown in Table 12.1, AAC systems are also often referred to as being either high- or low-technology systems. High-technology communication systems, or "high tech" (Sigafoos & Iacono, 1993) as they are commonly referred to, utilize microcomputers and specialized software. These have the capacity to provide printed and/or voice output. A device that has voice/speech output is referred to as an SGD. The speech may be digitized (i.e., natural speech that has been recorded) or synthesized (i.e., synthetic speech produced from stored digital data).

Low-technology communication systems, that is "low or light tech" (Sigafoos & Iacono, 1993), include symbol boards, books, and object boards that may be made commercially or by a service provider or family member. These systems also include devices operated by electromechanical switches. Low-tech systems are used by beginning communicators and those who are unable to access high-tech systems because of cost or severe physical disability and as backup systems when individuals' high-tech systems are under repair or unavailable.

Many people who use AAC, as well as families and professionals, favor high-tech devices because they not only offer the power of voice output but can also interface with other equipment (e.g., computers, environmental control systems). Furthermore, mobile technologies are used widely in the world and are, therefore, socially acceptable. They are relatively cheap to buy and allow the user to engage in a range of social, educational, and leisure activities. There is also a plethora of communication apps available. However, care must be taken when evaluating and selecting these as they are highly variable in quality and utility.

Mobile phones and iPads now claim a large part of the AAC market and have the advantage of being familiar to most people. For example, in some schools all work is done on

TABLE 12.1 | Summary of Features of Types of AAC Systems

	Features	
	Aided	*Unaided*
High technology	■ Utilizes microcomputers and specialized software ■ Synthesized or digitized speech, that is, voice output communication aids (SGDs) ■ May interface with a computer, environmental control system, or telephone ■ Accessed directly (e.g., using fingers or head pointer) or indirectly (e.g., scanning using a switch) ■ Requires a power source (battery) ■ Requires specialized repair ■ Expensive to purchase and maintain	
Low technology	■ No electronic parts but can include electromechanical switches ■ Accessed directly (e.g., finger pointing and eye gaze) or indirectly using another person to ask which symbol is required ■ Examples: Letter boards Chat books Object communication systems Schedules Symbol boards ■ Easy to maintain, but setup and maintenance can be costly in time	■ Manual signing ■ Examples: Amerind American Sign Language Signed English Auslan British Sign Language

a tablet or iPad. Mobile technologies have clearly changed the face of AAC (McNaughton & Light, 2013), but these authors have cautioned that communication, service provision, and implementation must be the focus for any individual needing an AAC system rather than the technology per se. Furthermore, high-tech systems are not suitable for everyone. Low-tech systems may be the best option for many individuals and also serve as backup communication systems in the event of device failure.

Regardless of the type of device(s) selected, decisions need to be made about the symbol systems to be used for communication. Symbol systems used on AAC systems vary in *transparency* (ease of deciphering what the symbol means) and *iconicity* (how closely it resembles what it represents). Researchers (Snodgrass, Stoner, & Angell, 2013) have demonstrated that children with severe intellectual disability (ID) can learn and use conceptually referenced symbols. Consequently, the idea of a *symbol hierarchy* relating to the learnability of symbols from easy to difficult, as proposed by Mirenda and Locke in 1989, is no longer well accepted. There are many symbol systems that are available commercially. These include pictures, line drawings, and symbol systems that are designed to provide fast and accurate access to language, such as Picture Communication Symbols (PCS)™, Minspeak (Baker, 1982), and Bliss symbols (Bliss, 1965). Symbols can also be thought of as static or dynamic. Static symbols do not change or move (i.e., printed language), whereas a dynamic symbol system does (i.e., ASL and some symbols on dynamic displays) (ASHA, 2002). Practitioners in AAC need to select the most appropriate system for an individual and be prepared to update the system if necessary. For example, early communicators might begin with an AAC system incorporating pictures and photos but progress to a literacy-based system as their literacy skills develop.

Many symbol sets or AAC systems are not true language systems but rather words and phrases from a language selected by caregivers or speech–language pathologists to support communication and meet an individual's immediate communication needs (Light, 1997). Unfortunately, these systems usually consist of mostly nouns, so the communication partner must use guessing, checks, and questions in order to assist the person who uses the system to complete a sentence (Balandin, 1994; Balandin & Iacono, 1993). Because these systems are developed by adults, they may incorporate graphics that are suitable for adults (e.g., "help" represented by a cross for the Red Cross) rather than developmentally appropriate graphics that better suit the cognitive and/or experiential level of the user (Light, 1997). Such symbols may be difficult for young children to relate to or understand or may be considered boring. In addition, research has indicated that preschool children aged 3 to 4 years have considerable difficulty transforming short spoken sentences into graphic symbol sequences, which is a skill expected of children who use AAC (Sutton, Trudeau, Morford, Rios, & Poirier, 2010). Furthermore, adults, including parents and educators, may be unaware of all the vocabulary that young children use and require in order to support their play and language development (Marvin, 1994; Marvin, Beukelman, & Bilyeu, 1994; Morrow, Mirenda, Beukelman, & Yorkston, 1993). Thus, for most children (and indeed adults who use AAC), the AAC system may not be adequate to meet all their communication needs. Despite studies that have indicated that AAC systems must be constantly updated and changed if they are to keep pace with the learner's needs (Balandin & Iacono, 1993; Beukelman, McGinnis, & Morrow, 1991), AAC systems are not always updated frequently enough for the user's needs. This is particularly problematic for children in the process of acquiring language, as it increases the risk of promoting a plateau in a child's language development rather than facilitating language advancement. When we consider the use of AAC systems for communication, we must bear in mind that no single system meets all an individual's communication needs. All of us rely on a variety of communication modes or multimodal communication to express our messages. The same consideration is important in thinking about children's AAC systems.

Multimodal Communication

Multimodal communication includes vocalizations, speech, facial expressions, gestures, movements, and body language, as well as written and electronic messages as a part of communication. It is important for service providers, family members, and people who use AAC to remember that no one mode of AAC will be optimal in all contexts. High-tech systems break down, low-tech systems may be lost or not contain needed vocabulary, and children who sign may need to communicate with others who do not understand the signs. In addition, many who rely on AAC are also able to use their voices in some situations. Such situations include emergencies when a cry signals that help is needed, in interactions with familiar people (e.g., family members), or when supplementing the use of AAC. Thus, those working with children with language disorders now emphasize the need for multimodal communication systems and encourage the speech and vocalizations in situations where these are understood by the communication partners (Blischak & Lloyd, 1996; Iacono, Mirenda, & Beukelman, 1993).

Not only does the use of multimodal communication help ensure that a person who uses AAC has a variety of systems that can be implemented as needed, it may foster further speech and language development. King, Hengst, and DeThorne (2013) demonstrated in a small, single-case design study that both the use of a multimodal AAC intervention and a speech intervention resulted in an increase in both speech quantity and quality. Iacono et al. (1993) suggested that the use of multimodal communication (signing and SGD) encouraged the two children with ID participating in their study to be more actively involved in communication. These researchers noted that multimodal communication was more effective in eliciting responses than an SGD alone for one child. And, van der Schuit and colleagues (2010) reported that an immersive, multimodal communication environment was beneficial to both speaking and nonspeaking children with ID.

Thus, recent research supports communication specialists to not only pay attention to multimodal communication but to also ensure the careful selection and ongoing modification of the AAC system. This is essential for a child's communication success. Researchers have identified a number of factors that can result in failure of an AAC system (Bailey, Paretter, Stoner, Angell, & Carroll, 2006; Baxter, Enderby, Evans, & Judge, 2012). One of the most common reasons for a child failing to use an AAC system is that the system is too difficult for the child to comprehend (Drager, Light, Speltz, Fallon, & Jeffries, 2003). Additional factors such as ease of use, reliability of the device, available support and time taken to learn the device and generate messages all impact whether a device will be used or abandoned (Baxter et al., 2012). Unfortunately, there has been a tendency for service providers to label children not using their systems as being unwilling to communicate rather than recognizing that the system may be unsuitable for the children. As we will discuss here, careful, ongoing assessment of a child's abilities and interests are of paramount importance when introducing AAC. In 2007, Light, Page, Curran, and Pitkin (2007) demonstrated that children whose help was solicited to design a device for a child with significant communication limitations generated ideas that met not only communication needs for the child but also addressed social needs, artistic expression, play, and telecommunication, ideas that help explain the success of mobile technologies with children who require AAC (van der Meer, Kagohara, et al., 2012; van der Meer et al., 2013).

Interprofessional Teams

There is agreement (Beukelman & Mirenda, 2014) that the implementation of successful AAC services requires input from interprofessional teams that include but are not limited to the following professions:

- Speech–language pathologist to provide communication assessment and intervention
- Occupational therapist to assist with seating and positioning
- Physical therapist to provide advice and therapy for motor problems
- Technical staff to assist with any high-tech systems and technology
- Rehabilitation engineers to customize equipment
- Regular/general and special educators to ensure that the child's educational and social needs are considered

Family members are, of course, part of every team. Other professionals (e.g., optometrist, audiologist) may also be involved if the child has additional sensory impairments that impact on language development and the use of an AAC system. Employing interprofessional collaborative teams to provide AAC interventions, particularly in inclusive classroom settings, not only increases the potential for both academic achievement and social participation for children who use AAC (Hunt, Soto, Maier, Muller, & Goetz, 2002) but also is consistent with U.S. federal education legislation and agreed on as good practice.

CHILDREN WHO BENEFIT FROM AAC SYSTEMS

People who use AAC have but one thing in common; they are unable to use speech as a primary functional communication mode, although the reasons why this is so may vary. Beukelman and Mirenda (2014) noted that there is no typical person who uses AAC. It is important to remember that there are many people, including children with language impairments, who benefit from the introduction of an AAC system.

It is not known how many children use AAC or how many might benefit from the introduction of an AAC system (Bax, Cockerill, & Carroll-Few, 2001). However, most children who do use AAC have a congenital disability, including ID, cerebral palsy, autism spectrum disorder (ASD), and/or severe developmental dyspraxia of speech (Binger & Light, 2006). Some children may need AAC after acquiring a communication disorder (e.g., traumatic brain injury [TBI]), and there has recently been interest in ensuring that children who are hospitalized have access to an AAC system if they are temporarily unable to speak because of extreme ill health or surgery (Costello, Patak, & Pritchard, 2010). Despite recognition of the effectiveness of AAC for improving communication, Cockerill et al. (2014) note that although 63 percent of young people with cerebral palsy in their study had impaired speech and/or language, only 32 percent had been provided with an AAC system, and of these only 25 percent used their systems at school and at home.

Since the late 1980s, it has been recognized that any child or individual who is unable to communicate using speech may benefit from the introduction of AAC and that no prerequisite skills are necessary (Kangas & Lloyd, 1988; Romski & Sevcik, 2005). Indeed, every child has the right to the services and technology that are needed to enhance communication and assist in participating in both academic and community activities (National Joint Committee for the Communication Needs for Persons with Severe Disabilities, 2002; United Nations, 2006).

The recognition that there are no prerequisite skills for the introduction of AAC (Kangas & Lloyd, 1988; Romski & Sevcik, 2005) was an important shift because people with a severe physical disability have reported spending many years in intervention working on speech production yet having no functional means of communication until they were introduced to AAC later in life (Merchen, 1984, 1990; Williams, 2000). For children with ID, including those with ASD, early introduction of AAC not only can provide a functional means of communication but can also reduce the likelihood of the use of disruptive and/or destructive behaviors as communicative acts (Beukelman & Mirenda, 2014; Sigafoos, Kerr, Roberts, & Couzens, 1994; Vicker, 1996). More recently, the preferences of children with disability have demonstrated that not only do these children learn to use AAC but they may prefer to use mobile technology if given the choice (van der Meer, Sigafoos, O'Reilly, & Lancioni, 2011).

Children with Challenging Behavior

There are some children with limited language and speech production who demonstrate challenging behavior. *Challenging behavior* or *behaviors of concern* are terms used to refer to socially unacceptable behavior that includes self-injury, aggression toward self and/or others (e.g., biting, scratching), and disruption (e.g., prolonged screaming). Many of these children have ID or ASD.

Since the mid-1980s, there has been recognition that challenging behavior is communicative (Carr & Durand, 1985; Donnellan, Mirenda, Mesaros, & Fassbender, 1984) and that such behavior should be treated as a communicative act. Challenging behavior can serve a variety of communicative functions:

- Escaping or avoiding an activity ("I don't like this place and want to leave now.")
- Having a break from situations ("I'm tired and want to take a rest before doing more.")
- Providing sensory stimulation to compensate for boredom or if a child is unable to occupy himself or herself in meaningful activities ("I'm bored and want something to do." "There's nothing else to do.")
- Gaining attention ("Hey, look.")
- Obtaining a desired object ("I want that.")

Many studies have demonstrated that it is possible to teach an acceptable communicative act using AAC to obtain a desired goal (O'Reilly, Edrisinha, Sigafoos, Lancioni, & Andrews, 2006; Sigafoos, Arthur-Kelly, & Butterfield, 2006; Sigafoos & Tucker, 2000; Walker & Snell, 2013). The acceptable AAC-based communicative acts then replace the unacceptable challenging behaviors as communication means.

When AAC techniques, including manual sign, communication boards, and SGDs, are used to reduce challenging behavior by providing effective and acceptable means of communication, this type of intervention is known as Functional Communication Training (FCT), which was introduced in Chapter 7 as one of several intervention approaches considered to be evidence based. FCT involves assessment of the function of the challenging behavior and systematic instruction of the new acceptable communicative behavior (Beukelman & Mirenda, 2014). New behaviors must be taught in natural contexts, and it is important that there be immediacy in the response of communication partners when the new behavior is first instigated. Behavior teams need to include an AAC specialist with experience in assessing the communicative function of challenging behaviors and with knowledge of a variety of communication systems. This helps ensure that the child with challenging behavior is furnished with a system suitable for his or her needs and level of skill. It is beyond the scope of this chapter and text to provide more detail on the variety of interventions available to deal with challenging behavior. There are, however, excellent resources devoted to this topic, including a systematic review of the outcomes of FCT (Walker & Snell, 2013).

Children with Language Impairments

In 2005, ASHA revised its definition of those served by AAC systems to include individuals with "severe disorders in speech-language production and/or comprehension, including spoken and written modes of communication" (ASHA, 2005). This definition expanded earlier perceptions that AAC systems are used exclusively by people with speech disorders. ASHA recognized AAC as being appropriate for use with individuals with language impairments, including children with language delay or disorder, ASD, ID, and acquired language disorders, who may use AAC systems to aid their comprehension and assist them in organizing and making sense of their activities (Mirenda & Brown, 2007). To date, the literature on children with language delay/disorder and no other concomitant disability (i.e., specific language impairment [SLI]) is scant, and further research is needed in this area.

Children with ASD

The use of AAC may benefit children with ASD who have no functional spoken language (approximately 50 percent) by supporting their receptive and expressive language needs (Cafiero, Acheson, & Zins, 2007; Light, Roberts, Dimarco, & Greiner, 1998; Mirenda, 2001). In the past, individuals with ASD have described their experiences as young children struggling to develop language and to make sense of the variety of stimuli that they experienced (e.g., sounds, smell, touch, movement) (Grandin, 1995). This scenario contrasts with what is now known about AAC being used successfully not only to improve communication but also to support language development and reduce challenging behavior in children with ASD (Cafiero & Delsack, 2007; Kagohara et al., 2012; Schlosser & Wendt, 2008).

As we saw earlier in this book, echolalia, literalness of meaning, and idiosyncratic use of words are all common in children with ASD who do develop speech. The use of AAC may be helpful in supporting more useful means of communication for children who exhibit these linguistic behaviors. Some children with ASD appear to have superior visual memory and visual spatial skills that may result in unusual reading or spelling skills and the ability to perform tasks that are at odds with their overall level of functioning (e.g., the ability to find particular words in the telephone book). Such skills may mask a child's receptive language impairment, resulting in high levels of frustration and limiting language and communication development. These children typically benefit from the use of AAC systems that allow them to make sense of their world by using visual symbols (e.g., photographs, words, signs) to help them order their day (MacDuff, Krantz, & McClannahan, 1993), support their language comprehension and literacy development (Norwell, 2007; Schlosser & Wendt, 2008), and help them be independent within the contexts of both school and home (Ganz et al., 2011).

Several AAC approaches have been used with children with ASD. One of these is Facilitated Communication (FC). FC claims to combine elements of physical support and positive expectations to allow individuals with ASD to communicate by typing messages (Biklen, 1990; Crossley, 1994). The technique involves a child with a disability typing messages with the support of a facilitator. The facilitator supports—but is not supposed to guide—the typist's arm. Calculator (1999) noted that "FC is portrayed as a method of unlocking undisclosed social, intellectual, and communicative skills that previously laid dormant in individuals" (p. 408).

FC is a controversial intervention because it is difficult to know who is actually typing the message—the facilitator or the child (Calculator, 1999). A recent systematic review has demonstrated that there is no scientific evidence to support FC (Schlosser et al., 2014) and clinicians are cautioned against recommending FC as an intervention. Despite the controversy, educators and clinicians report anecdotally that they have seen some children apparently using FC successfully and expressing their own thoughts.

Other forms of AAC used with children with ASD include visual support, SGDs, Picture Exchange Communication System (PECS), System for Augmenting Language (SAL), Aided Language Stimulation (ALS), and Natural Aided Language Stimulation (NALS) (Cafiero et al., 2007; Romski & Sevcik, 1996; Romski, Sevcik, & Forrest, 2000), several of which were introduced in Chapter 7. In ALS, the communication partner uses visual symbols coupled with the spoken word to support the message and assist comprehension. As described later, SAL (Romski & Sevcik, 1996; Romski et al., 2000) incorporates the use of an SGD and has been shown to facilitate both receptive and expressive language, including learning how to make requests. Schepis (2007) and Ganz, Davis, Lund, Goodwyn, and Simpson (2012) demonstrated that PECS and SGDs are effective in supporting individuals with ASD to engage in meaningful communication through requesting and social commentary and may increase use of vocalizations, words, and gestures. The aim of PECS is to teach children with ASD to use visual graphic symbols to make requests by exchanging the appropriate symbol for a preferred item (e.g., drink, cookie). Mirenda (2001) noted that the use of PECS may be helpful in facilitating speech development. Research in this area (Lerna, Esposito, Russo, & Massagli, 2009; Sulzer-Azaroff, Hoffman, Horton, Bondy, & Frost, 2009), has demonstrated some promising results. For example, research by Jurgens, Anderson, and Moore (2009) noted an increase in vocabulary and length of spoken utterances in free play of a 3-year-old with ASD who used PECS, and work by Yoder and colleagues (Yoder & Lieberman, 2010; Yoder & Stone, 2006a, 2006b) is suggesting that PECS may increase occurrences of a variety of communication behaviors in children with autism.

Studies (Flores et al., 2012; Schlosser et al., 2007; Thunberg, Sandberg, & Ahlsen, 2009) also support the use of SGDs for enhancing positive communication outcomes for children with ASD, and at the same time provide some evidence that children with ASD may prefer to use mobile technology such as iPads (van der Meer et al., 2011). Comparative research indicates similar outcomes for SGDs and PECS (Beck, Stoner, Bock, & Parton, 2008; Boesch, Wendt, Subramanian, & Hsu, 2013), with both systems resulting in an increase in requests by most of the children studied with ASD. As noted previously, FCT has been used to reduce challenging behaviors in children with ASD by replacing the behaviors with functionally equivalent communication skills (e.g., signing, using an SGD). Successful use of FCT was reported as early as 1985 (Horner & Budd, 1985) when a young boy with ASD was taught to use five manual signs to request items that he usually demanded by using challenging behaviors (e.g., yelling, grabbing). Since then, there has been a number of empirical studies that have demonstrated that FCT is an effective way to reduce challenging behavior and at the same time teach children with ASD to use functional communication (Mirenda, 1997, 2001). However, despite the emphasis on the need for communication partners to implement FCT strategies in order to promote successful and effective communication (Beukelman & Mirenda, 2014), there are few reports on the efficacy of training the communication partners of children with ASD. A systematic review of using telepractice in assessment and interventions for 46 children with ASD indicates that this area holds promise for this population and warrants further research (Boisvert, Lang, Andrianopoulos, & Boscardin, 2010). Regardless of the type of intervention selected for children with ASD, researchers have noted the importance of allowing children to choose the type of system (e.g., SGD, PECS) they prefer for communication (Lorah et al., 2013; van der Meer, Didden, et al., 2012; van der Meer et al., 2013).

Children with Intellectual Disabilities (ID)

One large group of children who can benefit from using AAC is those with ID. As with other disabilities discussed in this chapter, there is a broad range of cognitive function among those who are AAC users (Launonen, 2003).

Children with severe ID do not easily develop the symbolic underpinnings of language and may not produce spoken language (Beukelman & Mirenda, 2014). Those individuals with severe levels of ID or multiple and profound disabilities who are unable to speak and who are unintentional communicators are commonly referred to either as being "early communicators" (regardless of their chronological age) or as having nonsymbolic communication. They may communicate through a number of informal modes including facial expression, body posture, changes in breathing rate, movements, and vocalizations (e.g., crying, laughing) (Siegel & Cress, 2002). Children who begin with nonsymbolic communication may go on to develop the ability to learn a formal symbol system (e.g., sign, picture symbols, tangible symbols) (Rowland & Schweigert, 1990) or may remain at a nonsymbolic stage all their lives, depending on their level of cognitive ability and other factors, including levels of seizure activity, state of alertness, and nutritional status (Sigafoos et al., 2006). Ogletree and Pierce (2010) provide a comprehensive discussion of effective AAC practices with this group of children that includes ideas for implementing communication interventions.

One challenge in assisting these early communicators is to try to attribute meaning to different communicative acts and ensure that others involved with the individual respond to these acts appropriately (Beukelman & Mirenda, 2014). This not only helps children with ID learn that they can influence the environment but also fosters their development of meaningful communicative exchanges (Siegel & Cress, 2002). Those interacting with children who are early communicators need to support communication by attempting to interpret potential communicative acts (Keen, Woodyatt, & Sigafoos, 2002; Sigafoos et al., 2006). Personal communication dictionaries that describe idiosyncratic behaviors and the meaning of these are very helpful and assist in ensuring consistency in the responses of communication partners, including those who may be unfamiliar with the child. Such consistency is important in supporting the development of language and communication (Brady, Skinner, Roberts, & Hennon, 2006).

An additional challenge is to ensure that early communicators, whatever their chronological age, are provided with meaningful communicative experiences and that spoken language is supported by visual and tactile cues (Drager & Light, 2006; Goossens & Crain, 1986; Goossens, Crain, & Elder, 1992). As is the case with typically developing children, play and play activities foster communication, and it is important that parents and educators understand the potential of play to promote language and communicative acts in a functional setting (Drager & Light, 2006; Launonen, 2003; Trembath, Balandin, Togher, & Stancliffe, 2009). The use of AAC systems in play situations fosters communication and supports language development (Brady, Thiemann-Bourque, Fleming, & Matthews, 2013).

Some beginning communicators do not use their existing AAC systems because of motor and cognitive demands and insufficient quality, rate, and immediacy of reinforcement or response (Johnston, Reichle, & Evans, 2004). Thus, it is important that early communicators have access to a variety of appropriate AAC systems and that these systems are used by all those interacting in the situation to foster meaningful communication (Iacono, Chan, & Waring, 1998; Iacono & Duncum, 1995; Johnston et al., 2004; Romski et al., 2000). It is also important not to overlook trying out systems that may not immediately seem appropriate based on a child's diagnosis. For instance, parents have reported that some children with Angelman's syndrome can achieve success with some high-tech AAC systems as well as more commonly used low-tech systems (Calculator, 2013).

Children with Acquired Language Disorders

Although there is a growing body of literature that focuses on the use of AAC by adults with acquired language disorders, there is a dearth of information about AAC use with children with acquired aphasia, discussed in Chapter 10. Sieratzki, Calvert, Brammer, David, and Woll (2001) reported that a boy diagnosed at 5 years of age with Landau Kleffner syndrome (LKS), a type of acquired language impairment associated with seizures and severe communication impairment (Brown & Edwards, 1989), learned British Sign Language at 13, and this remained his most efficient mode of communication. Similarly, a girl diagnosed with LKS at 4½ years also used signed English as her preferred mode of communication. She was reported to have had an intact language system but severe phonological impairment. The authors suggested that this resulted from deprivation of auditory input due to chronic auditory agnosia associated with the syndrome (Baynes, Kegl, Brentari, Kussmaul, & Poizner, 1998). Pearce and Darwish (1984) reported that a boy with LKS learned Bliss symbols (Bliss, 1965) initially and, having learned 200 symbols, was introduced to sign language. By the age of 8 years, he was able to produce utterances that were 4 or 5 signs long, whereas he could produce only 10 to 15 monosyllabic words in a structured setting (Pearce & Darwish, 1984).

Despite some literature on children with LKS using AAC, within the AAC research there are no data-based studies that focus on AAC use with children with LKS, although the use of AAC to facilitate language is well recognized (Paul, 1997). Thus, the few cases in which successful use of AAC has been reported have been case studies or anecdotal reports (McNaughton, 1991).

Children with Physical Disabilities

It is important to remember that children with disabilities are as individual as typically developing children; it is important to avoid stereotypes and biases. For instance, it would be incorrect to assume that all children with physical disabilities have ID and/or language impairments. Some children with physical disabilities have intact language abilities but may not have the physical abilities to express their language through speech. Children with cerebral palsy make up the bulk of such children.

Nevertheless, there are challenges to speech and language development that are specific to children with severe speech and physical impairments (SSPI). For example, these children may have reduced mobility making them unable to walk or interact with their environment easily. Consequently, they are unable to explore their environment and learn by their own experience, two activities thought to be crucial to early language development (Light, 1997; von Tetzchner & Martinsen, 2000). Parents and caregivers of these children usually spend a great deal of time at medical centers, early intervention programs, and other appointments and so have little time for the activities that are known to be important in early language and reading development (e.g., play and activities that foster early literacy skills) (Beukelman & Mirenda, 2014; Light, 1997; Taylor & Iacono, 2003). Unfortunately, children with SSPI have been found to have difficulties with semantics, morphology, grammar, syntax, and spelling (Sturm & Clendon, 2004) despite their intact intellectual abilities.

When selecting an AAC system for a child with severe physical limitations, it is imperative to ensure that the system is flexible enough for the child to transition from one level of language complexity to another (Paul, 1997). Predicting the nature and rate of transitions for an individual child makes this a difficult task. Paul (1997) suggested that a communication device might be used to build on attempts at vocalization, thus providing a child with a means to transition from sounds to words. More research is needed on how children with physical disabilities using AAC make the transitions that are associated with typical language development.

Regardless of the physical limitations, the child with SSPI should be seen as a functional communicator, taking into account all the complex and dynamic communication needs of the child. In consideration of this important concept, Light (1997) posited that it is necessary to understand the physical, functional, language, social, and cultural contexts of language learning for the child who uses AAC in order to identify what facilitates and what impedes language learning. She noted that children who use AAC are not able to play and communicate at the same time, which means that the very act of using an AAC system requires that the play activity cease when the communicative act occurs (Light, Collier, & Parnes, 1985a, 1985b, 1985c). In addition, for children who use AAC, turn taking with natural-speaking partners is asymmetrical, with the speaking partners dominating conversations (Calculator & Dollaghan, 1982; Culp, 1987; Light et al., 1985a, 1985b, 1985c), taking more turns, and directing the child rather than following the child's lead (Light et al., 1985a, 1985b, 1985c; Sandberg & Liliedahl, 2008). This reduces a child's opportunity to practice language and learn new linguistic skills.

As a final point, access to a suitable AAC system that a child with a physical disability can use comfortably and without undue fatigue is of paramount importance. Many children have AAC systems that they cannot easily reach, that they are unable to switch on by themselves, or that are not always available. Clearly, these factors impact negatively on language use and language development. If children with physical disabilities are to develop language using AAC, they must have a suitable system, training in the use of the system, communication partners who understand how to interact using the system, experiences that foster language development, and the vocabulary in the system that enables them to express all the concepts and ideas that they generate. Furthermore, now that computers and mobile technologies are so commonplace in the home it is important that access to different technologies is integrated (Campbell, Milbourne, Dugan, & Wilcox, 2006; Pousada Garcia, Pereira Loureiro, Groba Gonzalez, Nieto Riveiro, & Pazos Sierra, 2011) while remembering that the child's communication needs should not be overlooked when considering the range of technology available (Light & McNaughton, 2013).

Children Who Are Temporarily Unable to Speak

There is now international recognition supported by a small body of research that when children are temporarily unable to speak, for example, when in intensive care units in the hospital, they are at risk of being confused and frightened and of being more likely to experience adverse events or medical errors (Costello et al., 2010; Fager & Spellman, 2010). Often, these children are too sick to learn to use an AAC system, and neither the child nor the family has time to consider or prepare such a system. Nevertheless, hospitals in the United States and in other parts of the world have mandated that communication should not be overlooked if patients are to remain safe and the number of adverse events occurring within the hospital system reduced (Costello et al., 2010; Hemsley & Balandin, 2014).

Costello and colleagues (2000, 2010) described a program used at the Boston Children's Hospital with young people who were scheduled for surgery and who had time to prepare for being unable to speak after surgery and during some part of recovery. Children were given the opportunity to learn to use a simple SGD that could be programmed with messages and vocabulary chosen by the patients and family members. A strength of this program was that the patients' own voices were used to program the messages before their surgery so that they could "speak" with their own voices on their SGDs. Preliminary evaluation of this program indicated not only that patients and families considered it beneficial but also that staff in the hospital believed that having a communication system available immediately after surgery resulted in better postoperative care and a speedier recovery. The impact on the language development of children who are in the hospital for long periods of time and who are unable to speak during this time (e.g., because they are intubated or have a tracheostomy) has yet to be explored. Nevertheless, the use of mobile technologies holds promise for this group as does the myriad of pictorial pain indicator systems that are easy to download from the Internet or include in mobile technology using an app.

AAC ASSESSMENT

Whatever is the cause or reason for a lack of or limited functional communication, an AAC assessment is the first step to successful AAC intervention. An AAC assessment involves more than assessing a child's current level of communication and suggesting a communication aid (Beukelman & Mirenda, 2014). The goal of AAC assessment is not only to identify a system that will be functional for a child but also to select one that will allow the child to develop language skills and meet future communication needs (Beukelman & Mirenda, 2014). It is also important to remember that assessment is but a part of any AAC intervention. Providing a suitable communication system does not, in itself, ensure that a child will use it or will communicate more effectively. As noted above, training of the child in the use of the system coupled with training of communication partners is important. The use of a biopsychosocial framework such as the ICF-CY[1] is now common practice in health services but it

1. The International Classification of Functioning, Disability, and Health (Children & Youth Version), developed by the World Health Organization (WHO).

TABLE 12.2 | An Outline of the Main Features of the Participation Model of AAC Assessment

Phases	Features
Phase I: Initial assessment for today	Aim: To gain a picture of the child's current level of functioning in order to develop a communication system that will meet the child's immediate needs ▪ Current communication needs assessed ▪ Physical, cognitive, language, and sensory skills assessed
Phase II: Detailed assessment for tomorrow	Aim: To develop a system that will serve the child in a variety of contexts with varied communication partners ▪ System needs to facilitate a variety of interactions (e.g., academic participation and social closeness) ▪ Future interactions and participation considered
Phase III: Follow-up assessment	Aim: To ensure that the system continues to meet the child's needs as he or she matures and becomes involved in different activities across a variety of contexts and partners ▪ Frequency of follow-up varies depending on the needs of the individual ▪ Young children developing language skills need more follow-up assessment; adolescents with developed language starting work need less frequent assessment

Source: Beukelman and Mirenda (2014).

is only gradually being used with children who use AAC. The ICF-CY takes into account the environment and communication partners, in other words, emphasizes that communication does not take place in a vacuum but is driven by and relevant to a range of other factors that are occurring in the person's daily context. The ICF-CY shows promise in supporting development of holistic goals for children who use AAC, but further research in this area is needed (Pless & Granlund, 2012; Rowland et al., 2012).

In common with any intervention using AAC, AAC assessment of children involves a team approach (Beukelman & Mirenda, 2014; Cockerill & Fuller, 2001; Costello, 2000; Proctor & Oswalt, 2008). Currently, the *Participation Model* of assessment (Beukelman & Mirenda, 2014) is used by many AAC teams. Table 12.2 describes the features of this model, which consists of three phases. As can been seen, this model stresses that assessment is an ongoing process, not an event that happens once for a child and the child's family.

Because many individuals with complex communication needs can and do use some speech or vocalizations, it is also important to assess a child's potential to use natural speech as well as to assess the child's language ability (Beukelman & Mirenda, 2014). Assessing language is, however, often problematic. For example, there are few norm-referenced tests that are appropriate to use with children with severe physical disability who are unable to speak, may be unable to manipulate objects, and/or may have additional sensory problems. A relatively recent systematic review (Geytenbeek et al., 2010) of language assessments used with young people with cerebral palsy identified that the Peabody Picture Vocabulary Test—Revised was the frequently used test which was suitable only for older children. The researchers suggested that a unique language test developed specifically for children with severe physical disability is needed (Geytenbeek et al., 2010). Morse (1988) suggested that norm-referenced assessment tools may be used but that care must be taken to note any changes and adaptations made to the testing procedures, and, of course, scores from norm-referenced tests would not be valid if adaptations were made. However, it is important to recognize that there are many individuals who use AAC who have been wrongly diagnosed, including being assessed as having an ID when they do not, because the testing materials were unsuitable or the individuals were physically unable to perform the tasks. In contrast to using norm-referenced tests, professionals experienced with AAC are able to complete a full and accurate assessment using skilled observation and in-depth interviewing. They may also focus on specific skills for targeted assessment (Wilkinson & Rosenquist, 2006).

Observations and interviews with communication partners form a major part of every AAC assessment (Beukelman & Mirenda, 2014; Cockerill & Fuller, 2001). It is important to observe how different communication partners interact with the child. In a study of 42 children with developmental disability, DeVeney, Hoffman, and Cress (2012) suggested that a communication-based developmental assessment may be more reliable than a developmental assessment in which cognitive and motor challenges may result in a skewed assessment of a child's abilities. As already discussed, it is essential that communication partners know how to interact effectively with a child who uses AAC and that they do not limit the child by being overly directive or by denying the child a wide range of communication experiences (Light, 1997). It may also be helpful to view videos of the child interacting in a variety of contexts.

AAC assessment is a complex and time-consuming process. It is likely to include a motor assessment as well as assessment of vision and hearing. Any child who uses AAC will require follow-up assessment to ensure that the system prescribed remains appropriate. With the rise of affordable mobile technology across the world, many children who previously could not access high-tech AAC now are able to do so and families may choose to sacrifice dedicated AAC systems in preference for mobile technology that is readily available and used by peers and others in the community. Further research is needed to explore if the influence of peer support and incidental learning in the community from others using similar mobile technology positively influences children's use of AAC.

AAC INTERVENTION

In this chapter, discussion has focused on a range of children with language disabilities who could benefit from use of an AAC system to enhance communication. Several methods of intervention have proven effective with specific populations of children. The next section highlights some of the methods and approaches used in targeting language development.

System for Augmenting Language (SAL)

The most comprehensive longitudinal research on the use of AAC to promote language and communication in children with ID has been conducted by Romski, Sevcik, and their colleagues. These researchers have used the SAL to successfully increase language production in elementary school children with ID, adolescents with ID in secondary school (Romski & Sevcik, 1996), and toddlers with ID (Romski et al., 2000). The SAL has five integrated components:

1. An SGD
2. A graphic symbol vocabulary individualized for each child and installed on the SGD
3. Functional communication experiences throughout the day that allow the child to use the SGD to communicate
4. An adult communication partner who uses the symbols on the SGD during communicative interaction
5. A detailed feedback mechanism for parents and teachers

A detailed description of the SAL is beyond the scope of this chapter, but interested readers can find more information in the work of Romski, Sevcik, Cheslock, and Barton (2006). A randomized control trial conducted by Romski and colleagues in 2010 indicated that augmenting children's language input or output increased children's vocabulary use and that augmented input/output interventions could be effectively implemented by parents (Romski et al., 2010). More recently, Barker, Akaba, Brady, and Thiemann-Bourque (2013) identified that when peers modeled the use of AAC for preschool children who used ACC, these children's language skills improved even if their teachers had had no specific training. Furthermore, treating the child who uses AAC as a competent communicator and using co-construction techniques rather than the natural speaker always leading the interaction may also be helpful when promoting communication (Sundqvist, Plejert, & Ronnberg, 2010).

Romski, Sevcik, and Adamson (1997) have suggested that children need to learn to understand the relationship not only between a spoken word and its referent but also between a visual symbol and the spoken word. Consequently, they have argued that children with limited comprehension must first learn the relationship between a visual symbol or manual sign and its referent before they can use AAC expressively.

Sign and Gesture

Results of several studies have indicated that gesture is a precursor of spoken language in typically developing young children (Rowe & Goldin-Meadow, 2009), and children's natural gestures may be used to foster interactions between children with disabilities and their communication partners (Calculator, 2002). Chan and Iacono (2001) reported that children with ID demonstrated similar use of gesture to typically developing children even though their speech development was delayed. Since that report, Stefanini, Caselli, and Volterra (2007) and Stefanini, Recchia, and Caselli (2008) have identified that children with Down syndrome make greater use of representational gestures than their peers without disability. This supports the argument that manual communication may be an advantage for children with Down syndrome given the strong association between gestures and language development within this group (Thal & Tobias, 1992, 1994; Zampini & D'Odorico, 2011).

The use of sign and gesture to support the language development of people with an ID is one of the earliest reported uses of AAC (Walker, 1976). It should be noted that some of the sign language systems used by the deaf community (e.g., American Sign Language) are not considered to be AAC systems but instead are languages in their own right. While people with ID are unlikely to become fluent users of a signed language, they may benefit from the use of sign to augment communication.

Key word signing (Beukelman & Mirenda, 2014; Tan, Trembath, Bloomberg, Iacono, & Caithness, 2014) is commonly used with children and adults who have language impairments. In key word signing, only the most important content words in the utterance are signed. In common with aided language stimulation, key word signing is always accompanied by speech and is sometimes termed *simultaneous communication* (Beukelman & Mirenda, 2014). For example, the sentence "It's time for us to go out now, go and get your coat" might be signed "time, out, you, get, and coat," but the whole sentence would be spoken. Thus, the child is exposed to complete sentences in spoken language and at the same time has visual cues in the form of sign to support comprehension and learning.

There have been a number of studies that have explored how best to select and teach signs to children who require a system other than speech to communicate (Fristoe & Lloyd, 1980; Spragale & Micucci, 1990). In order to encourage functional communication, signs should be selected that are most relevant and meaningful for a child and, therefore, most easily learned. This means that when working with young children, it is important to select signs and vocabulary that are developmentally appropriate. If signing is used as an aid to comprehension, it is important that all those interacting with the child use the signs consistently and that the child is rewarded for using sign.

Language and Speech Development

Many parents who are asked to consider using an AAC system with their children wonder if AAC will prevent or discourage the use of speech. Schlosser and Wendt (2008) conducted a review of literature from 1975 to 2007 and found results reporting the impact of AAC on speech to be variable in that some studies reported no gains in speech while others reported moderate gains. These differences were attributed to variability within this population of children. It is important to note that there was no evidence that AAC impeded speech performance. Other researchers have supported these findings (Millar et al., 2006). In fact, there is some evidence that AAC can facilitate language development (Blischak, Lombardino, & Dyson, 2003; King et al., 2013).

A suitable AAC system should be introduced as soon as it is probable that speech is not a functional communication mode for the child (Bax et al., 2001; Romski & Sevcik, 2005; Sevcik, Barton-Hullsey, & Romski, 2008). This includes children who are at risk for delayed language development (e.g., children with Down syndrome) and children who are at risk for problems with speech production (e.g., children with cerebral palsy). Because there are no reports of children preferring to use AAC to natural speech—and there are several reports that indicate that AAC may be used to support the development of natural speech (Bondy & Frost, 1994; Iacono & Duncum, 1995; Romski et al., 2000) and receptive language skills (Mirenda, 1997, 2001)—it is unwise to wait to see if children will develop speech and risk the children having no functional communication system. As Branson and Demchak (2009) identified through a systematic review of the literature, all infants and toddlers with disability demonstrated improvements in communication once AAC was introduced.

Romski and Sevcik (2005) addressed six myths and realities about the use of AAC with young children identified as being at risk for speech and language development. The first myth is that AAC should be viewed as a last resort when all other options have been exhausted. Based on the overwhelming evidence supporting early intervention for all types for children at risk for language development, AAC should be introduced during the period of language development to avoid communication failure in later years (Romski & Sevcik, 2005). The second myth is that AAC hinders or stops speech development. Once again, research has shown that children do not lose their motivation to speak because they have an AAC system in place. Some studies have shown that children actually increase use of speech (Beukelman & Mirenda, 2014; Romski & Sevcik, 2005). Children and families have been found to abandon AAC once purposeful speech developed (Romski & Sevcik, 2005). The third myth suggests that certain cognitive skills need to be in place before a child can be successful with AAC. As mentioned earlier in this chapter, it appears that many children may benefit from the introduction of an AAC system and that such a system may actually improve cognitive development (Romski & Sevcik, 2005). Similarly, the fourth myth addresses the idea that SGDs are appropriate only for children with intact cognition. Technical advances in device development and the means by which children interact with the devices have allowed children with a range of cognitive abilities to successfully have a voice through the use of technology. The fifth myth addresses the belief that chronological age is a factor in consideration for an AAC system. Current research supports the use of AAC with infants, toddlers, and preschoolers with a variety of disabilities (Romski & Sevcik, 2005). Finally, refutation of the sixth myth reveals that there is not a prescribed hierarchy of symbols from real objects to photographs to line drawings to abstract representations to written words, as once believed (Mirenda & Locke, 1989). The choice of a symbol system should be based on the abilities and level of functioning of the individual child. Research clearly supports the use of AAC systems as part of early intervention services. Indeed, Part C of the Individuals with Disabilities Education Act includes the use of AAC systems in its mandates to early interventionists.

In working with young children and families, it is important not to underestimate the importance of family involvement (Romski & Sevcik, 2005). Families become the primary environment in which the children communicate. They assume the role of "therapist" in addition to their parenting and caregiver roles. Many parents are still coming to terms with their child's disability and are seeking the best solutions for their children. All this suggests that parents of young children should be given extra support, information, and decision-making options when being introduced to an AAC system for their child (Romski & Sevcik, 2005). As mentioned in the section on assessment, there are limited tools available for assessment of children requiring AAC. This applies to assessment of infants, toddlers, and preschoolers as well. Care needs to be taken to conduct a comprehensive assessment over time, involving a number of sources and in a variety of contexts. Recommendations for AAC systems during early communication should take into consideration the eventual development and transitions that the child will encounter in the years preparing them for school-based services. That is, recommendations should take into account the expansion of communication partners and environments, along with the increased language demands that occur as a child progresses through the preschool years. Importantly, ongoing training of parents and professionals should accompany these changes and transitions (Romski & Sevcik, 2005).

There are several other issues that need to be taken into account when considering introducing AAC for a young child. The first is that using AAC is slow; the second is that AAC, no matter which system is introduced, will never provide the ease of communication enjoyed by those who speak. As Light (1997) noted, AAC systems rarely contain all the vocabulary or concepts that a child will need to communicate all of his or her thoughts or ideas. The use of AAC systems also alters some of what are usual pragmatic expectations of spoken communication, such as the timing of conversational turns, eye contact, and other aspects of nonverbal communication, such as the use of vocal tone, gestures, and facial expression. Adults with physical disabilities who use AAC have commented on the difficulty they experience when not only their vocal tone but also their facial expressions may be hard to control because of spasms and are consequently difficult to "read" (Merchen, 1990). On the other hand, the use of AAC does enable children to communicate, and there are many AAC users who succeed in mainstream education, complete postsecondary education, and lead fulfilling lives in the community. When considering AAC for children, parents and caregivers should be encouraged to focus on the child's opportunities for communication rather than speech. They should also be supported and encouraged to provide literacy experiences as early as possible. Increasingly, people who use AAC—researchers, clinicians, and educators—are stressing the importance of good literacy skills in supporting a positive quality of life and community involvement across the life span. For example, Stephenson (2010) pointed out the importance and relevance of picture book reading for children with severe ID, as it can provide a rich learning context for early symbol learning even if literacy is not a current goal.

Literacy Acquisition

Researchers have begun to recognize issues related to literacy acquisition for AAC users and explore the development of literacy (reading and writing) skills in people who use AAC. Failure to develop literacy restricts access to self-expression, independence, and more complex communication systems (Erickson & Clendon, 2005). The reasons for AAC users' failure to develop literacy are complex and go beyond their cognitive levels and/or language features. Nonetheless, some do go on to develop strong literacy skills, but a number does not. Sandberg, Smith, and Larsson (2010) studied the literacy skills of 28 children using AAC and found that 8 were classified as good readers, 10 as single-word readers, and, unfortunately, 10 as non-readers.

Smith (2006) identified a combination of factors as affecting poor acquisition of literacy skills in people who use AAC, including a lack of resources for the individual, limited literacy experiences, and a lack of instruction. Children's literacy development may also be affected by memory processes: research suggests that children who use AAC may have weaker phonological and visuospatial short-term memory and poorer phonemic awareness (Hart, Scherz, Apel, & Hodson, 2007; Larsson & Sandberg, 2008), skills known to be important for literacy development.

The use of traditional methods of literacy instruction may not be successful with these communicators. For example, several young people with cognitive delays who used AAC were instructed in phonological awareness and were found not to develop criteria for letter-sound correspondence and generalization in a story-reading activity (Truxler & O'Keefe, 2007). Bailey, Angell, and Stoner (2011) successfully trialed a structured intervention program that targeted sound-to-letter matching skills specifically with young adolescents who use AAC. The results were promising, but the authors cautioned that more research with a larger sample is required. Consequently, within the field of AAC there are recommendations that future research should focus on effective methods for literacy instruction specifically for AAC users.

In response to the need to attend to literacy development in children who use AAC, Smith (2006) and others have suggested several general principles for literacy instruction with AAC communicators:

1. Integrate all aspects of communication and encourage independent communication (Nunes da Ponte, 2002)
2. Encourage motivation and raise expectations for literacy development (McNaughton, 2002)
3. Provide intense, functional, meaningful, and real input over time (Gandell & Filippelli, 2002)
4. Integrate literacy skills across activities and goals (Wershing & Hughes, 2002)
5. Use SGD when available with opportunities for shared book reading (Jackson, Wahlquist, & Marquis, 2011)
6. Be flexible and willing to adapt and use trial-and-error approaches in meeting goals (Bialik & Seligman-Wine, 2002). Having multiple means for representation, expression and engagement are important when implementing literacy programs with children with disability (Browder, Mims, Spooner, Ahlgrim-Delzell, & Lee, 2008)

It is important that teachers and speech–language pathologists focus on the importance of literacy acquisition for children who use AAC and incorporate literacy development goals systematically into intervention programs. Table 12.3 shows one framework, SCRAWL, that Smith (2006) developed to help teach literacy to children who use AAC. As can be seen in the table, the components of SCRAWL include shared stories; comprehension; rapid word recognition; analysis and articulation; writing; and language, literacy, and literature. This framework can be altered to fit the needs of individual children who use AAC and the professionals with whom they interact.

TABLE 12.3 | The SCRAWL Framework for Teaching Literacy to Children Using AAC

	Description	Examples of Tasks
S	Shared stories Narratives of real events or fictional stories that reveal real experiences	Provide key words, phrases, and vocabulary items that are made accessible to children to allow them to tell a story about a trip to the farm
C	Comprehension Different levels of comprehension are important for reading and writing: word meaning, meaning relations across words in a sentence, contextual meaning, and nonliteral and inferential meaning (It is important to support vocabulary development.)	Sort the things seen at the zoo by categories (animals, equipment, and food) Retell the events emphasizing past tense
R	Rapid recognition Strengthen sight word recognition as well as phonological awareness and processing (sounding out words)	Post frequently occurring sight words on a wall and refer to them frequently throughout the day
A	Analysis and articulation Phonological awareness that allows the child to reflect on the sound structure of language, analyze patterns of sounds within words (e.g., recognize similar initial sounds or rhymes), and manipulate sounds within words	Identify number of syllables or initial phoneme for animals encountered on the farm
W	Writing Writing involves spelling individual words, constructing sentences, and creating texts	Write letters to the farmer thanking him or her for the visit
L	Language, literacy, and literature Reaching a stage of competence and enjoyment in written language, offering a chance to explore the wonder and richness of literacy	Establishing a reading corner that contains a variety of literature (picture books, poems, and references) about animals and farms

Source: Smith (2006).

SUMMARY

In this chapter we have seen that

- It is important for all children to have functional communication systems, whatever their levels of ability.
- AAC systems can augment or replace speech communication.
- AAC is a process that includes symbols.
- AAC can be effective for use with children with challenging behavior.
- All those working or interacting with children with a disability who use AAC have a responsibility to ensure that they are aware of the child's communication system, be it idiosyncratic gesture, body movements, sign, or an electronic communication system.
- AAC assessment is an ongoing process.
- Although relatively less is known about the impact of AAC on language development, a great deal is known about the effectiveness of AAC for those who are unable to communicate language using speech.
- There is no evidence that AAC use hinders language and speech development; there is some evidence that its use may facilitate language and speech development.
- The family needs to be included in all parts of the intervention, from discussion of a child's communicative needs to the development and introduction of the AAC system.
- Literacy instruction is an essential, valid, and nonnegotiable goal for children using AAC.

It is also important that professionals—and, in particular, speech–language pathologists as "communication experts"—have a solid, up-to-date working knowledge of AAC and AAC assessment and intervention. All children have a right to communicate, and AAC can provide the means for many, not only to better understand, but also to be "heard."

13

Assessment

LEARNING OBJECTIVES

After reading this chapter, you should be able to

- Discuss approaches to and purposes of the language assessment process
- Describe the tools and procedures typically used in language assessment
- Discuss the role of intelligence testing as part of the assessment process for children with language disorders and the several intelligence tests that might be used

The assessment process is the first step in helping children with language disorders. Information obtained from the process is used to identify those children for whom language intervention is appropriate and to provide initial directions for that intervention. As Shipley and McAfee (2009) write,

> Ultimately, all initial clinical decisions are based on information derived from an assessment process. . . . Completing an assessment involves gathering relevant information, assimilating it, drawing conclusions, and then sharing the findings and recommendations. (p. 4)

An overarching aim of assessment is to help professionals determine if a child's language reflects age-expected performance or if a language delay exists. If a delay exists, then assessment needs to help professionals determine if the reason for the delayed language is due to a language impairment or, as we learned in Chapter 9, a possible language difference or both, or a language delay attributable to other factors.

In this chapter, a number of procedures and tools employed in the language assessment process is reviewed.

APPROACHES TO AND PURPOSES OF THE LANGUAGE ASSESSMENT PROCESS

Some approaches to assessment emphasize the description, appraisal, and consequences of a child's language behaviors. With these approaches, aims are to identify problematic areas in the child's language performance and specify the patterns of language performance that the child possesses and those that are missing from the child's repertoire. The outcomes of such an approach are guidelines for developing appropriate intervention strategies. It is possible that in describing a child's language behaviors, other underlying or associated problems may be identified. That is, language behaviors may be indicators of primary or secondary etiological factors for which intervention, beyond just intervention for the language problem, is necessary. However, a search for an etiology is not a primary focus of the assessment. And, for children discussed in some of the previous chapters, the state of our science does not yet permit identification of cause.

Other approaches place more emphasis on looking for a cause of a child's language problem. Implied in these approaches is that knowing the etiology of the problem can lead to specific intervention plans. This approach is allied with the medical model, and the aim is to identify the etiology of a child's language disorder. Although the more descriptive or appraisal approach may lead to the identification of an underlying cause, the focus of the two approaches differs. With the causative approach, there is an emphasis on the "diagnosis" of the language disorder and its etiology. In reality, however, it may not always be possible to diagnose the etiology of a child's language disorder. In other instances, the etiology may indicate a larger condition of which a language disorder is only a part, as in the case of microcephaly and concomitant brain damage that result in intellectual disability and an accompanying language disorder. Such a diagnosis of the cause falls within the realm of medical practice. Knowing the etiology may not alter a language intervention program significantly, or it might make intervention more effective, as many language characteristics overlap from one primary etiology to another.

There are, however, instances when diagnosing the cause of a problem—or at least identifying causal-related factors—can affect the intervention strategies and the professionals involved in implementing a coordinated intervention program. One obvious example is a language disorder stemming from a hearing loss. In another situation, recognizing a child's language behaviors as being characteristic of a specific "diagnostic category," such as those communication behaviors observed in children with autism spectrum disorder, can lead to appropriate diagnostic team efforts and ultimately to effective medical, therapeutic, and/or educational intervention. Given what we are learning about genetics and potential implications for language performance, identifying the cause of a child's language disorder in other situations may lead to involving different teams of professionals and different directions for intervention. From this viewpoint, diagnosis and causation and the activities that go into searching for possible underlying causes are seen as important parts of the process albeit not to the exclusion of describing a child's language behavior.

Within the framework of these approaches, the assessment process aims to address several purposes. Because U.S. federal education legislation requires (and good practice in the absence of legal mandate indicates) that a child's assessment be carried out by a team of professionals, the different professionals will work together and bring together their information to achieve the same purposes. These include deciding whether a child has a language problem and/or whether a child qualifies for intervention, identifying what might be possible reasons or causes for a language problem if it exists or what factors might be contributing to and/or maintaining it, determining what language skills are and are not present in a child's language repertoire, profiling the child's strengths and weaknesses, and deciding what to recommend and directions for intervention if appropriate.

Determining if a Child Qualifies for Services

Not all children about whom several professionals might agree have language disorders qualify to receive intervention services. Whether a child is eligible to receive services from an agency or organization depends on the criteria set by that agency or organization. Consequently, this objective of assessment is, to some extent, separate from other objectives of the process because it considers the interests and policies of the service provider in addition to those of the child and his or her family. In contrast, the other objectives of the assessment process are child and family oriented. Issues such as standards for comparison, definitions of language impairment, normed cutoff scores, and what particular procedures and tests can be used to provide evidence for or against qualification for services come into play. Many of these issues have been discussed in other chapters.

The procedures needed to address this purpose often involve the use of norm-referenced tests. In fact, use of norm-referenced tests is sometimes mandated by federal education legislation and/or service providers' guidelines. Although there have also been some attempts in the past to mandate use of *specific tests* to demonstrate that children do or do not qualify for services, this practice has run up against issues of professional ethics (the professional needing to be the one who determines what tests are most appropriate for individual children), professional autonomy (the professional as the one who has the expertise and training to evaluate the quality of the tests and make appropriate selections), and legal issues. Consequently, the importance of these tools and, more importantly, their quality in the assessment process, cannot be underestimated. In fact, of the purposes of assessment, determining if a child qualifies for services is one for which norm-referenced tests, along with other procedures, are applicable and for which they are most used. It is essential that professionals know the characteristics of available norm-referenced tests, know what evidence is available about the tests, and critique tests by applying sound psychometric principles in order to choose the appropriate tests to use.

In recent years, there has been an increasing awareness of the need for authentic assessment and the importance of using results from more authentic approaches in deciding if a child can qualify for services. Consequently, decisions about qualifying children for services now regularly include information about a child's performance during real-life situations. These reflect best practices; these are also often legally mandated.

Deciding if a Child Has a Language Impairment, Delayed Language, or Language Difference

Another purpose of assessment is to determine if a language impairment exists because not all children who are seen for assessment have language impairments. Some children may have been referred by other professionals (e.g., physicians, psychologists, and/or general or special education teachers) or by their parents. Other children may have been identified as part of a screening program. Some may be exposed to a language in addition to English. Other children might have language delays but not language impairment. Some of the children seen for assessment will end up being identified as having a language impairment, others will end up having normal language development, others may have variations in their language performance due to language differences but not language disorders, and others may have both language disorders and language differences. A purpose of assessment is to differentiate among these possibilities for an individual child.

Screening. A screening typically involves a brief examination of several parameters of communication. Screening procedures are generally superficial and designed to serve large numbers of children in a short amount of time. Therefore, results of a screening cannot determine whether a child has a language problem. Rather, the purpose of a screening is to detect children whose language performances during this brief examination differ sufficiently from normal expectations to warrant concern and additional investigation or to raise red flags that individual children might be at risk for later language and/or academic difficulties. The results of a screening may raise concerns, but it can neither confirm nor reject those concerns. Having concerns raised, however, leads to referral for full assessment and diagnosis.

Before progressing further in our discussion, however, perhaps a comment based in common sense is in order. It is not necessary to have all children participate in a language screening. Screenings are designed to identify children whose language might be a concern when there are no other apparent disabilities. They are not for children who exhibit other conditions for which we know presence of language impairment is relatively predictable, such as intellectual disability.

One problem with screenings, which we encountered briefly in several previous chapters, is the degree to which professionals can have confidence that a screening program is detecting the "right" children for further assessment. This issue involves the following related concepts:

- *Sensitivity* (degree to which tested children with language problems were correctly identified)
- *Specificity* (degree to which tested children without language problems were accurately identified)
- *Positive predictive value* (the likelihood that children identified as language impaired will subsequently turn out to be language impaired)
- *Negative predictive value* (the likelihood that children identified as not being language impaired will subsequently turn out not to be language impaired)

In other words, children with normal language skills are not identified as candidates for full assessment, yet children with language problems are. When children with normal language skills are identified by a screening process as potentially language disordered, these results are termed *false positives*, and when children who do have language disorders are not identified, these results are termed *false negatives.*

No one screening procedure is infallible. An issue, therefore, becomes the direction of error with which we might be more professionally comfortable. A process that leads to too many false positives has the potential to swamp the service delivery system. As Tomblin, Hardy, and Hein (1991) point out, a screening process that results in a 60 percent false-positive error rate will generate, from a mass screening that identified 1,800 children as suspect and requiring full assessments, 1,350 children who turn out to have normal language skills and 900 who are found to have impaired language skills. A full assessment process takes a considerable amount of a professional's time. Therefore, completing full assessments on children who really did not need them consumes valuable professional resources. False negatives, on the other hand, risk missing children who need language intervention. If 1,000 children were screened but the screening process had a false-negative error rate of 10 percent, 100 children who had language impairments would be thought to have adequate language skills and likely not be provided with intervention. Given the now well-established relationship between language impairments and academic and social problems, this is a significant failure on the part of the system and has negative consequences for the children.

Another problem with screening processes is the degree to which less severe language problems that can interfere with academic performance are detected. Most screening procedures consist of relatively gross and superficial measures of language performance. Otherwise, the screening procedures become too lengthy for professionals to see large numbers of children in a short amount of time. A recurring theme in this text has been the need to stress or challenge a child's language performance if these problems are to be identified. When screening procedures fail to challenge children's language performances, professionals run the risk of increasing the false-negative rate. On the other hand, even normal children's language performances will deteriorate under conditions that stress their language systems too much. In such cases, professionals run the risk of increasing the false-positive rate. The answer is, of course, to determine the balance between too little and too much challenge to the child's system. Unfortunately, we do not know exactly what that balance should be or how to achieve it, although, as we have indicated previously in this text, narrative production or expository discourse for adolescents may provide some of the answers to this dilemma. It does not, however, provide all the answers. Therefore, including as part of screenings brief assessments of children's and adolescents' performances on tasks involving the possible clinical markers of language impairment that have been noted in earlier chapters, that is, nonword repetition, sentence recall, and verb tense morphology, may increase the accuracy of screening results.

Evaluation. Although a screening process might help as a first step in determining if a child has a language problem or is at risk for later academic problems, a more complete evaluation that examines many different aspects of the child's abilities and considers the child's environment (e.g., home, school, or preschool) is essential. Earlier we made the point that not all children referred for assessment have language impairments. We know that in some cases children may be seen for assessment because of false positives from screening processes. In other cases, a child may be referred by another professional as part of that individual's eliminative diagnostic process. That is, the referral source's operational plan may be that if a child does not have a language disorder, then the child does not have some other condition. Certain etiologies may then be eliminated from further consideration. Referrals may also come from people who are concerned about a child's communicative behavior but who are unaware of the language expectations for children at different ages. Some children seen for assessment may be "late bloomers," that is, children who are showing early but temporary delays in language development and who will outgrow their delays and do so without leaving residual problems.

In addressing the purpose of determining whether a child has a language problem, it is necessary as part of the more comprehensive assessment process to find out whether a specific child is demonstrating language behaviors that deviate from those typically evidenced by children of that age and to ascertain whether any differences, if they exist, are significant ones that are likely not to be resolved if left alone. This helps evaluators decide if a language delay is or is not present; it does not address the issue if, in the case of a language delay, there is a language impairment.

Procedures often involve exploring a child's performances on a variety of language tasks and in a variety of situations and comparing the performances to some standards or norms. These procedures can assist in deciding in deviations from standards or norms suggest the presence of language impairment or if the deviations are due to language delay alone. Parental/caregiver reports of children's language performances are additionally important tools used to determine the presence or absence of a language disorder. Different assessment procedures contribute different information about language delay and language disorders. For example, norm-referenced procedures can address the issue of language delay compared to peers, and criterion-referenced measures such as nonword repetition can contribute information to help decide if language impairment is present in the context of language delay.

Again a commonsense comment is in order. If a child's language performance does not reflect a delay or lag from the performance of age-level peers, then there is no language disorder, because if there is no language delay there can be no language disorder. However, it is possible that there can be language delay in the absence of language disorder. This last statement means we need to do more than compare a child's performance to those of his or her typically achieving same-age peers.

Several of the points raised in the section above on screening apply to the evaluation process. These are those related to sensitivity, specificity, positive and negative predictive values, and false-positive and false-negative aspects of our evaluation procedures and tools. Another is the need to include evaluation of children's nonword repetition abilities, sentence recall, verb tense morphology, and connected discourse abilities (e.g., narrative abilities, expository skill). Botting, Faragher, Simkin, Knox, and Conti-Ramsden (2001) found that for 7-year-olds with specific language impairment (SLI) measures of their expressive syntax, as well as narrative, were strongly predictive of their language levels when the children were 11 years old. We also know that older children and adolescents struggle with advanced syntax. Therefore, it is important to ensure that syntax, along with other language and language-related abilities, are also assessed during the evaluation process.

Identifying the Cause of the Problem

A third purpose—to identify the cause of the problem—refers to our previous discussion of etiologies and the diagnostic approach, and we will not repeat it here. Information supplied by others, such as from interviews with a child's primary caregivers and/or teachers, a case history questionnaire form, reports from other professionals, and/or information obtained from achieving other purposes of the assessment process, are usual methods of satisfying this objective—if it is possible to do at all. In some instances, attention to possible causes or causal-related factors can alert professionals to the need to make referrals to other professionals for additional examination.

In some instances, instead of being able to identify a cause or causal-related factors, it may be more realistic to identify maintaining factors. Although maintaining factors cannot be said to have caused or contributed to having caused a child's language problem, there are factors that can hinder a child's progress in language growth, even if intervention is commenced. One example of a maintaining factor might be recurring ear infections. Another might relate to child–parent/caregiver interactions. Still another might be a particular educational context of the child. Even though the assessment process might not result in causal or causal-related factors being identified, highlighting maintaining factors that can be addressed in intervention may be an important outcome of the process.

Identifying Deficit Areas

Another objective is directed at determining the parameters of language, both spoken and written, that may be deficits for a child and the mode(s)—comprehension and/or production—in which the deficits occur. Some children may have more difficulties comprehending and producing age-appropriate sentences, although they may have fewer problems comprehending and using most aspects of the semantic and pragmatic systems. Other children may evidence problems in all aspects of language. Norm-referenced and criterion-referenced approaches to testing and observation in all parameters of language are the procedures typically employed to accomplish this objective. Knowledge of a child's specific deficit areas can help determine the focus or foci of an appropriate intervention plan for an individual child.

Describing the Regularities in the Child's Language

Although achieving the above purpose may identify broad areas of language deficits, more specific, descriptive information about a child's language skills is necessary to develop an effective and comprehensive intervention plan. A further purpose is aimed at describing patterns of language skills within each of the parameters of language. These are the regularities that make up the child's language system in terms of both the patterns present in the child's system and those absent from the system. Rarely can the results of norm-referenced tests lead to a description of a child's language patterns (Huang, Hopkins, & Nippold, 1997; Merrell & Plante, 1997), and examining a child's performance on items within tests does not necessarily lead to correct decisions about the regularities in the child's language, in part because items on tests represent samples of particular skills that are too small to make valid conclusions. There is evidence that item-analysis approaches using norm-referenced tests do not yield consistent results, with children passing some items and failing others that examine the same linguistic structure (Merrell & Plante, 1997). As Merrell and Plante (1997) point out from looking at the results of their investigation, "Inappropriately deriving therapy objectives from a child's item-level performance would lead to unnecessary social and economic costs" (p. 57).

Analyses of a child's language behaviors when communicative situations and stimuli are systematically varied typically result in information that is more useful in developing intervention strategies than that which comes from norm-referenced testing. To achieve this objective, criterion-referenced and un-normed procedures, such as observation of the child in context followed by in-depth analyses of the results, are likely more revealing procedures to employ. These procedures also permit a baseline of a child's abilities to be determined from which the child's future progress, with or without intervention, can be measured.

Another aspect of this purpose is discovering a child's potential to improve performance, the extent to which a child can improve performance, and the circumstances under which improved performance can be obtained. In other words, the child's *ability to learn language* is assessed. This is a different focus from finding out what a child knows about language, for example, what the child knows with regard to syntax, by assessing the complexity of sentences he or she uses, or what the child knows in terms of vocabulary, by assessing the number of different words the child knows. These are examples of *language knowledge* and represent the child's current status with aspects of language. In contrast, assessing a child's ability to learn new language skills provides information about how good the child is at learning new language skills, not what the child already knows. A child might have a language delay for any number of different reasons, for example, an impoverished home environment or exposure to a language other than English, which means language knowledge is lower than it should be, but the child's ability to learn language might be quite good. For example, if provided exposure to new experiences and the vocabulary associated with these, the child quickly adds those words to his or her vocabulary. Many norm-referenced language tests, as well as language sampling, assess a child's language knowledge, but these do not provide information about the child's ability to learn language. For this purpose we need to engage in *dynamic assessment* (*DA*). DA has been discussed in previous chapters, particularly Chapter 9 about linguistically-culturally diverse children, and will be discussed in more detail later in this chapter because the applicability of DA is not limited to assessment of children from diverse backgrounds.

Deciding What to Recommend

The last purpose is addressed by bringing together the information gained by the team of professionals involved in a child's assessment and involves more than just deciding whether a child needs intervention. The views, beliefs, and values of families and others involved in a child's education and care need to have significant influence in the decision about what to recommend. Again, not only does federal legislation require that the input of families be considered, but it is good professional practice that can help increase the possibility that the child's family will be active participants in an intervention plan if intervention is recommended.

If intervention is warranted, part of deciding what to recommend involves deciding on the form of intervention (e.g., direct intervention delivered by a professional, indirect intervention delivered through another agent such as parents or teachers and guided and monitored by the professional, or a combination). It also involves deciding on the appropriate setting for intervention (e.g., in a separate room such as a resource room or clinic room, in a special class, in the classroom or preschool working in conjunction with the teacher, in the home, or in a combination of settings) and, if in a separate resource/clinic room, whether the child should be seen individually, in a group, or a combination of both. When intervention is necessary, specific, sequential language goals that evolve directly from a child's deficit areas, the regularities in the child's language system, those needed for academic and social success, and the types of context/cues that result in improved performance and that take into account the possible causal and/or maintaining factor(s) must be identified. The goals form the framework of an intervention plan designed for an individual child. Recommendations need to specify a series of goals to be incorporated into a comprehensive plan if the intervention is to be successful. This should include time lines for achievement of goals as well as identifiable links with the child's academic, social, emotional, and/or vocational functioning. Recommendations may also include referrals to other professionals who can assist the child or the child's caregivers. When intervention is not recommended, the plans for follow-up need to be determined. Children's progress without intervention is then monitored at regular intervals to ensure that the children are progressing adequately. The recommendations from the assessment process specify the follow-up times and the criteria against which progress will be evaluated. *It is not enough simply to recommend or not recommend intervention.*

Assessment is a continuing process. Those recommendations identified as a result of an initial diagnostic and assessment process cannot be considered "etched in stone." In situations where intervention has been recommended, it may be very inappropriate to adhere unbendingly to such recommendations once intervention commences. We learn more about a child as we work with that child over time than we can learn in the few hours spent during an initial assessment process. The child also changes. Because assessment is an ongoing process throughout intervention, we need to be prepared to change our minds or change our hypotheses as new information about a child comes to light. When intervention has not been initially recommended or when one form of intervention has been recommended, we also need to be prepared to change that initial recommendation if it is not working for the child.

Part of the ongoing nature of assessment is documenting the effectiveness of intervention. We need to monitor regularly how well the child is or is not meeting the intervention objectives. If the child is not making significant changes in language as a result of intervention, we need to do something different. Therefore, progress monitoring is essential.

During intervention, a child's performance on intervention goals is probed at regular intervals in systematic ways on tasks that have not been directly targeted in intervention, that is, on exemplars of the desired behavior that have not been presented during intervention and performance in authentic contexts, such as classrooms. The child's performance on some behaviors that have not been intervention goals is also measured regularly. If performance improves on intervention objectives but not on behaviors that have not been targeted in intervention, the changes on the target objectives can be viewed as resulting from intervention and not from other factors. Determining whether a change is real or random is more difficult. It involves issues of using valid and reliable procedures to measure performance. However, the same norm-referenced tests cannot be administered to a child repeatedly over short periods of time because the child's performance on the test is likely to improve just from practice with the test, not because the ability or skill being measured has itself improved. The tests therefore no longer measure the behavior in question accurately, assuming that they were an accurate measure initially. Professionals may need to use procedures they develop themselves, for which they cannot always ensure validity and reliability. Factors to consider in determining if a change is important include how the changes in language performance impact the child's life and what significant others think about the child's language behavior before and after intervention on targeted skills.

From the foregoing discussion, we can see that assessment is not truly distinct from intervention. Assessment and intervention are *dynamic, interactive processes* in all our efforts to assist children with language disorders.

TOOLS AND PROCEDURES

A variety of tools and procedures is employed in the assessment process for children with suspected language disorders. In combination, the results obtained from these procedures and tools are used to accomplish the purposes of the process. One procedure or tool is insufficient for a thorough assessment. Instead, it is from analyzing and synthesizing information obtained from a number of tools and procedures that the goals for an effective and comprehensive intervention program can be determined.

Gathering Information from Others

Gathering information about the child from others can help identify antecedent factors that might help resolve the questions about whether the child has a problem, the possible reasons for the problem, and/or what might be contributing to maintaining the problem. In many instances, the information can assist in helping to determine what to recommend, what needs to be included in an intervention plan, and what might be the predicted outcome for the child over time. Parents (or other caregivers) are an obviously important source of information—for information about the child's birth history and early developmental milestones, about past and ongoing health problems, and about other assessments the child may have had. Given the increasing knowledge about familial and possible genetic factors associated with child language impairments and syndromes that affect language ability, information about the presence of communication or learning difficulties in other members of the child's immediate and extended family is important. Parents and caregivers are also an important source of information about cultural and linguistic influences that might be affecting the child's performance and what beliefs and values are factors to consider in planning for the child. These individuals are essential partners early in the assessment process. In fact, in the early identification of language impairments in young children there is increasing use of parent report methods to provide information about their children's language (Klee, Pearce, & Carson, 2000; O'Neill, 2007; Rescorla & Achenbach, 2002). Information from parents can be obtained in a variety of ways, often used in combination. These include interviews, completion of child-related checklists (Klee et al., 2000; O'Neill, 2007; Rescorla & Achenbach, 2002), and/or completion of case history questionnaires, of which there are many different forms.

Teachers are also essential professionals who can provide invaluable information about how a child's language does or does not affect what the child can do academically and socially. Good practice, as well as mandated practice as a result of federal education laws, leads to their involvement in assessment. These professionals understand the curriculum demands, see the child try to deal with those demands given his or her language ability, and watch as the child interacts with peers and other adults. Experienced teachers also have encountered a large number of children over the years to whom they can compare how an individual child performs. These individuals can complete checklists in order to structure the information provided as well as being involved in discussions as members of an assessment team and as a member of an individual education plan (IEP) team.

Information from all members of an assessment team is important in order to bring together assessment information. In some instances, professionals who are not members of a current team have evaluated and/or worked with a child, and their reports become valuable pieces of information in assessment. Examples of these might be psychologists' previous reports, those of medical practitioners (e.g., neurologists or pediatricians), or those of audiologists.

What to Assess

Before assessment information is obtained from interaction with or observation of a child, an initial plan about what behaviors, skills, and interactions to assess needs to be determined. Such a plan needs to map how information is going to be obtained about: (a) the child's language knowledge with relevant aspects of language, (b) the ease or difficulty with which the child is able to learn new language skills, and (c) an area of functioning we have not mentioned frequently, that is, the child's abilities in selected areas of language processing. *Language processing* is associated with concepts of information processing that we encountered initially in Chapter 1. A review of that portion of the first chapter might be helpful here. One example of assessing an aspect of language processing might be to ask children to repeat increasing longer strings of random numbers, which is a task often used to explore children's auditory working (short-term) memory. Asking children to participate in nonword repetition (NWR) tasks is another example of assessing aspects of language processing, and we have seen in several places in this text suggestions that NWR ability might be a clinical marker of SLI. It is important, however, that as an assessment progresses, the plan is modified as needed.

Most assessment procedures include evaluating a child's abilities with the syntactic, semantic, morphological, phonological, and pragmatic components of the language system in terms of both the child's comprehension and production skills in these. For school-age children and adolescents, abilities in a number of these areas are assessed for both spoken and written language. For the most part, the procedures assess language knowledge. During the assessment, the situations in which the child demonstrates his or her skills with these different language parameters are systematically varied to provide a broad base of information regarding the child's areas of deficit and specific patterns of language competencies. Additionally, the effects of one component of language on the other language components, as the first component is assessed under several conditions, are examined. Trade-offs among the different aspects of language have been recognized both in children's normal language development and in children with language disorders, for example, Masterson and Kamhi (1992), Reed (1992), Schwartz, Leonard, Folger, and Wilcox (1980), and information about these patterns in a child's language profile can likely assist in planning intervention.

It should be no surprise that a child's performance on tasks that represent possible clinical markers should be assessed, and readers are referred to previous chapters, in particular to Chapter 3, for a review. Above, NWR was identified primarily as a task that taps into children's language processing abilities. Sentence recall tasks are probably more closely aligned to language knowledge (syntactic knowledge) assessment than language processing, even though there is a memory component involved (varying length of sentences). The argument that sentence recall is largely a language knowledge task is bolstered by the fact that children can repeat longer sentences for which they have the syntactic skills contained in the sentences but not shorter sentences for which the syntax exceeds their developmental level.

Observation of a child in a variety of settings is an essential feature of the assessment process. Because a child's language-learning environment can affect a child's language skills, an assessment of that environment is often included in the process. We indicated that information about a child's environment may provide clues as to the effectiveness or ineffectiveness of that environment for language learning. Observations of child–caregiver interactions and visits to the child's home may be included in the assessment process. Dialectal and sociological influences on a child's communicative behaviors need to be identified, and information on a child's code-switching abilities can provide important insights into the child's competency with language. Recall from Chapter 9 that a child who can successfully code switch is unlikely to have a language impairment. Observations of a child in the classroom and during peer interactions can yield valuable information about possible matches and mismatches between school demands and the child's language abilities and for making valid decisions about a child's communicative performance. Observation helps ensure that decisions about intervention and what intervention emphasizes are socially and ecologically valid for children.

Information about a child's abilities in areas other than language can help clarify the nature of the child's language problem and delineate a number of the recommendations to include in an intervention plan. For these reasons, a child's behavior and developmental gross and fine motor, perceptual, cognitive, adaptive, and general social skills may be assessed as part of the process. With teams of professionals involved in the assessment process, others may contribute considerable information about the child's abilities in these areas. Recall also from Chapter 3 that several of these areas of functioning may have predictive value in helping to know which toddlers with slow expressive language development are likely to catch up in their language development without intervention and which are not.

Methods of Assessment

Several methods of obtaining information about the language behaviors of children in an assessment process are typically employed. Norm-referenced tests, language sampling, and other criterion-referenced procedures are among the common methods. However, it is important that one method not be used to the exclusion of the other, and professionals need to be cognizant of the weaknesses of the procedures they are using as well as what the procedures can contribute to their decisions.

Norm-Referenced, Standardized Testing. A standardized test is one in which there is a procedure for administration and analysis of responses is specified by the test developers in an attempt to achieve uniformity across individuals using the test in order to ensure reliability and validity. The idea is to reduce unwanted variations in procedures that could confound interpretation of results. For most standardized language tests, the stimuli for obtaining responses from a child are developed by the author(s) of the test and are included with the test itself. The procedures for using the stimuli, recording responses, and judging the adequacy of responses are specified in the administration instructions.

Most standardized tests are also norm referenced. They provide a means for comparing a particular child's score to some standard or norm that is based on a derived distribution of many individuals' performances assumed to represent a normal distribution of abilities. That is, a representative group of children has typically been given the test, and their performances are those against which a specific child's score is then compared. To allow for comparison, the child's raw score (usually the number of correct responses or the number of errors) is generally converted to one or more other types of scores that reflect some sort of ranking or norm (e.g., age equivalencies, percentile ranks, or standard scores). The idea behind raw-score conversion is to give some indication of the child's performance compared to that of peers so that an individual child's performance can be judged as falling within or outside the limits of a normal range. Norm-referenced tests are generally considered to be tests of static language performance because they provide information about the child's language knowledge at a specific point in time.

There has been a proliferation of norm-referenced standardized language tests for use with young children. Numerous tests to measure children's comprehension of various aspects of the morphological, semantic, and syntactic systems are on the market. Tests designed to examine children's use of these systems are also available, as are tests to measure children's skills with the phonological system. There are fewer norm-referenced standardized tests in the area of pragmatics. Because the nature of pragmatics means that performance needs to change according to many different communicative variables interacting at one time, there are inherent difficulties in developing norm-referenced standardized procedures to assess pragmatics and, therefore, fewer tests to tap this area than areas of syntax, morphology, and semantics.

There are several reasons for test proliferation. The assessment process for a child suspected of having a language disorder is a demanding, time-consuming task. Consequently, there is an ongoing search to find easier and quicker methods of achieving the objectives of the process. The use of tests is often viewed, incorrectly, as a way of easing the assessment task. The emphasis on accountability, documentation, and qualifying children for services has also provided an impetus for test development in the belief that numbers and norms suffice as evidence of fulfilling these responsibilities. Although good assessment requires the ability to make judgments based on extensive knowledge about a child's performance, those who lack the knowledge or the confidence in their knowledge and abilities to make these judgments may turn to tests as the answers to their dilemmas, thus creating a demand for norm-referenced standardized tests.

Although there are problems in an overdependence on the use of norm-referenced standardized tests in the assessment process, these tools do serve several purposes. If selected carefully and employed correctly and if the results are interpreted properly, language tests can help determine whether a child has a language delay and, if a delay is present, help contribute to a professional's conclusion about whether a language impairment is or is not present, can assist in qualifying a child for services when appropriate, and, in some instances, can provide preliminary information about language areas that might be deficit. However, tests must be selected that are appropriate to the individual child in terms of the characteristics of the norming population to which the child's performance is going to be compared. Careful consideration of the norming population is essential in selecting appropriate tests to use.

Tests must demonstrate validity and reliability if they are to be useful at all. In addition, issues of specificity and sensitivity regarding accurate identification of language impairment in children, as discussed previously, are important in determining the validity and reliability of tests. None of these are aspects of test selection that can be taken lightly. Several authors have provided guidelines that can be used in selecting norm-referenced standardized tests, and what is currently a small body of empirical literature that explores the several validity and reliability characteristics of child and adolescent norm-referenced language tests is growing (e.g., Friberg, 2010; Hoffman, Loeb, Brandel, & Gillam, 2011; Plante & Vance, 1994, 1995). However, even when tests might meet what are considered acceptable standards for acknowledged guidelines, they may not demonstrate acceptable diagnostic accuracy and therefore adequate validity. As an example from one study (Plante & Vance, 1994), only 38 percent of 21 child language tests met half of what are typically recognized psychometric criteria. Of the four tests that met the most of these criteria, only one adequately discriminated between children who did and those who did not have language impairments (Plante & Vance, 1994). As a further example, in an investigation of four vocabulary tests (Gray, Plante, Vance, & Henrichsen, 1999), the four tests did not equally identify children with specific language impairment from those with normal language, and the children's scores varied across the tests. Some norm-referenced tests have better diagnostic accuracy than others (Friberg, 2010; Greenslade, Plante, & Vance, 2009; Pankratz, Plante, Vance, & Insalaco, 2007; Perona, Plante, & Vance, 2005). It is concerning, therefore, that research indicates professionals select the norm-referenced standardized language tests they use with children and adolescents on the basis of publication date (the more recent the publication the more likely to be selected) rather than the psychometric properties of the tests (Betz, Eickhoff, & Sullivan, 2013) and about half of school-based SLPs consider norm-referenced standardized tests as the most important assessment elements in their language assessment procedures (Eickhoff, Betz, & Ristow, 2010).

Savvy professionals regularly check the research literature for information about the various tests they are considering. In addition to the research literature, databases (which can often be accessed electronically), such as *Tests in Print* and *Mental Measurements Yearbooks*, provide information about tests and expert reviews of the tests to aid in informed test selection. There is no question that norm-referenced standardized tests must be chosen carefully, used carefully, and interpreted carefully. As Eisenberg, Fersko, and Lundgren (2001) remind us, "Ultimately, valid use of any assessment tool is up to the user" (p. 339).

Norm-referenced standardized tests are tools. They do not direct or determine the assessment process. We select and use them because we want to accomplish an objective and because we believe that they will assist us with that objective. We do not use a particular test or any tests just because they are available. As an analogy, we use a hammer because we want to accomplish a carpentry objective, and we believe that the hammer is the tool we need to complete our objective. We are also aware that there are varying qualities of different hammers and choose the hammer with the qualities we know are best for our objective. As another analogy, we use a measuring cup because we want to accomplish a cooking objective, and we believe that the cup is the tool we need. However, it could be that a saw of a particular quality would be a better tool for our carpentry objective or a food processor with particular features and of a particular quality would be better for our cooking objective. In the same way, a tool other than a norm-referenced standardized test or a different test could be better for accomplishing our specified objectives. Sometimes, we might have to use more than one tool to accomplish our objective (e.g., a hammer and a saw to complete the carpentry objective or a measuring cup and a food processor to complete our cooking objective). This means, of course, that we must know clearly what our objectives are before selecting the tools to accomplish them. Some of the common errors and misconceptions about norm-referenced standardized test use are listed in Table 13.1. When it comes to using norm-referenced standardized tests, Lieberman and Michael's (1986) quote, "Let the clinician beware" (p. 71) of 30 years ago has stood the test of time and is as apropos now as it was then. However, even though there are serious concerns about many of the norm-referenced standardized tests and the ways in which they are used, Apel (1999) concedes that their use is unlikely to disappear, in large part because of the pressure to have numbers to describe children's language performances in order to qualify them for services.

Norm-referenced standardized tests alone do not yield enough information to describe a child's patterns or regularities of language behavior or to decide on the specifics of an intervention plan. For the most part, such tests do not contain a sufficient number of items examining a single feature in a wide variety of contexts to describe the content of performance or determine whether that feature should be a target for intervention. What norm-referenced standardized tests may indicate are those skills that appear to be suspect and that need to be examined in more detail. Because these tests rarely provide us with sufficient information to develop intervention objectives, a more detailed description of the child's language is needed. To accomplish the purposes of describing a child's language patterns and determining the specific intervention recommendations for the child, we use different tools, such as language sampling and/or other criterion-referenced procedures.

TABLE 13.1 | Common Errors and Misconceptions in Using Norm-Referenced Standardized Tests

1. Assuming that test scores demonstrate professional accountability
2. Using tests to cover for insufficient knowledge or confidence
3. Misinterpreting various types of test scores
4. Using tests with children who are not represented in the norming sample
5. Administering tests with inadequately demonstrated validity and reliability
6. Using tests that do not measure the desired skills or abilities
7. Employing tests without being clear about the objectives to be accomplished by using the tests
8. Using tests to identify specific intervention objectives for children

Language Sampling. Our discussion here focuses on general principles of language sampling and much of the discussion focuses on procedures used with younger children. Readers are referred to Chapters 4 and 5 for more information about language sampling with older children and adolescents.

Language sampling is almost universally touted by expert child language professionals and scholars as perhaps the most valuable ecologically valid tool that can be used in assessment. Many states' departments of education either recommend or stipulate that language sampling be one of the assessment procedures used in assessing children's language. Despite the value placed on language sampling as an assessment tool, there is no one method for eliciting and analyzing a language sample. Research has, however, provided a number of evidence-based and best-practice guidelines for helping professionals make informed decisions about the variety of different methods and approaches that can be used for collecting and analyzing samples.

Eliciting the Sample. One of the principles related to obtaining language samples is that the sample used for analysis must, as much as possible, be an accurate representation of what the child does and can do with language. We know from previous chapters, that different methods of eliciting language samples can affect results in different ways. Therefore, clinicians need to think through what the pros and cons are of the different methods and attempt to match methods to the characteristics of the specific child. Age is an important factor in deciding on elicitation method. Play and conversation are two of the methods frequently used with young children. Clinicians need to keep in mind that young children with language impairment may be reticent to talk, especially to someone who is not familiar to them. Several studies have reported varying results with regard to the effect that the degree of examiner familiarity has on a child. Some of the studies have involved normally developing children, and others have involved children with language disorders. What is uncertain is whether children with language impairments might be more susceptible to various degrees of familiarity of their conversational partners than children whose language is developing normally.

If play is selected as an activity to elicit language from a child, there are differing opinions about what might be the better types of activities to use during play to elicit representative samples from children. Some suggest that using items that can be manipulated by children may reduce their talking because they become engrossed in the activity. Others advise using such items and activities because a child might be more apt to communicate when the focus is on activities rather than on talking, when the activities are unstructured and of the child's own choosing, and when the adult's language relates to the child's utterances and the activities and contains few yes/no question forms and imperatives, such as "Tell me. . . ." The differing advice need not be too disconcerting. The choice of activities and even whether to present several toys or activities at a time to the child or only one at a time really depends on the child. Some children become overwhelmed, distracted, and therefore silent if too many activities or too many toys are available, whereas other children need several alternatives, especially if some are not interesting to them. If one strategy is not working, change to the other, remembering that it is always easier to add activities and toys than to take some away. Whatever activities are used, however, they need to be appropriate for a child's age and cognitive level. However, we can see how advice to be flexible in eliciting a sample could play havoc when consistency of sample elicitation across children or across examiners would be important, such as when wishing to compare a particular child's performance on some metric obtained from a sample to samples obtained from other children of similar age. Another issue in selecting activities is the degree to which they can promote talk beyond the here and now, including past events, since professionals need to explore a child's decontextualized language abilities and tense verb use, including past-tense marking.

For younger children, one appropriate scenario might be for the examiner and child to play and talk together in a relaxed, natural, child-directed free-play situation. The examiner can comment on what he or she is doing and what the child is doing, respond in a spontaneous way to the child's attempts at communication and to the child's activities, ask occasional open-ended questions about the child's activities and intentions, and even be silent periodically while engaging in play with the child. With older children, an appropriate scenario might be one in which there is greater emphasis on conversation, interview, and/or narrative and expository discourse, which can take place around activities but with much less emphasis on play.

Another caution about what materials and activities to use when eliciting a language sample comes from our knowledge about the effects of shared knowledge between listener and speaker on the level of language children use. When listeners do not share the same knowledge as a speaker, even child speakers, and when there is a limited number of contextual cues to use, speakers provide more information and tend to use more complex linguistic means to do so.

Although the examiner's language should be natural for the situation, the examiner needs to attempt to elicit increasingly more complex language from the child by introducing more complex forms into his or her own language and creating situations in which a child's usual and logical responses would include these forms. This, of course, has the possible effect of introducing more structure into the sampling scenario. Some of the above discussion has suggested that low structure may encourage more reticent children to talk. However, there are other views that more structured contexts for eliciting language may be effective, particularly in eliciting certain types of language behaviors, and in some instances may result in higher-level language use by a child while being more time efficient. Evans and Craig (1992) found that an interview technique as opposed to free play elicited more and longer utterances from school-age children. The level of semantic and syntactic complexity of language that was elicited was not compromised, with indications that the interview situation tended to elicit more of the more advanced structures. Previously in this text, we have seen that samples elicited via conversation, different types of narrative, and different types of expository discourse have differing effects on the samples produced, for example, Huber, Reed, Patchell, and Conrad (2011); Nippold, Hesketh, Duthie, and Mansfield (2005); Nippold, Mansfield, Billow, and Tomblin (2008); Taliaferro, Reed, and Patchell (2015); Wetherell, Botting, and Conti-Ramsden (2007), which can yield different results regarding children's and adolescents' language.

An examiner also cannot always be sure that a sufficient number of occurrences of specific communicative behaviors will occur during a child-directed free play or even interview sample to allow for analysis. For example, in one study, occurrences of past-tense marking, an important language characteristic for determining presence or absence of language impairment, did not show up in the samples of toddlers until at least 200 utterances had been obtained (Tommerdahl, 2010). Eliciting and analyzing samples of this size are generally not feasible in common practice. Consequently, it may be necessary to use contrived situations or impose certain linguistic forms and activities on the child to elicit these language behaviors. This can sometimes be accomplished by such techniques as an examiner setting up a repetitive play routine with accompanying models of a desired verbalization (repeatedly extracting toys one at a time from a bag and saying "I have a . . ." and then handing the bag to the child with the expectation that the child would continue the pattern), puppet role-playing of familiar scripts, or familiar guessing or requesting games ("Do you have a . . ." in "Go Fish"). Contrived situations may also be helpful to assess a child's abilities to comprehend and use the range of intentions and the forms by which the intentions are conveyed. Sets of intentions and functions can be used as guidelines in examining how many different intentions and functions are present in a child's communicative patterns. Because intentions can be expressed by nonverbal and/or linguistic means, the manner by which a child codes the range of functions and intentions also needs to be determined. The degree of explicitness a child employs to express these, such as direct imperatives, permission directives, or hints, can also be examined. Contrived situations, such as giving a child broken pencils or only one part of a toy to use or by putting desired objects in a closed, clear plastic container, may create opportunities to examine a child's range of communicative intentions and the degree of sophistication in expressing the intentions.

At some point during a sampling procedure, it is necessary to challenge the child's language system. Although we may initially want to create a relaxed environment for a child with the idea of encouraging the child to "open up," such an environment may not place sufficient language demands on the child to tap the child's maximum potential or stress the language system to determine what, if any, linguistic breakdowns emerge. This means that the examiner will need to modify expectations and/or the language sample elicitation tasks for the child in order to encourage the child to use higher levels of language in more communicatively demanding contexts. This is particularly true for school-age children, some of whose language problems, particularly in the case of higher-level language difficulties, may be more subtle and not so readily apparent and detectable.

One way to increase language demands, as we know from previous chapters, is to ask the child to produce a narrative or some type of expository discourse. Use of a narrative task also has the advantage of allowing an examiner to analyze a child's use of narrative structure, which we discuss later in this chapter. Additionally, some language sample analysis procedures are based on narrative and/or expository samples of children's language and several include reference databases that can be valuable resources to which to compare an individual child's or adolescent's performance (Miller, Andriacchi, & Nockerts, 2015; Petersen, Gillam, & Gillam, 2008).

All narrative and expository elicitation tasks, however, are not equal in the ways they challenge a child's or adolescent's language system. For example, a child's ability to retell a favorite fictional story is heavily influenced by the amount of exposure the child has had to the story as well as by the child's language ability and knowledge of the narrative genre. Asking a child to retell a story after the examiner's telling of the story is affected by how well the child can remember the story and can utilize the examiner's model. This task may not, however, tap as much knowledge about narrative structure because a model was provided. If the person to whom the child is to retell the story is the same as the original storyteller, there is considerable shared knowledge between child and listener, so less complexity and detail may characterize the retelling in terms of both narrative complexity and linguistic complexity. Asking a child to make up a story and tell it is a very hard task that places considerable demands simultaneously on the child's language system, so if breakdowns occur, the examiner may not know what part of the process was problematic. In contrast, asking a child to tell about a familiar routine or script or about something that happened to him or her (personal narrative) may be much easier but insufficiently challenging to the child's language system, depending on the child's age. While telling or retelling a story from a book reduces memory demands and addresses some of the story's familiarity issues, there can be considerable cues available to the child about narrative structure and sequence so that knowledge of narrative genre may not be well tapped.

There is no one correct or universally accepted method for eliciting narratives or expository text from children and adolescents, and as we know, different approaches can yield different results. Hughes, McGillivray, and Schmidek (1997) have provided guidelines for narrative elicitation based on children's ages. For example, from preschool through about grade 6, personal narratives (descriptions of events experienced by the child) and scripts (descriptions of usual or typical routines, such as getting ready for school in the morning) might be appropriate. At these ages, fictional narratives (stories) might also be elicited, but the amount of support provided to the child for this type of narrative in terms of pictures and whether the context of the narrative is or is not shared with the listener can be systematically varied depending on the child's age. Hughes et al. (1997) suggest that story generation (making up a novel story) not be elicited until a child is school age. Beyond grade 6, personal narratives might no longer be appropriate, but between grades 7 and 9, scripts might continue to be elicited. For fictional narratives, both story generation and story retelling with varying degrees of picture support with and without shared context might elicit narratives appropriate for the children's ages. Beyond grade 9, however, these authors (Hughes et al., 1997) recommend that narrative elicitation be limited to story generation and story retelling. Recall from Chapter 5 that Nippold (2014) used fables because of her concern that usual story elicitation methods are often inappropriately juvenile for older children and adolescents. Ebert and Scott (2014) found that narrative correlated more closely with language test scores for younger school-age children than older students, which suggests that for older school-age children and adolescents it might be appropriate to decrease use of narratives for sample elicitation. Furthermore, we know that expository discourse takes on increasing importance as children age, so it might be reasonable to use more expository tasks than narrative tasks for sample elicitation. It is important to remember that what an examiner is trying to ascertain is information about a child's language, and the child's age needs to serve as a major factor in deciding which method is selected.

Principles of dynamic assessment might be helpful in assisting an examiner to find out what a child or adolescent is able to do, for example, with narrative or exposition, rather than just what the child or adolescent does. For example, Gummersall and Strong (1999) found that in a story retelling task, after an examiner had told the entire story to the children, asking the children to imitate the examiner's model of each sentence in the narrative resulted in an increase in the children's complexity of several syntax measures when the children told the story again by themselves. The positive effect of the syntactic complexity of the examiner's repetition on the story and of the children's practice by repeating the sentences applied to the story retellings both of normally developing school-age children and of school-age children with language disorders. In contrast, Ukrainetz and Gillam (2009) found that the SLI children in their study did not take full advantage of adult models as presented in the research to improve their narratives, although their narratives improved from their first to second story. Hughes (1998) used a different form of dynamic assessment. She employed a 1-minute wait period between children's, adolescents', and adults' exposure to a pictured story and their tellings of the story. When subjects utilized this wait period, not only was the overall length of the storytellings longer, but syntactically the utterances were longer than those of subjects who did not utilize the wait time but instead told their stories immediately after viewing the pictures for the story.

Because of the nature of language in interactions, the examiner's language and the activities will place constraints on what language will be elicited from a child. As a result, some important aspects of language may not be elicited, especially with older children. This is always one of the real dangers in language sampling. However, busy professionals may not always feel they can devote the time needed to elicit multiple language samples from a child. Hadley (1998) developed a protocol in an attempt to ensure that several text-level discourse genres of school-age children could be sampled systematically in a time-efficient way. This approach was also designed to tax children's language abilities so that their abilities under different language performance conditions could be evaluated. The text-level discourse samples in this protocol were conversation and, not surprisingly, narrative, including different forms of narrative (personal narrative and fictional retelling) and expository discourse (explaining or giving instructions, such as how to play a game). In her description of the protocol, Hadley (1998) provides considerable details about its application, and further information can be found in her description. She writes,

> If elicitation methods do not sufficiently tax older children's production systems, specific areas of weakness might not surface, and therefore, would not be "checked." Thus, the advantage of using these protocols, or other protocols based on these principles, lies in the comparison of strengths and weaknesses across different discourse types and under different situational task conditions, regardless of the analysis method used. (p. 139)

And, because we know that different disciplines use language in different ways, an examiner might want to obtain expository samples from several disciplinary areas.

Whatever approaches an examiner ultimately selects, however, it is important to remember that one of the main principles of language sampling elicitation is that the materials, activities, and tasks are chosen on the basis of what we want to learn about the child's or adolescent's language rather than letting the materials, tasks, and activities tell us what we do learn.

Sample Length. There is no one correct answer to the question of how long a sample should be for an adequate analysis or whether length should be measured in time or by number of utterances. This situation prompted Heilmann, Nockerts, and Miller (2010) to write that, "currently, there is a discontinuity in the literature regarding reliability of language sample measures and recommended sample sizes" (p. 394). The length of the sample may depend on the child's language level, age, willingness to talk, and fatigue level as well as the time that can be devoted to the task, the specific analysis techniques to be used, and the databases to which a child's sample might be compared. Historically, recommendations regarding the number of utterances that should be included in a sample have ranged from 50 to 100 (Lahey, 1988; Lee, 1974; Miller, 1981; Retherford, 2000; Tyack & Venable, 1999), and 50 utterances have been more or less agreed on as the acceptable *minimum* (Miller, 1996). Generally, a time of 30 minutes has been suggested as approximately the amount of time to spend obtaining a language sample (Crystal, Fletcher, & Garman, 1989; Lahey, 1988; Miller, 1981). Whether time or number of utterances, the bottom-line issue is the validity and reliability of the sample so that professionals can make good decisions on behalf of the children and adolescents. Children with language disorders may not talk very much, so it may take longer to obtain a minimum number of utterances, and obtaining a sufficient number of utterances to have confidence in the sample from which assessment recommendations are going to be made is essential.

There are purported problems of validity and reliability of using sample sizes that do not consist of at least 50 utterances, and Gavin and Giles (1996) have reported that there is even a risk of low retest reliability with samples that do not consist of at least 100 utterances. Although low sample length is an important concern for accurate assessment, long samples do not necessarily ensure that more complex language is elicited, and there is some suggestion that samples beyond 100 utterances may not increase what can be learned about a child's language. However, we do need to keep in mind that it is important to ensure that there are adequate opportunities for a child to use linguistic and communication features of interest in assessment, such as verb tenses. Recall that earlier we noted that in one study (Tommerdahl, 2010), verb tense marking did not show up in language samples of toddlers until about 200 utterances had been elicited. Unfortunately, in one report, only 15 percent of the SLPs surveyed used samples of 100 or more utterances (Kemp & Klee, 1997), and in two other reports, 25 percent (Hux, Morris-Friehe, & Sanger, 1993) and 43 percent (Loeb, Kinsler, & Bookbinder, 2000) of the SLPs surveyed indicated that they used sample sizes consisting of fewer than 50 utterances. Unfortunately, it does not appear that SLPs' sampling practices have changed in important ways since these studies. In a 2016 study (Pavelko, Owens, Ireland, & Hahs-Vaughn, 2016), the results indicated that only about one third of the school-based SLPs surveyed across the United States used samples consisting of 50 to 100 utterances, with 42 percent using samples with fewer than 50 utterances.

To the extent that short samples can compromise results, findings regarding language sampling practices are concerning. SLPs also report that time is a major issue that affects their language sampling practices (Kemp & Klee, 1997; Pavelko et al., 2016). Shorter samples might reduce the time associated with language sampling procedures, so the question arises as to whether there are ways to elicit valid and reliable shorter samples. Eisenberg and Guo (2015) compared a global score that measured the grammaticality of utterances (percent grammatical utterances—PGU) of the talk of 3-year-olds with and without language delay that was elicited by a set of 15 pictures versus a 7-picture set. The researchers concluded that the shorter sets were sufficient to result in trustworthy broad judgments about the language level of the children. In a related investigation, Guo and Eisenberg (2015) found that, for 3-year-old children both with and without language impairment, conversational samples of 7 to 10 minutes resulted in reliable samples for other global language measures, such as length of utterances and number of words in the samples. These authors did not investigate specific language measures, such as verb tense or complex sentence use. Heilmann, Nockerts, et al. (2010) also examined the reliability of shorter samples, measured in time (1-, 3-, and 7-minute samples) for several measures of language use in conversation and self-selected narratives, such as a favorite storybook. Reliability for more general language measures (e.g., total utterances in the sample) and more specific linguistic features (e.g., bound morphemes) were examined. Across normally developing children from 2;8 years to 13;3, the mean number of utterances produced in 7-minute samples was about 97, a number that falls easily within the historically recommended range of 50 to 100. While shorter samples were found to be reliable for the more global language measures, they were less so for the more specific linguistic measures, which we know are likely measures of linguistic features, such as verb morphology, that can signal the presence of language impairment. Validity of the samples elicited was not explored. Heilmann, Nockerts, et al. (2010) suggested it was possible that shorter samples for children who are less talkative, that is, likely those with language disorders, might not be appropriate since "reduced rates of talking can have large effects on short samples" (p. 401). These authors conclude that "blanket recommendations for sample length are inappropriate" (p. 402). It may be that shorter samples might provide metrics sufficient enough to determine language delay versus normal language, but they may not provide the levels of detail about a child's language (e.g., verb morphology, sentence complexity) that are robust enough for differentiating language disorder from language delay or for development of intervention objectives. Professionals need to make informed decisions based on evidence and best practice when deciding on sample length; the degree of assurance in the accuracy of the conclusions and decisions that are made about a child or adolescent need to guide what length of sample is used.

Recording the Sample. Rarely is it possible for an examiner who is busy interacting with a child to record in writing what the child says and does as the events are happening, yet a verbatim transcription that includes contextual information is essential for analysis. The usual method is to audio- or video record the interactions to preserve the events for later transcription and analysis. If audio recording is used, it is essential that the examiner make handwritten notes on the contexts in which a child's utterances occur. These notes should contain information about the objects in the environment; the child's nonverbal behaviors; the events that happen before, during, and after the child's statements; and the time of each interaction. The information is used later to interpret the child's utterances in terms of communicative behaviors, such as the functions, intentions, and semantic relations expressed. The smaller, digital, and easier-to-use video-recording equipment can reduce the need to hand record contextual information and increase the accuracy with which pragmatically relevant information can be retained for later analyses. In fact, Nelson (1998) has written that "videotaping is *essential* [emphasis added] to capture the nonlinguistic context for very young or physically impaired children" (p. 303). Unfortunately, it appears that clinicians do not regularly employ audio/video recording to preserve children's language samples for later analysis but instead attempt to transcribe in "real time" (Kemp & Klee, 1997; Pavelko et al., 2016). The accuracy of results arising from such transcription methods needs to be considered with healthy suspicion.

Transcription and Utterance Segmentation. Once a language sample is recorded, one of the first tasks that need to be completed is transcription of the recorded sample and the separation of the sample into units for analysis. The units used for analysis are typically referred to as *utterances*, and there are different definitions of what constitutes an utterance, many of which are specific to particular analysis approaches, with different language sample analysis approaches using different definitions to guide utterance segmentation. Given the varieties of language sample analysis approaches, it is important to know what type of information is being sought from a procedure and what might be the reference data (norms) that will be used so that these can be married with an appropriate approach. This also means that different ways of segmenting utterances may be used.

Four commonly used definitions of utterance that guide how language samples are separated into utterances for analysis are the following:

- Tone unit (prosodic unit)
- Sentence, per Developmental Sentence Scoring (DSS)
- C-unit
- T-unit

The *tone unit* is an utterance segmentation approach commonly associated with the analysis technique known as the Language Assessment, Remediation and Screening Procedure (LARSP) (Crystal, 1982; Crystal et al., 1989), several of Miller's (1981) language sample analysis procedures, and to some extent Lee's (1974) Developmental Sentence Types (DST) analysis procedures for presentence utterances. This segmentation approach depends heavily on prosodic features of language (e.g., intonation patterns, and pausing) as well as speakers' turns to determine where utterances end and begin. This approach to utterance segmentation is often used with young children in their early stages of language development. Because there is no specified syntactic component to the definition of what constitutes an utterance, single words, phrases, and syntactic structures that contain a subject and finite verb (i.e., sentence or clause) can all be considered as individual utterances. The *DSS sentence procedure* (Lee, 1974) applies to segmentation of samples that consist primarily of utterances with subject–predicate structures (i.e., complete sentences), corresponding with the DSS utterance definition and forming the basis of sample analysis according to DSS procedures. Hunt (1965) devised the *T-unit* as a way of segmenting samples of school-age children's written work into units for analysis. One T-unit consists of an independent or main clause with all its modifiers, including any dependent, or subordinate, clauses attached to it. This aspect of the T-unit definition is similar to the DSS definition in that each utterance contains a subject and finite verb. In contrast, the *C-unit* was used by Loban (1976) to analyze spoken language. The definition of a C-unit is the same as that for the T-unit except that in transcription of a sample, single words and phrases (i.e., not clauses, which have a subject and a finite verb) can be included in the sample to be analyzed if they are appropriate responses to an examiner's statements or questions. The T-unit and DSS definitions exclude these responses from analysis. T-unit and C-unit utterance definitions require that any utterance that contains a coordinating conjunction (e.g., *and*, *so*, or *but*) used to conjoin two or more independent clauses be broken into separate utterance units for analysis. For example, "But the boy didn't like the pie and he ordered a different one the next time" would be two analysis units: "But the boy didn't like the pie" and "And he ordered a different one the next time." Therefore, with T- and C-unit approaches, no analysis unit can technically consist of a compound sentence. This contrasts with the DSS procedure, which permits compound sentences as single utterances in specific situations. Although these different definitions of utterance and the resulting utterance segmentation procedures can be associated with particular analysis procedures, they are also often used to obtain common metrics of language ability, such as the average length of utterances, proportions of different types of clauses, or proportions of different words to number of words used.

The definition of utterance is not a trivial issue because the different definitions have the potential to affect a number of the metrics of interest obtained from language samples (Reed, MacMillan, & McLeod, 2001). If the definition of utterance—and therefore the segmentation of utterances—is tied to a particular type of sample analysis and even possibly some reference databases (norms), then segmenting a sample in a different way from the utterance definition specified by the procedure potentially invalidates the results and interpretations that can be made about the sample. The definitions can also affect a number of the more generic metrics. Reed et al. (2001) examined the effects of the four commonly used definitions of utterance noted above (tone unit, DSS sentence, C-unit, and T-unit) in an attempt to illustrate some of the ways that frequently used metrics derived from language samples can vary based on the definitions of utterance. The difference in definition with regard to whether utterances could consist of two or more independent clauses was an issue that could be expected to affect language sample analysis results. This issue did, in fact, show up in the results of the study by Reed et al. (2001) with regard to metrics obtained for (1) length of utterances, (2) number of utterances derived from the same spoken samples of children that were considered to comprise samples for analysis, and (3) numbers of dependent and independent clauses per utterance. Because segmentation of utterances according to the definition of the DSS procedure (Lee, 1974) permitted some compound sentences to be included in a sample, this resulted in longer utterances and fewer numbers of utterances in samples and affected calculation of metrics based on number of utterances in the sample (e.g., average length of utterances and average number of dependent clauses used per utterance). That different definitions of utterance had a considerable impact on the number of utterances that ultimately made up a sample is an important issue for validity, an issue we have noted above. Reliability of utterance segmentation across different examiners was another issue that emerged in the study. Reliability of utterance segmentation according to DSS, T-unit, and C-unit utterance definitions was high but was sufficiently low for the tone unit definition to be concerning. As can be seen, decisions on how to segment utterances need to be made carefully and ensure the decisions are consistent with specific analysis procedures and any norm-referenced databases to which a child or adolescent's language is to be compared.

TABLE 13.2 | Brown's Rules for Calculating MLU

A. Preferably use 100 utterances, although 50 may suffice for an estimate.
B. Determine total number of morphemes in language sample.
   1. Count as one morpheme:
      - Repetitions of words used for emphasis (*yes, yes, yes*)
      - Compound words (*birthday*)
      - Proper names (*Billy Boy* or *Sally Jones*)
      - Ritualized reduplications (*choo-choo*)
      - Diminutives (*doggie*)
      - Auxiliary verbs (*is* or *will*)
      - Irregular past-tense verbs (*ran* or *ate*)
      - Catenatives (*wanna* or *gonna*)
   2. Count as two morphemes all grammatical inflections, including:
      - Plural nouns (*dogs*)
      - Third-person singular present-tense verbs (*runs*)
      - Present progressive *-ing* (*running*)
      - Possessive nouns (*baby's*)
      - Regular past-tense verbs (*jumped*)
   3. Do not count:
      - Stutterings or dysfluencies, except for the one complete form (*I, I, I*)
      - Fillers (*um* or *oh*), except for *no, yeah, hi*
C. Divide the total number of morphemes by the number of utterances in the language sample.

Source: Brown (1973).

Analysis. Other decisions that need to be made once the sample is recorded are how the sample is going to be analyzed and what particular analysis approaches might be used. These decisions depend, in part, on the child's level of language and what types of samples have been elicited. We also need to have some metric of a child's language to guide us, and this frequently comes from the sample(s) obtained.

Mean Length of Utterance. Length of utterances increases from about one year of age through adolescence. However, length of utterance can be measured in different ways, resulting in different metrics. An often-used metric to guide an examiner in selecting other language sample analysis approaches to use, particularly when assessing young children, is mean length of utterance (MLU), which is based on morpheme, not word, measures, that is, MLU. MLU is based on Brown's (1973) early work that measured length in terms of morphemes and linked length of utterance to the emergence of specific grammatical morphological features (e.g., contractible copula and regular past tense). Brown's rules for calculating MLU are shown in Table 13.2. Miller (1981) subsequently developed stages of syntactic development to which the morphemes included in Brown's work could be assigned, that is, the Assigning Structural Stage procedure. Not only is MLU used as an indicator of how an examiner might analyze a sample, but it is also used as a metric itself in deciding on a child's language ability.

Although MLU is a frequently used clinical metric, Eisenberg et al. (2001) raised serious issues about the purposes for which MLU is used and the lack of standardization underpinning its use. These authors suggest that it may not be a valid and reliable measure and recommend that its use probably best be limited to the trait that it was originally intended to measure, that is, length of utterance, as opposed to purposes for which it is sometimes used (e.g., as an indicator of syntactic complexity). Johnston (2001) found that, even as a measure of length, varying what kinds of utterances (e.g., discourse-dependent utterances such as elliptical responses and imitations) are included and what are excluded from analysis can change MLU measures by 3 to 49 percent and can change sample sizes by 20 percent. Johnston's (2001) work reflects one of the differences regarding what constitutes an utterance according C-unit and T-unit definitions that was also noted by Reed et al. (2001) in their study. MLU has been described as particularly susceptible to variation depending on the context used to sample the language, and as a measure of language development, MLU in morphemes may be less reliable for children older than 3 to 3½ years of age. Dollaghan et al. (1999) also found that children's MLUs vary as a function of their mothers' level of education. Johnston's (2001) work also raised other concerns about the validity of MLU as a metric of children's language. In reference to the use of MLU in identifying language impairment, Eisenberg et al. (2001) write that "low MLU may be used as one piece of evidence supporting a diagnosis of language impairment in preschool children, but should never be used alone for this purpose" (p. 339).

Because of concerns about MLU in morphemes as a reliable measure of language development for children in the late preschool years and beyond, measuring length using words rather than morphemes has gained relative acceptability for children about 4 years of age and older. As a metric, MLU in words appears regularly in descriptions of the language of both language-impaired and typically developing children and adolescents. However, because length of utterance is particularly susceptible to variations in sampling contexts and sample elicitation approaches, clinicians need to be careful to control for these so that comparisons can be made to available databases, children's performance across time, and children's performances to other children (Miller et al., 2015). This is one reason that the questionable language sampling practices of SLPs revealed in several studies (Hux et al., 1993; Kemp & Klee, 1997; Pavelko et al., 2016) is a concern.

Analysis Approaches. In addition to MLU, a number of other features of language are frequently analyzed in language samples. What is included in analyses is generally guided by what information a professional wants to know about a child's language performance. For children at lower levels of language development, approaches that provide for analyses of the child's lexicon, semantic relations, grammatical morphemes, semantic intentions, and pragmatic functions reflected in the sample might be used. These might include, for example, Lahey's (1988) semantic relational analysis and/or Lee's (1974) DST presentence analysis procedure. To gather information about a child's lexical diversity from a language sample, two common approaches are a type-to-token ratio (TTR) (total number of different words divided by total number of words) and total number of different words (NDW). Use of a computer program (VOCD, a program of the CHILDES computerized language analysis system) (MacWhinney, 2000) provides for repeated random sampling of parts of a child's language sample to calculate multiple TTRs that are reported as D values. The idea is to find out the likelihood of a child using new vocabulary words in longer language samples. Because each sample yields multiple D values with this approach, a single, average D is reported. The D approach to estimating a child's lexical diversity has the purported advantages of being independent of sample size and addressing other problems related to usual TTR and NDW metrics. However, the findings of Owen and Leonard (2002) suggest that the measure is not completely free of the influence of the size of the language sample obtained.

For children at more advanced language levels, a child's lexicon again might be specified, and analyses of semantic intentions, semantic relations, grammatical morphemes, and pragmatic functions could be included. More in-depth analyses of advanced forms of syntax and morphology (e.g., clause types and clausal connectors, morphological complexity of vocabulary words) become increasingly important for older children and adolescents (Miller et al., 2015; Nippold, 2014; Ram, Marinellie, Benigno, & McCarthy, 2013). Table 13.3 lists a number of different language sample analysis approaches that are available. An emphasis on analysis of syntactic and morphological features of language is notable among these approaches, although several also include some procedures for analysis of semantic and pragmatic aspects of language, such as Retherford's (2000) *Guide to Analysis of Language Transcripts*.

From the above discussions, the prominence of analyzing language samples to determine what grammatical morphemes are present in children's language is evident. There are several reasons that most analyses include an analysis of grammatical morphemes. Previously in this text, we have seen that difficulties with use of grammatical markers—and

TABLE 13.3 | Some Language Analysis Procedures

Author/Developer	Procedure
Crystal, Fletcher, and Garman (1989)	Language Assessment, Remediation, and Screening Procedure—2 (LARSP—2)
Hannah (1977)	Applied Linguistic Analysis II
Lee (1974)	Developmental Sentence Analysis: Developmental Sentence Types (DST) Developmental Sentence Scoring (DSS)
MacWhinney (2000)	The CHILDES System, 3rd Edition
Miller et al. (2015)	Systematic Analysis of Language Transcripts (SALT)
Mordecai and Palin (1982)	Lingquest 1 & 2
Nippold (2014)	Language Sampling with Adolescents: Implications for Intervention
Pye (1987)	Pye Analysis of Language (PAL)
Retherford (2000)	Guide to Analysis of Language Transcripts, 3rd Edition
Scarborough (1990)	Index of Productive Syntax (IPSyn)
Tyack and Venable (1999)	Language Sampling, Analysis, and Training—3

in particular those related to tense marking—are characteristics of children and possibly even adolescents with language impairments and that these difficulties may even constitute a clinical marker of specific language impairment. The work of Brown (1973), de Villiers and de Villiers (1973), and Miller (1981), which linked children's MLU development and the emergence of grammatical morphemes, has been used frequently in the identification of children with language disorders, and often a discrepancy between MLU and the presence or absence of particular grammatical morphemes is employed as an indicator of impairment (Leonard, 2014).

There are, however, some problems with grammatical morpheme analysis in the identification of language impairment that professionals need to take into account in their language sampling and analysis procedures. Among these are (1) the considerable variability from child to child in the acquisition of grammatical morphemes, in particular the 14 examined by Brown (1973), which has been identified more recently, and (2) the evidence that language samples may not contain sufficient instances of obligatory contexts for each of the morphemes to occur in order to judge accurately whether children have acquired the individual grammatical markers. In describing the findings of their study, Balason and Dollaghan (2002) wrote that the results "indicate that previous interpretations of relationships among age, language levels, and GM [grammatical morpheme] production based on group mean data are suspect, given the substantial variability in frequency of OCs [obligatory contexts] and percentage of GM production" (p. 967). Lahey (1994) has even questioned if we really know what the course and sequence is for children's acquisition of grammatical morphemes, although Hadley and Short's (2005) work on the onset of tense marking in young children adds considerable and useful information with regard to the early emergence of tense marking.

What this means is that in analyses of children's use of grammatical morphemes in their language samples, particularly in comparing morpheme acquisition to their MLUs, we need to be very careful that we have obtained sufficient evidence about a child's use of grammatical morphemes and that we are interpreting the evidence in relation to MLU thoughtfully. We may need to probe using contrived situations to elicit multiple opportunities for obligatory contexts of individual grammatical morphemes (Rice, Wexler, & Cleave, 1995; Rice, Wexler, & Hershberger, 1998), such as the 52-item task developed by Marchman, Wulfeck, and Ellis Weismer (1999) to assess past-tense marking and the 12-item task developed by Simkin and Conti-Ramsden (2001) to assess third-person singular verb marking. One standardized test, the Rice/Wexler Test of Early Grammatical Impairment (Rice & Wexler, 2001), which is based on the probes used in the authors' research, may include sufficient numbers of exemplars for each grammatical morpheme to make judgments about a child's use of each morpheme. In Chapter 5, the use of contrived situations in assessment of adolescents was also suggested as an effective way of ensuring adequate sampling.

Whatever analysis procedures an examiner chooses to use, the regularities in the child's communicative behaviors must be abstracted in order to identify the specific target skills that need to be included in a language intervention plan. Different procedures provide different types of information, and it may be necessary to use several analyses.

Analysis of Mazes and Disruptions. Recall from Chapter 2 that in Loban's (1976) longitudinal study of the language development of school-age children and adolescents, at all grade levels from grades 1 to 12, students who had poor language skills exhibited more maze behavior than those who had advanced language skills. The amount and type of maze behavior that occurs in language samples of younger children and adolescents are aspects of language performance that are frequently included in analyses and that can "supplement traditional language testing of children" (Nettelbaldt & Hansson, 1999, p. 495) with language impairment. As Hadley (1998) points out, "One indicator of linguistic vulnerability is excessive use of maze behavior (i.e., false starts, pauses, repetitions, and revisions)" (p. 134). Guo, Tomblin, and Samelson (2008) found that the fourth-grade children with SLI in their study demonstrated greater maze behavior in narratives than their typically developing peers. Thordardottir and Ellis Weismer (2002) suggest that different types of mazes, such as filled pauses and content mazes, may indicate different areas of vulnerability for children so that not all mazes are interpreted similarly in terms of what they inform about a child's language.

Dollaghan and Campbell (1992) developed a taxonomy of various disruptions or mazes that can occur in children's language samples and procedures to calculate them as a ratio of the number of disruptions to the number of unmazed words that occur in a sample. This ratio was used to control for samples of differing lengths. Four major types of disruptions are included in the taxonomy, with subtypes within each of the major types. Table 13.4 summarizes the types of disruptions identified by these authors. In a preliminary study investigating the utility of the taxonomy, Dollaghan and Campbell (1992) found that, in language samples elicited via a structured interview technique, the most frequently occurring types of disruptions for both normally achieving students and those with language impairment due to traumatic brain injury were pauses and repetitions, which together accounted for about 70 percent of all disruptions. Revisions and orphans (disruptions that lacked an obvious relationship to other elements in the utterance) each accounted for 15 percent of the remaining 30 percent of disruptions. However, only the frequency with which silent pauses of 2 seconds or more were used differentiated the two groups at a statistically significant level, with the students with language impairment using significantly more silent pauses than the normally achieving students. Although not significant, the data suggested a trend toward the students with language impairment using all types of pauses more frequently than the normally achieving students.

Hadley (1998) reminds us, however, that "different discourse types have been shown to tax children's language systems to different degrees" (p. 134), and we know that narratives can particularly stress children's language abilities. In explaining her protocol for sampling children's language in several text-level discourse contexts, the child in one case study that was presented clearly demonstrated a greater number of mazes during two narrative tasks (fictional retelling to a naive listener and relating a known story to a naive listener) than during conversation (interview), relating a personal narrative, and expository discourse (explanation of games or sports). Given that Dollaghan and Campbell (1992) used samples obtained from interviews (conversations) rather than narratives, their sample-elicitation task may not have been sufficiently demanding to reveal greater differences in maze behavior

TABLE 13.4 | Descriptions of Dollaghan and Campbell's Taxonomy for Classifying Disruptions/Mazes Occurring in School-Age Children's Utterances Produced during Language Samples Elicited Using Interview/Conversation

Major Type	Subtypes	Definitions/Examples
Pauses		
	Filled pauses	One-syllable, nonlexical vocalizations (e.g., *um*)
	Silent pauses	Silence for 2 seconds or longer
	Pause strings	Occurrence of more than one filled and/or silent pause in succession
Repetitions		
	Forward repetitions	Repeats an incomplete element and then completes it (e.g., "I said we thought about it")
	Partial repetitions	Repeats an incomplete element but does not complete it (e.g., "I said we thought thought . . .")
	Exact repetitions	Repeats an already completed element (e.g., "I said we thought about it thought about it")
	Backward repetitions	Insertion of an element between an unaltered repetition (e.g., "I said I know I said we thought about it")
Revisions		
Each also coded for aspect(s) of language being revised (lexical, grammatical, phonological, or multiple aspects)	Correction of error	Correction of grammatical error (e.g., "I said we thinked thought about it")
	Addition of information	Addition of lexical information (e.g., "I said firmly said we thought about it")
	Deletion of information	Deletion of lexical information (e.g., "I firmly said I said we thought about it")
	Unknown	Reasons for revisions that affect several elements not apparent
Orphans		
(No apparent relationship to other elements)	Phonemes	"I said frrrr we thought about it"
	Words	"I said we girl thought about it"
	Strings (words or words and phonemes)	"I said frrrr girl we thought about it"

Source: Dollaghan and Campbell (1992).

between students with language impairments and those with normal language. In contrast, Thordardottir and Ellis Weismer (2002) used narrative samples, with their results indicating differences in the types of mazes of SLI and normally developing children.

Another aspect of analyzing mazes from which examiners might obtain useful information involves the grammatical elements of utterances associated with the occurrences of mazes. If, as Hadley (1998) suggests, mazes reflect aspects of language performance that are vulnerable or wobbly, it is possible that the elements of language reflected in the mazes are those parameters of language with which a child may be struggling. For example, in Reed and Evernden's (2001) investigation comparing verb morphological performances of students with reading and language problems with their normally achieving peers, none of the mazes that occurred in the language samples of the normally achieving students involved verbs. This contrasted with the students with reading/language problems, for whom 13.5 percent of their mazes involved verbs, even though both students with reading/language problems and normally achieving students used about the same amount of maze behavior overall. Examiners might want to note what elements of language are involved in children's mazes as well as what types of mazes are involved because it is possible that these may be clues as to what could be specific weaknesses in a child's language system.

Narrative, Expository, and Presuppositional Analyses. Several different approaches are available for narrative and expository analyses, some of which may be more helpful for analyzing attempts of younger children, perhaps in the preschool years, whereas others might be more appropriate for use with older school-age children and adolescents. Different forms of analyses are also likely more appropriate for different types of narratives and expository text than others. Chapters 1 and 2 introduced readers to different types of expository text and the information there can guide approaches to use in expository text analyses. With regard to narrative analyses. Table 13.5 lists a number of approaches and highlights features of each. These analysis approaches provide different information about children's abilities with narrative production, so it is important for an examiner to select the analysis approach that fits what information is being sought.

TABLE 13.5 | Examples of Approaches for Analyzing and Assessing Narratives

Approach	Author(s)	Features
Narrative levels	Applebee (1978)	Six developmental levels in children's narratives 2 to 5 years old: heaps (no organization, bits of random information from whatever comes to a child's mind; approximately 2 years of age), sequences, primitive narratives, unfocused chains, focused chains, true narratives (plot with chain of events, themes or morals emerging; about 20% of 5-year-olds show evidence of true narratives) Additional levels identified in older children's narratives (6 to 17 years) Hutson-Nechkash's (1990) summary of Applebee's (1978) extensions: ■ Provide summaries and characterizing stories (about 7 to 11 years) ■ Provide analysis of narratives (approximately 13 to 15 years) ■ Provide generalizations about theme or moral of narrative (16+ years)
Story grammar	Stein and Glenn (1979) Glenn and Stein (1980)	Focuses on development of the structural patterns and structural properties of narratives (i.e., types of sequences, types and number of episodes) Seven stages (in order from least to most complex): ■ Descriptive sequence (preschool): chain of setting statements with no temporal or causal links ■ Action sequence (preschool): setting statement with action statements functioning as attempts; action statements are chronologically but not causally chained ■ Reaction sequence (preschool): setting statement, an initiating event, and several action (attempt) statements in order of direct cause-and-effect relation (i.e., first action directly causes next action but with no goal direction) ■ Abbreviated episode (about 6 years of age): setting statement and either an initiating statement followed by a consequence or an event statement followed by a consequence; goal direction is either explicit or implicit ■ Complete episode (about 7 to 8 years of age): setting statement and two of three components (initiating event, internal response, attempt) followed by a consequence; goal direction is present ■ Complex episode (about 11 years of age): multiple episodes or expansion of complete episodes; reaction statements and internal plans may be included ■ Interactive episode (11+ years): more than one character and separate episodes with each influencing the others

(Continued)

TABLE 13.5 | *Continued*

Approach	Author(s)	Features
Story grammar decision tree	Westby (1998)	A decision tree based on Stein and Glenn's (1979) story grammar At each stage, in developmental sequence, a decision is made as to whether a child's narrative represents the particular stage; if not, the stage assigned is the lower stage in the sequence; if yes, a decision is made about the next-higher stage As an example, does the narrative evidence explicit planning or intentional behavior, characteristic of "abbreviated episode," per above; if not, child's stage is "reaction sequence"; if yes, the child's stage is either at the "abbreviated episode" stage or higher
Narrative stages	Westby (1998)	Four sequential stages of narrative development Stages in order of development: ▪ Additive chain (events that can occur in any order) ▪ Temporal chain (event presented in temporal order) ▪ Causal chain (cause-and-effect relationships presented in order) ▪ Multiple causal chain (multiple causal relationships presented) Subcategories considered for narratives at or above causal chain stage: ▪ Initiating event ▪ Setting ▪ Reaction ▪ Internal response (states or thoughts of characters) ▪ Attempt ▪ Resolution/consequence
Holistic analysis	McFadden and Gillam (1996)	Focuses evaluation of narrative on general impressions Not dependent on preset criteria or characteristics Narratives scored as "weak," "adequate," "good," or "strong" Elements at text level (e.g., connectives, constituents) as opposed to sentential level (length of utterance, predicate types) contribute to evaluation of quality Numerical values assigned, if needed, from 1 (weak) to 4 (strong)
Strong Narrative Assessment Procedure	Strong (1998)	Quality evaluation referenced to age of child Criterion-referenced, standardized procedure Uses story retelling tasks Initial model via audiotape of story and wordless picture book Retell to naive listener without pictures Appropriate for elementary and middle school students Procedures for analyzing length and fluency of narrative production, cohesion, syntax, and story grammar
Story Construction Subtest, Detroit Tests of Learning Aptitude—4	Hammill (1998)	Norm-reference, standardized subtest Three story creations each from a colored picture stimulus Stories scored for number and complexity of semantic themes Scores reflect story content rather than story form Percentile ranks, standard scores, age equivalents available Norms available for ages 6 to 17 years
Test of Narrative Language	Gillam and Pearson (2004)	Norm-referenced, standardized test Uses three narrative formats: no picture, sequence picture cues, single picture cue Assesses children (5 to 12 years of age) in their ability to remember and tell stories

TABLE 13.5 | *Continued*

Approach	Author(s)	Features
		Measures how well children use aspects of their language as they engage in narrative tasks Percentile ranks, standard scores available
Index of Narrative Complexity (INC)	Petersen, Gillam, and Gillam (2008)	Criterion-referenced measures of important features of good narratives: ■ Characters ■ Setting ■ Initiating Events ■ Internal Responses ■ Plans ■ Action/Attempts ■ Complications ■ Consequences ■ Formulaic Markers (mark beginning/end of narrative) ■ Temporal Markers ■ Causal Adverbial Clauses ■ Knowledge of Dialogue ■ Narrator Evaluations Awards points 0 to 2–3 for each feature, with 3 being most complex indicator of a feature; points summed for INC score Can be used with different narratives, but similar narrative type needs to be used for comparisons Sensitive to changes in narrative ability as a result of narrative intervention
Narrative Scoring Scheme	Heilmann, Miller, Nockerts, and Dunaway (2010)	Scores elementary school students' narrative elicited as a retell of a story from a wordless picture book Judges seven key story grammar and literate language features: ■ Introduction ■ Conflict Resolution ■ Conclusion ■ Mental State Verbs ■ Character Development ■ Referencing ■ Cohesion 0 to 5 points award for each feature, ranging from not present to proficient
Memory-for-Stories Subtest, Test of Memory and Learning	Reynolds and Bigler (1994)	Norm-referenced, standardized subtest Three story retells each after examiner reads a story Includes a delayed story retelling condition; the three stories retold after a wait of about 30 minutes Stories scored for characters and actions included the retells Scores reflect story content rather than story form Percentile ranks, standardized scores, and scaled scores available Norms available for ages 5 through 19 years

Measures of cohesion for features that occur within narratives and expository text and that tie the elements together in meaningful ways can contribute to estimates of the quality and complexity of children's narratives and expository discourse. Some of the linguistic cohesive devices that occur in connected discourse are pronouns following initial nomination of the referent ("The boy ran. . . . *He* caught. . . ."), conjunctions and adverbial connectives ("*Unfortunately*, the boy. . . ."), and indefinite versus definite articles ("*A* child found. . . . *The* child returned. . . ."). Paul and her co-researchers (Paul, Hernandez, Taylor, & Johnson, 1996) reported that one of the distinguishing features between the narratives of normally

TABLE 13.6 | Examples of Manipulating Antecedent Events

Types of Manipulation	Explanations/Examples
Modality change	Present stimuli in a visual rather than auditory form.
Progressive addition of modalities	Present stimuli in one modality (e.g., auditory), add a second modality for bimodality stimuli (e.g., auditory plus visual), add a third modality for multimodality stimuli (e.g., auditory plus visual plus tactile).
Multiple presentations of stimuli before child response	Present stimuli one or more times (e.g., say the word or sentence several times) before asking the child to respond; can be combined with previous approach.
Provide models/hints for target response	Present an example of expected response for child to imitate; present first part (or last part) of the expected response; tell the child to think about producing the target before asking the child to produce it; tell the child a critical feature of the correct response.

Source: Olswang and Bain (1991).

developing school-age children and their peers with language impairments was the use of linguistic devices that provided cohesive ties across the propositions presented in the narratives. Liles (1985) developed a system to score the use of cohesive ties in children's narratives as a measure of narrative performance. This system uses a metric that is the proportion of complete (appropriate and accurate) cohesive ties to all cohesive devices attempted in a narrative sample. The Narrative Scoring Scheme (Heilmann et al., 2010), listed in Table 13.6, provides for explicit scoring of cohesion in narratives. McFadden and Gillam (1996) found that the quality of children's narratives judged according to the author's holistic scoring procedure (Table 13.6) was associated with the text-level features (e.g., connectives) that appeared in the narratives but not the sentence-level features (e.g., length of utterance). Such information suggests that an examiner might want to include analysis procedures that look at the quality and quantity of cohesive ties that children use in their narratives.

In the same way that dynamic assessment procedures can be used with other aspects of language assessment, these procedures can be applied to narratives. For example, Gillam, Peña, and Miller (1999) have described a mediated learning experience, a form of the test–teach–retest method of dynamic assessment, to ascertain how much and what kinds of changes to elements of narrative production (e.g., increasing complexity of episodes and/or adding information about the characters) a child can make with only two intervention sessions. The amount of teaching effort that was required for the child to change is also evaluated. These authors suggest that children who make relatively rapid gains with short-term, mediated teaching are less likely to be language disordered.

One of the aspects of narratives that make them particularly demanding language tasks is that they require that the needs of the listener be considered and attended to so that the right amount of information unknown to the listener is provided but information that the listener knows is not made explicit. That is, children need to demonstrate *presupposition* abilities. However, presupposition is not limited to narrative tasks but is an essential feature of interpersonal communication generally. Appropriate skills with presupposition can be assessed by systematically varying the conditions in which a child needs to communicate, that is, who the partners are and what they might know about what the child needs to communicate. The discussion thus far has focused on spoken narrative and exposition. Increasingly, analyses of older children's and adolescents' written discourse is emerging as an important piece of the assessment picture, especially with implementation of Response to Intervention (RtI) models of intervention and emphases on educational relevance for the services provided to students. In Chapter 5, analyses of students' written language in students' portfolios were recommended as part of assessment, and Nippold's (2014) approaches were identified as one way to approach analyses of such samples. In their tutorial, Price and Jackson (2015) outline a number of procedures for obtaining and analyzing samples of students' written language that can be used to complement spoken language sampling. In both Nippold's and Price and Jackson's approaches, there are considerable parallels in processes, procedures, and elements for analyses to those used in spoken language sample analysis. In fact, in one study of the written persuasive discourse of children, adolescents, and young adults, Nippold, Ward-Lonergan, and Fanning (2005) used the computerized analysis program, Systematic Analysis of Language Transcripts (SALT) (Miller et al., 2015), which was originally developed for analysis of spoken language, to analyze the written samples.

Analyses of Organization of Social Discourse. One aspect of assessing a child's pragmatic abilities is to assess the child's ability to participate as a partner in conversational interchanges. Specific behaviors to evaluate are the amount of a child's social speech (speech addressed to a listener) versus nonsocial speech (speech that does not obligate a listener to respond, such as monologues) and the child's abilities to maintain a topic of conversation, to initiate and terminate conversations, and to repair communication breakdowns. A child's turn-taking skills are also assessed. Dyadic communication portions of a language sample may provide the necessary information to assess many of these skills.

Several guides are available to assist in analyzing a child's discourse skills. In Chapter 3, we learned about a method of assessment that can be used with young children in group situations to examine, in real time, their social, interactive communication with peers (Rice, Sell, & Hadley, 1990). Recall that Fey's (1986) interactionist approach (Chapter 3) emphasizes how children use language in social-conversational situations. Fey developed a coding system based on those of Dore (1979) and Chapman (1981) to describe and classify each conversational act a child produces during an interactive interchange, with some acts reflecting assertiveness and others reflecting responsiveness. Examples from this coding system are requests for information (RQIN), requests for attention (RQAT), statements (ASST), disagreements (ASDA), responses to requests for information (RSIN), responses to requests for clarification (RSCL), and responses to requests for attention (RSAT). The proportion with which these different acts occur during the interchange is used to classify a child into one of four profiles of social-conversational participation (e.g., active conversationalist, passive conversationalist, inactive communicator, or verbal noncommunicator) (*see* Chapter 3). Retherford (2000) also presents systematic procedures for conversational analysis that examiners might find helpful.

The Breakdown Coding System (BCS) (Yont, 1998; Yont, Hewitt, & Miccio, 2000) was developed to provide a tool for analyzing preschoolers' communication breakdowns as these occurred in naturalistic interactions with their mothers. This system describes what is in a child's language that caused the listener (in this case mother) to signal a communication failure on the child's part. This system differs from others, therefore, in that it looks at the source of a child's communication breakdown, not the child's ways of attempting or not attempting to repair communication breakdown. What the child did that caused a breakdown is determined by what the listener communicates to the child about the nature of the breakdown. That is, the classification of the problem is based on what the listener did not understand. There are five ways in which mothers can request clarifications of what their children tried unsuccessfully to communicate and seven types of child communication failures that the mothers could identify with their clarification requests. In a preliminary study using this coding system, differences between children with specific language impairment and normally developing children were apparent in the types and frequency of breakdowns the children had (Yont & Hewitt, 1999). Yont et al. (2000) suggested that the system can assist in identifying individual children's profiles of communication breakdown and potentially point the way to developing intervention objectives.

When samples of "naturalist" dyadic communication have failed to elicit discourse elements of interest, role-playing and contrived communicative situations may be needed to create opportunities to assess a child's skills. For example, an examiner may purposefully give vague instructions to a child or use a nonverbal cue indicating a lack of understanding, such as a puzzled expression, to evaluate a child's reactions.

Computer-Assisted Analysis. Several computer programs have been developed to assist in analyzing language samples and creating language sample databases. Among these are *Systematic Analysis of Language Transcripts (SALT)* (Miller et al., 2015), *Lingquest 1 & 2* (Mordecai & Palin, 1982), the *CHILDES* system (MacWhinney, 1996, 2000), *Pye Analysis of Language* (Pye, 1987), and *Computerized Profiling* (Long, 2010; Long, Fey, & Channell, 2000). These programs generally provide for access to and/or analyses of a variety of morphosyntactic aspects of language, and several also provide for analyses of some semantic and pragmatic characteristics. Some, like SALT (Miller et al., 2015), also have databases that permit comparison of results to norms.

In using most of the computerized programs, the utterances for analysis are entered into the computer according to the format specified by the program. The advantage of computerized analyses is that these can be performed more quickly and generally more accurately than by hand (Long, 1999a). Long and Channell (2001) write that "all of these programs have the ability to produce detailed analyses far faster than they could be done by hand" (p. 180), which means that an argument for not using language sampling—that is, that it took more time for analyses than busy professionals could devote to the process—is no longer valid.

The primary difference between different computerized analysis programs deals with what the examiner needs to do and what the computer does (Long, 1999b). Some of the programs assist mostly by retrieving, counting, and categorizing data after a human examiner has entered a transcript into the computer with necessary codings for the utterances. The examiner uses his or her metalinguistic knowledge, such as segmenting utterances, identifying mazes, and coding occurrences of morphological markers, in assigning the requisite codes. This means that some degree of analysis of each utterance is required by the examiner as it is entered. Unless these structures are coded initially, the computer cannot perform further analyses accurately. Accuracy in entering the initial data is essential. Other programs can assist the examiner by interacting symbiotically with the human transcriber so that the program analyzes many aspects of the transcript, such as word boundaries, word types, and syntactic categories. More recently, computer programs have used algorithms to increase the level of automatic analyses that they are able to do so that the human effort can be decreased further (Channell, 1998; Channell & Johnson, 1999). This approach means that the computer programs simulate and execute some of a human's "metalinguistic knowledge." Long and Channell (2001) examined the accuracy of results for automatically generated metrics for four analyses—MLU, LARSP, DSS, and IPSyn. Results were promising, suggesting that generally the generated analyses were equally as accurate as a human completing the analyses. These authors (Long & Channell, 2001) concluded that

> at least for certain procedures, software can produce analysis results that rival those achieved by hand. This should not be seen as cause for alarm. Rather, it should impel us to reconsider the purpose of clinical language analysis. Now, and increasingly in the future, the burden of generating an analysis will become lighter. This will, thankfully, permit us to focus our attention on *how* that information should be used in our evaluation and treatment decisions. (p. 187)

Future developments, including those in voice recognition, should add to the benefits offered by computerized language sampling analyses.

Dynamic Assessment and Criterion-Referenced Testing. Criterion-referenced testing is designed to probe whether a child's performance with regard to a particular language skill, such as ability to mark regular past-tense verbs with different allomorphs appropriately, attains a specified level of performance—the criterion. In some instances, the child is compared to his or her own performance at different times, such as before targeting an intervention objective and then at some time later after a period of intervention; in other instances, as McCauley (1996) writes, a child's performance might be "interpreted in terms of established performance levels" (p. 122), such as when a child's MLU is compared to Brown's (1973) stages. In fact, language sampling is perhaps the most common criterion-referenced procedure used in child language assessment, but is likely not often recognized or at least not labeled as a criterion-referenced procedure (McCauley, 1996). It is important to recognize that even though criterion-referenced procedures are not norm-referenced, they are typically administered in standardized ways and some are formally standardized.

Criterion-referenced testing in child language assessment is not really new. Some time ago, at least in terms of the history of the study of child language disorders, Leonard, Prutting, Perozzi, and Berkley (1978) wrote about the value of this type of testing and proposed three reasons for employing criterion-referenced, clinician-constructed tasks as a supplement to norm-reference testing:

1. *Few norm-reference tests assess a sufficient number of items for a specific linguistic feature to determine whether that feature is truly present or absent in the child's language patterns.* For example, the Patterned Elicitation Syntax Test with Morphological Analysis (Young & Perachio, 1993) contains only two items that examine regular plural morphemes and one item that examines irregular past tense.

   Therefore, criterion-reference testing might be used as a form of *extension testing*. In using a criterion-referenced approach to assessing a child's skills with morphological markers, for example, with regular noun plural morphemes, more regular noun plural items could be selected so that root word endings are varied and more opportunities to respond to items examining all three regular allomorphs are provided for the child. Items might include *drums, dogs, cakes, lips, horses*, and *dishes*. Tasks could be designed in an attempt to be as consistent as possible with the format of the test, which prompted extension criterion testing.
2. *A range of norm-referenced tests is not available to examine some aspects of language, so choice of what to use is limited.* For example, assessment of pragmatic skills and narrative abilities are areas relatively less tapped by norm-referenced tests. Several of the approaches previously discussed in this chapter would be examples of using criterion-referenced tests to fill a gap in the range of available tests.
3. *The tasks or stimuli used to assess a feature may create problems for the child rather than the child actually having a problem with the feature itself.* This is what Sabers (1996) referred to as the techniques used to measure a trait affecting the degree to which the intended trait is actually measured. For example, previously in this chapter, we discussed how different approaches to assessing children's narrative skills might place different forms of constraints on what skills with narrative the child might be able to demonstrate. The same issue applies to norm-referenced tests.

In order to discern the reasons for a child's problem, a task or stimulus different from the ones used on a norm-referenced test to assess the feature can be devised. This is actually a form of dynamic assessment. For example, the pictures provided with a test may be unclear or confusing. It is also possible that changing the pictorial stimuli may elicit correct responses. In one study (Barrow, Holbert, & Rastatter, 2000) of the effects of colored versus black-and-white stimuli on the picture-naming speed and accuracy of normally developing children 4 to 8 years of age, the addition of color increased naming speed for vocabulary words that were within an emerging period for the children (i.e., words most likely to be in the process of being learned). When the vocabulary words were well within the repertoires of the children or beyond their developmental level, colored pictures held no advantage over black-and-white pictures. For more advanced vocabulary words, the addition of color helped the children name the pictures depicting the words more accurately. As another example, a child may not be able to deal with sentence-completion tasks, such as "Here is a dog. Here are two . . .," which are types of tasks used in several norm-referenced tests. However, the same child may be able to use the same morphological forms in other types of tasks.

We have seen several times elsewhere in this text that nonword repetition ability has gained prominence as a potential clinical marker of SLI in children. It is important, therefore, that assessment includes tasks designed to evaluate children's abilities to repeat nonsense words of increasing complexity. Standardized criterion-referenced tasks, such as those of Dollaghan and Campbell (1998) and Gathercole, Willis, Baddeley, and Emslie (1994), are frequently used. Because these tasks have typically been used with school-age children, Gray (2003) explored the "usefulness of nonword repetition as a diagnostic measure of SLI in younger children" (p. 134) and, in particular, preschool children. As noted in Chapter 3, others are also working on developing standardized nonword repetition tasks for use with toddlers and preschoolers (Chiat & Roy, 2007; Roy & Chiat, 2004; Stokes & Klee, 2009; Thal, Miller, Carlson, & Vega, 2005). As this aspect of assessment has become more important, increasing numbers of formal measurement tools, such as the Comprehensive Test of Phonological Processing—2 (CTOPP-2) (Wagner, Torgesen, Rashotte, & Pearson, 2013), which includes nonword repetition tasks, are also being developed.

Dynamic assessment addresses how facilely children can learn language. Children who have typical ability to learn language do not have language impairment, although they could have language delay in terms of what they know about aspects of language because of events extrinsic to the children. Therefore, the principle behind dynamic assessment is to explore how quickly a child can learn one or more new language skills or how quickly a child can positively modify his or her language under "ideal," short-term language learning. Thus, dynamic assessment is concerned with a child's or adolescent's language-learning ability rather than what he or she knows about a particular language ability (e.g., a score on a norm-referenced test of verb morphology) or how he or she processes language and/or language-related tasks (e.g., nonword repetition). Although dynamic assessment is a relatively well-known type of criterion-referenced testing, it is not a new concept. The basis for dynamic assessment procedures is Vygotsky's (1978) concept of *zone of proximal development* (ZPD). The idea is that learning for a child occurs when the child attempts to function in this zone, which is the area of functioning between what the child is able to do without assistance from more capable individuals (e.g., parents, clinicians, teachers, higher-functioning peers) and what the child can do with different levels of assistance from these individuals. According to Gutiérrez-Clellen and Peña (2001), in dynamic assessment, "the goal is to determine the 'size' of the [child's] zone of proximal development" (p. 212), with the aim of learning the *modifiability* of the child's language performance. There are several dynamic assessment approaches that have been described to ascertain the degree of modifiability (Gutiérrez-Clellen & Peña, 2001; Peña, 1996). Among these are the following:

1. *Test–teach–retest,* in which
    - A child's initial performance without prompts, as in a norm-reference testing situation, is determined
    - Essential components of the skill or task are taught, often in a brief teaching situation
    - The child's performance after teaching is tested again to determine change, if any, in performance
2. *Graduated prompting,* in which
    - A hierarchy of prompts in order of least amount of assistance to most amount of assistance is determined
    - Each prompt is provided one at a time, beginning with the least assistance, and the child's response to each is determined
3. *Limits testing,* in which
    - Usual procedures and instructions as to how to deliver stimuli during testing are modified in order to provide a child with a considerable amount of additional cues and reinforcement
    - Some of these modifications can include explaining the test tasks to the child and even providing some rationale as to how to approach them
    - The child's responses to the additional assistance are determined, in part to determine if the child understands the task itself

The activities related to short-term intervention/teaching, providing supports, or prompting are commonly referred as *mediated learning experiences* (*MLEs*).

These several dynamic assessment approaches recognize that different contexts with differing amounts of cues and support can elicit better (or worse) language performance from a child and that the professional can systematically manipulate contextual support and/or cues for a child and observe what conditions, if any, result in more advanced (or lower-level) responses. Ways to manipulate context are to change the antecedent events that occur before asking a child for a response, to change what happens after a child's response, or to change the task. It is possible that of these methods, changing the antecedent events is likely the most frequently used, the one that often results in changed performance, and the one that may provide the most information about what situations produce (Olswang & Bain, 1991). Common ways in which antecedent events can be manipulated are shown in Table 13.6. The information gained from these procedures helps in knowing which children may benefit the most from intervention and change their behaviors most easily and what methods might best be used to facilitate change.

INTELLIGENCE TESTING

Results of intelligence quotient (IQ) tests administered by qualified psychologists are often part of a comprehensive assessment process for a child with a suspected language disorder, and in previous chapters we have discussed relationships among children's cognitive abilities, mental age, and language. The use of IQ tests has been inextricably tied to identification of children with language disorders and frequently to qualifying children with language impairments for intervention services. As we have seen, in most cases the concept of match/mismatch between intellectual ability/cognitive ability and language ability is core to these identification and qualifying procedures. However, the practice of using IQ tests in these ways has increasingly been seen as untenable, in part because of the recognition that factors that affect performance on IQ tests probably also affect language abilities. In fact, federal education policy now discourages this practice known as cognitive referencing. Nevertheless, it is likely that changes in practice will be slow to come.

What is surprising is that the extent to which IQ testing has become so established in assessment, identification of children with language disorders, and practices to qualify children for services given its dubious past record for accomplishing these purposes. For example, in the past, children with normal or above cognitive abilities but with language differences or disorders—such as hearing-impaired children and linguistically-culturally diverse children with cerebral palsy—have been misdiagnosed as intellectually disabled and placed in classrooms for cognitively low-functioning children. A major reason for these misdiagnoses stems from the nature of some of the intelligence tests that were used. Historically, the Stanford-Binet Intelligence Scale (Terman & Merrill, 1973) originally yielded a single IQ score and was recognized as heavily based on language and language-related abilities. When given to a child with a language problem or difference, the resulting IQ score reflected more directly the child's language skills rather than the child's cognitive level. More recent editions have led to separate verbal and nonverbal/performance subtests, such as the fifth edition, the Stanford-Binet V. The Wechsler Intelligence Scale for Children—V (WISC-V) (Wechsler, 2014) and the Wechsler Preschool and Primary Scale of Intelligence—IV (WPPSI-IV) (Wechsler, 2012) also yield separate IQ scores for performance and verbal portions, as well as a full-scale combined IQ score, which at least try to address some of the issues surrounding IQ testing with children with language impairments. As with the Stanford-Binet, the verbal scale tends to reflect a child's language abilities or disabilities. The performance scale may be a more accurate indication of a language-disordered child's intellectual level, although cautions are even appropriate in interpreting the performance IQ as valid. One reason for caution—but not the only reason—is that instructions are given orally, and a child with language comprehension problems can be at a severe disadvantage in completing the performance tasks accurately because the instructions may not be understood. For example, in one study involving a previous version of the WISC, WISC-R performance IQ scores of hearing-impaired children increased about 20 points when the examiner's oral instructions were supplemented with manual communication (Sullivan, 1978). In another example, Braden (1994) has reported that, on performance IQ tests where hearing-impaired children are shown what to do, their scores do not differ from those of children without hearing losses, but when the instructions on performance IQ tests need to be presented orally to the children, they score significantly poorer than their hearing peers, even though their scores can still be within normal limits.

An extremely unfortunate situation for language-different and language-disordered children was the description and subsequent use of an early edition of the Peabody Picture

Vocabulary Test (PPVT) (Dunn, 1965) as a measure of intellectual functioning. Rather than assessing intellectual level, the PPVT and its newer edition, the Peabody Picture Vocabulary Test—IV (PPVT-IV) (Dunn & Dunn, 2007), actually assess receptive single-word vocabulary. Fortunately, the authors of the PPVT-IV no longer refer to the test as a measure of intelligence, although some texts on psychological assessment continue to list it as an intelligence test. The Kaufman Assessment Battery for Children—2 (Kaufman & Kaufman, 2004a) and its shorter version, the Kaufman Brief Intelligence Test—2 (K-BIT-2) (Kaufman & Kaufman, 2004b) are increasingly becoming popular intelligence tests, especially their nonverbal scales. These assess individuals' abilities to problem solve using simultaneous or sequential mental processes. Restrictions on whom is qualified to administer the K-BIT-2 are more lenient than for many other tests of intelligence, making it a more accessible tool for a variety of professionals trained in norm-referenced, standardized testing procedures.

There are several alternative intelligence tests that minimize the language loading seen in some of the tests. Two such tests are the third edition of the Columbia Mental Maturity Scale (Burgemeister, Blum, & Lorge, 1971) and the Universal Nonverbal Intelligence Test—2 (UNIT-2) (Bracken & McCallum, 2016). Based on their review of the psychometric characteristics of nonverbal intelligence tests, with a particular focus on their use with children with possible language impairment, DeThorne and Schaefer (2004) suggested the UNIT might be the best choice in what they termed "high-stakes assessments" (p. 287) for these children. Other tests of nonverbal intelligence include the Test of Nonverbal Intelligence—IV (Brown, Sherbenou, & Johnsen, 2010) and the Comprehensive Test of Nonverbal Intelligence—2 (Hammill, Pearson, & Wiederholt, 2009). The Raven's Coloured Progressive Matrices (Raven, 2003), a set of tests based mostly on visual perception, are also sometimes used with communicatively impaired or language-different children. Where children with language impairments are concerned, Conti-Ramsden, Botting, Simkin, and Knox (2001) suggest that the use of the Raven's matrices as tests of children's intellectual functioning may have some particular advantages over other nonverbal or performance intelligence tests that can include timed tasks and those requiring memory skills. Because the tasks in the Raven's matrices rely primarily on visual perception and reasoning/logic tasks and are not timed, children with language impairment, who are frequently believed to have problems with working memory and/or slowed general processing abilities, may be better able to demonstrate their intellectual abilities when these matrices are used rather than other nonverbal intelligence tests (Conti-Ramsden et al., 2001).

Although norm-referenced tools for assessment of intelligence are supposed to be given in very specific ways with little room for deviation from stated protocols, their uses with language-disordered or language-different children may require special precautions in giving the tests or modifications of instructions, materials, or administration procedures if relatively accurate estimates of intelligence are to be obtained. For example, for a child with cerebral palsy with severe oral and motor involvements, testing materials may need to be cut apart and placed so that the child can respond only by having to look at the stimuli to respond. Or the examiner may need to change the procedures to allow for multiple-choice responses instead of oral or motor target responses. A number of intelligence tests has timed subtests that are inappropriate for children with motor handicaps, and many of the tests that minimize language loading emphasize the visual modality, rendering them unsuitable for children with visual impairments. In some cases, children with sensory impairments may be given only one scale of the WISC-V or the WPPSI-IV, such as the verbal scale to children with visual impairments and the performance scale to children with hearing impairments. For a hearing-impaired child who is visually oriented, appropriate visual cues may help the child perform optimally, but distracting visual information may adversely affect the child's performance. In administering test items that use a picture–response format, an examiner should avoid looking at any specific picture after giving a test stimulus or placing his or her hand in such a way as to direct inadvertently the hearing-impaired child's responses. These are only a few examples of the modifications and precautions necessary when testing these special children. Of course, most intelligence tests are standardized, so changing administration procedures to accommodate these children potentially invalidates the results. On the other hand, to administer tests to children whose communicative and other abilities spuriously affect results about their intellectual functioning is equally invalid. Given the intertwining of language with intelligence tests, children with language impairments are exceptionally special.

SUMMARY

In this chapter we have seen that

- Language assessment needs to accomplish a number of purposes, and several procedures and tools are employed to achieve these purposes.
- Screenings are brief examinations of children's communicative performances, the results of which can raise concerns about children's language but cannot determine if children have language problems; issues of test sensitivity, specificity, positive predictive value, negative predictive value, and false-positive and false-negative results are important issues in assessment and test use.
- The regularities in a child's language need to be identified to develop intervention objectives; language sampling, dynamic assessment, and other forms of criterion-referenced testing, including clinician-constructed tasks, are valid procedures to use in achieving this.
- Assessment is an ongoing process; evaluation of intervention efficacy is part of this ongoing process.
- Norm-referenced tests are tools and do not suffice as sole methods to be used in achieving the objectives of assessment; professionals must be careful not to misuse nor misinterpret norm-referenced tests.
- Factors to consider in language sampling include methods used to elicit the sample, the settings and communicative partners involved in eliciting the sample, the length of the sample, the ways to record the sample, and transcription and analysis procedures to be used.
- Assessing interactive discourse, pragmatic, and narrative skills is essential as part of the assessment process and may require using un-normed, but often standardized, approaches.
- Intelligence testing is generally a part of a child's total assessment; obtaining valid results when children have language problems is a challenging task for professionals and requires careful test selection and may involve modification of usual procedures.

The language assessment process for a child with a suspected language problem involves gathering information about the child from a variety of sources and procedures. All these lead to accomplishing the purposes of the assessment process. One of these purposes is determining the directions that intervention for a child with a language problem should take.

14

Considerations for Language Intervention

LEARNING OBJECTIVES

After reading this chapter, you should be able to

- Discuss considerations in planning and implementing intervention
- Describe methods of highlighting intervention targets
- Describe procedures and techniques designed to facilitate children's learning of language targets
- Discuss various approaches to intervention
- Describe how the pieces of the intervention puzzle are put together

*I*n previous chapters, we discussed a number of intervention considerations. Many of these intervention strategies are appropriate for other children and situations and should be viewed as having applications beyond the specific instances cited. However, no two language-disordered children are exactly alike in the language abilities and disabilities they manifest. Therefore, each child's language intervention plan is developed individually and is initially based on the results of the assessment process and later on the ongoing assessment that is part of any intervention program. There is no one recipe for language intervention. Instead, multiple factors and approaches must be considered in planning.

Fey and Proctor-Williams (2000) list four aims of intervention for grammatical targets:

1. Attend to a new or unmastered language form or operation in the input.
2. Recognize the semantic, pragmatic, and/or grammatical functions of the new form.
3. Relate the new form or operation to their existing grammatical systems and modify their grammars accordingly.
4. Access and produce the new structure more quickly and reliably after it is generated by their underlying grammars. (p. 178)

It seems that these aims could as easily apply to intervention for pragmatic or semantic targets. The following sections provide guidelines for how these aims of intervention might be achieved for children with language impairments regardless of the specific targets for a child at a particular point in time.

Health care and education sectors are increasingly calling for, and even mandating that, intervention practices be based in scientifically documented evidence. Even though professionals might express interest in providing interventions that are grounded in evidence, for whatever reasons research has suggested that they may not always engage in behaviors that involve seeking out evidence (Hoffman, Ireland, Hall-Mills, & Flynn, 2013). This state of affairs might be perceived as unsettling when considering the possible negative effects on the efficacy and effectiveness of interventions provided for children with language disorders. A more sobering situation is that, even if they do regularly attempt to seek out language intervention evidence, there would only be a small body of scientifically based evidence available for them to unearth (Cirran & Gillam, 2008), and what they do unearth is not part of a well-organized or integrated framework (Turkstra, Norman, Whyt, Dijkers, & Hart, 2016). However, the few available individual intervention studies are generally of high quality, which led Cirran and Gillam (2008) to suggest that professionals "can have some confidence in the specific language intervention practices" (p. S110) described in the literature. Against this backdrop, Cirran and Gillam (2008) advise professionals (1) to use the evidence that is available to the best advantage for children, (2) to consider the perspectives of parents and teachers in planning and implementing intervention, and (3) to monitor closely each child's progress in intervention so that, if the child is not progressing in authentic ways that impact the child's life and not just for isolated, short-term objectives, intervention approaches are changed. The volume of intervention research is growing, and it will, over time, fill the evidence-based intervention "toolbox." Readers are advised to stay tuned—and to engage in behaviors that lead to seeking out developments in evidence-based practices. What follows in this chapter is a combination from the literature of evidence-based intervention approaches and those arising from expert opinion, which are generally informed by experience and research, albeit not intervention research per se.

CONSIDERATIONS IN INTERVENTION

Normal versus Not-So-Normal Processes

Many approaches in language intervention are based on language behaviors and developmental patterns observed in normal children. This implies that what is good and works for children who are acquiring language normally is good and will work for children with language disorders. The problem is, of course, that children with language problems are not learning language normally, and it is possible that what works for normal language-learning children may not work for language-disordered children and vice versa. One example of differential responsiveness to different interventions arose in the findings of a study conducted by Throneburg, Calvert, Sturm, Paramboukas, and Paul (2000). These researchers compared different service delivery models for teaching curricular vocabulary to elementary school students with speech-language impairment and those not receiving special services, that is, typically developing children. The typically developing children increased their vocabulary knowledge with exposure to either a collaborative or classroom-based intervention whereas for the children with speech-language impairment the collaborative approach was the most effective intervention.

Several approaches to intervention place an emphasis on naturalistic child-directed environments that resemble normal language-learning interactions of mothers and their children. These approaches are based, in large part, on the knowledge that normal children learn language by actively exploring their environments and communicatively interacting with others. However, it is possible that not all language-impaired children will benefit optimally from such a strategy because some children with language problems begin intervention as passive or unresponsive and/or whatever is the reason for their language problems it affects their ability to make efficient use of the ambient language-learning environment. These children may not be able to take good advantage of such a "naturalist" environmental strategy. It is likely that at least some language- disordered children need "not-so-normal" intervention approaches in order to benefit most from intervention. What this means is that we may need to modify the "normal process" of intervention somewhat in order to effect language change as efficaciously as possible. Doing more of what is normal by applying the "normal process" model fully to language intervention for language-disordered children may not be entirely appropriate.

Developmental and Nondevelopmental Intervention

A consideration of intervention somewhat related to the previous discussion is that of using normal child language-development information to guide planning and implementation of intervention. Language intervention plans are often heavily grounded in normal language development. We have encountered this notion elsewhere in this text. Normal language-developmental patterns can guide the sequences of objectives planned for language-disordered children. A rationale behind a developmental approach is that a particular language skill has antecedents that provide the bases for the acquisition of the higher-level skill. New language skills are built on previously acquired skills, and earlier-acquired abilities influence the learning of later-developing skills. Information from normal language development assists us, therefore, in deciding what skills need to be learned before other skills can be acquired.

In many cases, a developmental approach to language intervention is warranted. Besides providing a rationale for selecting initial goals of intervention, it serves as a way of guiding ongoing intervention for children. Examples of using a developmental approach in choosing intervention goals for syntax or morphology include (1) focusing on relative clauses to modify objects of sentences before relative clauses to modify subjects of sentences for which an embedding process is required, (2) emphasizing the present progressive verb inflection (*-ing*) before past-tense verbs or third-person present-tense regular verb inflections (*runs*), or (3) introducing the allomorph /z/ to pluralize nouns before the allomorphs /s/ and /əz/. Because normal language-learning children generally use semantic relations that express nomination, recurrence, and nonexistence before those indicating attributes of objects, we might use this information to guide intervention goals in the semantic area; thus, we might emphasize the former types of semantic relations in intervention before entity + attributive ("car big") and attributive + entity ("big car") relations. For intervention focusing on pragmatic aspects of language, utterances that encode only one function per utterance might be stressed before asking children to encode two or more functions per utterance. Intervention for conversational turn-taking skills might begin with the language precursors of reciprocal interactions at the nonverbal level, if the child lacks these skills, before introducing verbal turn-taking activities. In helping children learn to maintain a topic in conversation, intervention might first include objectives aimed at having the children use one, possibly two, contingent responses and later include objectives for several contingent responses. Furthermore, contingent responses involving repetitions of part of an adult's previous utterance (focus/imitation devices) might be encouraged before contingent responses involving the addition of new information (substitution/expansion devices).

Normal developmental data need to be viewed, however, as providing guidelines rather than prescriptions for language intervention. Furthermore, although a developmental approach is probably the more frequently used strategy for planning intervention, there may be occasions when deviations from usual developmental sequences are appropriate. Age of the children for whom intervention is being planned might be an important factor. Older children are more apt to have gaps in their language knowledge and world knowledge so that these need to be filled by intervention. Younger children might be more likely to follow developmental sequences. And, research has not yet established developmental sequences for all language skills. In these cases, it is not possible to follow developmental sequences in intervention. Intervention with children with autism spectrum disorder frequently does not follow developmental sequences, and individual characteristics of other children with language disorders, such as a child's cognitive level, level of comprehension for a particular language skill, or response to intervention, may indicate the use of nondevelopmental strategies. In other instances, a child or the child's parents/caregivers or teachers may have immediate communication needs that support the choice of a nondevelopmental approach.

Rules and Regularities

In Chapter 5, Kamhi's (2014) points about distinguishing between performance and learning were raised to emphasize the notion that children with language disorders need to learn language, not just respond to narrow, context-specific objectives. Intervention objectives are used as road maps to guide the learning process, but they should not be confused with the destination, that is, what we want the children to learn. The task of intervention is to help the children discover, that is learn, the rules and regularities of language so that the language behaviors can be used in context-independent situations without prompts from intervention or education agents. Learning the rules and regularities promotes generalization, especially when the language abilities that are learned are useful and functional for the children. Thus, intervention needs to emphasize the learning of broad-based rules and regularities (Fey, Long, & Finestack, 2003).

Children with language disorders seem to have particular difficulties figuring out the principles, rules, and regularities of language (e.g., semantic maps of super- and subordinate classifications of words, use of verb allomorphs, preposing and transposing patterns for question forms, and appropriate and inappropriate conversational topics with teachers). The aim of intervention is, therefore, to create and/or capitalize on situations and experiences so that the child can discover the regularities. Presenting multiple repetitions of systematically controlled but varied exemplars of intervention targets may help facilitate the desired discoveries. Even if the source of a child's problem is not in figuring out the rule and regularities but instead in limitations or difficulties in processing information, the use of multiple and systematically controlled exemplars can be an effective intervention strategy. In this case, the repetitious patterning associated with this intervention approach can reduce the processing demands for these children and therefore reduce the complexity of the task demands for them.

To illustrate, if a goal is to help a child discover the meaning of *more* to express recurrence, one activity might involve a musical jack-in-the-box controlled by an adult. After an initial presentation of the toy's action (hopefully to the child's delight) the adult allows the child to play with it momentarily, then closes the lid, gives it back to the child for a moment, and finally asks the child, *More? More?* After a slight pause, the adult repeats the sequence. After the whole process is repeated several times, the adult can begin to pause for longer periods of time between saying *more* and opening the box, with the aim that the child will request *more.* Should that happen, the adult immediately opens the box. Although the child may begin to use *more* in this situation, we cannot be sure exactly what the child has discovered about the meaning. The intervention scenario is still quite context bound. It may be that the child has linked the little doll, the action of popping up, or the action of winding the handle with the word. Consequently, other events that highlight the regularities of *more* need to be introduced into intervention. The jack-in-the-box activity might be followed by a treat, such as juice, during which the child is given sip-sized amounts of juice in a glass. After the child drinks the juice, the adult asks *More?*—and more is poured. The intention is that the child will start to use the expression appropriately after the adult begins to pause between asking if the child wants more and supplying it. Additional events clearly illustrating the desired discoveries are also necessary. (The intervention context is gradually increasing and becoming less context bound.) A pragmatic emphasis is inherent in such an intervention approach. In this example, the inclusion of communicative intents in the form of Halliday's (1975) regulatory function or Dore's (1975) requesting action intention is obvious. The child discovers that the behaviors of others can be regulated and that desires can be met through the appropriate use of language.

To discover the rules and regularities, a child will probably need to be helped to use both inductive and deductive processes. *Induction* involves discovering a general rule from observing multiple individual cases; *deduction* is applying a general or known rule to a new or unknown situation. However, different types of intervention objectives (e.g., semantic objectives, morphological or syntactic objectives, and pragmatic objectives) may require different approaches in helping children discover the rules and regularities. Connell (1989), for instance, reported that an intervention approach that employed induction facilitated semantic objectives, but an intervention approach that employed deduction, facilitated a morphosyntactic target.

Although this principle of assisting children to discover the regularities applies to language intervention for preschoolers, school-age children, and adolescents alike, it is especially applicable for younger children who have not acquired metalinguistic skills in order to talk about and analyze language. For older children and adolescents with some metalinguistic abilities, explanations of the regularities to be discovered may help them focus on the rules. Incorporating some use of writing or written practice may even assist older children in identifying the regularities and reinforce the interaction between oral and written language (Fey et al., 2003). However, these explanations and analyses complement, not substitute for, actual practice in systematically expanding but contextually appropriate situations. The idea of expanding the contexts in which children are learning the rules and regularities of a particular language skill is consistent with what Kamhi (2014) referred to as the instructional factor that suggests "the conditions of instruction and practice should be varied" (p. 94) because the "information becomes linked with a greater range of contextual cues and encoded in more than one way" (p. 94).

Controlling and/or Reducing Language Complexity

If we are going to focus on rules and regularities, it makes some sense to try to control complexity in such a way that a child can figure out what the rules and regularities are. In the previous discussion, the procedures used to help children discover the rules and regularities of language were also described as potentially helping to reduce the complexity of the task of learning language for them. Given the thrust in the literature indicating that many children with language impairments may have limited or impaired processing capacities, it seems that important considerations in intervention should be controlling and reducing the complexity of the language demands of a language target we are asking children to acquire.

With regard to controlling the complexity of the language demands for the child, when intervention focuses on one aspect of language, it is important to control the complexity of the other aspects that are simultaneously included. We do not expect a language-disordered child to use a new word in a multiword utterance containing a new syntactic form to express a new function all at the same time. Even children who are acquiring language normally do not do this. They tend to use simpler, earlier-acquired syntactic structures to encode new ideas or content and to express earlier-acquired content in new syntactic structures and newly acquired intentions and functions in old, well-established linguistic forms to express well-known content. There is substantial evidence that aspects of language interact with each other and that there are trade-offs in what children can do with the demands of language of various language tasks at any point in time, depending on the degree of difficulty of the combination of tasks, the robustness of the children's knowledge of the tasks, and/or the facility of their mental operations are at handling the tasks.

In using this information for intervention, we would make an attempt to reduce the complexities seen in usual language-learning situations so that the children's tasks in identifying the rule and regularities for the intervention target and in being able to use the target are simplified. For example, a new morphological or syntactic structure would initially be presented in a situation where the child could use well-established words in highly stabilized, perhaps even routinized, contexts. For semantics, intervention would first involve new words or new semantic relations used in familiar morphosyntactic forms and contexts. For improvement of pragmatic skills, the child would initially be encouraged to apply the new pragmatic skills in situations when the child could use old linguistic forms in familiar interactions. Even controlling the phonological content of words being taught in intervention focusing on semantics may influence how easily the words are acquired. As a child starts to demonstrate acquisition of the new target language behavior, it is important to gradually and systematically introduce less established aspects of the other language components. This last statement refers back to our point in the previous section about systematically expanding the contextually appropriate situations in which the new language skill is expected to be used. This promotes generalization.

There is evidence indicating that it is also important to control the complexity of the language input or stimuli we provide to the child as we are attempting to assist the child to acquire a particular feature of language. Some of this evidence comes from studies of mothers talking to their normally developing children. Not only do mothers reduce their rates of speech and vary prosodic features of the language, they also reduce the overall complexity of their language by using short, simple utterances. From an intervention perspective, for example, in a program to help toddlers between about 2 and 2½ years of age with slow expressive language development but most with age-appropriate receptive language vocabulary to acquire new lexical targets (words), Girolametto, Pearce, and Weitzman (1996) taught the children's mothers to reduce their rate of speech to their children, the length of utterances they used, and their lexical diversity as well as to increase the frequency with which they modeled lexical targets. The children whose mothers reduced the complexity of their language input made gains not only with the intervention targets but in a variety of other language areas. Similar gains were not evidenced in children whose mothers had not made these changes in their interactions with their children. Such approaches to reducing input complexity may also be effective in highlighting the systematic patterns from which a child is to learn the guiding rules and regularities if the child is having difficulties figuring these out. Instead of adults using long, complex utterances that can hide the elements to be discerned or overload a child's processing facilities, pairing short, simple utterances with appropriate content and context appears to be a logical approach. In addition to controlling the length and morphosyntactic complexity of language models, an adult needs to use words in the utterances that are well within a child's semantic repertoire. If the child does not understand the meaning of an adult's model, it is doubtful the child will discern much of anything from the utterance. The point is that complexity matters, and controlling it matters even more. However, a note of caution is important. Even though the complexity of language models and language input to the children may be reduced, it needs to be grammatically, semantically, and pragmatically complete and appropriate. As Kamhi (2014) writes, "Telegraphic utterances (e.g., *push ball, mommy sock*) should not be provided as input for children with limited language" (p. 92). Even parents talking to their young, typically developing children do not do this; instead they would, for example, use complete noun phrases (e.g., *push the ball*) or inflect the verb (e.g., *pushes the ball*) or inflect the possessive noun (e.g., *mommy's sock*) or even use a short complete sentence that comments on the children's meaning, (e.g., *Yes, that's mommy's sock*).

Comprehension or Production

Most children with language disorders have problems both using and comprehending language. Therefore, a common issue is whether to focus first on comprehension and then move to production or to start with areas of production that need to be addressed. We need to recall that comprehension does not always precede production. Another important consideration is that the process of working on production, if carried out in meaningful contexts and with pragmatically appropriate grounding, is likely to bring along comprehension and knowledge of the language target. As Leonard (1998) suggests, "In gaining practice in the production of the target forms, the children are also learning the appropriate contexts in which they are used" (p. 194). It is hard to see how helping children to discern rules and regularities, as discussed above, could be carried out without helping a child to understand. However, having children produce specific forms by rote, without understanding the utterances' meanings or purposes, certainly does not lay the groundwork for generalization to everyday use. We also need to recall that there is now some thinking that rarely do children have expressive language problems in the absence of comprehension deficits (Leonard, 2009; Tomblin & Zhang, 2006), even if the comprehension problems have not been identified. This would support the notions of developing intervention that focuses on both expression and comprehension.

Although it might be defensible to decide to focus on production with the aim of concurrently developing comprehension, there is some evidence suggesting that comprehension work alone is not sufficient to result in production for children with language disorders, even though such an approach might work for normally developing children. Here we can see the relevance of our discussion at the beginning of this chapter about "normal versus not-so-normal processes." Three studies chosen from across several decades and representing different intervention aims can be used to illustrate this point. In one of these studies, Dollaghan (1987) investigated normal and language-impaired children's abilities to fast map the meanings of words. She found that both the normal and language-impaired children were equally able to infer word meaning from limited, structured exposures. However, the language-impaired children could not produce the words following limited exposure, whereas the majority of the normal language-learning children could. Connell and Stone's (1992) study focused on morphological acquisition. In their study, normal and language-impaired children were taught several morphemes. Both the normal and the language-disordered children learned to comprehend the meaning of the morphemes. Unlike the normal children, however, the language-impaired children were able to use the morphemes only if they had previously been asked to produce utterances containing the morphemes. The effectiveness of two grammatical morphological treatment procedures used with 5-year-old children with specific language impairment (SLI) was the focus of the study by Smith-Lock, Leitão, Prior, and Nickels (2015). One of the treatment approaches used a cueing hierarchy that elicited a correct response following a child's incorrect production of a targeted grammatical morphological marker and the other treatment approach used a recasting procedure that occurred following a child's incorrect response but did not require the child to then make a correct response. (Recasting as an intervention technique is discussed later in this chapter.) The procedure that required the children to make a correct response following their incorrect response was more effective in facilitating the children's progress than the procedure not requiring the children to correct their errors. These studies suggest that children with language impairments need to be given opportunities to produce intervention targets in order for them to be realized in their expressive language. For these children, it seems that training involving comprehension results in comprehension of the targets, training involving comprehension alone did not result in production, and production practice resulted in using the targets.

We are not sure why this may be so for children with language disorders. It may be that the task of production requires more practice, experience, more effort, and/or time with intervention targets generally. In drawing on the works of E. Bjork (2004) and R. Bjork (2011), Kamhi (2014) summarizes that

> retrieving information from memory facilitates long-term retention. . . . [and] that the more difficult the act of a successful retrieval, the greater the learning benefit . . . and, conversely, the easier it is to retrieve something, the less long-term learning there will be. (p. 94)

Recall from Chapter 3 that Gray (2003) found, compared to normally developing children, that children with SLI needed two times as many opportunities to hear new words in order to learn their meanings and before being able to produce them also needed another two times as many opportunities to use them while continuing to be exposed receptively to the words. Together, these findings suggest that intervention may need to quadruple receptive exposures, compared to those provided for normal-language children, for language-impaired children to add new words to their expressive lexicons. This suggests a quantity factor. That is, the quantity of work with the targets needs to be greater because the children must do something more than they might if work were limited to comprehension.

Having suggested that production might actually aid acquisition compared to comprehension work alone, it is also possible the act of production itself might require too many resources for a child. That is, the act of production may be sufficiently taxing for the current abilities of a child so that it is beyond what the child is able to do. This might apply particularly in the early stages of learning a new language skill, and results from dynamic assessment processes might help us sort out if this is the case. If this is the case, considerations related to reducing complexity might take precedence, and we would choose to focus initially on comprehension and move to production later in intervention, recognizing the need to move to production and not leave it at a comprehension stage too long.

Comprehension difficulties, however, are major problems for some children and adolescents. These may be more debilitating for the children and adolescents than their expressive language delays and may even be more recalcitrant to intervention (Boyle, McCartney, O'Hare, & Forbes, 2009; Law, Garrett, & Nye, 2004). In a meta-analysis of the efficacy of intervention for young children with developmental speech and language delays and disorders, the researchers were unable to substantiate the effectiveness of intervention for children with receptive language problems (Law et al., 2004). Of course, if intervention programs focus more heavily on facilitating expressive language growth, either to the exclusion or minimization of emphases on at least concurrent development of receptive language, then from our previous discussion here we should not be surprised by suggestions that receptive language might be less responsive to intervention.

Comprehension difficulties can be particularly problematic for school-age children. If they cannot comprehend easily and quickly what their teachers say, they cannot learn, and if they cannot comprehend what their teachers or peers say, they are likely to respond inappropriately and sometimes say or do some very strange things as a result. Even for preschoolers, comprehension problems are seen to affect interpersonal relationships with peers. Gertner, Rice, and Hadley (1994) found that for preschoolers with SLI, their level of receptive vocabulary knowledge predicted their being named or not named as a friend by their preschool peers, and those with lower comprehension vocabulary were less likely to be nominated as friends. Recall also from Chapter 4 that elementary school children with receptive language involvements are less likely than those with expressive language problems to receive intervention. The comprehension problems seem overlooked even though they are significant negative factors in academic and social success (Zhang & Tomblin, 2000). From this perspective, intervention must include attention to comprehension abilities.

Focus of Intervention and Picking Intervention Targets

Decisions about whether the language targets or objectives of initial intervention focus on a child's pragmatic, semantic, and/or morphosyntactic skills depend on an individual child's needs as identified through the assessment process. Very young, prelinguistic children may first need to develop intentional and nonverbal communicative interactions and cognitive skills associated with language learning, such as participation in joint action and joint attention routines or symbolic play with accompanying symbolic gestures, or gestural requests for objects. For other children, developing social interactive discourse skills may be most immediate. Discovering morphological or syntactic rules and regularities may be the appropriate focus of intervention for other language-disordered children, whereas developing semantic skills may be most important for still others. Children often need intervention in more than one area and/or need to strengthen their associations among the areas (Fey et al., 2003). Intervention for the specific language patterns presented by a child is individualized for each child.

Results from dynamic assessment procedures can help in decisions about what to target and often in what order. If the concepts associated with Vygotsky's (1978) zone of proximal development are used, then those skills that fall within this zone for the child, determined as a result of dynamic assessment, will be probable candidates as intervention targets. Skills that might fall in this zone might include ones for which the child was stimulable during dynamic assessment, had receptive knowledge of but did not produce, or used only some of the time. However, if a child is using targets correctly in more than half of the opportunities to do so, then those skills might not be as high of a priority for intervention as others that the child uses sometimes but not the majority of the time. The logic is that the child is likely to acquire skills in the former category with less intervention, whereas those in the latter category might be within the zone of proximal development and amenable to improvement with adequate intervention. For intervention for grammatical forms, we might be able to select from either those that children use some of the time or do not use at all since, according to the findings of Nelson, Camarata, Welsh, Butovsky, and Camarata (1996), either responds to intervention about equally as well. A caveat, however, might be that a child's receptive knowledge of targets, even if they are not used, could affect the suitability of those as the focus of intervention.

Although it may be appropriate to focus intervention on one aspect of language, this does not preclude attention to the other aspects of language. Intervention plans need to attend to all aspects of language simultaneously, even though one aspect may receive greater emphasis. It also makes little sense in intervention to have a child produce syntactic sequences, for example, that contain words whose meanings are unknown to the child or to use sentences in which the semantic relations among the words are normally nonsensical (e.g., "The tree is walking."). It is also likely that language targets taught using nonsense forms will not generalize very well. Intervention with a syntactic focus also needs to help a child realize the ways in which linguistic forms can be used for communication. Even when intervention has a pragmatic focus, form and content must match the aspects of use being emphasized. Similarly, intervention with a semantic focus must include relationships among meanings of words as expressed in morphological and syntactic forms and use of the word meanings in appropriate contexts. When all aspects of language are kept in mind in planning and executing intervention, a primary focus on one aspect may well facilitate a child's learning of other, secondary aspects concurrently. This is likely to be true, however, only if intervention is not limited solely to "drill work." Instead, intervention needs to encourage a child's use of a specific target in human interactions (Fey et al., 2003).

Although intervention may begin with a greater focus on one aspect of language than others, the focus and targets of intervention may shift several times during a child's continuing intervention program. Ongoing intervention for a child is a fluid process, the focus of which changes to meet the child's changing needs. This means that it is essential to probe regularly and to reassess systematically along the way. And, as the focus of intervention changes for a child, the strategies must also change.

Usefulness of Intervention Content

Language-disordered children must learn to communicate, not just learn the forms and content of language, and for school-age children intervention needs to focus on the language skills the children need to survive and succeed in learning environments, that is, educationally and socially relevant intervention. Almost all individuals working with children with language impairments agree that intervention needs to have as much of a pragmatic focus that demonstrates the usefulness of particular language targets as possible. Among the many helpful principles of intervention that Paul and Norbury (2012) lists are several that reinforce the importance of making the content of intervention useful. Among these are the following:

- Make the language informative (p. 78)
- Increase the motivation to communicate within the task (p. 78)
- Obligate pragmatically appropriate responses (p. 82)

Regardless of what specific language skills are targets of intervention, we want children to learn that, with appropriate language, they can better control their environments and what happens to them, influence other people, establish and maintain relationships with others, gain information, and succeed.

In planning content and forms to stress in intervention, the ways in which children can employ them in their daily environments are always considered. Teaching children about how to communicate may, in fact, be the primary focus of intervention in some instances. Recall that some language-impaired youngsters seem to be uninterested in communication and communicative interactions. Helping these children to discover that language is useful for a variety of functions and intentions and then teaching them how to employ language to accomplish these purposes can be important intervention objectives in and of themselves.

When it is appropriate to emphasize syntax and morphology in intervention, the usefulness of the forms for the child is an equally important consideration in selecting what grammatical features to teach. This includes the unique and definitive meanings the forms can encode for a child, the efficiency with which certain forms can accomplish communication (e.g., one utterance encoding two ideas, as in a sentence with a relative clause, "I like the boy who plays nicely," rather than two utterances to express the ideas, "I like the boy. He plays nicely"), and the variety of ways the forms can provide for encoding functions and intentions (e.g., direct versus indirect requests).

Child Characteristics

Most certainly, the individual characteristics of each child influence not only what the focus of intervention will be but many of the other decisions that are made about intervention as well. For a child with attention difficulties, we may decide that a nondistracting intervention environment may be appropriate. For a child with communicative interactive difficulties without attention problems, we may decide that a group setting, classroom, or preschool setting may be appropriate. The combinations are numerous, but among the child characteristics often considered, beyond the children's profiles for specific language skills, are age, nonverbal intelligence level, and amount of verbal behavior generally, in addition to types of language needs or the focus of intervention. Clearly, these are not discrete child characteristics but can instead be expected to interact. For example, older children can be expected to have greater language functioning and have implications for academic success that are increasingly important, and therefore intervention might need to focus on morphosyntactic structures. Similarly, more cognitively advanced children can be expected to have greater language functioning. Unfortunately, we have only limited empirically derived information to provide guidelines for matching specific child characteristics with intervention approaches and/or strategies, and for the present, we do not know exactly how level of functioning, type of intervention objective, and intervention approach may interact. We do know, however, that we need to consider such interactions in making decisions about intervention for individual children.

Another child characteristic to be considered in intervention relates to the child's interests, which affect the activities to be employed. Activities need to reflect the child's interests and cognitive level. When a child is presented with alternative toys and situations, it may be possible for the adult to follow the child's lead in what is interesting and stimulating for the child at the moment and create logical opportunities for use of a targeted language skill in that context. In what has become a classic example of taking advantage of children's interests, Holland (1975) wrote,

> I observed a therapy session in which a gifted clinician was teaching "more." She had prepared for the session by amassing quantities of similar small items to use in conjunction with her own utterance "more ________" and had plans eventually to demand the word from the child. However, the child, hyperactive and of limited verbal skills, became fascinated by a box of Kleenex in the room. The clinician began pulling tissues from the box, accompanying each pull with her utterance "more Kleenex." Eventually, when clinician and child had scattered tissues around the room the clinician introduced the utterance "more throw," accompanied by the two of them creating a snowfall of tissues. In this manner the child learned "more." (pp. 517–518)

Unfortunately, some language-disordered children demonstrate so little interest in their environments that an approach focusing on child-centered activities is useless, at least in early stages of intervention. For these children, the adult may need to create the interesting or rewarding situations artificially through structured reinforcement schedules, parallel and intersecting play activities, and/or careful control of stimuli presentations. In other instances, specific targeted language behaviors, such as some morphosyntactic structures, may necessitate more adult-centered activities. The point is that both child-centered and adult-centered activities can be appropriate, depending on the individual child's status and the language behavior to be emphasized. Successful language intervention depends, in part, on the ability to determine which approach is appropriate under particular circumstances, a willingness to employ each as the situations demand, and a recognition and willingness to change these when they are not working.

Metalinguistics

We have seen that toddlers and to some extent preschoolers possess only rudimentary metalinguistic skills and that the beginning of relatively sophisticated metalinguistic skills emerges in the early school years—or late preschool years. Therefore, for young children, it is inappropriate to base intervention strategies solely on metalinguistic skills. That is, we do not teach a word's meaning, a discourse rule, or a morphosyntactic structure only by explaining the meaning or the rule to a toddler or preschooler. Rather, we teach by example. This does not mean, however, that we avoid referring to a regularity. In fact, such reference may actually help a young child focus on the regularity, focus intervention on learning rather than just responses, and promote development of metalinguistic skills, as well as provide direct instruction about a language feature. Such reference is not unusual in parent–preschooler interactions, although it may not correspond to parent–toddler interactions. Parents of normal preschoolers often comment to their children that certain words have specific meanings, some things can be said to some people and not others, and some ways of saying a sentence are right and others are wrong. What the developmental information about toddlers' and preschoolers' metalinguistic skills does imply is that intervention strategies that depend only on metalinguistic skills are not appropriate. In contrast, intervention for school-age children and adolescents not only may include metalinguistics as an intervention strategy but may actually focus on improving metalinguistic abilities as intervention objectives themselves.

Reinforcement, Generalization, and Learning

Reinforcement is a powerful factor in language intervention, and several different types of reinforcement can promote language learning. Note here the emphasis on language learning and not solely language performance. Some of these are natural consequences of a communicative act. In our earlier example with *more*, using the word *more* can have natural and very reinforcing consequences for children. In intervention, we can both capitalize on the natural reinforcing consequences of communicative acts and create opportunities for reinforcing consequences to occur. The more these can be employed in intervention, the more likely it is that children will find what they are doing useful and be inclined to do more of it. Naturally occurring reinforcers or consequences of communicative events are often referred to as *intrinsic reinforcement* because these are inherent to the interaction. Another kind of reinforcement occurs outside usual communicative interactions in situations where a child might be given a star, tally mark, stamp, or verbal praise ("Good word," "Nice sentence," or "Nice asking"). These are *extrinsic reinforcers*, which can be used as effectively in language intervention as they are in other aspects of children's lives, such as parents' praise, school, and grades. There are also occasions in language intervention with some children when only extrinsic reinforcers are effective. On a long-term basis, language intervention should probably not depend solely on extrinsic reinforcers. Because they are artificial, it is unlikely that they will retain their reinforcing properties, in contrast to naturally occurring intrinsic reinforcers.

If extrinsic forms of reinforcement are employed in language intervention, there needs to be a consistent move toward eventually replacing them with more natural intrinsic ones. This can be accomplished either by gradually fading the extrinsic reinforcements and introducing the naturalistic reinforcements or by pairing the extrinsic and intrinsic reinforcers so that the naturalistic forms take on the characteristics of the extrinsic reinforcers. Achieving generalization of targets can also be more difficult with extrinsic than intrinsic reinforcers because naturalistic reinforcers tend to facilitate generalization, which is one reason for the general preference for emphasizing intrinsic reinforcers with their natural consequences of communication. Kamhi (2014) actually cautions against using too much evaluative feedback, suggesting that feedback, such as "Nice sentence" or "Good ending on the word," can both disrupt the natural flow of interactions and lead to a reduction in the power of the reinforcement because it becomes less meaningful to the children. Behaviorism theory also tells us that, while 1:1 reinforcement schedules (1 response to 1 reinforcement) are helpful in initially establishing responses to requests in intervention, they are not powerful for extending or maintaining performances. Extension and maintenance are best served by intermittent, random, and mostly intrinsic reinforcers. Thus, intervention needs to move to these patterns of reinforcement as quickly as possible.

Generalization of language skills learned in intervention to effective use in everyday situations is the major objective in developing language intervention plans. Unfortunately, a lack of generalization is too frequently a problem. All too often, children are observed to use language skills focused on in intervention only in those situations and not to use the same skills in other contexts. Not surprisingly, the types of reinforcements employed, as just discussed, may be one reason that generalization fails to occur. Another problem that can limit generalization is lack of deep learning of targeted language skills; overlearning is needed for children with language disorders, and without it, they may not generalize. Still another issue often occurs because of a focus on performance related to intervention objectives and targets rather on meaningful learning of the language skills. Lack of continuity in building language skills systematically across years of intervention and intervention plans that lack social validity are other barriers to generalization. Generalization needs to be considered at all stages of intervention and from the beginning of intervention.

It is possible that children will spontaneously generalize use of specific language skills to other skills that closely resemble the skill emphasized in intervention and to contexts that differ only slightly from the situation used in intervention to teach a language skill. For example, a child who receives intervention targeting the auxiliary *is* may generalize its use to auxiliary *are* if used in similar syntactic constructions (Leonard et al., 2002; Leonard et al., 2000). Although some limited spontaneous response class generalization and generalization to slightly different contexts may be observed for some language skills, attention needs to be given to several specific aspects of intervention to promote generalization. That is, intervention needs to use the following:

1. Different stimuli to elicit the targeted language behavior.
2. A variety of contexts in which the targeted language behavior is to be used.
3. Different people with whom the targeted behavior is to be used. These people may include other children, parents, classroom teachers, and other adults.

In effectively employing parents and other adults in an intervention plan, it is likely that these people will need specific training in how best to facilitate generalization. As we have seen previously in this text, parents/caregivers and teachers are essential partners in intervention.

HIGHLIGHTING INTERVENTION TARGETS

For whatever reasons, language-disordered children have not learned and do not learn language incidentally in the same ways as normal children. When a specific language feature is chosen as a target for intervention, it may be necessary to highlight the regularities of the feature in order for a language-disordered child to discover the general rule from exposure to particular instances and/or keep the feature in the child's immediate environment long enough for the child to process and/or retain it. The aim is to enhance the saliency of the language patterns. There are several techniques that can be employed to increase the salience of language features. Earlier we indicated that some use of techniques involving metalinguistic skills might help to emphasize the critical features for a child. Other techniques discussed here are multiple exposures to the language feature targeted, suprasegmental and rate variations, and input modality variations.

Multiple Exposures

Paul and Norbury (2012) cleverly used the adage, "If I've said it once, I've said it a hundred times" (p. 80), to make the point about the need for children with language disorders to be exposed to multiple exemplars of whatever the language target is. More exposure to exemplars is better; redundancy is essential. In reviewing the research on the efficacy of treatment for children with SLI, Leonard (1998) concluded that "the most successful approaches were those that encouraged production and provided *multiple* [emphasis added] yet natural cues for the desired response" (p. 203).

Research related to one intervention technique that we discuss later in this chapter illustrates the point about frequency of exposure. (The technique is *recasting,* in which an adult's response after a child's utterance is referentially contingent with the child's but adds or modifies one or more language elements to what the child said.) The combination of findings from several studies and the literature that have looked at the use of this particular technique led Proctor-Williams, Fey, and Loeb (2001) to write that "for children with SLI . . . increased exposure to recasts may indeed be necessary for language development to proceed at rates that approach those of their typically developing peers" and that "unless rates of target-specific recasts approach .8 per minute, the rate used in the experiment of Camarata, Nelson, and Camarata (1994), it may be unreasonable to expect success" (p. 166) in intervention. This is basically one recast per minute during adult–child interactions. With training aimed at parents of preschool children with language impairment, researchers have shown that they can increase the frequency of parental recasts to rates up around two per minute (Fey, Cleave, & Long, 1997; Fey, Cleave, Long, & Hughes, 1993; Fey, Krulik, Loeb, & Proctor-Williams, 1999). This compares to other research that has suggested that estimates of the average number of parents' recasts in their interactions with their young, typically developing children range from 0.06 to about 1 per minute (Conti-Ramsden, 1990; Conti-Ramsden, Hutcheson, & Grove, 1995; Farrar, 1990; Fey et al., 1999). In summarizing, Fey and Proctor-Williams (2000) write that, if intervention for young children with language impairments is to have a significant impact, then

> it appears not to be enough just to recast the children's utterances at rates found in their environment. Instead, successful intervention efforts involving recasts have increased the rates by approximately 2–4 times those observed in naturalistic contexts. (p. 180)

This line of reasoning is consistent with the findings of Gray (2003) in her research on word learning of preschoolers with SLI, which was mentioned previously in this chapter and in Chapter 3.

Clearly, for language-disordered children, controlling their exposure to exemplars of the desired language targets and increasing the frequency of the children's exposures to these are ways to enhance salience. The technique of multiple exposures can be used for any aspect of language targeted for intervention in order to assist a child to discover the appropriate rules or retain and process the information from the exemplars. To illustrate, in targeting the early developing regulatory function, a game similar to "Simon Says" can be employed. The adult can first direct the activities of the child via utterances such as "You hop," "You jump," or "Hop," "Jump." After multiple examples, the child becomes the director and orders the adult, who obeys readily. A subsequent activity can employ dolls, one for the child and one for the adult. During play, the adult repeatedly tells the doll to perform acts, such as "Go to bed," and follows each command with the consequent action, such as putting the doll in a cradle. After multiple sequences, the adult can cue the child by asking, "What do you want your doll to do? Tell him" or "Tell my doll what to do."

Gentle sabotage can be an effective intervention technique. When things do not go just according to plan, the most efficient and effective way of correcting the situation is with language. A caution is warranted, however. Although gentle sabotage may work, sabotage that creates frustration in the child will not work and is unfair to the child. Gently sabotaging a child's play with cars and trucks by moving another vehicle to block the movement of the child's can help the child realize that his or her verbalizations can regulate the adult's behavior. The adult can say "Move" or "Don't" and then move the vehicle. Desirable toys can be placed in sight but out of reach of the child. The adult can even talk about the seen but unreachable toys. If the child points to one of them, a gestural regulatory behavior, the adult can reach for a toy, pause, cue the child with "Get the toy?" and pause again to wait momentarily for the child's order. In a 30-minute period with activities such as these, it may be possible to generate 60 to 100 examples of the regulatory function paired with linguistically appropriate structures and corresponding content, or a rate of two to three exposures per minute.

The examples given at the beginning of this chapter to illustrate discovery of the meaning of *more* can also be used to demonstrate the technique of multiple exposures in semantically focused intervention. In a morphological or syntactic focus to intervention, such as one targeting the copula *is* to form interrogatives, multiple exposures to the target can be accomplished during guessing games ("Is it a dog?" or "Is it red?"). For example, the adult and child can take turns hiding objects in a box. After each object is hidden, the adult can engage in a sequence, such as asking "Is it blue?"; looking in the box; saying "No"; asking "Is it red?"; looking again; saying "No"; asking "Is it green?"; looking again; saying "Yes"; and finally removing the green object. (This activity assumes, of course, that the child knows colors.)

Another way to increase children's exposures to language targets is to increase the number of intervention opportunities or sessions they receive. However, very little is known about what is the optimal number of sessions (that is, intervention intensity or dose) children with language impairments need to receive in order to facilitate the greatest amount of progress in the least amount of time. And the relationship between amount of progress and intervention intensity (or dose) is not necessarily straightforward (Yoder, Fey, & Warren, 2012). One study does, however, provide us with some preliminary guidance. Jacoby, Levin, Lee, Creaghead, and Kummer (2002) found that the more intervention sessions young children received, the greater their progress was. Of particular interest was the finding that, for about 75 percent of the children, 20 hours of intervention was needed for them to improve at least one functional communication level, and no children improved more than two levels with fewer than 20 hours. These findings suggest a relationship between amount of intervention and amount of progress; we suspect that the greater the amount of intervention, the more exposure children have to language targets.

Distributed versus Massed Trials and Exposures

Although "more matters" is probably one of the more important principles of intervention, the effectiveness of "more" might be enhanced, or even decreased, by how the "more" trials are scheduled. In fact, Yoder et al. (2012) suggest that how intervention sessions are distributed and spaced may be more important for children's learning progress than the dose or intensity of intervention. A child can be exposed to many learning trials in mass or a fewer number of trials/exposures that are spaced over a particular amount of time, that is, massed versus distributed learning opportunities. For example, a child might have 30 minutes of intervention twice a week, during which 30 exposures/trials of a target occur in each of the sessions. Over a period of 10 weeks, there would have been 600 exposures/trials (60 trials/exposures per week × 10 weeks). Alternatively, the intervention could be spaced out or distributed so that the child is seen for 15 minutes, 4 times a week, with 15 exposures/trials occurring in each session. Over a period of 10 weeks, the child would have received an equivalent 600 exposures/trials.

The work of a few researchers has provided some evidence that children with SLI generally show greater progress in acquisition of intervention targets (e.g., new vocabulary words and verb forms) when intervention is planned for distributed exposures/trials instead of massed exposures/trials (Childers & Tomasello, 2002; Riches, Tomasello, & Conti-Ramsden, 2005; Schwartz & Terrell, 1983). As Riches et al. (2005) comment, children with SLI evince "rapid forgetting" (p. 1397). Delivery of intervention needs to try to counter this rapid forgetting by setting up intervention schedules that best facilitate remembering over time, and it appears that distributed intervention schedules are generally better than massed intervention for facilitating learning.

Suprasegmental and Rate Variations

Suprasegmental or prosodic features, such as stress, and modifying rate of input to a child are suggested as influencing children's language learning. Varying these may increase the salience of a selected language target. Some of the suggestions have been based on observations of mothers' talk to their normally developing children, in which they have been found to speak more slowly and increase the number of words that receive primary stress in their utterances.

The findings from the work of Ellis Weismer and her colleagues (Ellis Weismer, 1997; Ellis Weismer & Hesketh, 1993, 1996, 1998; Ellis Weismer & Schraeder, 1993) have suggested that several different prosodic modifications in an adult's language during intervention, such as increased vocal stress on language targets and slower speech rate in presenting language targets, have positive effects in facilitating the language learning of children with language impairments for lexical and possibly grammatical targets. Ellis Weismer and Schraeder (1993) also found that increased wait time between requests to a child and the child's response facilitated children's narrative production. This finding with regard to wait time improving narrative performance is consistent with that of (Hughes, 1998), which we presented in the previous chapter on assessment. Wait time was also suggested as an intervention strategy for adolescents in Chapter 5. Although Evans, Viele, and Kass (1997) did not find that a response latency (pause) before formulating their response in their turn during conversation predicted the length of the response used by school-age children with SLI, the children's use of a verbal filler (e.g., *um*, *uh*) before their responses, which was another way of "buying" response formulation time, did predict their use of longer responses. Recall also that earlier in this chapter we reported that Girolametto et al. (1996) found that when mothers reduced their rate of speech to their toddlers with language delay, along with making other changes in their language stimulation techniques, the toddlers made more progress than toddlers whose mothers did not make this and other changes in their language input. An important aspect of the work of Ellis Weismer and colleagues is that the suprasegmental and rate variations investigated tended to be more effective in improving children's language performances when the language tasks were more challenging or difficult for them, that is, when the tasks were more taxing on the children's language abilities and resources and/or increased the language-processing demands for the children. Often, this was in tasks where the children were asked to use the targets rather than simply indicating their comprehension of them. Again, we see level of complexity implicated as an aspect to consider in language intervention.

We could use the target of interrogative reversal and answer sequences to illustrate how stress might be used in intervention to increase salience of the target. For example, an adult could stress the *is* in the syntactic sequence ("*Is* it blue? Yes it *is*"; "*Is* it red? Yes it *is*"; "*Is* it green? Yes it *is*") both to highlight its presence and to contrast its location in the utterances. A finding from one study (Swanson & Leonard, 1994) about the duration of what is a frequent target of intervention for young children, the uncontracted copula *is*, could also be helpful in manipulating duration—and therefore stress and saliency—to assist children's language learning. In this study, when the verb was in the final position of sentences, its length in mothers' speech to young children was 250 milliseconds (ms), compared to the much shorter duration of 60 ms for the verb when the mothers used it in sentence initial positions, as in "*Is* it blue?" or in the middle of sentences, as in "The baby *is* big." Some morphological markers, such as possessive, plural, and third-person singular present-tense verb inflections that we know have both low semantic and perceptual salience, lend themselves well to being prolonged as well as being stressed in intervention.

It may also be important to control stress in another way to increase effectiveness of intervention. We know that many of the language features that are especially challenging for children often occur in relatively unstressed contexts, such as the *is* in "*Jim*my is *eat*ing," in which italics indicate the two stressed syllables that make up the five-syllable utterance. Yet, for children learning English, there seems to be a bias for better production when weak syllables come after stressed ones (Gerken, 1994; Gerken & McGregor, 1998; McGregor, 1997). Because, as McGregor (1997) suggests, "manipulation of prosodic-phonological contexts should aid grammatical morpheme acquisition" (p. 63), initially we might ask children to produce a particular language target in contexts where it follows a stressed syllable, such as the *is* in "*Jim* is *eat*ing" rather than "*Jim*my is *eat*ing" (Bedore & Leonard, 1995; Gerken & McGregor, 1998). However, children need to maintain their use of the targets in other contexts. This means that there may be a logical way to build in extension and generalization by manipulating the stress patterns of required utterances so that the children are gradually asked to use the targets in the less facilitating and less supportive stress patterns, such as when the targets follow an unstressed syllable, as in "*Kat*ie is *runn*ing" and "The *ba*by is *cry*ing."

Input Modality Variations

In Chapter 5, we suggested that, for adolescents with language disorders, use of intransient and stable visual or graphic stimuli in intervention could reduce the information-processing demands of language-learning tasks by keeping information needed to complete the tasks in the immediate environment while processing could take place. We have also seen elsewhere in this text (e.g., Chapter 1 describing aspects of normal communication process and Chapter 12 on augmentative and alternative communication) that communication is, in fact, multimodal. These ideas can be applied to language intervention for younger children. Some children can benefit from intervention that employs input modalities in addition to the auditory modality. For example, adults' use of gestures paired with specific linguistic forms has been shown to increase language-impaired schoolchildren's comprehension of novel words (Ellis Weismer & Hesketh, 1993).

The words *here*, *there*, and *give* provide excellent examples of how meaning can be enhanced by the combined use of the words and supporting gestures. Gestures can highlight a number of pragmatic intents and functions, such as reaching for desired objects as "I want the . . ." is said. Gestures can also reinforce turn-taking skills. In intervention designed to pair "all gone," "no, no," or "gone" with the object relations of disappearance and nonexistence, an adult can raise his or her hands in the classic "I don't know"/"Where is it?" gesture, adopt a puzzled facial expression, and move his or her head in a searching manner as the appropriate linguistic forms are modeled. Recall that children will often follow an adult's eye gaze. Negative headshakes can also highlight negative markers in targets such as "The dog is *not* big."

Graphically displayed symbols have also been used occasionally to enhance the salience of a specific target. The symbols are typically presented in conjunction with auditory input and then gradually faded as a child begins to demonstrate awareness of the target. One classic example is the Fokes Sentence Builder (Fokes, 1976, 1977). However, such an approach is probably most appropriately used with older language-disordered children and for morphosyntactic intervention goals, ensuring that sentences that are created are semantically plausible.

PROCEDURES AND TECHNIQUES TO FACILITATE CHILDREN'S LEARNING OF LANGUAGE TARGETS

Consistent with the previous discussion in this chapter that children need to learn rules and regularities in language intervention, the word "learning" is used in the title of this chapter section. And, in reading about the following procedures, it is important to keep in mind the notion of "learning" as the aim of intervention. The techniques presented are only mechanisms to help the children discover the rules and regularities. In reading about the following procedures and techniques, it is also important to keep in mind that the previous discussion of ways to highlight language targets can be used with these facilitating techniques.

On a continuum, illustrated in Figure 14.1, these techniques can range from those that are quite indirect and "natural" (i.e., used by parents naturally with their normally developing children), unintrusive (not interfering with or interrupting the flow of a normal adult-child interaction), and quite child centered to those that are more didactic and directive, intrusive on the flow of adult–child interactions, and adult centered. Some of the techniques

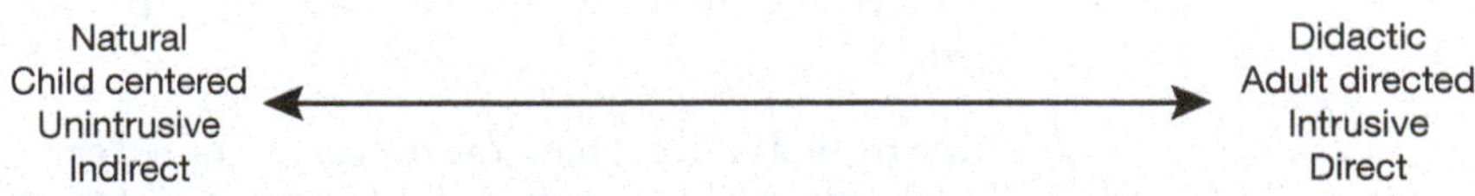

FIGURE 14.1 | Continuum Representing Degrees of Naturalness and Directiveness of Procedures and Techniques to Facilitate Children's Learning of Language Targets

have evolved from observations of parents' verbal behaviors that seem to promote language learning in their normally developing children; others come from behavioral orientations and related learning theories.

These techniques can be divided into those that are used before a child's response, in order to set up or stimulate the occurrence of the response, and those that occur after a child's utterance, in order to modify or encourage the child toward the desired target for the next time the child has an opportunity to use it. Thus, the following sections divide the techniques into those that are *a priori* and those that are post hoc to a child's utterance. There is no preferential or hierarchical order in the presentation of the techniques. More often than not, intervention utilizes combinations of the techniques, and in some instances, various labels have been used in the literature to refer to what are essentially the same or similar techniques. Examples of each technique are given below. However, because the examples are designed to illustrate a specific technique, they may appear here more stilted and exaggerated than their uses would be in language intervention situations and child–adult interactions.

Before the Child's Utterance

Self-Talk and Parallel Talk. In using self-talk, an adult talks aloud about objects in the immediate environment and about actions that are occurring at the moment. It is important that the topics for the talk be in context at the moment, to parallel the situations in which children typically first begin to talk. The language the adult uses needs to correspond closely to the child's language level in terms of both grammatical and semantic complexity. In other words, the adult's vocabulary and linguistic structures should neither greatly exceed the child's language capacity nor be at a level too simplistic for the child.

Self-talk can emphasize very specific aspects of language that a child needs to acquire, or it can be used as a more general language stimulation approach. The idea is for the child to hear the target language behaviors frequently. However, the purpose of self-talk is not to have the child repeat the targets. Therefore, the child is not overtly directed to talk. The following three examples illustrate how self-talk might be utilized during interactions with a child. In the first two examples, a specific language target is emphasized. The targets are repeated many times although in slightly different ways. The last example represents a more general self-talk activity. The language level in the last example is aimed at using two- and occasional three-word combinations.

Example 1

TARGET: *am* + verb + *ing*

SITUATION: Adult and child are looking at a book.

Oh, I am looking at the book. . . . I am opening the book . . . I am opening the book. . . . I am looking at the picture. . . . I am pointing to the dog. . . . I am turning the page. . . . Oh, there is a new picture. . . . I am pointing to the ball. . . . I am looking at the cat. . . . I am pointing to the cat. . . . I am closing the book now. . . . Now, I am putting the book away . . . I am putting the book away. . . . I am putting the book away.

Example 2

TARGET: The color "red"

SITUATION: Adult and child are playing with toys of various colors, many of which are red.

I see the red car. . . . I have the red car . . . the red car. . . . My car is red . . . red. . . . Oh, here is a red ball. . . . The red ball. . . . My ball is red. . . . Like the apple. . . . The apple is red, too. . . . I want the red apple. . . . Oh, here is a red block. . . . I'll put my red block with my red apple . . . and my red car. . . . These are all red. . . . Red toys. . . . The toys are red.

Example 3

TARGET: Two- and three-word combinations

SITUATION: Adult and child are cleaning up a room.

Clean the room. . . . Put toys away. . . . Put the toys away. . . . The ball's away. . . . Find the book. . . . Where's the book? . . . Where's the book? . . . Oh . . . the book's over there. . . . There's the book. . . . Put the book away. . . . Now, where's the glue? . . . Put the glue away. . . . There, the glue's away. . . . All gone. . . . What now? . . . I see the paper. . . . I'll get the paper. . . . The paper's put away. . . . Where's the block? . . . Oh . . . I see blocks. . . . Blocks on the table. . . . On the table. . . . There's the block. . . . Blocks are on the table. . . . Get the blocks. . . . Put the blocks away.

In contrast to self-talk, in which adults describe what they are doing, parallel talk emphasizes what the child is doing or what is about to happen to the child or is in the child's environment. Again, the purpose is not to have the child repeat the utterances used by the adults but to put the language, at the appropriate complexity level, in the child's auditory environment as the child is acting on the environment. Like self-talk, parallel talk activities can be used to emphasize specific language skills or to encourage language learning more generally. The following two examples illustrate parallel talk.

Example 1

TARGET: Use of elliptical responses to maintain conversation

SITUATION: Adult and child are playing with dolls, a dollhouse, and its furnishings.

Who has the chair? . . . Oh, she does. . . . Here it is. . . . Where is the table? . . . Oh yes, over there. . . . You get it. . . . Who wants it? . . . You do? . . . Me, too. . . . We'll both get it. . . . Where was it? . . . Oh, over there. (In this example, we also see the adult using deictic terms—*here* and *there*—and presuppositions in the form of the pronoun *it*.)

Example 2

TARGET: Three- and four-word phrases

SITUATION: Child is putting an animal puzzle together.

You have a horse. . . . You're putting the horse there. . . . Putting the horse there. . . . Good, the horse goes there. . . . Oh, you have a dog. . . . A little dog. . . . Oh, oh, the dog fell down. . . . Picking up the dog. . . . Putting the dog in the puzzle. . . . The dog is in the puzzle. . . . Looking for the duck. . . . Where's the duck? . . . Can't find the duck. . . . Oh, there's the duck. . . . Putting the duck in the puzzle. . . . All done now. . . . The puzzle is done. . . . All done now. . . . The puzzle is done.

Self-talk and parallel talk can be used together during adult–child intersecting and cooperative interactions. The next example incorporates both language facilitation techniques.

Example

TARGET: Performative intents encoded with "going to"

SITUATION: Adult and child are playing with various toys.

Oh, I'm going to get the toy. . . . You're going to get the car. . . . Going to get the car. . . . You're going to get the car. . . . You're going to go. . . . I'm going to color. . . . You're going to color. . . . You're coloring. . . . I'm going to cut. . . . You're going to cut. . . . You are going to fall. . . . Oops, you fell. . . . You are going to get up.

Imitation, Modeling, and Priming. A number of terms has been used to refer to imitation and modeling. As a result, some confusion as to their meanings has arisen. For our purposes, *imitation* and *mimicry* can be used synonymously. These terms refer to responses that are basically similar, if not identical, to a previously presented stimulus and that occur temporally in close proximity to the stimulus. The use of mimicry or imitation implies, according to Courtright and Courtright (1976), a "one-to-one process of literal matching" (p. 655). An interchange, such as the following one, involves imitation on a child's part:

> **ADULT:** Look at what the girl is doing now. Tell me, "The girl is running."
>
> **CHILD:** Girl is running.

Imitation can prove to be a valuable facilitating technique (Camarata & Nelson, 1992; Courtright & Courtright, 1976; Fey & Proctor-Williams, 2000), particularly in the early stages of language intervention for a specific targeted language behavior. Dependence on imitation, however, needs to be reduced as a child becomes more able to use the targets (Fey & Proctor-Williams, 2000). From this perspective, imitation can be seen as a facilitating technique that may be helpful to start a child's acquisition of a language target but not a technique that is continued once the path to acquisition is under way. Some have also objected to imitation because it violates normal language-learning interactions. This objection is not really true, however. Very young, normal language learners have been observed to imitate the language of adults, and imitation has been seen as an early developing mechanism that young language learners use to maintain topics of conversation across turns. Another counterargument to objections of using imitation as an intervention technique is that children with language impairments have not been successful in learning language via normal child–adult interaction. It is also possible to create situations where imitation can be used in reasonably pragmatically appropriate interchanges and interactions.

In contrast to imitation, *modeling* is a technique in which an adult (or sometimes other children) provides several examples of slightly different utterances, each of which contains the same critical language feature to be acquired by a child. This is one of the several techniques commonly included in an approach to intervention that is often referred to as *focused stimulation*. The expected response to these models may not match the models exactly, but the aim is that it will contain the common critical element(s) in the models. The following interchange represents a modeling approach:

> **ADULT:** This dog is big. That cat is big. The elephant is big. That lion is big. Oh look, a pig.
>
> **CHILD:** Pig is big.

Many exemplars are provided for a child before a situation is created to which a child might respond. There is no hard-and-fast rule about how many exemplars should be provided before moving on, but some suggest 10 to 20 (Fey & Proctor-Williams, 2000). In some uses of modeling, there is no direct request or command (or a mand) for the child to respond, although it is certainly hoped that the child will. And we saw in the research of Smith-Lock et al. (2015) that eliciting a response from a child was more effective than not requiring a correct response and only recasting the child's incorrect response. In other uses of modeling, an evoked response may be part of the technique. That is, the child is directed to respond, as in the example below, which is a modification of the example above:

> **ADULT:** This dog is big. That cat is big. The elephant is big. That lion is big. Oh look, a pig. Tell me about this pig.
>
> **CHILD:** Pig is big.

We can see from the child's response in both of these examples that common elements of the adult's utterances have been included to produce a similar but not exact response. Often, at least one other person (adult or child) may be included in intervention when a modeling approach is used. The third person models the target behaviors in response to the adult's stimuli. This makes the techniques particularly applicable to use in groups of children. Positive reinforcements may be provided for the third person's appropriate responses, as the child observes both the responses and the reinforcements. Such an approach is consistent with social learning theory (Bandura, 1971, 1977). If we examine the examples for self-talk and parallel talk, we can see how much modeling of target language behaviors occurs. The following examples illustrate how modeling can be used. In light of our previous discussion about increasing the saliency of the target, the models of the target language behavior might receive a little extra stress as the examples are modeled and/or might be presented at a slightly slower rate.

Example 1

TARGET: *a* + noun

SITUATION: Adult and child are looking at picture cards.

ADULT: Oh look, *a* dog! This is *a* dog. Look, *a* dog. This is *a* cat. This is *a* cat. This is *a* cat. *A* ball. Here is *a* ball. Oh, *a* top! *A* top. This is *a* top. This is *a* cup. Oh, *a* new picture. What is this?

CHILD: A coat.

Example 2

TARGET: Meaning and use of *in*

SITUATION: Adult and child are playing with a number of small toys and a paper bag, a box, and an old purse.

ADULT: Here's a block. Let's put the block *in* the purse. Look *in* the purse. Put the block *in* the purse. Where's the block?—Oh, look *in* the purse (both adult and child look). *In* the purse. Look, here's a ball. We'll put the ball *in* the bag. Look *in* the bag. The ball's *in* the bag. Where's the ball?—Look *in* the bag. *In* the bag. Now, let's put the car *in* the box. Good, you put it *in* the box. *In* the box. Here's a spoon. Here it goes. *In* the box. Where's the spoon?—See, *in* the box. Oh, here's a horse. I'll put the horse *in* the box. Where's the horse?

CHILD: In box.

Basing their work on that of Bock and colleagues (Bock & Loebell, 1990; Bock, Loebell, & Morey, 1992), Leonard et al. (2000, 2002) examined the role of structural *priming* in increasing the likelihood that the language of children with language impairment will include particular features if their previous utterance contained the same features. One of the scenarios used to elicit responses from the children in this research required the children first to imitate a sentence containing a specific target (e.g., uncontractible auxiliary *is* in present progressive sentences, such as "The mouse is eating the cheese") in response to a picture and then to provide a spontaneous (nonimitated) response to a new picture that also requires the same structure, although a plural subject could be depicted (e.g., uncontractible auxiliary *are* in present progressive sentences, such as "The dogs are chasing the ball"). Results confirmed the tendency of children to be more accurate in using the target forms under the priming condition as opposed to situations where they first produced a sentence with a different target structure, such as a past-tense verb.

These investigations were not intervention studies per se. However, Miller and Deevy (2006) designed an intervention study to explore the effectiveness of priming in facilitating SLI children's syntax. The positive effects of priming that had been observed in the earlier studies of Leonard et al. (2000, 2002) were confirmed, that is, the increased likelihood that children with SLI would produce particular syntactic structures after having just repeated a sentence with a similar syntactic form. Manipulating situations in which children are first required to imitate a targeted structure and then to provide an immediately subsequent nonimitated, novel response with the same essential grammatical constituents might be an effective intervention approach. Suprasegmental variations could be used in presenting the target to be imitated in order to increase its saliency. Further research is needed, however, to confirm or reject the effectiveness of priming as an intervention technique and, in particular, the additive effects, if any, of other facilitating techniques. The following example illustrates how a dialogue between an adult and child might incorporate priming.

Example

TARGET: *are* + verb + *ing*

SITUATION: Adult and child are looking at pictures.

Adult: Look at this picture. Tell me what is happening. Tell me, The boys *are chasing* the ball.

Child: Boys are chasing the ball.

Adult: Now tell me about the horse.

Child: Horse is jumping the fence.

Adult: Tell what is happening here. Tell me. The mouse *is eating* the cheese.

Child: Mouse is eating cheese.

Adult: Tell about the cats.

Child: Cats are catching the bug.

After the Child's Utterance

Reauditorization. Reauditorization is a language stimulation technique in which an adult repeats a child's correct response immediately after the correct response. In contrast to the previous language-facilitating techniques, which are employed before a child responds, reauditorization occurs in response to the child's statements. The concept behind this approach is to keep the auditory models of target language behaviors in a child's auditory environment a bit longer. This language-facilitating technique is rarely used by itself. Instead, it is typically combined with other techniques, such as modeling. Following is an example of reauditorization combined with modeling using an evoked-response technique. In this example, positive verbal reinforcement is also incorporated with the language stimulation techniques.

Example

TARGET: *are* + verb + *ing*

SITUATION: Adult and child are on a playground.

Adult: You *are swinging.* We *are swinging.* I like it. Oh, now you *are running.* You *are running.* We *are running.* We *are jumping* now. You *are jumping.* We *are jumping.* Now, you *are hopping.* Me, too. What are we doing?

Child: We are hopping.

Adult: We *are hopping* (reauditorization). Good. We *are hopping* up and down. You *are hopping.* We *are hopping* (reauditorization).

Recasting. In the above example, recasts occurred in the adult's two utterances following the positive verbal reinforcement, *Good*, and before the second reauditorization. As we indicated earlier, recasting is a facilitating technique in which an adult's response after a child's utterance maintains the topic, content, and reference of the child's utterance (i.e., is referentially contingent) but in some way adds or modifies one or more language elements to what the child said. This technique has also been seen in the literature variably as *expansion* or sometimes *expatiation.* (The differences between techniques are not always obvious.) The adult models for the child a slightly more complex or linguistically appropriate way of saying what the child has said and/or extends what the child has said to a slightly different context with slightly different content by adding information. What the adult chooses to include in the recast is typically the target of intervention for the child. The overall complexity of the recast, however, cannot be so difficult that the aspects of language that are the targets of intervention get lost in the adult's response. Recasting is often used with other language stimulation techniques, such as imitation, modeling, and reauditorization. The following three examples show various combinations of recasting, modeling, and reauditorization, as well as positive verbal reinforcement.

Example 1

TARGET: Attributive *big* + noun

SITUATION: Adult and child are putting toys away.

ADULT: We need to clean up. We need to put our toys away. Clean up now. Put the *big ball* away. No, not the little ball—the *big ball*. The *big ball*. I'll take the little ball. Good, you put the *big ball* away. Now, you have the *big truck*. I'll take the little truck. You put the *big truck* away. Good. Now, what do you have?

CHILD: Big car.

ADULT: *Big car* (reauditorization). That's right. You have the *big car* (recast). The *big car* (recast). I want the *big car* (recast). *Big car* (reauditorization). The *big car* (recast). Now, I'll take the *big boat* (model). Here's the *big boat* (model). You take the *big boat* (model). Put the *big boat* away (model). Good. What do you have now?

Example 2

TARGET: Regular past-tense verbs

SITUATION: Child and adult are looking at a storybook of "Jack and the Beanstalk."

CHILD: He climb up.

ADULT: He *climbed* up (recast). Jack *climbed* up the tree (recast). He *looked* around (model). He *looked* for a house (model). Jack *called* for help (model). He *called* and he *called* (model). He *yelled* and he *yelled* (model). He *wanted* to go home (model). He *climbed* down the beanstalk (model). What did he do?

CHILD: He climbed down.

ADULT: He *climbed* down (reauditorization). Yes, he *climbed* down the beanstalk (recast).

Example 3

TARGET: *will* + verb

SITUATION: Adult and child are decorating a bulletin board for Valentine's Day.

ADULT: I *will put* a heart here (model). I *will put* it here (model). I *will pin* it here (model). Where will you put your heart? (Notice the adult's question contains a varied form of the target and is also phrased so that the child's response could include the target.)

CHILD: I put it here.

ADULT: You *will put* it here? (recast) You *will pin* it here? (recast) That *will be* a good place. I *will glue* my arrow there, too (model). I *will glue* it on (model). Where will you glue yours?

CHILD: Will glue there.

ADULT: *Will glue* there (reauditorization). Good, that's right. You *will glue* it. (recast). You *will glue* your arrow there (recast). I *will get* the glue and I *will get* the other arrow (model and recast). And, I *will get* another arrow (model). Now, we *will glue* our arrows (model). What will we do?

CHILD: We *will glue* arrows.

ADULT: We *will glue* arrows (reauditorization). Good. You *will glue* your arrow and I *will glue* mine (recast).

Response Dialogues

When a child's specific language response is inadequate in terms of a target response, engaging the child in systematic types of interchanges may help elicit a response that more closely approximates the target. Lee, Koenigsknecht, and Mulhern (1975) have proposed seven different interchange techniques: complete model, reduced model, expansion request, repetition request, repetition of error, self-correction request, and rephrased question. These interchanges, or response dialogues, were originally developed as part of the Interactive Language Development Teaching (ILDT) (Lee et al., 1975) strategy. This language-teaching strategy is built around stories, usually with accompanying pictures, with different stories facilitating various aspects of language. These response dialogues are not completely unrelated to some of what we saw in the work of Leonard et al. (2000, 2002) and Miller and Deevy (2006) on priming effects because the stories set up the grammatical structure for the child and then systematically respond to the child's attempt in such a way to try to prime the child to use a correct structure in the next attempt. Fey and Proctor-Williams (2000) cite ILDT as one example of the way some of the less "natural" facilitating techniques, such as imitation and modeling, might be made more pragmatically appropriate for children.

In this approach, which is often used with a small group of children, the professional presents a small portion of a story and, using specific targeted language features, questions the children about the story. Additional portions of the story are then presented and dialogue routines completed. Each question is designed to elicit a specific structure. In reviewing the ILDT, Leonard (1998) wrote that the stories not only focused on "particular grammatical forms but also served as a means of teaching new lexical items, narrative cohesion, and other grammatical forms" (p. 206).

Some children need more assistance than others to modify initially inadequate responses in the direction of more complete responses. Therefore, these different interchange techniques are designed to provide varying amounts of help. Some give children considerable assistance in modifying initial responses; others offer very little help. These interchange techniques are described below. They are presented in decreasing order of assistance given to children in approximating target responses.

Complete Model. In light of our previous discussion of modeling as a facilitating technique, this use of the term *model* is a misnomer. As used to describe this interchange technique, it requests an imitative or mimicked response from the child. After an inadequate response from the child, an adult provides an example of the exact target utterance that the child is expected to duplicate. Following is an example of this interchange technique.

Example

TARGET: Past-tense verbs formed by adding the allomorph /t/ (*kicked*)

ADULT: Yesterday, we read a story about a rabbit. What did the rabbit do in the story?

CHILD: He hop into a basket.

ADULT: *He hopped into a basket.*

CHILD: He hopped into a basket.

ADULT: Good. What else did the rabbit do?

CHILD: The rabbit kick the fence.

ADULT: *The rabbit kicked the fence.*

CHILD: The rabbit kicked the fence.

ADULT: Good. What else did the rabbit do?

Reduced Model. In a reduced model, the elements of a target utterance that have been omitted are included in an adult's response. The partial model cues a child as to the exact element(s) that need special focus in a reformulation. As Lee et al. (1975) explain, a partial model is "not imitation but rather reformulation of an utterance" (p. 18). The following example illustrates an interchange using reduced, or partial, models.

Example

TARGET: Noun + *is* + verb + *ing*

ADULT: What is the boy doing?
CHILD: Boy jumping.
ADULT: *Is*
CHILD: Boy jumping.
ADULT: *Is jumping.*
CHILD: Boy is jumping.
ADULT: Good. Boy is jumping (reauditorization).

Partial models can include only the missing parts of the target or the missing elements plus closely associated grammatical units, as in the adult's second partial model in the example above. The last adult utterance provides a reauditorization of the child's correct response. Such an utterance could additionally include a recast.

Expansion Request. In an expansion request, the adult informs the child that the response is not adequate and that more information is needed. However, the adult does not provide the missing information. The child must decide, without the adult identifying the missing element(s), what has been omitted and then supply a complete structure on reformulation. There are several ways of requesting an expansion. These include "Tell me the whole thing," "Tell me more," "I didn't hear all of it," or "There's more." The following example illustrates expansion requests.

Example

TARGET: *Do* + subject + verb ("Do you want some food?")

ADULT: We are going to pretend we're in a restaurant. You are the waiter. You have to ask us what we want to eat.
CHILD: You want hamburger?
ADULT: *Tell me the whole thing.*
CHILD: Do you want hamburger?
ADULT: Good. Yes, I do want hamburger.
CHILD: Want milk?
ADULT: *Say the whole thing.*
CHILD: You want milk?
ADULT: *More.*
CHILD: Do you want milk?
ADULT: Good. Yes, I do want milk. I do want milk to drink (recast). I do want milk to drink with my hamburger (recast). What else do you have?

Repetition Request. According to Lee et al. (1975), a repetition request does not let a child know whether the response was adequate. As such, this interchange can be used to stabilize a correct response by having the child say it again or to reformulate adequately an incorrect response. In this latter use, a child has to reauditorize internally the first utterance, compare it to an internal standard auditory model, and restructure the utterance. We see examples of repetition requests in the following.

Example

TARGET: Use of polite requests

CHILD: Close the door.
ADULT: *What did you say? Say that again.*
CHILD: Close the door.
ADULT: *What did you say?*
CHILD: Can you close the door?
ADULT: Good. Yes, I will close the door now.

Repetition of Error. In some ways, this appears to be a form of providing a stimulus for a child to imitate. However, the adult is actually supplying an incorrect model. This is often accompanied by a questioning intonation or an unpleasant facial grimace. The child's task is to recognize the nonverbal cues that the response was inadequate, identify the error, and reformulate the response. However, if this interchange is used too early in intervention with a child, the child might mistakenly interpret the adult's utterance as a correct model to be imitated (Lee et al., 1975). Consequently, accurate interpretation of this approach is a more complex task than those listed earlier. Following is an example of this interchange technique.

Example

TARGET: Use of *red* to describe objects appropriately

ADULT: I have an apple. What color is the apple?
CHILD: The apple green.
ADULT: *The apple is green?*
CHILD: Apple green.
ADULT: *Green?*
CHILD: Apple red.
ADULT: You're right. The apple is red (recast).

Self-Correction Request. As the name of this technique implies, the adult asks a child to self-evaluate an utterance. In some instances, this approach may be employed even though a child's response was correct. The purpose is to reinforce and stabilize use of the target. In other instances, the technique can be used when the child's response is inaccurate. Despite the situation in which it is utilized, the purpose is to have the child self-monitor language productions in much the same way as adult speakers monitor their own productions. Use of self-correction interchanges is illustrated in the following example.

Example

TARGET: Irregular third-person present-tense singular verbs

CHILD: He haves some toys.
ADULT: *Is that right?*
CHILD: He has some toys.
ADULT: *Is that okay?*
CHILD: Yes.
ADULT: What else does he have?
CHILD: He has some shoes.
ADULT: *Is that right?*
CHILD: Yes.

Rephrased Question. This interchange may be especially effective when a number of other interchanges have occurred in order to elicit an adequate target response from a child (Lee et al., 1975). Rephrasing the original question may help the child stabilize use of the target language behavior. The following example shows this technique used in combination with the techniques of repetition request and repetition of an error.

Example

TARGET: *is* + verb + *ing*

ADULT: What is the boy doing?

CHILD: Boy crying.

ADULT: Boy crying? (repetition of error)

CHILD: Boy is crying.

ADULT: Good. Tell me again (repetition request).

CHILD: Boy is crying.

ADULT: *Is the boy laughing?*

CHILD: No, boy is crying.

In many instances, several of these techniques are used in combination in any one set of successive utterances between child and adult, as the last example illustrates. As we indicated earlier, other language-facilitating techniques, such as modeling, reauditorization, and recasts, can also be incorporated. The following example demonstrates several interchange techniques and language-facilitation approaches. An important feature in this example is that every time the child gave an inadequate response, the adult's subsequent interchange technique was one that provided more help or that is lower in the hierarchy. It is important that a child not become frustrated as a result of giving several inaccurate responses in a row. The adult must be aware of this possibility and modify the situation so that the child will succeed.

Example

TARGET: Interrogative reversal of copula *is*

SITUATION: Adult and child are guessing the contents of a large box filled with various toys.

ADULT: What is in the box? (self-talk) Let's guess. Is it a ball? (model) I don't know (self-talk). Is it a ball? (model) Yes, it is a ball (self-talk). What else is in the box?

CHILD: It a car?

ADULT: What did you say? (repetition request)

CHILD: It a car?

ADULT: Is it (reduced model)

CHILD: Is it a car?

ADULT: Is it a car? (reauditorization) Good. Let's look to see if you guessed right. Yes, it is a car (recast). It is a big, red car (recast). Is it a big, red car? (recast) Yes, it is a big, red car (self-talk). It is my turn to guess (self-talk). Let's see (self-talk). Is it a . . . (model). Is it a horse? (model) No, it is not a horse (self-talk). Your turn.

CHILD: It a pig?

ADULT: It a pig (repetition of error—accompanying facial grimace).

CHILD: Is it a pig?

ADULT: Is it a pig? (reauditorization) Good. Let's see if it is a pig. Is it a pig? (reauditorization) Yes, it is a pig (recast). It is a little pig (recast). Is it a little pig? (recast) Yes, it is a little pig (self-talk). My turn (self-talk). Is it a . . . (model). Is it a duck? (model) No, it is not a duck (self-talk). Your turn.

CHILD: It a truck?

ADULT: Did you say that right? (self-correction request)

CHILD: It a truck?

ADULT: Tell me the whole thing (expansion request).

CHILD: Is it a truck?

ADULT: Did you say that right now? (self-correction request)

CHILD: Yes.

ADULT: What is in the box? (rephrased question)

CHILD: Is it a truck?

ADULT: Is it a truck? (reauditorization) Good question. Let's look.

So Which Ones Should We Use?

To date, we have no clear evidence as to the superiority of one technique over others for different language targets at children's different stages of communicative development. Different techniques have been subjected to empirical scrutiny, and there have been studies that have tried to match children's characteristics with particular techniques, such as level of nonverbal intelligence and imitation versus techniques involving recasting. However, as Leonard (1998) summarizes for us, we are not yet at the point in the state of the science where we can match children and their characteristics with language targets with particular facilitating techniques and procedures. What we do know, however, is that intervention works, and we should probably try to elicit responses, that is, get the children to talk and to use their targets rather than settle for letting the children only listen to their targets. For the most part, however, the decisions about which of the techniques may be effective are left to the adult facilitating language learning for a specific child. Certainly, some approaches seem more appropriate for some children at specific points in an intervention sequence than others. There needs to be sufficient flexibility so that when one technique or combination of techniques is not working, other techniques can be selected. And several techniques are typically used with a child at a time.

APPROACHES TO INTERVENTION

In this section, we discuss various approaches to intervention. Although we divide this section into four subsections, it will become apparent that the topics are not completely discrete. Rather, aspects of each discussion interact with aspects of the others. Among additional factors that need to be kept in mind and that need to interact with the approaches to intervention presented here are the several legislative mandates and initiatives, in particular the Individuals with Disabilities Education Act (IDEA), No Child Left Behind (NCLB) legislation, and Response to Intervention (RtI) frameworks, that affect service delivery strategies for children and adolescents with language disorders. These were discussed more fully in several previous chapters.

Direct and Indirect Intervention

Previously in this text, reference has been made to direct and indirect approaches to intervention. The basic difference between the two approaches is who acts as the primary agent of language change for a child. In *direct intervention*, the professional assumes the role as the primary change agent. The professional plans the objectives of intervention and the strategies to be employed in accomplishing the objectives and implements the strategies by direct interaction with the child or children. Others, such as parents/caregivers and teachers, are typically involved in the planning and may even assist the professional in implementation, but the professional retains the role as the major change agent. In *indirect intervention*, the professional also plans the objectives of intervention, again typically with the involvement of parents/caregivers and/or teachers and/or assistants/aides and decides on specific strategies for implementation. However, individuals other than the language professional, such as parents/caregivers, teachers, or aides/assistants, carry out the plans. The professional works with these individuals to show them how to carry out the plans and monitors the implementation and the child's progress. The professional generally does not work directly with the child or children. In Chapter 3, we discussed the necessity to train parents/caregivers for indirect intervention with toddlers and preschoolers. The same is true if assistants or aides are involved (Dickson et al., 2009), and it is true when teachers or day-care providers are the primary agents of change. In some cases, a combination of direct and indirect intervention may be warranted, or intervention may change from one approach to another as the objectives of intervention and the child's language behavior change.

There are few empirical data to help us in deciding which approach is most effective under what conditions. However, in two studies, outcomes of language intervention for school-age children with language impairments delivered by speech–language pathologists (SLPs) and by speech–language pathology assistants (SLPAs) were examined in terms of both effectiveness (degree of children's progress on intervention objectives) and costs (Boyle et al., 2009; Dickson et al., 2009). In both studies, outcomes for intervention by SLPs and SLPAs were comparable, but costs for the services were less for intervention delivered by the assistants. In the studies, the SLPAs were well trained. The SLPs made the decisions about the children's treatment objectives and general intervention methods and supervised the work of the assistants, and an intervention manual that both the professionals and the assistants used had been developed. Nevertheless, there were notable cost savings for similar outcomes when indirect intervention (the assistants) was implemented.

As we saw in Chapter 3, parents can be powerful partners in helping to deliver intervention to young children. There are several parent training programs, such as the *Hanen Early Language Parent Program* (Girolametto, Greenberg, & Manolson, 1986), although the effectiveness of only a few have been subjected to extensive, independent empirical study. However, in one randomized controlled study (Buschmann et al., 2009), the effectiveness of short-term, structured, parent-delivered language intervention used with toddlers with slow expressive language development (SELD) was compared to a nonintervention group. The SELD toddlers who received parent-delivered intervention made major language gains over a 1-year period. Since the toddlers were identified as language delayed and not language impaired, we cannot know if similar results would be obtained for children with SLI. Nevertheless, the study does highlight that parents can be positive assets in indirect intervention approaches. As another example (Starling, Munro, Togher, & Arciuli, 2012)), in a study focused on adolescents with language impairment, Starling, an SLP, trained eighth-grade regular/general education teachers from a variety of academic disciplines to modify their use of instructional spoken and written classroom language in ways that better supported the learning of the language-impaired adolescents who were in an inclusive, mainstream classroom setting. Results indicated that the trained teachers modified their instructional language in ways consistent with the training, whereas there was no change in the spoken and written instructional language of the untrained secondary school teachers. Furthermore, the changes in the teachers' instructional language were associated with significant improvements in the written expression and listening comprehension of the adolescents with language impairment. The language-impaired adolescents in the classes of the untrained teachers did not show such language growth.

These examples suggest that indirect intervention has the potential to be effective and possibly cost effective. What the studies have in common, however, is the necessity to provide training for the agents of intervention, when those individuals are not the language professionals, and for the professionals to provide oversight and monitoring of children's progress. To some, the idea that agents other than language professionals might provide equally effective intervention could be disconcerting and threatening to professional boundaries and identities. On the other hand, findings such as these could be viewed as a way of providing intervention to children who otherwise might not receive it because there are not sufficient numbers of language professionals or resources to serve all the children who need assistance. It is also possible that direct and indirect intervention might be more appropriate at different points in a child's intervention trajectory. Olswang and Bain (1991b) have suggested that direct intervention may be more appropriate when the aim is to establish a new language behavior and that indirect intervention may be more appropriate when the aim is to stabilize, generalize, or extend a language behavior that the child already demonstrates or that has been established as a result of direct intervention.

Group and Individual Intervention

In Chapter 5, we suggested that, for adolescents with language impairment, group intervention may be more effective than individual, or one-to-one, intervention. This belief is somewhat counter to a more traditional view that a one-to-one setting is the more effective format for language intervention. With a one-to-one format, extraneous environmental distractions can be controlled to allow a child to focus attention on the desired stimuli. Language learning, it is believed, will be promoted quickly.

The rationale behind a one-to-one structure for language intervention may, in part, be valid. Reducing distractions can increase the salience of the provided stimuli, and more opportunities for exemplars and responses might be possible. However, language is an interactive, interpersonal behavior. As such, many of the reasons cited for employing group intervention for language-disordered adolescents apply to intervention for younger children (Bunce, 1995; Rice & Wilcox, 1995; Swenson, 2000). Young children learn language by interacting with their environments and the people in them. A one-to-one intervention format often limits the number of events and contexts in which language teaching can occur and restricts the number of people with whom the language can be used. In contrast, small-group intervention formats for young language-disordered children can provide situations for language learning that are not present in individual intervention settings. In light of our previous discussions of reinforcement and generalization, we can see how a group format might furnish opportunities for naturalistic reinforcers to occur and promote generalization. Each child in a small group is exposed to a variety of stimuli, experiences, contexts, and people that are not available in one-to-one situations. A number of adults, including parents, often participate with the children in group situations, thereby providing the children opportunities to use language with different adults as well as with other children. Such a format can also be used to help train parents and teachers in strategies to be employed in indirect intervention.

In the two studies referenced above about the effectiveness of direct versus indirect intervention modes, group versus individual intervention was also examined (Boyle et al., 2009; Dickson et al., 2009). Recall that in these studies, the children were of school age. Individual intervention did not show an advantage in terms of outcomes compared to group intervention. And, not surprisingly, group intervention modes were more cost effective than individually delivered intervention.

The decision as to whether a child will benefit more from a group setting or an individual format depends on the specific child. Some children, particularly those who are hyperactive, distractible, or inattentive or those who show little interest in interacting with people, may initially require one-to-one intervention. For other children, a small-group setting may be the most appropriate. Furthermore, the type of setting from which a specific child will benefit more may change as the child's behaviors and language skills change. Children who initially required individual intervention can progress so that a group setting is warranted. Children initially seen in a group setting may progress to needing intervention for very specific skills best accomplished in an individual format. Again, there is no fixed rule as to which format must be used throughout a child's entire intervention program. Instead, flexibility in providing a child with the appropriate setting at a particular point in intervention is the key.

The decision regarding the structure of a child's intervention does not always have to involve a choice between a group or individual format. In many instances, a combination of the two can be effective (Cleave & Fey, 1997). Targeted language skills can be presented in an undistracting, one-to-one situation and then extended to a variety of contexts with a variety of people present in a group setting.

Three Language-Teaching Methods

Beyond considering the degree of "naturalism" of facilitating techniques that can be used in language intervention, as illustrated in Figure 14.1, the larger structure of intervention can vary along a continuum of "naturalness." Some can be quite didactic, while others are quite unstructured and focus exclusively on child-centered approaches. Each, however, has strengths and weaknesses, so many professionals have tried to adopt methods somewhere between the extremes. Fey (1986) terms these "hybrid" methods. These attempt to bring to intervention environments and/or activities that are as natural as possible but that still provide sufficient opportunities for the adults to control and manipulate the teaching situations in order to ensure adequate exemplars, opportunities for response, practice, and generalization.

Olswang and Bain (1991a) have described three commonly adopted language-teaching methods: milieu teaching, joint action routines, and inductive teaching. As the authors explain, these methods share some similar features and incorporate procedures found in other methods as well. However, they vary in terms of the degree of structure involved. The various facilitating techniques discussed in the previous section will be used within the formats of these three language-teaching methods. However, it is logical to assume that some techniques will be more compatible with one or two of the teaching approaches than another.

Milieu Teaching. Of the three methods, milieu teaching employs the least amount of structure. Natural consequences of communication as reinforcements, activities determined by the child's interests and attention, conversational contexts for teaching, and intervention in the child's usual environment (home, preschool, and classroom) are characteristics of the milieu teaching approach. Opportunities for targeted language behaviors are dispersed throughout a session. Three procedures are used in milieu teaching, although these procedures can also be employed in other teaching approaches. The procedures are incidental teaching, mand-model teaching, and delay.

Incidental Teaching. In incidental teaching, the child determines the activity or topic and the adult works the language teaching into it. The activity or topic lasts only as long as the child is interested in and reinforced by it. During the activity, the adult may use a variety of the facilitating techniques discussed previously to elicit specific language behaviors.

Mand Model. Unlike incidental teaching, a mand-model approach is a more adult-directed procedure. The adult chooses a time to direct the child's attention to an object or activity and asks for (mands) a response from the child or provides a prompt for a response. If the child gives an appropriate response verbally, the adult reinforces the child's response and then gives the child the desired object or allows the activity to proceed. If the child's response is incomplete or incorrect, models of the target response or other elicitation techniques are used.

Delay. When a child wants an object out of reach or desires certain events to occur, the adult looks questioningly at the child but waits, usually for about 15 seconds, before responding to the child. Obviously, the adult is waiting for an appropriate response from the child before complying. If the child does not respond, the adult may provide a model of the target response or use other elicitation techniques and wait again. Generally, the sequence is repeated only twice before complying with the child's desires. Too many repetitions without a successful outcome may do nothing more than increase a child's frustration. However, if too many unsuccessful outcomes are occurring, immediate reevaluation of the teaching approaches and strategies being employed is warranted.

Delay is an important intervention procedure even when it is used with other language-teaching methods. Language-disordered children may not be able to respond as quickly as normal language-learning children. They may very well need more time to understand what is expected, to process the stimuli, and/or to retrieve and generate a response.

Joint Action Routines. This teaching method is sometimes known as *script therapy.* The idea behind joint action routines is to create interactive, systematic repetitions of events in which each partner has predictable language and behavioral patterns to complete. The routines can reflect usual events in a child's environment, or they can be created. These routines are socially based and incorporate the need to communicate. They focus on specific themes or topics, such as craft activities in which the adult and child interact and the child has to ask for needed materials, or they may be centered around pretend play routines. Joint action routines are purported to reduce demands on a child so that the child can focus on the language tasks required (Ellis Weismer, 2000). As the child becomes familiar with specific routines, the expectations for language use gradually change to more advanced skills. A problem with the joint action routine method of language teaching is the manner in which the routines are or are not modified to increase the level of language expected from a child and the strategies employed to elicit the higher-level language behaviors. Generalizing the routines to novel situations can sometimes also be problematic.

Inductive Teaching. Inductive teaching is the most structured and adult-centered method discussed here. The adult manipulates meaningful communicative interactions so that the child begins to identify patterns (or regularities). The three elements of inductive teaching are the following (Olswang & Bain, 1991a):

1. The communicative interactions are arranged to allow the child to discover that a pattern exists.
2. The child discovers that the meaningful context or communicative interaction is associated with the pattern and, in fact, explains the pattern.
3. The child learns that the patterns involved affect meaning.

The child hypothesizes "the rule that captures the nature of the correspondence between the observed pairs of stimuli. The assumption of this procedure is that the induction process is an innate one so that by this step, if the preceding ones have been arranged correctly, hypothesizing the rule will occur automatically" (Olswang & Bain, 1991a, pp. 81–82).

In practice, it is not unusual to see professionals using elements of all three methods. Each has its merits and its drawbacks. The merits need to be matched to the child and the intervention objectives. The different methods or elements of the methods may suit different children and different language objectives. What we do not know yet is how to match these variables unfailingly. We do know that we need to try.

Service Delivery Models

Previously in this text, we introduced ideas related to different models of delivering language intervention services to children. In addition to findings from research, forms of service delivery are influenced by the setting in which intervention is to occur, policies and orientations of different service providers, and legislative mandates.

Increasingly, however, it is clear that the trend has been to provide language intervention in children's classrooms or their other usual environments. Settings consistent with this trend are sometimes referred to as *inclusive, integrated*, or *mainstreamed.* These services are sometimes delivered by an adult other than the professional, in which case they can be considered indirect interventions, per our previous discussion. These also probably fall into the category of consultation services because of the consultative role that the language professional plays. In some situations, children may be provided language intervention by the language professional in the children's classrooms during activities taking place at various times of the day, such as free reading time, art, and group discussions. These services are considered direct intervention and not necessarily consultative. In still other cases, the language professional delivers the services in the classrooms, generally in collaboration with the general/regular educator or other professionals, aides, or parents/caregivers in the environment, that is, collaborative service delivery. Forms of delivery in these instances may include team teaching or turn teaching with the teachers. Strengths that have been attributed to collaborative—and even consultative—service delivery models are the ecological validity of the language intervention and the promotion of generalization. However, there is considerable variation in how different service delivery models are implemented.

In the midst of the trend toward increasing use of collaborative and/or consultative service delivery models, use of what has come to be known as the "traditional pullout" model of service delivery, even in school settings, has not been abandoned, even in settings where collaborative/consultation models have also been implemented. A 2008 survey of the American Speech-Language-Hearing Association (ASHA) indicated that the predominant service delivery model used by school SLPs was the pullout model (American Speech-Language-Hearing Association, 2008). Pullout means that a child leaves the activities of the typical educational routine to receive services from a specialist. At the extreme, the pullout might be complete, in which case the child receives all of his or her education in a self-contained classroom or more recently even in self-contained schools, given an increase in the number of such special schools, from which the child might again be pulled out for other special services, such as language intervention (Conti-Ramsden, Botting, Simkin, & Knox, 2001; Hirst & Britton, 1998). More often, however, pullout means that the child participates in the usual educational routine for most of the time, leaves it temporarily for special services, and then returns. In Chapter 5, we discussed why this model was not appropriate at the secondary school level for adolescents with language disorders. Two of the biggest criticisms of the model relevant to language intervention have been the limited contextual support for language learning and the difficulties in generalizing language skills into a naturalistic environment.

Others have interpreted pullout to mean that a child is seen individually by the professional. However, pullout does not equate to individual intervention and does not preclude group intervention, which can take place within a pullout model. Therefore, the issues related to pullout are not essentially issues related to individual versus group intervention approaches. It is likely that some language-disordered children at certain times during their language intervention benefit from language teaching that takes place in a less distracting environment in which the targeted rules and regularities can be made more salient and language-teaching techniques can be used more consistently. Most professionals now agree that, as a sole model of intervention, a pullout model is inadequate. It can, however, be used successfully in combination with both consultative and collaborative models.

Unfortunately, the state of the science does not provide sufficient evidence that a particular service delivery model is more effective than another (Cirrin et al., 2010). There is, however, some suggestion in the research that "classroom-based direct services are at least as effective as pullout intervention for some intervention goals" (Cirrin et al., 2010, p. 233). Until research is able to provide more guidance about the relative effectiveness of specific models for particular language goals and children, a perspective that service delivery does not have to be "all or nothing" with regard to models is likely the currently sufficing approach. Intervention needs to be viewed as requiring several service delivery models, with each contributing differently to different children with differing language needs at different times.

PUTTING IT TOGETHER

We have reviewed many of the factors that go into planning and implementing language intervention. Each of these represents a decision point in the planning process, but each decision is not independent. We have seen that the factors frequently interact with each other. The decisions, therefore, interact. Figure 14.2 illustrates some of these factors and the interactions as well as the complexity involved in the intervention decision-making process. There is no claim that the model includes all the factors affecting intervention decisions. Furthermore, as we learn more about intervention and children with language disorders, more factors will probably be added. It is also possible that some factors will combine with others. Ultimately, the factors and the decisions will combine to produce an individual child's intervention plan. Planning and implementing language intervention for individual children is a complex decision-making process.

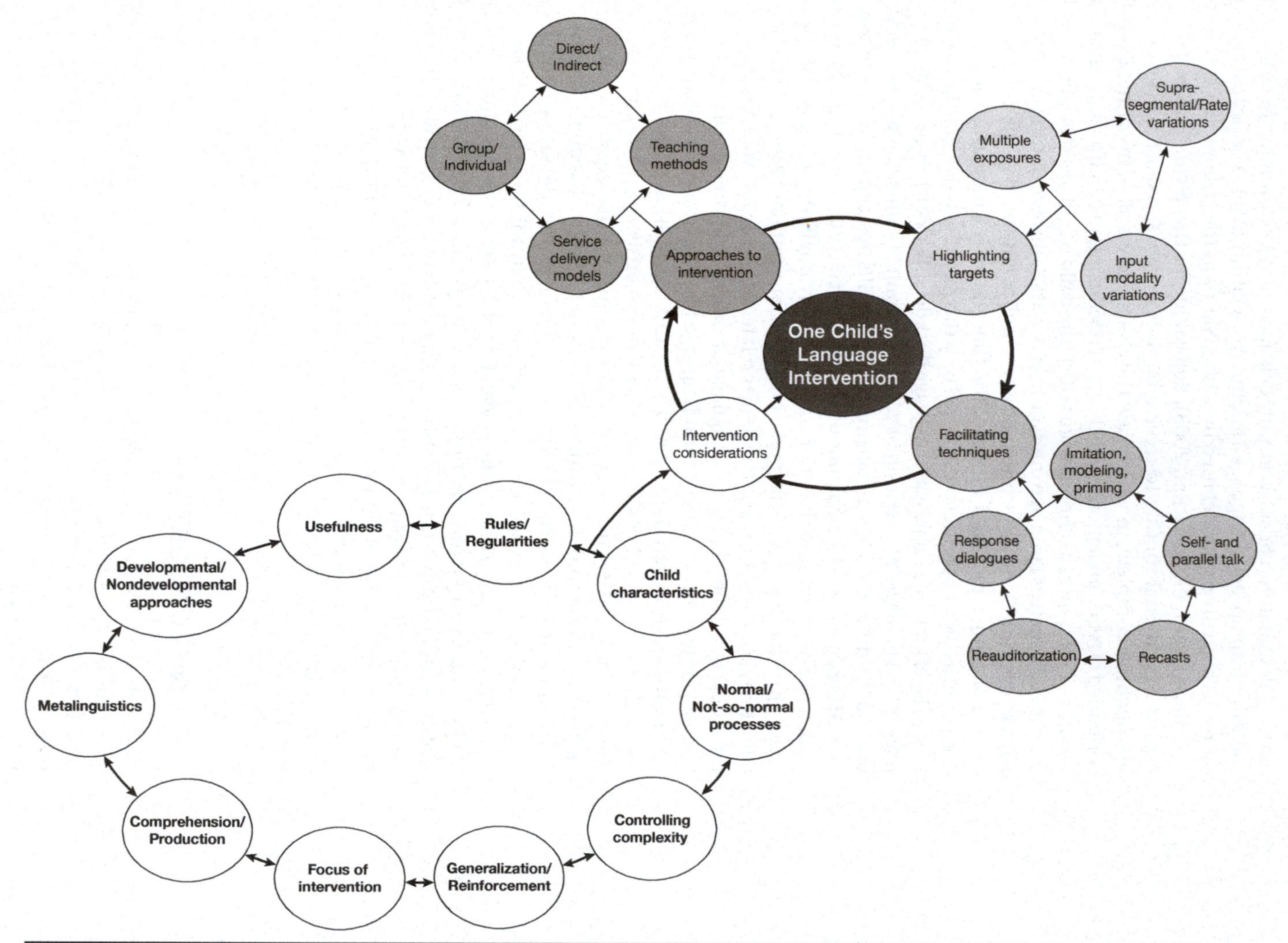

FIGURE 14.2 | A Model of Language Intervention

SUMMARY

In this chapter we have seen that

- Normal language processes generally guide much of what we do in language intervention, but there are indications that children with language disorders may need intervention that modifies normal processes in order to realize language features productively.
- Language intervention aims to help children discover rules and regularities and/or provide opportunities for the children to process relevant information about what it is they need to learn.
- Language intervention needs to stress the usefulness of language.
- Developmental approaches are more frequently used to guide the sequencing of intervention objectives, although nondevelopmental approaches may sometimes be appropriate.
- Comprehension of a language target is sometimes emphasized before production; in other instances, comprehension and production are emphasized concomitantly. It may be that language-disordered children need to have practice in producing targeted language behaviors in order to learn to use them most efficiently.
- The focus of intervention depends on an individual child's needs and likely changes throughout the child's total intervention program.
- It is important to control all aspects of language complexity when planning for and requiring a response from a child.
- Reinforcement and generalization are important considerations in planning intervention; generalization may be promoted more successfully when naturalistic reinforcers and varied contexts are incorporated into the implementation of intervention.
- The characteristics of each child affect the intervention approaches and strategies chosen, but we still do not know how to match most efficaciously child characteristics and intervention approaches and/or strategies.
- Language intervention for young children does not depend heavily on metalinguistic approaches but does not avoid incorporating metalinguistics. In contrast, for older children, improving their metalinguistic abilities may be a focus of intervention, and metalinguistic approaches are sometimes employed as teaching strategies.
- Intervention can be direct or indirect and can be provided via several language-teaching strategies and service delivery models.
- Exposure to language targets needs to be more frequent, made more salient for children with language impairment, and likely delivered in spaced, distributed schedules.
- Many direct and indirect facilitating and elicitation techniques can be employed.
- Planning and implementing language intervention is a complex decision-making process in which multiple factors interact.

Each language-disordered child has unique needs that require flexibility in planning intervention. Unless intervention is viewed as an individually designed, dynamic, fluid process, language-disordered children will be fortunate if their needs are met at least some of the time.

References

Chapter 1

Axtell, R. (1991). *Gestures: The do's and taboos of body language around the world*. Baltimore: John Wiley & Sons.

Bandura, A. (1971). *Psychological modeling*. Chicago: Aldine-Atherton.

Baron-Cohen, S. (1989). The autistic child's theory of mind: A case of specific developmental delay. *Journal of Child Psychology and Psychiatry, 30*, 285–297.

Baron-Cohen, S. (2000). Theory of mind and autism: A fifteen-year review. In S. Baron-Cohen, H. Tager-Flusberg, & D. Cohen (Eds.), *Understanding other minds: Perspectives from developmental cognitive neuroscience* (pp. 3–20). New York: Oxford Press.

Bates, E. (1979). *The emergence of symbols: Cognition and communication in infancy*. New York: Academic Press.

Bates, E., Benigni, L., Bretherton, I., Camaioni, L., & Volterra, V. (1977). From gesture to the first word: On cognitive and social prerequisites. In M. Lewis & L. Rosenblum (Eds.), *Interaction, conversation, and the development of language*. New York: John Wiley & Sons.

Bloom, L. (1988). What'is language? In M. Lahey (Ed.), *Language disorders and language development*. Columbus, OH: Merrill/Macmillan.

Chomsky, N. (1965). *Aspects of the theory of syntax*. Cambridge, MA: MIT Press.

Chomsky, N. (1981). *Lectures on government and binding*. Dordrecht, Holland: Foris.

Coady, J., & Evans, J. (2008). Uses and interpretations of nonword repetition tasks in children with and without specific language impairments (SLI). *International Journal of Language and Communicative Disorders, 43*, 1–40.

Ellis Weismer, S., & Evans, J. (2002). The role of processing limitations in early identification of specific language impairment. *Topics in Language Disorders, 22*, 15–29.

Ellis Weismer, S., Evans, J., & Hesketh, L. (1999). An examination of verbal working memory capacity in children with specific language impairment. *Journal of Speech, Language, and Hearing Research, 42*, 1249–1260.

Finneran, D., Francis, A., & Leonard, L. (2009). Sustained attention in children with specific language impairment (SLI). *Journal of Speech, Language, and Hearing Research, 52*, 915–929.

Graf Estes, K., Evans, J., & Else-Quest, M. (2007). Differences in nonword repetition performance of children with and without specific language impairment: A meta-analysis. *Journal of Speech, Language, and Hearing Research, 50*, 177–195.

Hall, E. (1990). *The silent language*. New York: Anchor Books.

Hayakawa, S. (1964). *Language in thought and action* (2nd ed.). New York: Harcourt, Brace & World.

Hillis, A., & Bahr, D. (2001). Neurological and anatomical bases. In D. Bahr (Ed.), *Oral motor assessment and treatment: Ages and stages*. (pp. 1–41). Needham Heights, MA: Allyn & Bacon.

Joos, M. (1976). The style of the five clocks. In N. Johnson (Ed.), *Current topics in language: Introductory readings*. Cambridge, MA: Winthrop.

Kuhl, P. (1990). Auditory perception and the ontogeny and phylogeny of human speech. *Seminars in Speech and Hearing, 11*, 77–91.

Kuhl, P., & Meltzoff, A. (1988). Speech as an intermodal object of perception. In A. Yonas (Ed.), *Perceptual development in infancy. The Minnesota symposia on child psychology* (Vol. 20, pp. 235–266). Hillsdale, NJ, England: Lawrence Erlbaum Associates.

Ladefoged, P. (2006). *A course in phonetics* (5th ed.). Boston: Thomson, Wadsworth.

Langacker, R. (1968). *Language and its structure: Some fundamental linguistic concepts*. New York: Harcourt, Brace & World.

Leonard, L., Ellis Weismer, S., Miller, C., Francis, D., Tomblin, J. B., & Kail, R. (2007). Speed of processing, working memory, and language impairment in children. *Journal of Speech, Language, and Hearing Research, 50*, 408–428.

Luria, A. (1961). *The role of speech in the regulation of normal and abnormal processes in the child*. Baltimore: Penguin.

Luria, A., & Yudovich, F. (1971). *Speech and the development of mental processes in the child*. Baltimore: Penguin.

Miller, C., Kail, R., Leonard, L., & Tomblin, J. B. (2001). Speed of processing in children with specific language impairment. *Journal of Speech, Language, and Hearing Research, 44*, 416–433.

Miller, J., & Paul, R. (1995). *The clinical assessment of language comprehension*. Baltimore: Paul H. Brookes.

Montgomery, J. (2000). Verbal working memory and sentence comprehension in children with specific language impairment. *Journal of Speech, Language, and Hearing Research, 43*, 293–308.

Montgomery, J., Evans, J., & Gillam, R. (2009). Relation of auditory attention and complex sentence comprehension in children with specific language impairment: A preliminary study. *Applied Psycholinguistics, 30*, 123–151.

Piaget, J. (1954). *The origins of intelligence*. New York: Basic Books.

Prutting, C. (1982). Pragmatics as social competence. *Journal of Speech and Hearing Disorders, 47*, 123–134.

Rice, M. (1983). Contemporary accounts of the cognition/language relationship: Implications for speech-language clinicians. *Journal of Speech and Hearing Disorders, 48*, 347–359.

Skinner, B. (1957). *Verbal behavior*. Englewood Cliffs, NJ: Prentice-Hall.

Thurlow, C. (2005). Deconstructing adolescent communication. In Williams, A., & Thurlow, C. (Eds.), *Talking adolescence: Perspectives on communication in the teenage years* (pp. 1–20). New York: Peter Lang Publishing.

Ukrainetz, T. (2006). *Contextualized language intervention: Scaffolding PreK–12 literacy achievement*. Eau Claire, WI: Thinking Publications.

Vygotsky, L. (1962). *Thought and language*. Cambridge, MA: MIT Press.

Wiig, E., & Semel, E. (1984). *Language assessment and intervention for the learning disabled* (2nd ed.). New York: Merrill/Macmillan.

Windsor, J., Milbrath, R., Carney, E., & Rakowski, S. (2001). General slowing in language impairment: Methodological considerations in testing the hypothesis. *Journal of Speech, Language, and Hearing Research, 44*, 446–461.

Chapter 2

Achenbach, T. (1970). Standardization of a research instrument for identifying associative responding in children. *Developmental Psychology, 2*, 283–291.

Applebee, A. N. (1978). *The child's concept of story: Ages two to seventeen*. Chicago: University of Chicago Press.

Armour-Thomas, E., & Allen, B. (1990). Componential analysis of analogical-reasoning performance of high and low achievers. *Psychology in the Schools, 27*, 269–275.

Bates, E. (1976). *Language and context: The acquisition of pragmatics*. New York: Academic Press.

Berko, J. (1958). The child's learning of English morphology. *Word, 14*, 150–177.

Bloom, L. (1970). *Language development: Form and function in emerging grammars*. Cambridge, MA: MIT Press.

Bloom, L., & Lahey, M. (1978). *Language development and language disorders*. New York: Macmillan.

Bloom, L., Rocissano, L., & Hood, L. (1976). Adult-child discourse: Developmental interaction between information processing and linguistic knowledge. *Cognitive Psychology, 8*, 521–552.

Brinton, B., & Fujiki, M. (1984). Development of topic manipulation skills in discourse. *Journal of Speech and Hearing Research, 27*, 350–357.

Brown, R. (1973). *A first language: The early stages*. Cambridge, MA: Harvard University Press.

Burnett Heyes, S., Jih, Y.-R., Block, P., Hiu, C.-F., Holmes, E., & Lau, J. (2015). Relationship reciprocation modulates resource allocation in adolescent social networks: Developmental effects. *Child Development, 86*, 1489–1506.

Burnett, S., & Blakemore, S.-J. (2009). The development of adolescent social cognition. *Annals of the New York Academy of Sciences, 1167*, 51–56.

Chall, J. (1996). *Stages of reading development*. Fort Worth, TX: Harcourt Brace.

Crystal, D., & Davy, D. (1975). *Advanced conversational English*. London: Longman.

Doell, E. H., & Reed, V. A. (2007, July). *Teachers' question scaffolds: Potential contexts for language facilitation or elaborate guessing games?* Paper presented at the 5th Asia Pacific Conference on Speech, Language, and Hearing, Brisbane, Australia.

Dollaghan, C. (1987). Fast mapping in normal and language-impaired children. *Journal of Speech and Hearing Disorders, 52*, 218–222.

Dore, J. (1975). Holophrases, speech acts and language universals. *Journal of Child Language, 2*, 21–40.

Ehren, B. (2010). Reading comprehension and expository text structure: Direction for intervention with adolescents. In M. Nippold & C. Scott (Eds.), *Expository discourse in children, adolescents, and adults: Development and disorders* (pp. 215–240). New York: Psychology Press.

Fowles, B., & Glanz, M. (1977). Competence and talent in verbal riddle comprehension. *Journal of Child Language, 4*, 417–432.

Gardner, H. (1974). Metaphors and modalities: How children project polar adjectives into diverse domains. *Child Development, 45*, 84–91.

Gardner, H., Kircher, M., Winner, E., & Perkins, D. (1975). Children's metaphoric productions and preferences. *Journal of Child Language, 2*, 125–141.

Golinkoff, R., Mervis, C., & Hirsh-Pasek, K. (1994). Early object labels: The case for a developmental lexical principles framework. *Journal of Child Language, 21*, 125–155.

Halliday, M. (1974). A sociosemiotic perspective on language development. *Bulletin of the School of Oriental and African Studies, 37*, Part 1.

Halliday, M. (1975). *Learning how to mean: Explorations in the development of language*. London: Edward Arnold.

Hass, W., & Wepman, J. (1974). Dimensions of individual difference in the spoken syntax of school children. *Journal of Speech and Hearing Research, 17*, 455–469.

Hughes, D. L., McGillivray, L., & Schmidek, M. (1997). *Guide to narrative language: Procedures for assessment*. Eau Claire, WI: Thinking Publications.

Johnson, C. (1995). Expanding norms for narration. *Language, Speech and Hearing Services in Schools, 26*, 326–341.

Johnson, C., & Anglin, J. (1995). Qualitative developments in the content and form of children's definitions. *Journal of Speech and Hearing Research, 38*, 612–629.

Justice, L., & Ezell, H. (2002). Use of storybook reading to increase print awareness in at-risk children. *American Journal of Speech-Language Pathology, 11*, 17–29.

Justice, L., Weber, S., Ezell, H., & Bakeman, R. (2002). A sequential analysis of children's responsiveness to parental print references during shared book-reading interactions. *American Journal of Speech-Language Pathology, 11*, 30–40.

Keenan, E. (1975). Evolving discourse: The next step. *Papers and Reports on Child Language Development, 10*, 80–87.

Kessel, F. (1970). The role of syntax in children's comprehension from ages six to twelve. *Monographs of the Society for Research in Child Development, 35*, 1–95.

Lahey, M. (1988). *Language disorders and language development*. Columbus, OH: Macmillan.

Larson, V., & McKinley, N. (1998). Characteristics of adolescents' conversations: A longitudinal study. *Clinical Linguistics and Phonetics, 12*, 183–203.

Larson, V., & McKinley, N. (2003). *Communication solutions for older students*. Eau Claire, WI: Thinking Publications.

Lazar, R., Warr-Leeper, G., Nicholson, C., & Johnson, S. (1989). Elementary school teachers' use of multiple meaning expressions. *Language, Speech and Hearing Services in Schools, 20*, 420–430.

Limber, J. (1973). The genesis of complex sentences. In T. Moore (Ed.), *Cognitive development and the acquisition of language* (pp. 169–185). New York: Academic Press.

Loban, W. (1976). *Language development: Kindergarten through grade twelve*. Urbana, IL: National Council of Teachers of English.

Longacre, R. (1983). *The grammar of discourse*. New York: Plenum.

Markman, E. (1989). *Categorization and naming in children*. Cambridge, MA: MIT Press.

Markman, E., & Wachtel, G. (1988). Children's use of mutual exclusivity to constrain the meaning of words. *Cognitive Psychology, 20*, 121–157.

McLean, J., & Snyder-McLean, L. (1999). *How children learn language*. San Diego, CA: Singular.

McLeod, S., van Doorn, J., & Reed, V. A. (2001a). Consonant cluster development in two-year-olds: General trends and individual differences. *Journal of Speech, Language, and Hearing Research, 44*, 1144–1171.

McLeod, S., van Doorn, J., & Reed, V. A. (2001b). Normal acquisition of consonant clusters. *American Journal of Speech-Language Pathology, 10*, 99–110.

Menn, L., & Stoel-Gammon, C. (2008). Phonological development: Learning sounds and sound patterns. In J. Berko-Gleason (Ed.), *The development of language* (7th ed., pp. 58–103). Boston: Allyn & Bacon.

Menyuk, P. (1972). *Sentences children use*. Cambridge, MA: MIT Press.

Mervis, C., & Bertrand, J. (1994). Acquisition of the novel name-nameless category (N_3C) principle. *Child Development, 65*, 1646–1662.

Moran, M. (1975). *Verb inflections of normal and learning disabled children*. University of Kansas, Lawrence.

Nippold, M. (Ed.). (1988). *Later language development: Ages nine through nineteen*. Boston: Little Brown.

Nippold, M. (1991). Evaluating and enhancing idiom comprehension in language-disordered students. *Language, Speech and Hearing Services in Schools, 22*, 100–106.

Nippold, M. (1993). Developmental markers in adolescent language: Syntax, semantics, and pragmatics. *Language, Speech and Hearing Services in Schools, 24*, 21–28.

Nippold, M. (1994a). Persuasive talk in social contexts: Development, assessment, and intervention. *Topics in Language Disorders, 14*, 1–12.

Nippold, M. (1994b). Third-order verbal analogical reasoning: A developmental study of children and adolescents. *Contemporary Educational Psychology, 19*, 101–107.

Nippold, M. (1995). School-age children and adolescents: Norms for word definition. *Language, Speech and Hearing Services in Schools, 26*, 320–325.

Nippold, M. (1999). Word definition in adolescents as a function of reading proficiency: A research note. *Child Language Teaching and Therapy, 15*, 171–176.

Nippold, M. (2000). Language development during the adolescent years: Aspects of pragmatics, syntax, and semantics. *Topics in Language Disorders, 20*, 15–28.

Nippold, M. (2007). *Later language development: School-age children, adolescents, and young adults.* Austin, TX: PRO-ED.

Nippold, M., Allen, M., & Kirsch, D. (2001). Proverb comprehension as a function of reading proficiency in preadolescents. *Language, Speech and Hearing Services in Schools, 32*, 90–100.

Nippold, M., Cuyler, J., & Braunbeck-Price, R. (1988). Explanation of ambiguous advertisements: A developmental study with children and adolescents. *Journal of Speech and Hearing Research, 31*, 466–474.

Nippold, M., Hegel, S., Sohlberg, M., & Schwarz, I. (1999). Defining abstract entities: Development in pre-adolescents, adolescents, and young adults. *Journal of Speech, Language, and Hearing Research, 42*, 473–481.

Nippold, M., Hegel, S., Uhden, L., & Bustamante, S. (1998). Development of proverb comprehension in adolescents: Implications for instruction. *Journal of Children's Communication Development, 19*, 49–55.

Nippold, M., Hesketh, L., Duthie, J., & Mansfield, T. (2005). Conversational versus expository discourse: A study of syntactic development in children, adolescents, and adults. *Journal of Speech, Language, and Hearing Research, 48*, 1048–1064.

Nippold, M., Leonard, L., & Kail, R. (1984). Syntactic and conceptual factors in children's understanding of metaphors. *Journal of Speech and Hearing Research, 27*, 197–205.

Nippold, M., Mansfield, T., & Billow, J. (2007). Peer conflict explanations in children, adolescents, and adults: Examining the development of complex syntax. *American Journal of Speech-Language Pathology, 16*, 179–188.

Nippold, M., Mansfield, T., Billow, J., & Tomblin, J. B. (2008). Expository discourse in adolescents with language impairments: Examining syntactic development. *American Journal of Speech-Language Pathology, 17*, 356–366.

Nippold, M., Mansfield, T., Billow, J., & Tomblin, J. B. (2009). Syntactic development in adolescents with a history of language impairments: A follow-up investigation. *American Journal of Speech-Language Pathology, 18*, 241–251.

Nippold, M., & Martin, S. (1989). Idiom interpretation in isolation versus context: A developmental study with adolescents. *Journal of Speech and Hearing Research, 32*, 59–66.

Nippold, M., Moran, C., & Schwarz, I. (2001). Idiom understanding in preadolescents: Synergy in action. *American Journal of Speech-Language Pathology, 10*, 169–179.

Nippold, M., & Rudzinski, M. (1993). Familiarity and transparency in idiom explanation: A developmental study with children and adolescents. *Journal of Speech and Hearing Research, 36*, 728–737.

Nippold, M., Schwarz, I., & Undlin, R. (1992). Use and understanding of adverbial conjuncts: A developmental study of adolescents and young adults. *Journal of Speech and Hearing Research, 35*, 108–118.

Nippold, M., & Sun, L. (2008). Knowledge of morphologically complex words: A developmental study of older children and young adolescents. *Language, Speech and Hearing Services in Schools, 39*, 365–373.

Nippold, M., & Taylor, C. (1995). Idiom understanding in youth: Further examination of familiarity and transparency. *Journal of Speech and Hearing Research, 38*, 426–433.

Nippold, M., & Taylor, C. (2002). Judgments of idiom familiarity and transparency: A comparison of children and adolescents. *Journal of Speech, Language, and Hearing Research, 45*, 384–391.

Nippold, M., Taylor, C., & Baker, J. (1996). Idiom understanding in Australian youth: A cross-cultural comparison. *Journal of Speech and Hearing Research, 39*, 442–447.

Nippold, M., Uhden, L., & Schwarz, I. (1997). Proverb explanation through the lifespan: A developmental study of adolescents and adults. *Journal of Speech, Language, and Hearing Research, 40*, 245–253.

Pan, B., & Uccelli, P. (2008). Semantic development: Learning the meanings of words. In J. Berko-Gleason (Ed.), *The development of language* (7th ed., pp. 104–138). Boston: Allyn & Bacon.

Paul, R. (1981). Analyzing complex sentence development. In J. Miller (Ed.), *Assessing language production in children: Experimental procedures* (pp. 36–40). Baltimore: University Park Press.

Pine, J. (1999, July). *Tense optionality and children's use of verb morphology: Testing the optional infinitive hypothesis.* Paper presented at the International Association for the Study of Child Language, San Sebastian, Spain.

Pollio, M., & Pollio, H. (1979). A test of metaphoric comprehension and some preliminary developmental data. *Journal of Child Language, 6*, 111–120.

Poole, E. (1934). Genetic development of articulation of consonant sounds in speech. *Elementary English Review, 11*, 159–161.

Power, R., Taylor, C., & Nippold, M. (2001). Comprehending literally-true versus literally-false proverbs. *Child Language Teaching and Therapy, 17*, 1–18.

Prutting, C. (1979). Process: The action of moving forward progressively from one point to another on the way to completion. *Journal of Speech and Hearing Disorders, 44*, 3–30.

Reed, V. A. (1990, March). *Differences in the language skills of 8- and 14-year-old children.* Paper presented at the annual conference of the Australian Association of Speech and Hearing, Sydney, Australia.

Reed, V. A. (1991). What Crocodile Dundee never told us. *American Journal of Speech-Language Pathology, 1*, 11–12.

Reed, V. A., Griffith, F., & Rasmussen, A. (1998). Morphosyntactic structures in the spoken language of older children and adolescents. *Clinical Linguistics and Phonetics, 12*, 163–181.

Reed, V. A., McLeod, K., & McAllister, L. (1999). Importance of selected communication skills for talking with peers and teachers: Adolescents' opinions. *Language, Speech and Hearing Services in Schools, 30*, 32–49.

Rescorla, L., Alley, A., & Christine, J. (2001). Word frequencies in toddler's lexicons. *Journal of Speech, Language, and Hearing Research, 44*, 598–609.

Schober-Peterson, D., & Johnson, C. (1989). Conversational topics of 4-year-olds. *Journal of Speech and Hearing Research, 32*, 857–870.

Scott, C. M. (1984). Adverbial connectivity in conversations of children 6 to 12. *Journal of Child Language, 11*, 423–452.

Scott, C. M., & Rush, D. (1985). Teaching adverbial connectivity: Implications from current research. *Child Language Teaching and Therapy, 1*, 264–280.

Scott, C. M., & Stokes, S. (1995). Measures of syntax in school-age children and adolescents. *Language, Speech and Hearing Services in Schools, 26*, 309–319.

Shatz, M., & O'Reilly, A. (1990). Conversational or communicative skill? A reassessment of two-year-olds' behaviour in miscommunication episodes. *Journal of Child Language, 17*, 131–146.

Shultz, T., & Horibe, F. (1974). Development of the appreciation of verbal jokes. *Developmental Psychology, 10*, 13–20.

Shultz, T., & Pilon, R. (1973). Development of the ability to detect linguistic ambiguity. *Child Development, 44,* 728–733.

Skibbe, L., Justice, L., Zucker, R., & McGinty, A. (2008). Relation among maternal literacy belief's, home literacy practices, and the emergent literacy skills of preschoolers with specific language impairment. *Early Education and Development, 19,* 68–88.

Smit, A., Hand, L., Freilinger, J., Bernthal, J., & Bird, A. (1990). The Iowa articulation norms project and its Nebraska replication. *Journal of Speech and Hearing Disorders, 55,* 779–798.

Snow, C., Burns, M., & Griffin, P. (Eds.). (1998). *Preventing reading difficulties in young children.* Washington: National Academy Press.

Spector, C. (1990). Linguistic humor comprehension of normal and language-impaired adolescents. *Journal of Speech and Hearing Disorders, 55,* 533–541.

Spector, C. (1996). Children's comprehension of idioms in the context of humor. *Language, Speech and Hearing Services in Schools, 27,* 307–313.

Stein, N., & Glenn, C. (1979). An analysis of story comprehension in elementary school children. In R. Freedle (Ed.), *New directions in discourse processing* (Vol. 2, pp. 53–120). Norwood, NJ: Ablex.

Stenner, A., Burdick, H., Sanford, E., & Burdick, D. (2006). How accurate are lexile text measures? *Journal of Applied Measurement, 7,* 307–322.

Stenner, A., Burdick, H., Sanford, E., & Burdick, D. (2007). *The Lexile Framework for Reading Technical Report.* Durham, NC: MetaMetrics, Inc.

Sturm, J., & Nelson, N. (1997). Formal classroom lessons: New perspectives on a familiar discourse event. *Language, Speech and Hearing Services in Schools, 28,* 255–273.

Tager-Flusberg, H., & Zukowski, A. (2008). Putting words together: Morphology and syntax in the preschool years. In J. Berko-Gleason (Ed.), *The development of language* (7th ed., pp. 139–191). Boston: Allyn & Bacon.

Templin, M. (1957). *Certain language skills in children: Their development and interrelationships.* Minneapolis: University of Minnesota Press.

Ukrainetz, T. (2006). *Contextualized language intervention: Scaffolding PreK-12 literacy achievement.* Eau Claire, WI: Thinking Publications.

Van den Bos, W., Westenberg, M., van Dijk, E., & Crone, E. (2010). Development of trust and reciprocity in adolescence. *Cognitive Development, 25,* 90–102.

van Kleeck, A., Gillam, R., Hamilton, L., & McGrath, C. (1997). The relationship between middle-class parents' book-sharing discussion and their preschoolers' abstract language development. *Journal of Speech, Language, and Hearing Research, 40,* 1261–1271.

Warden, D. (1976). The influence of context on children's use of identifying expressions and references. *British Journal of Psychology, 67,* 101–112.

Wegner, J., & Rice, M. (1988, November). *The acquisition of verb-particle constructions: How do children figure them out?* Paper presented at the Annual Convention of the American Speech-Language-Hearing Association, Boston.

Wiig, E. (1982). *Identifying language disorders in adolescents.* Paper presented at the Gunderson Clinic, La Crosse, WI.

Wiig, E. (1989). *Steps to language competence: Developing metalinguistic strategies.* San Antonio, TX: The Psychological Corporation.

Wiig, E., Gilbert, M., & Christian, S. (1978). Developmental sequences in the perception and interpretation of lexical and syntactic ambiguities. *Perceptual and Motor Skills, 44,* 959–969.

Wiig, E., & Semel, E. (1984). *Language assessment and intervention for the learning disabled* (2nd ed.). New York: Merrill/Macmillan.

Winner, E., Rosenstiel, A., & Gardner, H. (1976). The development of metaphoric understanding. *Developmental Psychology, 12,* 289–297.

Chapter 3

Accardo, P., Capute, A., Bennett, A., Keshishian, E., O'Connor Leppert, M., Montgomery, T., & Whitman, B. (2005). *The Capute Scales: Cognitive Adaptive Test and Clinical Linguistic and Auditory Milestone Scale.* Baltimore: Paul H. Brookes.

Achenbach, T. (1991a). *Manual for the Child Behavior Checklist/4–18.* Burlington: University of Vermont Press.

Achenbach, T. (1991b). *Manual for the Teacher Report Form.* Burlington: University of Vermont Press.

Achenbach, T. (1992). *Manual for the Child Behavior Checklist/2–3 and 1992 Profile.* Burlington: University of Vermont, Department of Psychiatry.

American Psychiatric Association (APA). (2013). *Diagnostic and statistical manual of mental disorder* (5th ed.). Washington: Author.

Applebee, A. (1978). *The child's concept of story: Ages two to seventeen.* Chicago: University of Chicago Press.

Archibald, L., & Joanisse, M. (2009). On the sensitivity and specificity of nonword repetition and sentence recall to language and memory impairments. *Journal of Speech, Language, and Hearing Research, 52,* 899–914.

Ash, A., & Redmond, S. (2014, June). *An exploratory analysis of social (pragmatic) communication symptoms in young school age children.* Paper presented at the Symposium on Research on Child Language Disorders, Madison, WI.

Asher, S., & Gazelle, H. (1999). Loneliness, peer relations, and language disorder in childhood. *Topics in Language Disorders, 19,* 16–33.

Baker, L., & Cantwell, D. (1982). Psychiatric disorder in children with different types of communication disorders. *Journal of Communication Disorders, 15,* 113–126.

Baker, L., & Cantwell, D. (1983). Developmental and behavioral characteristics of speech and language disordered children. In S. Chess & T. Thomas (Eds.), *Annual progress in children development* (pp. 205–216). New York: Brunner-Mazel.

Baltaxe, C., & Simmons, J. (1988). Communication deficits in preschool children with psychiatric disorders. *Seminars in Speech and Language, 8,* 81–90.

Bayley, N. (2006). *Bayley Scales of Infant and Toddler Development (Bayley-III)* (3rd ed.). San Antonio, TX: Pearson.

Beitchman, J., Wilson, B., Brownlie, E., Walters, H., & Lancee, W. (1996). Long-term consistency in speech/language profiles: I. Developmental and academic outcomes. *Journal of the American Academy of Child and Adolescent Psychiatry, 35,* 804–814.

Beitchman, J., Wilson, B., Brownlie, E., Walters, H., Inglis, A., & Lancee, W. (1996). Long-term consistency in speech/language profiles: II. Behavioral, emotional, and social outcomes. *Journal of the American Academy of Child and Adolescent Psychiatry, 35,* 815–825.

Beitchman, J., Wilson, B., Johnson, C., Atkinson, L., Young, A., Adlaf, E., & Douglas, L. (2001). Fourteen-year follow up of speech/language-impaired and control children: Psychiatric outcome. *Journal of the American Academy of Child and Adolescent Psychiatry, 40,* 75–82.

Bishop, D. V. M. (1994). Grammatical errors in specific language impairment: Competence or performance limitations? *Applied Psycholinguistics, 15,* 507–550.

Bishop, D. V. M. (1997). *Uncommon understanding: Development and disorders of language comprehension in children.* East Sussex, UK: Psychology Press.

Bishop, D. V. M. (2000). Pragmatic language impairment: A correlate of SLI, a distinct subgroup, or part of the autistic continuum? In D. V. M. Bishop & L. Leonard (Eds.), *Speech and language impairment in children: Causes, characteristics, intervention and outcome.* East Sussex, UK: Psychology Press.

Bishop, D. V. M. (2006). What causes specific language impairment? *Current Directions in Psychological Science, 15,* 217–221.

Bishop, D. V. M., Adams, C., & Norbury, C. (2006). Distinct genetic influences on grammar and phonological short-term memory deficits: Evidence from 6-year-old twins. *Genes, Brain and Behavior, 5*, 158–169.

Bishop, D. V. M., & Edmundson, A. (1987). Language-impaired 4-year-olds: Distinguishing transient from persistent impairment. *Journal of Speech and Hearing Disorders, 52*, 156–173.

Bishop, D. V. M., Price, T., Dale, P., & Plomin, R. (2003). Outcomes of early language delay: II. Etiology of transient and persistent language difficulties. *Journal of Speech, Language, and Hearing Research, 46*, 561–575.

Black, B., & Hazen, N. (1990). Social status and patterns of communication in acquainted and unacquainted preschool children. *Developmental Psychology, 26*, 379–387.

Black, B., & Logan, A. (1995). Links between communication patterns in mother-child, father-child, and child-peer interactions and children's social status. *Child Development, 66*, 255–271.

Brinton, B., & Fujiki, M. (2014). Social and affective factors in children with language impairment: Implications for literacy learning. In C. A. Stone, E. Silliman, B. Ehren, & G. Wallach (Eds.), *Handbook of language and literacy: Development and disorders* (2nd ed., pp. 173–189). New York: The Guilford Press.

Brinton, B., Fujiki, M., & McKee, L. (1998). Negotiation skills of children with specific language impairment. *Journal of Speech, Language, and Hearing Research, 41*, 927–940.

Brownlie, E., Beitchman, J., Escobar, M., Young, A., Atkinson, L., Johnson, C., Douglas, L. (2004). Early language impairment and young adult delinquent and aggressive behavior. *Journal of Abnormal Child Psychology, 32*, 453–467.

Bunce, B. (1995). *Building a language-focused curriculum for the preschool classroom: A planning guide* (Vol. II). Baltimore: Paul H. Brookes.

Bzoch, K., League, R., & Brown, V. (2003). *Receptive-expressive emergent language test—3* (3rd ed.). Austin, TX: Pearson.

Cabell, S., Justice, L., Zucker, T., & McGinty, A. (2009). Emergent name-writing abilities of preschool-age children with language impairment. *Language, Speech and Hearing Services in Schools, 40*, 53–66.

Carrow, E. (1974). *Carrow Elicited Language Inventory*. Austin, TX: Learning Concepts.

Catts, H. (1997). The early identification of language-based reading disabilities. *Language, Speech and Hearing Services in Schools, 28*, 86–89.

Catts, H., Fey, M., Zhang, X., & Tomblin, J. B. (2002). A longitudinal investigation of reading outcomes in children with language impairments. *Journal of Speech, Language, and Hearing Research, 45*, 1142–1157.

Chiat, S., & Roy, P. (2007). The Preschool Repetition Test: An evaluation of performance in typically developing and clinically referred children. *Journal of Speech, Language, and Hearing Research, 50*, 429–443.

Chiat, S., & Roy, P. (2008). Early phonological and sociocognitive skills as predictors of later language and social communication outcomes. *Journal of Child Psychology and Psychiatry, 49*, 635–645.

Chiat, S., & Roy, P. (2013). Early predictors of language and social communication impairments at ages 9–11 years: A follow-up study of early-referred children. *Journal of Speech, Language, and Hearing Research, 56*, 1824–1836.

Choudhury, N., & Benasich, A. (2003). A family aggregation study: The influence of family history and other risk factors on language development. *Journal of Speech, Language, and Hearing Research, 46*, 261–272.

Cleave, P., & Fey, M. (1997). Two approaches to the facilitation of grammar in children with language impairments: Rationale and description. *American Journal of Speech-Language Pathology, 6*, 22–32.

Clegg, J., Hollis, C., Mawhood, L., & Rutter, M. (2005). Developmental language disorders – a follow-up in later adult life: Cognitive, language and psychosocial outcomes. *Journal of Child Psychology and Psychiatry, 46*, 128–149.

Coady, J., & Evans, J. (2008). Uses and interpretations of non-word repetition tasks in children with and without specific language impairments (SLI). *International Journal of Language and Communicative Disorders, 43*, 1–40.

Coggins, T. (1991). Bringing context back into assessment. *Topics in Language Disorders, 11*, 43–54.

Connell, P. (1986). Teaching subjecthood to language-disordered children. *Journal of Speech and Hearing Research, 29*, 481–492.

Connell, P., & Stone, C. (1992). Morpheme learning of children with specific language impairment under controlled instructional conditions. *Journal of Speech and Hearing Research, 35*, 844–852.

Conti-Ramsden, G. (1990). Maternal recasts and other contingent replies to language-impaired children. *Journal of Speech and Hearing Disorders, 55*, 262–274.

Conti-Ramsden, G. (2003). Processing and linguistic markers in young children with specific language impairment (SLI). *Journal of Speech, Language, and Hearing Research, 46*, 1029–1037.

Conti-Ramsden, G., & Botting, N. (1999). Classification of children with specific language impairment: Longitudinal considerations. *Journal of Speech, Language, and Hearing Research, 42*, 1195–1204.

Conti-Ramsden, G., Botting, N., & Faragher, B. (2001). Psycholinguistic markers for specific language impairment (SLI). *Journal of Child Psychology and Psychiatry, 42*, 741–748.

Conti-Ramsden, G., Botting, N., Simkin, Z., & Knox, E. (2001). Follow-up of children attending infant language units: Outcomes at 11 years of age. *International Journal of Language and Communication Disorders, 36*, 207–219.

Conti-Ramsden, G., Crutchley, A., & Botting, N. (1997). The extent to which psychometric tests differentiate subgroups of children with SLI. *Journal of Speech, Language, and Hearing Research, 40*, 765–777.

Conti-Ramsden, G., & Dykins, J. (1991). Mother-child interactions with language-impaired children and their siblings. *British Journal of Disorders of Communication, 26*, 337–354.

Conti-Ramsden, G., Falcaro, M., Simkin, Z., & Pickles, A. (2007). Familial loading in specific language impairment: Patterns of differences across proband characteristics, gender, and relative type. *Genes, Brain and Behavior, 6*, 216–228.

Conti-Ramsden, G., Hutcheson, G., & Grove, J. (1995). Contingency and breakdown: Children with SLI and their conversations with mothers and fathers. *Journal of Speech and Hearing Research, 38*, 1290–1302.

Coplan, J. (1993). *Early language milestone scale—2*. Austin, TX: PRO-ED.

Corriveau, K., Pasquini, E., & Goswami, U. (2007). Basic auditory processing skills and specific language impairment: A new look at an old hypothesis. *Journal of Speech, Language, and Hearing Research, 50*, 647–666.

Craig, H., & Gallagher, T. (1986). Interactive play: The frequency of related verbal responses. *Journal of Speech and Hearing Research, 29*, 375–383.

Dale, P., Price, T., Bishop, D. V. M., & Plomin, R. (2003). Outcomes of early language delay: I. Predicting persistent and transient language difficulties at 3 and 4 years. *Journal of Speech. Language, and Hearing Research, 46*, 544–560.

Dale, P., Simonoff, E., Bishop, D. V. M., Eley, T., Oliver, B., Price, T., & Plomin, R. (1998). Genetic influences on language delay in two-year-old children. *Nature Neuroscience, 1*, 324–328.

Deevy, P., Wisman Weil, L., Leonard, L., & Goffman, L. (2010). Extending use of the NRT to preschool-age children with and without specific language impairment. *Language, Speech, and Hearing Services in Schools, 41*, 277–288.

DeKroon, D., Kyte, C., & Johnson, C. (2002). Partner influences on the social pretend play of children with language impairments. *Language, Speech, and Hearing Services in Schools, 33*, 253–267.

Delgado, C., Mundy, P., Crowson, M., Markus, J., Yale, M., & Schwartz, H. (2002). Responding to joint attention and language development: A comparison of target locations. *Journal of Speech, Language, and Hearing Research, 45*, 715–719.

Dick, E., Wulfeck, B., Krupa-Kwiatkowski, M., & Bates, E. (2004). The development of complex sentence interpretation in typically developing children compared with children with specific language impairments or early unilateral focal lesions. *Developmental Science, 7*, 360–377.

Dockrell, J., & Messer, D. (2007). Language profiles and naming in children with word finding difficulties. *Folio Phonatrica et Logopaedica, 59*, 318–323.

Dollaghan, C., & Campbell, T. (1998). Nonword repetition and child language impairment. *Journal of Speech, Language, and Hearing Research, 41*, 1136–1146.

Dollaghan, C., & Campbell, T. (2009). How well do poor language scores at ages 3 and 4 predict poor language scores at age 6? *International Journal of Speech-Language Pathology, 11*, 358–365.

Dollaghan, C., Campbell, T., Paradise, J., Feldman, H., Janosky, J., Pitcairn, D., & Kurs-Lasky, M. (1999). Maternal education and measures of early speech and language. *Journal of Speech, Language, and Hearing Research, 42*, 1432–1443.

Donlan, C., Cowan, R., Newton, E., & Lloyd, D. (2007). The role of language in mathematical development: Evidence from children with specific language impairments. *Cognition, 103*, 23–33.

Eisenberg, S., Fersko, T., & Lundgren, C. (2001). The use of MLU for identifying language impairment in preschool children: A review. *American Journal of Speech-Language Pathology, 10*, 323–342.

Ellis Weismer, S. (1991). Hypothesis-testing abilities of language-impaired children. *Journal of Speech and Hearing Research, 34*, 1329–1338.

Ellis Weismer, S. (2007). Typical talkers, late talkers, and children with specific language impairment: A language endowment spectrum? In R. Paul (Ed.), *Language disorders from a developmental perspective* (pp. 83–101). Mahwah, NJ: Erlbaum.

Ellis Weismer, S., & Evans, J. (2002). The role of processing limitations in early identification of specific language impairment. *Topics in Language Disorders, 22*, 15–29.

Ellis Weismer, S., Evans, J., & Hesketh, L. (1999). An examination of verbal working memory capacity in children with specific language impairment. *Journal of Speech, Language, and Hearing Research, 42*, 1249–1260.

Ellis Weismer, S., Murray-Branch, J., & Miller, J. (1994). A prospective longitudinal study of language development in late talkers. *Journal of Speech and Hearing Research, 37*, 852–867.

Ellis Weismer, S., Plante, E., Jones, M., & Tomblin, J. B. (2005). A functional magnetic resonance imaging investigation of verbal working memory in adolescents with specific language impairment. *Journal of Speech, Language, and Hearing Research, 48*, 405–425.

Ellis Weismer, S., Tomblin, J. B., Zhang, X., Buckwalter, P., Chynoweth, J., & Jones, M. (2000). Nonword repetition performance in school-age children with and without language impairment. *Journal of Speech, Language, and Hearing Research, 43*, 865–878.

Evans, J., Viele, K., & Kass, R. (1997). Response latency and verbal complexity: Stochastic models of individual differences in children with specific language impairments. *Journal of Speech, Language, and Hearing Research, 40*, 754–764.

Felsenfeld, S., & Plomin, R. (1997). Epidemiological and offspring analyses of developmental speech disorders using data from the Colorado Adoption Project. *Journal of Speech and Hearing Research, 40*, 778–791.

Fenson, L., Dale, P., Reznick, J., Hartung, J., & Burgess, S. (1990). *Norms for the MacAurthur Communicative Development Inventories*. Paper presented at the International Conference on Infant Studies, Montreal.

Fenson, L., Marchman, V., Thal, D., Dale, P., Reznick, J., & Bates, E. (2007). *MacArthur-Bates communicative development inventories (CDIs)* (2nd ed.). Baltimore: Paul H. Brookes.

Fey, M. (1986). *Language intervention with young children*. San Diego, CA: College-Hill Press.

Fey, M., Cleave, P., Long, S., & Hughes, D. (1993). Two approaches to the facilitation of grammar in language-impaired children: An experimental evaluation. *Journal of Speech and Hearing Research, 36*, 141–157.

Fey, M., Krulik, T., Loeb, D., & Proctor-Williams, K. (1999). Sentence recast use by parents of children with typical language and specific language impairment. *American Journal of Speech-Language Pathology, 8*, 273–286.

Flax, J., Realpe-Bonilla, T., Hirsch, L., Brzustowicz, L., Bartlett, C., & Tallal, P. (2003). Specific language impairment in families: Evidence for co-occurrence with reading impairments. *Journal of Speech, Language, and Hearing Research, 46*, 530–543.

Friedrich, M., & Friederici, A. (2006). Early N400 development and later language acquisition. *Psychophysiology, 43*, 1–12.

Fujiki, M., Brinton, B., & Clarke, D. (2002). Emotion regulation in children with specific language impairment. *Language, Speech and Hearing Services in Schools, 33*, 102–111.

Fujiki, M., Brinton, B., Hart, C. H., & Fitzgerald, A. (1999). Peer acceptance and friendship in children with specific language impairment. *Topics in Language Disorders, 19*, 34–48.

Gathercole, S., Hitch, G., Service, E., & Martin, A. (1997). Phonological short-term memory and new word learning in children. *Developmental Psychology, 33*, 966–979.

Gathercole, S., Willis, C., Baddeley, A., & Emslie, H. (1994). The Children's Test of Nonword Repetition: A test of phonological working memory. *Memory, 2*, 103–127.

German, D. (1979). Word-finding skills in children with learning disabilities. *Journal of Learning Disabilities, 12*, 176–181.

German, D. (2000). *Test of word finding—2*. Austin, TX: PRO-ED.

Gertner, B., Rice, M., & Hadley, P. (1994). Influence of communicative competence on peer preferences in a preschool classroom. *Journal of Speech and Hearing Research, 37*, 913–923.

Girolametto, L. (1997). Development of a parent report measure for profiling the conversational skills of preschool children. *American Journal of Speech-Language Pathology, 6*, 25–33.

Girolametto, L., Pearce, P., & Weitzman, E. (1996). Interactive focused stimulation for toddlers with expressive vocabulary delays. *Journal of Speech and Hearing Research, 39*, 1274–1283.

Girolametto, L., & Weitzman, E. (2002). Responsiveness of child care providers in interactions with toddlers and preschoolers. *Language, Speech and Hearing Services in Schools, 33*, 268–281.

Girolametto, L., Weitzman, E., & Greenberg, J. (2000). *Teacher interaction and language rating scale*. Toronto, Canada: The Hanen Centre.

Girolametto, L., Weitzman, E., van Lieshout, R., & Duff, D. (2000). Directiveness in teachers' language input to toddlers and preschoolers in day care. *Journal of Speech, Language, and Hearing Research, 43*, 1101–1114.

Girolametto, L., Weitzman, E., Wiigs, M., & Pearce, P. (1999). The relationship between maternal language measures and language development in toddlers with expressive vocabulary delays. *American Journal of Speech-Language Pathology, 8*, 364–374.

Girolametto, L., Wiigs, M., Smyth, R., Weitzman, E., & Pearce, P. (2001). Children with a history of expressive vocabulary delay: Outcomes at 5 years of age. *American Journal of Speech-Language Pathology, 10*, 358–369.

Gladfelter, A., & Leonard, L. (2013). Alternative tense and agreement morpheme measures for assessing grammatical deficits during the preschool period. *Journal of Speech, Language, and Hearing Research, 56*, 542–552.

Goodyer, I. (2000). Language difficulties and psychopathology. In D. V. M. Bishop & L. Leonard (Eds.), *Speech and language impairment in children: Causes, characteristics, intervention and outcome* (pp. 227–244). East Sussex, UK: Psychology Press.

Gopnik, M. (1990). Feature-blind grammar and dysphasia. *Nature, 344*, 715.

Graf Estes, K., Evans, J., & Else-Quest, N. (2007). Differences in the nonword repetition performance of children with and without specific language impairment: A meta-analysis. *Journal of Speech, Language, and Hearing Research, 50*, 177–195.

Gray, S. (2003a). Diagnostic accuracy and test-retest reliability of nonword repetition and digit span tasks administered to preschool children with specific language impairment. *Journal of Communication Disorders, 36*, 129–151.

Gray, S. (2003b). Word-learning by preschoolers with specific language impairment: What predicts success? *Journal of Speech, Language, and Hearing Research, 46*, 56–67.

Gray, S. (2005). Word learning by preschoolers with specific language impairment: Effect of phonological or semantic cues. *Journal of Speech, Language, and Hearing Research, 48*, 1452–1467.

Gualtieri, C., Koriath, U., Van Bourgondien, M., & Saleeby, N. (1983). Language disorders in children referred for psychiatric services. *Journal of the American Academy of Child Psychiatry, 22*, 165–171.

Hadley, P. (1999). Validating a rate-based measure of early grammatical abilities: Unique syntactic types. *American Journal of Speech-Language Pathology, 8*, 261–272.

Hadley, P., & Rice, M. (1991). Conversational responsiveness of speech- and language-impaired preschoolers. *Journal of Speech and Hearing Research, 34*, 1308–1317.

Hadley, P., & Rice, M. (1996). Emergent uses of BE and DO: Evidence from children with specific language impairment. *Language Acquisition, 5*, 209–243.

Hadley, P., Rispoli, M., & Hsu, N. (2016). Toddlers' verb lexicon diversity and grammatical outcomes. *Language, Speech, and Hearing Services in Schools, 47*, 44–58.

Hadley, P., & Schuele, C. M. (1998). Facilitating peer interaction: Socially relevant objectives for preschool language intervention. *American Journal of Speech-Language Pathology, 7*, 25–36.

Hadley, P., & Short, H. (2005). The onset of tense marking in children at risk for specific language impairment. *Journal of Speech, Language, and Hearing Research, 48*, 1344–1362.

Hart, B., & Risley, T. (1995). *Meaningful differences in the everyday experience of young American children*. Baltimore: Paul H. Brookes.

Hazen, N., & Black, B. (1989). Preschool peer communication skills: The role of social status and interaction context. *Child Development, 60*, 867–876.

Hedrick, D., Prather, E., Tobin, A., Allen, D., Bliss, L., & Rosenberg, L. (1984). *Sequenced inventory of communication development—revised*. Los Angeles: Western Psychological Services.

Hresko, W., Reid, D. K., & Hammill, D. (1999). *Test of early language development—3* (3rd ed.). San Antonio, TX: Pearson.

Ingram, D. (1989). *First language acquisition: Method, description, and explanation*. Cambridge, UK: Cambridge University Press.

Jerome, A., Fujiki, M., Brinton, B., & James, S. (2002). Self-esteem in children with specific language impairment. *Journal of Speech, Language, and Hearing Research, 45*, 700–714.

Johnson, C., Beitchman, J., Young, A., Escobar, M., Atkinson, L., Wilson, B., & Wang, M. (1999). Fourteen-year follow up of children with and without speech/language impairments: Speech/language stability and outcomes. *Journal of Speech, Language, and Hearing Research, 42*, 744–760.

Johnston, J. (1994). Cognitive abilities of children with language impairment. In R. Watkins & M. Rice (Eds.), *Specific language impairments in children* (pp. 107–121). Baltimore: Paul H. Brookes.

Kail, R., Hale, C., Leonard, L., & Nippold, M. (1984). Lexical storage and retrieval in language-impaired children. *Applied Psycholinguistics, 5*, 37–49.

Kelly, D. (1998). A clinical synthesis of the "late talker" literature: Implications for service delivery. *Language, Speech, and Hearing Services in Schools, 29*, 76–84.

Klee, T., Carson, D., Gavin, W., Hall, L., Kent, A., & Reece, S. (1998). Concurrent and predictive validity of an early language screening program. *Journal of Speech, Language, and Hearing Research, 41*, 627–641.

Lahey, M. (1988). *Language disorders and language development*. Columbus, OH: Macmillan.

Lahey, M. (1990). Who shall be called language disordered? Some reflections and one perspective. *Journal of Speech and Hearing Disorders, 55*, 612–620.

Law, J., Rush, R., Schoon, I., & Parsons, S. (2009). Modeling developmental language difficulties from school entry into early adulthood: Literacy, mental health, and employment outcomes. *Journal of Speech, Language, and Hearing Research, 52*, 1401–1416.

Law, J., Tomblin, J. B., & Zhang, X. (2008). Characterizing the growth trajectories of language impaired children between 7 and 11 years of age. *Journal of Speech, Language, and Hearing Research, 51*, 739–750.

Lee, L. L. (1971). *Northwestern Syntax Screening Test*. Evanston, IL: Northwestern University Press.

Leonard, L. (1987). Is specific language impairment a useful construct? In S. Rosenberg (Ed.), *Advances in applied psycholinguistics: Disorders of first-language development (Volume 1)* (pp. 1–39). New York: Cambridge University Press.

Leonard, L. (1991). Specific language impairment as a clinical category. *Language, Speech, and Hearing Services in Schools, 22*, 66–68.

Leonard, L. (1998). *Children with specific language impairment*. Cambridge, MA: MIT Press.

Leonard, L. (2009). Is expressive language disorder an accurate diagnostic category? *American Journal of Speech-Language Pathology, 18*, 115–123.

Leonard, L. (2014). *Children with specific language impairment* (2nd ed.). Cambridge, MA: MIT Press.

Leonard, L., Bortolini, U., Caselli, M., McGregor, K., & Sabbadini, L. (1992). Morphological deficits in children with specific language impairment: The status of features in the underlying grammar. *Language Acquisition: A Journal of Developmental Linguistics, 2*, 151–179.

Leonard, L., Deevy, P., Miller, C., Rauf, L., Charest, M., & Kurtz, R. (2003). Surface forms and grammatical functions: Past tense and passive participle use by children with specific language impairment. *Journal of Speech, Language, and Hearing Research, 46*, 43–55.

Leonard, L., Eyer, J., Bedore, L., & Grela, B. (1997). Three accounts of the grammatical morpheme difficulties of English-speaking children with specific language impairment. *Journal of Speech, Language, and Hearing Research, 40*, 741–753.

Leonard, L., McGregor, K., & Allen, G. (1992). Grammatical morphology and speech perception in children with specific language impairment. *Journal of Speech and Hearing Research, 35*, 1076–1085.

Leonard, L., Miller, C., Deevy, P., Rauf, L., Gerber, E., & Charest, M. (2002). Production operations and the use of nonfinite verbs by children with specific language impairment. *Journal of Speech, Language, and Hearing Research, 45*, 744–758.

Leonard, L., Miller, C., & Finneran, D. (2009). Grammatical morpheme effects on sentence processing by school-aged adolescents with specific language impairment. *Language and Cognitive Processes, 24*, 450–478.

Leonard, L., Miller, C., & Gerber, E. (1999). Grammatical morphology and the lexicon in children with specific language impairment. *Journal of Speech, Language, and Hearing Research, 42*, 678–689.

Leonard, L., Nippold, M., Kail, R., & Hale, C. (1983). Picture naming in language-impaired children. *Journal of Speech and Hearing Research, 26*, 609–615.

Leonard, L., Schwartz, R., Chapman, K., Rowan, L., Prelock, P., Terrell, B., . . . Messick, C. (1982). Early lexical acquisition in children with specific language impairment. *Journal of Speech and Hearing Research, 25*, 554–564.

Loeb, D., & Leonard, L. (1991). Subject case marking and verb morphology in normally developing and specifically language-impaired children. *Journal of Speech and Hearing Research, 34*, 340–346.

Long, S., Olswang, L., Brian, J., & Dale, P. (1997). Productivity of emerging word combinations in toddlers with specific expressive language impairment. *American Journal of Speech-Language Pathology, 6*, 34–47.

Mack, A., & Warr-Leeper, G. (1992). Language abilities in boys with chronic behavior disorders. *Language, Speech, and Hearing Services in Schools, 23*, 214–223.

MacLachlan, B., & Chapman, R. (1988). Communication breakdowns in normal and language learning-disabled children's conversation and narration. *Journal of Speech and Hearing Disorders, 53*, 2–7.

Marchman, V., Wulfeck, B., & Ellis Weismer, S. (1999). Morphological productivity in children with normal language and SLI: A study of the English past tense. *Journal of Speech, Language, and Hearing Research, 42*, 206–219.

Marvin, C., & Privratsky, A. (1999). After-school talk: The effects of materials sent home from preschool. *American Journal of Speech-Language Pathology, 8*, 231–240.

Masterson, J. (1997). Interrelationships in children's language production. *Topics in Language Disorders, 17*, 11–22.

McArthur, G., Atkinson, C., & Ellis, D. (2009). Atypical brain responses to sounds in children with specific language and reading impairments. *Developmental Science, 12*, 768–783.

McArthur, G., & Bishop, D. V. M. (2005). Speech and non-speech processing in people with specific language impairment: A behavioural and electrophysiological study. *Brain and Language, 94*, 260–273.

McGregor, K. (1997). The nature of word-finding errors of preschoolers with and without word-finding deficits. *Journal of Speech, Language, and Hearing Research, 40*, 1232–1244.

McGregor, K., Friedman, R., Reilly, R., & Newman, R. (2002). Semantic representation and naming in young children. *Journal of Speech, Language, and Hearing Research, 45*, 332–346.

McGregor, K., Newman, R., Reilly, R., & Capone, N. (2002). Semantic representation and naming in children with specific language impairment. *Journal of Speech, Language, and Hearing Research, 45*, 998–1014.

McGregor, K., Oleson, J., Bahnsen, A., & Duff, D. (2013). Children with developmental language impairment have vocabulary deficits characterized by limited breadth and depth. *International Journal of Language and Communication Disorders, 48*, 307–319.

Menyuk, P. (1964). Comparison of grammar of children with functionally deviant and normal speech. *Journal of Speech and Hearing Research, 7*, 109–121.

Merzenich, M., Jenkins, W., Johnston, P., Schreiner, C., Miller, S., & Tallal, P. (1996). Temporal processing deficits of language-learning impaired children ameliorated by training. *Science, 271*, 77–81.

Messer, D., & Dockrell, J. (2006). Children's naming and word-finding difficulties: Descriptions and explanations. *Journal of Speech, Language, and Hearing Research, 49*, 309–324.

Miller, C., Kail, R., Leonard, L., & Tomblin, J. B. (2001). Speed of processing in children with specific language impairment. *Journal of Speech, Language, and Hearing Research, 44*, 416–433.

Miller, C., & Leonard, L. (1998). Deficits in finite verb morphology: Some assumptions in recent accounts of specific language impairment. *Journal of Speech, Language, and Hearing Research, 41*, 701–707.

Miller, C., Leonard, L., & Finneran, D. (2008). Grammaticality judgments in adolescents with and without language impairment. *International Journal of Language and Communication Disorders, 43*, 346–360.

Montgomery, J. (2005). Effects of input rate and age on the real-time language processing of children with specific language impairment. *International Journal of Language and Communication Disorders, 1*, 177–188.

Montgomery, J., & Leonard, L. (1998). Real-time inflectional processing by children with specific language impairment: Effects of phonetic substance. *Journal of Speech, Language, and Hearing Research, 41*, 1432–1443.

Montgomery, J., & Windsor, J. (2007). Examining the language performances of children with and without specific language impairment: Contributions of phonological short-term memory and speed of processing. *Journal of Speech, Language, and Hearing Research, 50*, 778–797.

Moore, D. R. (2011). The diagnosis and management of auditory processing disorder. *Language, Speech, and Hearing Services in Schools, 42*, 303–308.

Nelson, K., Welsh, J., Camarata, S., Butkovsky, L., & Camarata, M. (1995). Available input for language-impaired children and younger children of matched language levels. *First Language, 15*, 1–17.

Newbury, D., & Monaco, A. (2010). Genetic advances in the study of speech and language disorders. *Neuron, 68*, 309–320.

Nippold, M., Mansfield, T., Billow, J., & Tomblin, J. B. (2009). Syntactic development in adolescents with a history of language impairments: A follow-up investigation. *American Journal of Speech-Language Pathology, 18*, 241–251.

Nippold, M., & Schwarz, I. (1996). Children with slow expressive language development: What is the forecast for school achievement? *American Journal of Speech-Language Pathology, 5*, 22–25.

Oetting, J., & Horohov, J. (1997). Past-tense marking by children with and without specific language impairment. *Journal of Speech, Language, and Hearing Research, 40*, 62–74.

Oller, D. K., Eilers, R. E., Neal, A. R., & Schwartz, H. K. (1999). Precursors to speech in infancy: the prediction of speech and language disorders. *Journal of Communication Disorders, 32*, 223–245.

Olswang, L., & Bain, B. (1991). Intervention issues for toddlers with specific language impairments. *Topics in Language Disorders, 11*, 69–86.

Olswang, L., & Bain, B. (1996). Assessment information for predicting upcoming change in language production. *Journal of Speech and Hearing Research, 39*, 414–423.

Olswang, L., Rodriguez, B., & Timler, G. (1998). Recommending intervention for toddlers with specific language learning difficulties: We may not have all the answers, but we know a lot. *American Journal of Speech-Language Pathology, 7*, 23–32.

Paul, R. (1991). Profiles of toddlers with slow expressive language development. *Topics in Language Disorders, 11*, 1–13.

Paul, R. (1993). Outcomes of early expressive language delay. *Journal of Childhood Communication Disorders, 15*, 7–14.

Paul, R. (1996). Clinical implications of the natural history of slow expressive language development. *American Journal of Speech-Language Pathology, 5*, 5–21.

Paul, R. (1997). Understanding language delay: A response to van Kleeck, Gillam, and Davis. *American Journal of Speech-Language Pathology, 6*, 40–49.

Paul, R. (2000). Predicting outcomes of early expressive language delay: Ethical implications. In D. V. M. Bishop & L. Leonard (Eds.), *Speech and language impairments in children: Causes, characteristics, intervention and outcomes* (pp. 195–209). East Sussex, UK: Psychology Press.

Paul, R., Hernandez, R., Taylor, L., & Johnson, K. (1996). Narrative development in late talkers: Early school age. *Journal of Speech and Hearing Research, 39*, 1295–1303.

Paul, R., Looney, S., & Dahm, P. (1991). Communication and socialization skills at ages 2 and 3 in "late-talking" young children. *Journal of Speech and Hearing Research, 34*, 858–865.

Paul, R., Murray, C., Clancy, K., & Andrews, D. (1997). Reading and metaphonological outcomes in late talkers. *Journal of Speech, Language, and Hearing Research, 40*, 1037–1047.

Paul, R., & Smith, R. (1993). Narrative skills in 4-year-olds with normal, impaired, and late-developing language. *Journal of Speech and Hearing Research, 36*, 592–598.

Pawłowska, M. (2014). Evaluation of three proposed markers for language impairment in English: A meta-analysis of diagnostic accuracy studies. *Journal of Speech, Language, and Hearing Research, 57*, 2261–2273.

Plante, E., Shenkman, K., & Clark, M. (1996). Classification of adults for family studies of developmental language disorders. *Journal of Speech and Hearing Research, 39*, 661–667.

Platt, J., & Coggins, T. (1990). Comprehension of social-action games in prelinguistic children: Levels of participation and effects of adult structure. *Journal of Speech and Hearing Disorders, 55*, 315–326.

Plomin, R., & Dale, P. (2000). Genetics and early language development: A UK study of twins. In D. V. M. Bishop & L. Leonard (Eds.), *Speech and language impairments in children: Causes, characteristics, intervention and outcomes* (pp. 35–51). East Sussex, UK: Psychology Press.

Plomin, R., DeFries, J., McClearn, G., & McGuffin, P. (2001). *Behavioral genetics* (4th ed.). New York: Worth.

Popescu, M., Fey, M., Lewine, J., Finestack, L., & Popescu, E.-A. (2009). N400 responses of children with primary language disorders: Intervention effects. *Neuroreport, 20*, 1104–1108.

Prizant, B., Audet, L., Burke, G., Hummel, L., Maher, S., & Theadore, G. (1990). Communication disorders and emotional and behavioral disorders in children and adolescents. *Journal of Speech and Hearing Disorders, 55*, 179–192.

Redmond, S. (2016a). Language impairment in the attention-deficit/hyperactivity disorder context. *Journal of Speech, Language, and Hearing Research, 59*, 133–142.

Redmond, S. (2016b). Markers, models, and measurement error: Exploring the links between attention deficits and language impairments. *Journal of Speech, Language, and Hearing Research, 59*, 62–71.

Redmond, S., & Rice, M. (1998). The socioemotional behaviors of children with SLI: Social adaptation or social deviance? *Journal of Speech, Language, and Hearing Research, 41*, 688–700.

Redmond, S., & Rice, M. (2001). Detection of irregular verb violations by children with and without SLI. *Journal of Speech, Language, and Hearing Research, 44*, 655–669.

Redmond, S., Thompson, H., & Goldstein, S. (2011). Psycholinguistic profiling differentiates specific language impairment from typical development and from attention-deficit/hyperactivity disorder. *Journal of Speech, Language, and Hearing Research, 54*, 99–117.

Redmond, S., & Timler, G. (2007). Addressing the social concomitants of developmental language impairments. In A. Kamhi, J. Masterson, & K. Apel (Eds.), *Clinical decision making in developmental language disorders* (pp. 185–202). Baltimore: Paul H. Brookes.

Reed, V. A. (1992). Associations between phonology and other language components in children's communicative performance. *Australian Journal of Human Communication Disorders, 20*, 75–87.

Reed, V. A., Conrad, T., & Patchell, F. (2006, June). *Verb morphological patterns of 16-year-old adolescents with and without specific language impairment.* Paper presented at the 11th Symposium of the International Clinical Phonetics and Linguistics Association, Dubrovnik, Croatia.

Reed, V. A., & Patchell, F. (2010, April). *Discerning differences in the verb morphology of adolescents with specific language impairment.* Paper presented at the Annual Conference of the New Zealand Speech-Language Therapy Association, Wellington, New Zealand.

Reed, V. A., Patchell, F., & Conrad, T. (2006, November). *Verb morphology of younger and older adolescents with SLI.* Paper presented at the Annual Convention of the American Speech-Language-Hearing Association, Miami.

Rescorla, L. (1989). The language development survey: A screening tool for delayed language in toddlers. *Journal of Speech and Hearing Disorders, 54*, 587–599.

Rescorla, L. (1991). Identifying expressive language delay at age two. *Topics in Language Disorders, 11*, 14–20.

Rescorla, L. (1993). *Outcome of toddlers with specific expressive delay at ages 3, 4, 5, 6, 7, & 8.* Paper presented at the Biennial Meeting of the Society for Research in Child Development, New Orleans, LA.

Rescorla, L. (2002). Language and reading outcomes to age 9 in late-talking toddlers. *Journal of Speech, Language, and Hearing Research, 45*, 360–371.

Rescorla, L., & Achenbach, T. (2002). Use of the Language Development Survey (LDS) in a national probability sample of children 18 to 35 months old. *Journal of Speech, Language, and Hearing Research, 45*, 733–743.

Rescorla, L., Alley, A., & Christine, J. (2001). Word frequencies in toddlers' lexicons. *Journal of Speech, Language, and Hearing Research, 44*, 598–609.

Rescorla, L., Dahlsgaard, K., & Roberts, J. (2000). Late-talking toddlers: MLU and IPSyn outcomes at 3;0 and 4;0. *Journal of Child Language, 27*, 643–664.

Rescorla, L., & Goossens, M. (1992). Symbolic play development in toddlers with expressive specific language impairment. *Journal of Speech and Hearing Research, 35*, 1290–1302.

Rescorla, L., Hadicke-Wiley, M., & Escarce, E. (1993). Epidemiological investigation of expressive language delay at age two. *First Language, 13*, 5–22.

Rescorla, L., & Lee, E. (2001). Language impairment in young children. In T. Layton, E. Crais, & L. Watson (Eds.), *Handbook of early language impairment in children: Nature* (pp. 11–55). Albany, NY: Delmar.

Rescorla, L., Ross, G., & McClure, S. (2007). Language delay and behavioral/emotional problems in toddlers: Findings from two developmental clinics. *Journal of Speech, Language, and Hearing Research, 50*, 1063–1078.

Rice, M. (2000). Grammatical symptoms of specific language impairment. In D. V. M. Bishop & L. Leonard (Eds.), *Speech and language impairment in children: Causes, characteristics, intervention and outcome* (pp. 17–34). East Sussex, UK: Psychology Press.

Rice, M. (2012). Toward epigenetic and gene regulation models of specific language impairment: Looking for links among growth, genes, and impairments. *Journal of Neurodevelopmental Disorders, 4*. doi: 10.1186/1866-1955-4-27.

Rice, M. (2013). Language growth and genetics of specific language impairment. *International Journal of Speech-Language Pathology, 15*, 223–233.

Rice, M., Hoffman, L., & Wexler, K. (2009). Judgments of omitted BE and DO in questions as extended finiteness clinical markers of specific language impairment (SLI) to 15 years: A study of growth and asymptote. *Journal of Speech, Language, and Hearing Research, 52*, 1417–1433.

Rice, M., Sell, M., & Hadley, P. (1990). The social interactive coding system (SICS): An on-line, clinically relevant descriptive tool. *Language, Speech, and Hearing Services in Schools, 21*, 2–14.

Rice, M., Sell, M., & Hadley, P. (1991). Social interactions of speech- and language-impaired children. *Journal of Speech and Hearing Research, 34*, 1299–1307.

Rice, M., Smith, S., & Gayán, J. (2009). Convergent genetic linkage and associations to language, speech and reading measures in families of probands with specific language impairment. *Journal of Neurodevelopmental Disorders, 1*, 264–282.

Rice, M., Spitz, R., & O'Brien, M. (1999). Semantic and morphosyntactic language outcomes in biologically at-risk children. *Journal of Neurolinguistics, 12*, 213–234.

Rice, M., & Wexler, K. (1996). Toward tense as a clinical marker of specific language impairment in English-speaking children. *Journal of Speech and Hearing Research, 39*, 1239–1257.

Rice, M., Wexler, K., & Cleave, P. (1995). Specific language impairment as a period of extended optional infinitive. *Journal of Speech and Hearing Research, 38*, 850–863.

Rice, M., Wexler, K., & Hershberger, S. (1998). Tense over time: The longitudinal course of tense acquisition in children with specific language impairment. *Journal of Speech, Language, and Hearing Research, 41*, 1412–1431.

Rice, M., Wexler, K., Marquis, J., & Hershberger, S. (2000). Acquisition of irregular past tense by children with specific language impairment. *Journal of Speech, Language, and Hearing Research, 43*, 1126–1145.

Rice, M., & Wilcox, K. (Eds.). (1995). *Building a language-focused curriculum for the preschool classroom: A foundation for lifelong communication* (Vol. I). Baltimore: Paul H. Brookes.

Riches, N. (2012). Sentence repetition in children with specific language impairment: An investigation of underlying mechanisms. *International Journal of Language and Communication Disorders, 47*, 499–510.

Riches, N. (2016). Complex sentence profiles in children with specific language impairment: Are they really atypical? *Journal of Child Language*, 1–28. doi: 10.1017/S0305000915000847

Rispoli, M., & Hadley, P. (2011). Toward a theory of gradual morphosyntactic learning. In I. Arnon & E. Clark (Eds.), *Experience, variation, and generalization: Learning a first language* (pp. 15–34). Amsterdam, the Netherlands: Benjamins.

Roberts, J., Rabinowitch, S., Bryant, D., Burchinal, M., Koch, M., & Ramey, C. (1989). Language skills of children with different preschool experiences. *Journal of Speech and Hearing Research, 32*, 773–786.

Robertson, S., & Ellis Weismer, S. (1997). The influence of peer models on the play scripts of children with specific language impairment. *Journal of Speech, Language, and Hearing Research, 40*, 49–61.

Robertson, S., & Ellis Weismer, S. (1999). Effects of treatment on linguistic and social skills in toddlers with delayed language development. *Journal of Speech, Language, and Hearing Research, 42*, 1234–1248.

Rossetti, L. (2006). *The Rossetti infant-toddler language scale*. East Moline, IL: LinguiSystems.

Roth, F. (1987). Temporal characteristics of maternal verbal styles. In K. Nelson & A. van Kleeck (Eds.), *Children's language* (Vol. 6). Hillsdale, NJ: Erlbaum.

Roy, P., & Chiat, S. (2004). A prosodically controlled word and nonword repetition task for 2- to 4-year olds: Evidence from typically developing children. *Journal of Speech, Language, and Hearing Research, 47*, 223–234.

Rutter, M. (2008). Diagnostic concepts and risk processes. In C. Norbury, J. B. Tomblin & D. V. M. Bishop (Eds.), *Understanding developmental language disorders: From theory to practice* (pp. 205–215). New York: Psychology Press.

Scarborough, H. (1990). Index of productive syntax (IPSyn). *Applied Psycholinguistics, 11*, 1–22.

Scarborough, H., & Dobrich, W. (1990). Development of children with early language delay. *Journal of Speech and Hearing Research, 33*, 70–83.

Schwartz, R., & Leonard, L. (1982). Do children pick and choose? An examination of phonological selection and avoidance in early lexical acquisition. *Journal of Child Language, 9*, 319–336.

Sheng, L., & McGregor, K. (2010a). Lexical-semantic organization in children with specific language impairment. *Journal of Speech, Language, and Hearing Research, 53*, 146–159.

Sheng, L., & McGregor, K. (2010b). Object and action naming in children with specific language impairment. *Journal of Speech, Language, and Hearing Research, 53*, 1704–1719.

Shriberg, L., Gruber, F., & Kwiatkowski, J. (1994). Developmental phonological disorders III: Long-term speech-sound normalization. *Journal of Speech and Hearing Research, 37*, 1151–1177.

Shriberg, L., & Kwiatkowski, J. (1988). A follow-up study of children with phonologic disorders of unknown origin. *Journal of Speech and Hearing Disorders, 53*, 144–155.

Shriberg, L., & Kwiatkowski, J. (1994). Developmental phonological disorders I: A clinical profile. *Journal of Speech and Hearing Research, 37*, 1100–1126.

Shriberg, L., Lohmeier, H., Campbell, T., Dollaghan, C., Green, J., & Moore, C. (2009). A nonword repetition task for speakers with misarticulations: The syllable repetition task (SRT). *Journal of Speech, Language, and Hearing Research, 52*, 1189–1212.

Shriberg, L., Tomblin, J. B., & McSweeny, J. (1999). Prevalence of speech delay in 6-year-old children and comorbidity with language impairment. *Journal of Speech, Language, and Hearing Research, 42*, 1461–1481.

Silliman, E., & Wilkinson, L. (2014). Policy and practice issues for students at risk in language and literacy learning: Back to the future. In C. A. Stone, E. Silliman, B. Ehren & G. Wallach (Eds.), *Handbook of language and literacy: Development and disorders* (2nd ed., pp. 105–126). New York: The Guilford Press.

Snowling, M., Bishop, D. V. M., Stothard, S., Chipchase, B., & Kaplan, C. (2006). Psychosocial outcomes at 15 years of children with a preschool history of speech-language impairment. *Journal of Child Psychology and Psychiatry, 47*, 759–765.

Snyder, L. (1984). Developmental language disorders: Elementary school age. In A. Holland (Ed.), *Language disorders in children*. San Diego, CA: College-Hill Press.

Sparrow, S., Cicchetti, D., & Saulnier, C. (2016). *Vineland adaptive behavior scales (Vineland III)* (3rd ed.). San Antonio, TX: Pearson.

Stanovich, K. (1986). Matthew effects in reading: Some consequences of individual differences in the acquisition of literacy. *Reading Research Quarterly, 21*, 360–364.

Stevens, C., Fanning, J., Coch, D., Sanders, L., & Neville, H. (2008). Neural mechanisms of selective auditory attention are enhanced by computerized training: Electophysiological evidence from language-impaired and typically developing children. *Brain Research, 1205*, 55–69.

Stevens, C., Sanders, L., & Neville, H. (2006). Neurophysiological evidence for selective auditory attention deficits in children with specific language impairment. *Brain Research, 1111*, 143–152.

Stokes, S., & Klee, T. (2009). The diagnostic accuracy of a new Test of Early Nonword Repetition for differentiating late talking and typically developing children. *Journal of Speech, Language, and Hearing Research, 52*, 872–882.

Storkel, H. (2003). Learning new words II: Phonotactic probability in verb learning. *Journal of Speech, Language, and Hearing Research, 46*, 1312–1323.

Stothard, S., Snowling, M., Bishop, D. V. M., Chipchase, B., & Kaplan, C. (1998). Language-impaired preschoolers: A follow-up into adolescence. *Journal of Speech, Language, and Hearing Research, 41*, 407–418.

Tallal, P., Miller, S., Bedi, G., Byma, G., Wang, X., Nagarajan, S., . . . Merzenich, M. (1996). Language comprehension in language-learning impaired children improved with acoustically modified speech. *Science, 271*, 81–84.

Thal, D., & Katich, J. (1996). Predicaments in early identification of specific language impairment: Does the early bird always catch the worm? In K. Cole, P. Dale, & D. Thal (Eds.), *Assessment of communication and language* (pp. 1–28). Baltimore: Paul H. Brookes.

Thal, D., Miller, S., Carlson, J., & Vega, M. (2005). Nonword repetition and language development in 4-year-old children with and without a history of early language delay. *Journal of Speech, Language, and Hearing Research, 48*, 1481–1495.

Thal, D., Oroz, M., Evans, D., Katich, J., & Leasure, K. (1995, June). *From first words to grammar in late-talking toddlers.* Paper presented at the Symposium on Research in Child Language Disorders, Madison, WI.

Tomblin, J. B. (2014). Educational and psychosocial outcomes of language impairment in kindergarten. In J. B. Tomblin & M. Nippold (Eds.), *Understanding individual differences in language development across the school years* (pp. 166–203). New York: Psychology Press.

Tomblin, J. B., Freese, P., & Records, N. (1992). Diagnosing specific language impairment in adults for the purpose of pedigree analysis. *Journal of Speech and Hearing Research, 35*, 832–843.

Tomblin, J. B., Hardy, J., & Hein, H. (1991). Predicting poor-communication status in preschool children using risk factors present at birth. *Journal of Speech and Hearing Research, 34*, 1096–1105.

Tomblin, J. B., Mainele-Arnold, E., & Zhang, X. (2007). Procedural learning in adolescents with and without specific language impairment. *Language Learning and Development, 3*, 269–293.

Tomblin, J. B., Records, N., Buckwalter, P., Zhang, X., Smith, E., & O'Brien, M. (1997). Prevalence of specific language impairment in kindergarten children. *Journal of Speech and Hearing Research, 40*, 1245–1260.

Tomblin, J. B., Records, N., & Zhang, X. (1996). A system for the diagnosis of specific language impairment in kindergarten children. *Journal of Speech and Hearing Research, 39*, 1284–1294.

Tomblin, J. B., Smith, E., & Zhang, X. (1997). Epidemiology of specific language impairment: Prenatal and perinatal risk factors. *Journal of Communication Disorders, 30*, 325–344.

Tomblin, J. B., & Zhang, X. (2006). The dimensionality of language ability in school-age children. *Journal of Speech, Language, and Hearing Research, 49*, 1193–1208.

Tomblin, J. B., Zhang, X., Buckwalter, P., & O'Brien, M. (2003). The stability of primary language disorder: Four years after kindergarten diagnosis. *Journal of Speech, Language, and Hearing Research, 46*, 1283–1296.

Trauner, D., Wulfeck, B., Tallal, P., & Hesselink, J. (1995). Neurologic and MRI profiles of language impaired children: Technical Report CND-9513. San Diego: Center for Research in Language, University of California.

Trauner, D., Wulfeck, B., Tallal, P., & Hesselink, J. (2000). Neurological and MRI profiles of children with developmental language impairment. *Developmental Medicine and Child Neurology, 42*, 470–475.

Ukrainetz, T., & Gillam, R. (2009). The expressive elaboration of imaginative narratives by children with specific language impairment. *Journal of Speech, Language, and Hearing Research, 52*, 883–898.

Ullman, M., & Gopnik, M. (1994). Past tense production: Regular, irregular and nonsense verbs. *McGill Working Papers in Linguistics, 10*, 81–118.

U.S. Department of Education. (2009). *Twenty-eighth Annual Report to Congress on the Implementation of the Individuals with Disabilities Education Act, 2006*. Washington: Author.

van Kleeck, A., Gillam, R., & Davis, B. (1997). When is "watch and see" warranted? A response to Paul's 1996 article, "Clinical implications of the natural history of slow expressive language development." *American Journal of Speech-Language Pathology, 6*, 34–39.

Vernes, A., Newbury, D., Abrahams, B., Winchester, L., Nicod, J., Groszer, M., ... Fisher, S. (2008). A functional genetic link between distinct developmental language disorders. *The New England Journal of Medicine, 359*, 2337–2345.

Viding, E., Price, T., Spinath, F., Bishop, D. V. M., Dale, P., & Plomin, R. (2003). Genetic and environmental mediation of the relationship between language and nonverbal impairment in 4-year-old twins. *Journal of Speech, Language, and Hearing Research, 46*, 1271–1282.

Walsh, I., Scullion, M., Burns, S., MacEvilly, D., & Brosnan, G. (2014). Identifying demographic and language profiles of children with a primary diagnosis of attention deficit hyperactivity disorder. *Emotional and Behavioural Difficulties, 19*, 59–70.

Warlaumont, A., & Jarmulowicz, L. (2012). Caregivers' suffix frequencies and suffix acquisition by language impaired, late talking, and typically developing children. *Journal of Child Language, 39*, 1017–1042.

Watkins, R., & Rice, M. (1991). Verb particle and preposition acquisition in language-impaired preschoolers. *Journal of Speech and Hearing Research, 34*, 1130–1141.

Watt, N., Wetherby, A., & Shumway, S. (2006). Prelinguistic predictors of language outcome at 3 years of age. *Journal of Speech, Language, and Hearing Research, 49*, 1224–1237.

Weiss, A., & Nakamura, M. (1992). Children with normal language skills in preschool classrooms for children with language impairments: Differences in modeling styles. *Language, Speech, and Hearing Services in Schools, 23*, 64–70.

Wetherby, A., & Prizant, B. (2002). *Communication and symbolic behavior scales—Developmental profile.* Baltimore: Paul H. Brookes.

Wetherby, A., & Prizant, B. (2003). *Communication and symbolic behavior scales—Normed edition.* Baltimore: Paul H. Brookes.

Wexler, K., Schütze, C., & Rice, M. (1998). Subject case in children with SLI and unaffected controls: Evidence for the Agr/Tns omission model. *Language Acquisition, 7*, 317–344.

Whitehurst, G., & Fischel, J. (1994). Early developmental language delay: What, if anything should the clinician do about it? *Journal of Child Psychology and Psychiatry, 35*, 613–648.

Whitehurst, G., Fischel, J., Arnold, D., & Lonigan, C. (1992). Evaluating outcomes with children with expressive language delay. In W. Warren & J. Reichle (Eds.), *Causes and effects in communication and language intervention* (pp. 277–314). Baltimore: Paul H. Brookes.

Whitehurst, G., Fischel, J., Lonigan, C., Valdez-Menchaca, M., Arnold, D., & Smith, M. (1991). Treatment of early expressive language delay: If, when, and how. *Topics in Language Disorders, 11*, 55–68.

Wiig, E., Semel, E., & Secord, W. (2013). *Clinical evaluation of language fundamentals—5*. San Antonio, TX: Pearson.

World Health Organization. (2016). *International Statistical Classification of Diseases and Related Health Problems* (10th ed.). Geneva: Author.

Zhang, X., & Tomblin, J. B. (2000). The association of intervention receipt with speech-language profiles and social-demographic variables. *American Journal of Speech-Language Pathology, 9*, 345–357.

Zimmerman, I., Steiner, V., & Pond, R. (2011). *Preschool language scales—5*. San Antonio, TX: Pearson.

Chapter 4

Abrahamsen, E., & Sprouse, P. (1995). Fable comprehension by children with learning disabilities. *Journal of Learning Disabilities, 28*, 302–308.

American Psychiatric Association. (2000). *Diagnostic and statistical manual of mental disorders* (4th ed.). Washington: Author.

American Speech-Language-Hearing Association (ASHA) Committee on Language Learning Disabilities. (1982). The role of the speech-language pathologist in learning disabilities. *ASHA, 24*, 937–944.

American Speech-Language-Hearing Association. (1993). *Definitions of communication disorders and variations* [Relevant Paper]. Available from www.asha.org/policy.

American Speech-Language-Hearing Association. (2005). (Central) auditory processing disorders: The role of the audiologist [Position statement]. Available from www.asha .org/policy.

Bashir, A. (1989). Language intervention and the curriculum. *Seminar in Speech and Language, 10*, 181–191.

Bashir, A., Kuban, K., Kleinman, S., & Scavuzzo, A. (1984). Issues in language disorders: Considerations of cause, maintenance and change. In J. Miller & R. Schielfelbusch (Eds.), *ASHA Reports, 12*, 92–106.

Boudreau, D. (2008). Narrative abilities: Advances in research and implications for clinical practice. *Topics in Language Disorders, 28*, 99–114.

Brinton, B., & Fujiki, M. (2014). Social and affective factors in children with language impairment: Implications for literacy learning. In C. Stone, E. Silliman, B. Ehren, & G. Wallach (Eds.), *Handbook of language and literacy: Development and disorders* (2nd ed., pp. 173–189). New York: Guilford Press.

Brozo, W. (2010). Response to intervention or responsive instruction? Challenges and possibilities of response to intervention for adolescent literacy. *Journal of Adolescent and Adult Literacy, 53*, 277–281.

Bryan, T., Bay, M., Lopez-Reyna, N., & Donahue, M. (1991). Characteristics of students with learning disabilities: A summary of the extant data base and its implications for educational programs. In J. Lloyd, N. Nirbhay & A. Repp (Eds.), *The regular education initiative: Alternative perspectives on concepts, issues, and models* (pp. 113–131). Sycamore, IL: Sycamore.

Burkard, R. (2009). Foreword. In A. Cacace & D. MacFarland (Eds.), *Controversies in central auditory processing disorder* (pp. vii–viii). San Diego, CA: Plural Publishing.

Campbell, W., & Skarakis-Doyle, E. (2007). School-aged children with SLI: The ICF as a framework for collaborative service delivery. *Journal of Communication Disorders, 40*, 513–535.

Carlisle, J., & Goodwin, A. (2014). Morphemes matter: How morphological knowledge contributes to reading and writing. In C. Stone, E. Silliman, B. Ehren, & G. Wallach (Eds.), *Handbook of language and literacy: Development and disorders* (2nd ed., pp. 265–282). New York: Guilford Press.

Catts, H., Bridges, M., Little, T., & Tomblin, J. B. (2008). Reading achievement growth in children with language impairments. *Journal of Speech, Language, and Hearing Research, 51*, 1569–1579.

Catts, H., Compton, D., Tomblin, J. B., & Bridges, M. (2012). Prevalence and nature of late-emerging poor readers. *Journal of Educational Psychology, 104*, 166–181.

Catts, H., Fey, M., Zhang, X., & Tomblin, J. B. (1999). Language basis of reading and reading disabilities: Evidence from a longitudinal investigation. *Scientific Studies of Reading, 3*, 331–361.

Catts, H., Fey, M., Zhang, X., & Tomblin, J. B. (2001). Estimating the risk of future reading difficulties in kindergarten children: A research-based model and its clinical implementation. *Language, Speech, and Hearing Services in Schools, 32*, 38–50.

Catts, H., & Kamhi, A. (2012). *Language and reading disabilities* (3rd ed.). Boston: Allyn & Bacon.

Christensen, C. (1992). Discrepancy definitions of reading disability: Has the quest led us astray? A response to Stanovich. *Reading Research Quarterly, 27*, 276–278.

Colozzo, P., Gillam, R., Wood, M., Schnell, R., & Johnston, J. (2011). Content and form in the narratives of children with specific language impairment. *Journal of Speech, Language, and Hearing Research, 54*, 1609–1627.

Coltheart, M. (2005). Analyzing developmental disorders of reading. *Advances in Speech-Language Pathology, 7*, 49–57.

DeBonis, D. (2015). It is time to rethink Central Auditory Processing Disorders protocols for school-aged children. *American Journal of Audiology, 24*, 124–136.

Dekemel, K. (2003). Building a power lexicon: Vocabulary acquisition in language-learning disabled students. In K. DeKemel, *Intervention in language arts: A practical guide for speech-language pathologists* (pp. 79–94). Philadelphia: Butterworth-Heinemann.

Dockrell, J. (2014). Developmental variations in the production of written text: Challenges for students who struggle with writing. In C. Stone, E. Silliman, B. Ehren, & G. Wallach (Eds.), *Handbook of language and literacy: Development and disorders* (2nd ed., pp. 505–523). New York: Guilford Press.

Dockrell, J., Lindsay, G., & Connelly, V. (2009). The impact of specific language impairment on adolescents' written text. *Exceptional Children, 75*, 427–446.

Donahue, M., (2014). Perspective-taking and reading comprehension of narratives: Lessons learned from "The Bean." In C. Stone, E. Silliman, B. Ehren, & G. Wallach (Eds.), *Handbook of language and literacy: Development and disorders* (2nd ed., pp. 323–338). New York: Guilford Press.

Duke, N. (2004). The case for informational text. *Educational Leadership, 61*, 40–44.

Ehren, B. (2009). Looking through an adolescent literacy lens at the narrow view of reading. *Language, Speech, and Hearing Services in Schools, 40*, 192–195.

Ehren, B. (2013, November). Helping older students meet Common Core Standards: Important work for SLPs. Workshop presented for the Corona-Norco School District. Norco, CA.

Ehren, B., Hatch, P., & Ukrainetz, T. (2012, November). SLPs: At the core of the Common Core State Standards (CCSS). Seminar presented at the American Speech-Language-Hearing Association Convention, Atlanta.

Ehren, B., Lenz, K., & Deshler, D. (2014). Adolescents who struggle and 21st century literacy. In C. Stone, E. Silliman, B. Ehren, & G. Wallach (Eds.), *Handbook of language and literacy: Development and disorders* (2nd ed., pp. 619–636). New York: Guilford Press.

Ehren, B., Murza, K., & Malani, M. (2012). Disciplinary literacy from a speech-language pathologist's perspective. *Topics in Language Disorders, 32*, 85–98.

Ehren, B., & Whitmire, K. (2009). Speech-language pathologists as primary contributors to response to intervention at the secondary level. *Seminars in Speech and Language, 30*, 90–104.

Ellis, E. (1997). Watering up the curriculum for students with disabilities: Goals of the knowledge dimension. *Remedial and Special Education, 18*, 326–347.

Fang, Z., Schleppegrell, M., & Moore, J. (2014). The linguistic challenges of learning across academic disciplines. In C. Stone, E. Silliman, B. Ehren, & G. Wallach (Eds.), *Handbook of language and literacy: Development and disorders* (2nd ed., pp. 302–322). New York: Guilford Press.

German, D. (1994). Word finding difficulties in children and adolescents. In G. Wallach & K. Butler (Eds.), *Language learning disabilities in school-age children and adolescents: Some principles and applications* (pp. 323–347). Boston: Allyn & Bacon.

Graham, S., & Herbert, M. (2010). Writing to read: Evidence for how writing can improve reading (A Carnegie Corporation Time to Act report). Washington: Alliance for Exceptional Education. Retrieved from http://all4ed.org/wp-content/uploads/2010/04/WritingToRead.pdf.

Green, L., & Roth, K. (2013). Increasing inferential reading comprehension skills: A single case treatment study. *Canadian Journal of Speech-Language Pathology and Audiology, 37,* 228–239.

Haager, D., & Vaughn, S. (2013). Common Core State Standards and students with learning disabilities: Introduction to the special issue. *Learning Disabilities Research and Practice, 28,* 1–4.

Hadley, P. (1998). Language sampling protocols for eliciting text-level discourse. *Language, Speech, and Hearing Services in Schools, 29,* 132–147.

Hall, L. (2012). How popular culture texts inform and shape students' discussions of social studies' texts. *Journal of Adolescent and Adult Literacy, 55,* 296–305.

Harcourt School Publishers. (2000). Harcourt Brace social studies: The early United States. Teachers edition, Grade 5 (Vol. 1). New York: Author.

IDEA. (2004). *Reauthorization of the Individuals with Disabilities Education Act.* http://idea.ed.gov/download/finalregulations.pdf.

Justice, L. (2006). Evidence-based practice, response to intervention, and the prevention of reading difficulties. *Language, Speech, and Hearing Services in Schools, 37,* 284–297.

Justice, L., & Ezell, H. (2004). Print referencing: An emergent literacy enhancement strategy and its clinical application. *Language, Speech, and Hearing Services in Schools, 35,* 185–193.

Kaderavek, J. (2015). *Language disorders in children: Fundamental concepts of assessment and intervention* (2nd ed.). Upper Saddle River, NJ: Pearson.

Kamhi, A. (2009). The case for the narrow view of reading. *Language, Speech, and Hearing Services in Schools, 40,* 174–177.

Keenan, J. (2014). The assessment of reading comprehension. In C. Stone, E. Silliman, B. Ehren, & G. Wallach (Eds.), *Handbook of language and literacy: Development and disorders* (2nd ed., pp. 469–484). New York: Guilford Press.

Koutsoftas, A., & Gray, S. (2012). Comparison of narrative and expository writing in students with and without language-learning disabilities. *Language, Speech, and Hearing Services in Schools, 43,* 395–409.

Lahey, M. (1990). Who shall be called "language disordered"? Some reflections and one perspective. *Journal of Speech and Hearing Disorders, 55,* 612–620.

Leonard, L. (1991). Specific language impairment as a clinical category. *Language, Speech, and Hearing Services in Schools, 22,* 66–68.

Lesaux, N., Kieffer, M., Faller, S., & Kelley, J. (2010). The effectiveness and ease of implementation of an academic vocabulary intervention for linguistically diverse students in urban middle schools. *Reading Research Quarterly, 45,* 196–228.

Lyon, G. (1998). *Overview of reading and literacy initiatives.* Washington: Committee on Labor and Human Resources.

Lyon, G., Shaywitz, S., & Shaywitz, B. (2003). A definition of dyslexia. *Annals of Dyslexia, 53,* 1–14.

Mason, L., Meadan, H., Hedin, L., & Corso, L. (2006). Self-regulated strategy development instruction for expository text comprehension. *Teaching Exceptional Children, 38,* 47–52.

McArthur, G., Hogben, J., Edwards, V., Heath, S., & Mengler, E. (2000). On the "specifics" of specific reading disability and specific language impairment. *Journal of Child Psychology and Psychiatry, 41,* 869–874.

McGregor, K., & Windsor, J. (1996). Effects of priming on the naming accuracy of preschoolers with word-finding deficits. *Journal of Speech and Hearing Research, 39,* 1048–1058.

McKeown, M., Beck, I., & Blake, R. (2009). Rethinking reading comprehension instruction: A comparison of instruction for strategies and content approaches. *Reading Research Quarterly, 44,* 218–253.

Moore, B., & Montgomery, J. (2008). *Making a difference for America' children: Speech-language pathologists in public schools.* Austin, TX: PRO-ED.

Nagy, W., & Anderson, R. (1984). The number of words in printed school English. *Reading Research Quarterly, 19,* 304–330.

National Governors Association Center for Best Practices and Council of Chief State School Officers (2010). *Common Core State Standards Initiative.* Retrieved August 29, 2016, from http://www.corestandards.org/read-the-standards/

National Joint Committee on Learning Disabilities (1991). Learning disabilities: Issues on definition. *ASHA, 33* (Suppl 5), 18–20.

Nelson, N. (2005). The context of discourse difficulty in classroom and clinic: An update. *Topics in Language Disorders, 25,* 322–331.

Newman, R., & German, D. (2002). Effects of lexical factors on lexical access among typical language-learning children and children with word-finding difficulties. *Language and Speech, 45,* 285–317.

Ness, M. (2011). Teachers' use of and attitudes toward informational text in K-5 classrooms. *Reading Psychology, 32,* 28–53.

Nippold, M. (2007). *Later language development: School-age children, adolescents, and young adults.* Austin, TX: PRO-ED.

Nippold, M. (2014). Language intervention at the middle school: Complex talk reflects complex thought. *Language, Speech, and Hearing Services in Schools, 45,* 153–156.

Nippold, M., & Scott, C. (Eds.). (2009). *Expository discourse in children, adolescents, and adults: Development and disorders.* New York: Taylor & Francis.

Ogle, D. (1986). K-W-L: A teaching model that develops active reading of expository text. *Reading Teacher, 39,* 564–570.

Owens, R. (2016). School-age literacy development: In R. Owens. *Language development: An introduction* (9th ed., pp. 359–395). Boston: Pearson.

Palincsar, A., Brown, A., & Campione, J. (1994). Models and practices of dynamic assessment. In G. Wallach & K. Butler (Eds.), *Language learning disabilities in school-age children and adolescents: Principles and Applications* (pp. 132–144). Boston: Allyn & Bacon.

Paul, R., & Norbury, C. (2012). *Language disorders from infancy through adolescence: Listening, speaking, reading, writing, and communicating* (4th ed.). St. Louis, MO: Elsevier Mosby.

Redmond, S. (2016a). Language impairment in the attention-deficit/hyperactivity disorder context. *Journal of Speech, Language, and Hearing Research, 59,* 133–142.

Redmond, S. (2016b). Markers, models, and measurement error: Exploring the links between attention deficits and language impairments. *Journal of Speech, Language, and Hearing Research, 59,* 62–71.

Redmond, S., Thompson, H., & Goldstein, S. (2011). Psycholinguistic profiling differentiates specific language impairment from typical development and from attention-deficit/hyperactivity disorder. *Journal of Speech, Language, and Hearing Research, 54,* 99–117.

Rees, N. (1973). Auditory processing factors in language disorders: The view from Procrustes' bed. *Journal of Speech and Hearing Disorders, 38,* 304–315.

Richard, G. (2011). Forum editor. The role of the speech-language pathologist in identifying and treating children with auditory processing disorder. *Language, Speech, and Hearing Services in Schools, 42,* 241–302.

Roth, F., & Troia, G. (2009). Applications of Responsiveness to Intervention and the speech-language pathologist in elementary school settings. *Seminars in Speech and Language, 30,* 75–89.

Scarborough, H. (2003). Connecting early language and literacy to later reading (dis)abilities: Evidence, theory, and practice. In S. Newman & D. Dickenson (Eds.), *Handbook of Early Literacy Research* (pp. 97–110). New York: Guilford Press.

Scarborough, H. (2009). Connecting early language and literacy to later reading (dis)abilities: Phonological awareness and some other promising predictors. In B. Shapiro, P. Accardo, & A. Capute (Eds.), *Specific reading disability: A view of the spectrum* (pp. 75–119). Baltimore: York Press.

Schuele, C., & Boudreau, D. (2008). Phonological awareness intervention: Beyond the basics. *Language, Speech, and Hearing Services in Schools, 31,* 3–20.

Scott, C. (2011). Assessment of language and literacy: A process of hypothesis testing for individual differences. *Topics in Language Disorders, 31,* 24–39.

Scott, C. (2014). One size does not fit all; Improving clinical practice in older children and adolescents with language and learning disorders. *Language, Speech, and Hearing Services in Schools, 45,* 145–152.

Scott, C., & Balthazar, C. (2010). The grammar of information: Challenges for older students with language impairments. *Topics in Language Disorders, 30,* 288–307.

Scott, C., & Koonce, N. (2014). Syntactic contributions to literacy learning. In C. Stone, E., Silliman, B. Ehren, & G. Wallach (Eds.), *Handbook of language and literacy: Development and disorders* (2nd ed.) (pp. 283–301). New York: Guilford Press.

Scott, C., & Windsor, J. (2000). General language performance measures of spoken and written narrative expository discourse of school-age children with language learning disabilities. *Journal of Speech, Language, and Hearing Research, 43,* 324–339.

Shanahan, T., & Shanahan, C. (2012). What is disciplinary literacy and why does it matter? *Topics in Language Disorders, 32,* 7–18.

Shaywitz, B., Fletcher, J., & Shaywitz, S. (1995). Defining and classifying learning disabilities and attention-deficit/hyperactivity disorder. *Journal of Child Neurology, 10,* S50–57.

Silliman, E., & Berninger, V. W. (2011). Cross-disciplinary dialogue about the nature of oral and written language problems in the context of developmental, academic, and phenotype profiles. *Topics in Language Disorders, 31,* 6–23.

Silliman, E., & Wilkinson, L. (2014). Policy and practice issues for students at risk in language and literacy learning: Back to the future. In C. Stone, E. Silliman, B. Ehren, & G. Wallach (Eds.). *Handbook of language and literacy: Development and disorders* (2nd ed., pp. 105–126). New York: Guilford.

Singer, B., & Bashir, A. (2004). Empower: A strategy for teaching students with language learning disabilities how to write expository text. In E. Silliman & L. Wilkinson (Eds.), *Language and Literacy Leaning in Schools* (pp. 239–272). New York: Guilford Press.

Singer, B., & Bashir, A. (2012, November). Self-talk: Its role in intervention and strategy learning. Seminar presented at the American Speech-Language-Hearing Association Conference, Atlanta.

Staskowski, M., & Rivera, E. A. (2005). Speech-language pathologist's involvement in Responsiveness to Intervention activities. *Topics in Language Disorders, 25,* 132–147.

Stone, C., Silliman, E., Ehren, B, & Wallach, G. (2014). Preface. In C. Stone, E. Silliman, B. Ehren, & G. Wallach (Eds.), *Handbook of language and literacy: Development and disorders* (2nd ed., pp. xv–xvi). New York: Guilford.

Stothard, S., Snowling, M., Bishop, D. V. M., Chipchase, B., & Kaplan, C. (1998). Language-impaired preschoolers: A follow-up into adolescence. *Journal of Speech, Language, and Hearing Research, 41,* 407–418.

Suddarth, R., Plante, E., & Vance, R. (2012). Written narrative characteristics in adults with language impairment. *Journal of Speech, Language, and Hearing Research, 55,* 409–420.

Sun, L., & Nippold, M. (2012). Narrative writing in children and adolescents: Examining the literate lexicon. *Language, Speech, and Hearing Services in Schools, 43,* 2–13.

Sun, L., & Wallach, G. (2013). Adolescent literacy: Looking beyond core language learning deficits. *Perspectives on Language Learning and Education, 20,* 57–66.

Sun, L., & Wallach, G. (2014). Language disorders ARE learning disabilities: Challenges on the divergent and diverse path to language learning disability. *Topics in Language Disorders, 34,* 25–38.

Tomblin, J. B., Zhang, X., Buckwalter, P., & O'Brien, M. (2003). The stability of primary language disorder: Four years after kindergarten diagnosis. *Journal of Speech, Language, and Hearing Research, 46,* 1283–1296.

Troia, G. (2005). Responsiveness to Intervention: Roles for speech-language pathologists in the prevention and identification of learning disabilities. *Topics in Language Disorders, 25,* 106–119.

Troia, G. (2014). Phonological processing deficits and literacy learning: Current evidence and future directions. In C. Stone, E. Silliman, B. Ehren, & G. Wallach (Eds.), *Handbook of language and literacy: Development and disorders* (2nd ed., pp. 227–245). New York: Guilford Press.

U.S. Department of Education, National Center for Education Statistics (NCES). (2006). Digest of educational statistics. 2005 (NCES) 2006-030). Chapter 2, http://nces.ed.gov/pubresearch/pubsinfo.asp?pubid=2006030.

U.S. Department of Education, National Center for Education Statistics (NCES). (2007). Back to school statistics. http://nces.ed.gov/fastfacts/display.asp/id=372.

van Kleeck, A. (1994). Metalinguistic development. In G. Wallach & K. Butler (Eds.), *Language learning disabilities in children and adolescents: Some principles and applications* (pp. 53–98). Boston: Allyn & Bacon.

Vermiglio, A. (2014). On the clinical entity in audiology: (Central) auditory processing and speech recognition in noise disorders. *Journal of the American Academy of Audiology, 25,* 904–917.

Wadman, R., Durkin, K., & Conti-Ramsden, G. (2011). Close relationships in adolescents with and without a history of specific language impairments. *Language, Speech, and Hearing Services in Schools, 42,* 41–51.

Wallach, G. P. (2008). *Language intervention for school-age students: Setting goals for academic success.* St. Louis, MO: Mosby/Elsevier.

Wallach, G. (2011). Peeling the onion of auditory processing disorder: A language/curricular-based perspective. *Language, Speech, and Hearing Services in Schools, 42,* 273–285.

Wallach, G. (2014). Improving clinical practice: A school-age and school-based perspective. *Language, Speech, and Hearing Services in Schools, 45,* 127–136.

Wallach, G., Charlton, S., & Christie, J. (2009). Making a broader case for the narrow view: Where to begin? *Language, Speech, and Hearing Services in Schools, 40,* 201–211.

Wallach, G., Charlton, S., & Christie, J. (2010). What do you mean by that? Constructive beginnings when working with adolescents with language learning disabilities. *Perspectives on Language Learning and Education, 17,* 77–84.

Wallach, G., Charlton, S., & Bartholomew, J. (2014). The spoken-written comprehension connection: Constructive intervention strategies. In C. Stone, E. Silliman, B. Ehren, & G. Wallach (Eds.), *Handbook of language and literacy: Development and* disorders (2nd ed., pp. 485–501), New York: Guilford Press

Ward-Lonergan, J. (2010). Supporting literacy development in adolescents through written language intervention. *Perspectives on Language Learning and Education, 17*, 85–92.

Ward-Lonergan, J., & Duthie, J. (2012, March). Expository discourse intervention for adolescents with language disorders. *Perspectives on Language Learning and Education, 20*, 44–56.

Westby, C. (1994). The effects of culture on genre, structure, and style of oral and written texts. In G. Wallach & K. Butler (Eds.), *Language learning disabilities in school-age children and adolescents: Some principles and applications* (pp. 180–218). Boston: Allyn & Bacon.

Westby, C. (2014). A language perspective on executive functioning, metacognition, and self-regulation in reading. In C. Stone, E. Silliman, B. Ehren, & G. Wallach (Eds.), *Handbook of language and literacy: Development and disorders* (2nd ed., pp. 339–358), New York: Guilford Press.

Whitmire, K., O'Rivers, K., Mele-McCarthy, J., & Staskowski, M. (2014). Building an evidence base for speech-language services in the schools: Challenges and recommendations. *Communication Disorders Quarterly, 35*, 84–92.

Wiig, E., Zureich, P., & Chan, H.-N. (2000). A clinical rationale for assessing rapid automatized naming in children with language disorders. *Journal of Learning Disabilities, 33*, 359–374.

Windsor, J., Scott, C., & Street, C. (2000). Verb and noun morphology in the spoken and written language of children with language learning disabilities. *Journal of Speech, Language, and Hearing Research, 43*, 1322–1336.

Wixson, K., Lipson, M., & Valencia, S. (2014). Response to Intervention for teaching and learning in language and literacy. In C. Stone, E. Silliman, B. Ehren, & G. Wallach (Eds.), *Handbook of language and literacy: Development and disorders* (2nd ed., pp. 637–653). New York: Guilford.

Wong, B., Graham, L., Hoskyn, M., & Berman, J. (Eds.). (2008). *The ABCs of learning disabilities*. Burlington, MA: Elsevier Academic Press.

Zhang, X., & Tomblin, J. B. (2000). The association of intervention receipt with speech-language profiles and social-demographic variables. *American Journal of Speech-Language Pathology, 9*, 345–357.

Chapter 5

Alt, M., Arizmendi, G., & Beal, C. (2014). The relationship between mathematics and language: Academic implications for children with specific language impairment and English language learners. *Language, Speech, and Hearing Services in Schools, 45*, 220–233.

Apel, K. (1999a). An introduction to assessment and intervention with older students with language-learning impairments: Bridges from research to clinical practice. *Language, Speech, and Hearing Services in Schools, 30*, 228–230.

Apel, K. (1999b). Checks and balances: Keeping the science in our profession. *Language, Speech, and Hearing Services in Schools, 30*, 98–107.

Aram, D., Ekelman, B., & Nation, J. (1984). Preschoolers with language disorders: 10 years later. *Journal of Speech and Hearing Research, 27*, 232–244.

Archwamety, T., & Katsiyannis, A. (2000). Academic remediation, parole violation, and recidivism rates among delinquent youths. *RASE: Remedial and Special Education, 21*, 161–170.

ASHA. (2009). *2009 Member Counts: Demographic profile of the ASHA constituents for the period January 1 through June 30, 2009: Table 7*. Rockville, MD: Author.

ASHA. (2016). ASHA summary membership and affiliation counts, year-end 2015. Rockville, MD: Author.

Asher, S., & Gazelle, H. (1999). Loneliness, peer relations, and language disorder in childhood. *Topics in Language Disorders, 19*, 16–33.

Beitchman, J., Adlaf, E., Douglas, L., Atkinson, L., Young, A., Johnson, C., & Wilson, B. (2001). Comorbidity of psychiatric and substance use disorders in late adolescence: A cluster analysis approach. *American Journal of Drug and Alcohol Abuse, 27*, 421–440.

Beitchman, J., Brownlie, E., Inglis, A., Wild, J., Ferguson, B., Schachter, D., & Mathews, R. (1996). Seven-year follow up of speech/language impaired and control children: Psychiatric outcome. *Journal of Child Psychology and Psychiatry, 37*, 961–970.

Beitchman, J., Wilson, B., Brownlie, E., Walters, H., Inglis, A., & Lancee, W. (1996). Long-term consistency in speech/language profiles: II. Behavioral, emotional, and social outcomes. *Journal of the American Academy of Child and Adolescent Psychiatry, 35*, 815–825.

Beitchman, J., Wilson, B., Brownlie, E., Walters, H., & Lancee, W. (1996). Long-term consistency in speech/language profiles: I. Developmental and academic outcomes. *Journal of the American Academy of Child and Adolescent Psychiatry, 35*, 804–814.

Beitchman, J., Wilson, B., Douglas, L., Young, A., & Adlaf, E. (2001). Substance use disorders in young adults with and without LD: Predictive and concurrent relationships. *Journal of Learning Disabilities, 34*, 317–332.

Beitchman, J., Wilson, B., Johnson, C., Atkinson, L., Young, A., Adlaf, E., & Douglas, L. (2001). Fourteen-year follow up of speech/language-impaired and control children: Psychiatric outcome. *Journal of the American Academy of Child and Adolescent Psychiatry, 40*, 75–82.

Betz, S., Eickhoff, J., & Sullivan, S. (2013). Factors influencing the selection of standardized tests for the diagnosis of specific language impairment. *Language, Speech, and Hearing Services in Schools, 44*, 133–146.

Bigelow, B. (2000). Delinquency. *Current Opinion in Psychiatry, 13*, 64–70.

Bjork, E. (2004). *Research on learning as a foundation for curricular reform and pedagogy*. Paper presented at the Reinvention Center's 2nd National Conference: Integrating research into undergraduate education: The value added, Washington, DC.

Botting, N., & Conti-Ramsden, G. (2000). Social and behavioural difficulties in children with SLI. *Child Language Teaching and Therapy, 16*, 105–120.

Bowers, L., Huisingh, R., & LoGiudice, C. (2007). *Test of problem solving—2 Adolescent*. East Moline, IL: LinguiSystems.

Bowers, L., Huisingh, R., & LoGiudice, C. (2009). *The listening comprehension test: Adolescent*. East Moline, IL: LinguiSystems.

Bowers, L., Huisingh, R., & LoGiudice, C. (2010). *Social language development test adolescent*. Moline, IL: Linguisystems.

Bowers, L., Huisingh, R., LoGiudice, C., & Orman, J. (2005). *The word test—2 Adolescent* (2nd ed.). Moline, IL: LinguiSystems.

Bowers, L., Huisingh, R., LoGiudice, C., & Orman, J. (2010). *The expressive language test—2* (2nd ed.). East Moline, IL: LinguiSystems.

Boyce, N., & Larson, V. (1983). *Adolescents' communication: Development and disorders*. Eau Claire, WI: Thinking Publications.

Bray, C. (1995). Developing study, organization, and management strategies for adolescents with language disabilities. *Seminars in Speech and Language, 16*, 65–83.

Brownlie, E., Jabbar, A., Beitchman, J., Vida, R., & Atkinson, L. (2007). Language impairment and sexual assault of girls and women: Findings from a community sample. *Journal of Abnormal Child Psychology, 35*, 618–626.

Bryan, K., Garvani, G., Gregory, J., & Kilner, K. (2015). Language difficulties and criminal justice: The need for earlier identification. *International Journal of Language and Communication Disorders, 50*, 763–775.

Buttrill, J., Niizawa, J., Biemer, C., Takahashi, C., & Hearn, S. (1989). Serving the language learning disabled adolescent: A strategies-based model. *Language, Speech, and Hearing Services in Schools, 20*, 185–203.

Camarata, S., Hughes, C., & Ruhl, K. (1988). Mild/moderate behaviorally disordered students: A population at-risk for language problems. *Language, Speech and Hearing Services in Schools, 19*, 191–200.

Carrow-Woolfolk, E. (2011). *Oral and Written Language Scales—II.* Torrance, CA: Western Psychological Services (WPS).

Carrow-Woolfolk, E. (2017). *Comprehensive assessment of spoken language—2.* Torrance, CA: Western Psychological Services (WPS).

Casner-Lotto, J., & Barrington, L. (2006). Are they really ready to work? Employers' perspectives on the basic knowledge and applied skills of new entrants to the 21st Century workforce. The Conference Board, Corporate Voices for Working Families, Partnership for 21st Century Skills and Society for Human Resource Management. Retrieved from http://www.p21.org/documents/Final_Report_PDF09-29-06.pdf

Catts, H., Fey, M., Zhang, X., & Tomblin, J. B. (2002). A longitudinal investigation of reading outcomes in children with language impairments. *Journal of Speech, Language, and Hearing Research, 45*, 1142–1157.

Catts, H., & Kamhi, A. (Eds.). (1999). *Language and reading disabilities.* Needham Heights, MA: Allyn & Bacon.

Cirrin, F., & Gillam, R. (2008). Language intervention practices for school-age children with spoken language disorders: A systematic review. *Language, Speech, and Hearing Services in Schools, 39*, S110–S137.

Clegg, J., & Henderson, J. (1999). Developmental language disorders: Changing economic costs from childhood into adult life. *Mental Health Research Review, 6*, 27–30.

Clegg, J., Hollis, C., Mawhood, L., & Rutter, M. (2005). Developmental language disorders—a follow-up in later adult life: Cognitive, language and psychosocial outcomes. *Journal of Child Psychology and Psychiatry, 46*, 128–149.

Clegg, J., Stackhouse, J., Finch, K., Murphy, C., & Nicholls, S. (2009). Language abilities of secondary age pupils at risk of school exclusion: A preliminary report. *Child Language Teaching and Therapy, 25*, 123–140.

Cohen, N., Davine, M., Horodezky, N., Lipsett, L., & Isaacson, L. (1993). Unsuspected language impairments in psychiatrically disturbed children: Prevalence and language and behavioral characteristics. *Journal of the American Academy of Child and Adolescent Psychiatry, 32*, 595–603.

Cohen, N., Farnia, F., & Im-Bolter, N. (2013). Higher order language competence and adolescent mental health. *Journal of Child Psychology and Psychiatry, 54*, 733–744.

Comkowycz, S., Ehren, B., & Hayes, N. (1987). Meeting classroom needs of language disordered students in middle and junior high schools: A program model. *Journal of Childhood Communication Disorders, 11*, 199–208.

Conti-Ramsden, G., & Botting, N. (2004). Social difficulties and victimization in children with SLI at 11 years of age. *Journal of Speech, Language, and Hearing Research, 47*, 145–161.

Conti-Ramsden, G., Botting, N., & Durkin, K. (2008). Parental perspectives during the transition to adulthood of adolescents with a history of specific language impairment (SLI). *Journal of Speech, Language, and Hearing Research, 51*, 84–96.

Conti-Ramsden, G., Botting, N., Simkin, Z., & Knox, E. (2001). Follow-up of children attending infant language units: Outcomes at 11 years of age. *International Journal of Language and Communication Disorders, 36*, 207–219.

Conti-Ramsden, G., & Durkin, K. (2008). Language and independence in adolescents with and without a history of specific language impairment (SLI). *Journal of Speech, Language, and Hearing Research, 51*, 70–83.

Conti-Ramsden, G., Durkin, K., & Simkin, Z. (2010). Language and social factors in the use of cell phone technology by adolescents with and without specific language impairment (SLI). *Journal of Speech, Language, and Hearing Research, 53*, 196–208.

Conti-Ramsden, G., Durkin, K., Simkin, Z., & Knox, E. (2009). Specific language impairment and school outcomes. I: Identifying and explaining variability at the end of compulsory education. *International Journal of Language and Communication Disorders, 44*, 15–35.

Conti-Ramsden, G., Durkin, K., & Walker, A. (2010). Computer anxiety: A comparison of adolescents with and without a history of specific language impairment (SLI). *Computers and Education, 54*, 136–145.

Conti-Ramsden, G., St Clair, M., Pickles, A., & Durkin, K. (2012). Developmental trajectories of verbal and nonverbal skills in individuals with a history of specific language impairment: From childhood to adolescence. *Journal of Speech, Language, and Hearing Research, 55*, 1716–1735.

Damico, J. (1993). Language assessment in adolescents: Addressing critical issues. *Language, Speech, and Hearing Services in Schools, 24*, 29–35.

Davis, A., Sanger, D., & Morris-Friehe, M. (1991). Language skills of delinquent and nondelinquent adolescent males. *Journal of Communication Disorders, 24*, 251–266.

Deshler, D., & Schumaker, J. (1988). An instructional model for teaching students how to learn. In J. Graden, J. Zins, & M. Curtis (Eds.), *Alternative educational delivery systems: Enhancing instructional options for all students* (pp. 391–411). Washington: National Association of Secondary Principals.

Deshler, D., Schumaker, J., Lenz, B., Bulgren, J., Hock, M., Knight, J., & Ehren, B. (2001). Ensuring content-area learning by secondary students with learning disabilities. *Learning Disabilities Research and Practice, 16*, 96–108.

Despain, A., & Simon, C. (1987). Alternative to failure: A junior high school language development-based curriculum. *Journal of Childhood Communication Disorders, 11*, 139–179.

Donlan, C., Cowan, R., Newton, E., & Lloyd, D. (2007). The role of language in mathematical development: Evidence from children with specific language impairments. *Cognition, 103*, 23–33.

Doren, B., Bullis, M., & Benz, M. (1996). Predicting arrest status of adolescents with disabilities in transition. *The Journal of Special Education, 29*, 363–380.

Dunn, L., & Dunn, D. (2007). *Peabody picture vocabulary test—4.* San Antonio, TX: Pearson.

Durkin, K., & Conti-Ramsden, G. (2007). Language, social behavior, and the quality of friendships in adolescents with and without a history of specific language impairment. *Child Development, 78*, 1441–1457.

Durkin, K., & Conti-Ramsden, G. (2010). Young people with specific language impairment: A review of social and emotional functioning in adolescence. *Child Language Teaching and Therapy, 26*, 105–121.

Durkin, K., & Conti-Ramsden, G. (2014). Turn off or tune in? What advice can SLTs, educational psychologists and teachers provide about uses of new media and children with language impairments? *Child Language Teaching and Therapy, 30*, 187–205.

Durkin, K., Conti-Ramsden, G., & Walker, A. (2011). Txt lang: Texting, textism use and literacy abilities in adolescents with and without specific language impairment. *Journal of Computer Assisted Learning, 27*, 49–57.

Durkin, K., Conti-Ramsden, G., Walker, A., & Simkin, Z. (2009). Educational and interpersonal uses of home computers by adolescents with and without specific language impairment. *British Journal of Developmental Psychology, 27*, 197–217.

Durkin, K., Simkin, Z., Knox, E., & Conti-Ramsden, G. (2009). Specific language impairment and school outcomes. II: Educational context, student satisfaction, and post-compulsory progress.

International Journal of Language and Communication Disorders, 44, 36–55.

Ehren, B. (1994). New directions for meeting the academic needs of adolescents with language-learning disabilities. In G. Wallach & K. Butler (Eds.), *Language-learning disabilities in school-age children and adolescents: Some principles and applications* (pp. 393–417). Boston: Allyn & Bacon.

Ehren, B. (2002). Speech-language pathologists contributing significantly to the academic success of high school students: A vision for professional growth. *Topics in Language Disorders, 22*, 60–80.

Ehren, B. (2009a). Looking through an adolescent literacy lens at the narrow view of reading. *Language, Speech, and Hearing Services in Schools, 40*, 192–195.

Ehren, B. (2009b). Response-to-Intervention: SLPs as linchpins in secondary schools. *The ASHA Leader, 14*, 10–13.

Ehren, B., & Lenz, B. (1989). Adolescents with language disorders: Special considerations in providing academically relevant language intervention. *Seminars in Speech and Language, 10*, 192–203.

Ehren, B., & Murza, K. (2010). The urgent need to address workforce readiness in adolescent literacy intervention. *SIG 1 Perspectives on Language Learning and Education, 17*, 93–99.

Ehren, B., Murza, K., & Malani, M. (2012). Disciplinary literacy from a speech-language pathologist's perspective. *Topics in Language Disorders, 32*, 85–98.

Ehren, B., & Whitmire, K. (2009). Speech-language pathologists as primary contributors to Response to Intervention at the secondary level. *Seminars in Speech and Language, 30*, 90–104.

Ellis, E. (1993). Integrative strategy instruction: A potential model for teaching content area subjects to adolescents with learning disabilities. *Journal of Learning Disabilities, 26*, 358–383, 398.

Evans, J., Viele, K., & Kass, R. (1997). Response latency and verbal complexity: Stochastic models of individual differences in children with specific language impairments. *Journal of Speech, Language, and Hearing Research, 40*, 754–764.

Fang, Z. (2012). Language correlates of disciplinary literacy. *Topics in Language Disorders, 32*, 19–34.

Fang, Z., & Schleppegrell, M. (2010). Disciplinary literacies across content areas: Supporting secondary reading through functional language analysis. *Journal of Adolescent and Adult Literacy, 53*, 587–597.

Fazio, B. (1994). The counting abilities of children with specific language impairment: A comparison of oral and gestural tasks. *Journal of Speech, Language, and Hearing Research, 37*, 358–368.

Fazio, B. (1996). Mathematical abilities of children with specific language impairment: A 2-year follow-up. *Journal of Speech, Language, and Hearing Research, 39*, 839–849.

Fey, M. (1988). Generalization issues facing interventionists: An introduction. *Language, Speech, and Hearing Services in Schools, 19*, 272–281.

Foley, R. (2001). Academic characteristics of incarcerated youth and correctional educational programs: A literature review. *Journal of Emotional and Behavioral Disorders, 9*, 248–259.

Fujiki, M., Brinton, B., & Clarke, D. (2002). Emotion regulation in children with specific language impairment. *Language, Speech, and Hearing Services in Schools, 33*, 102–111.

Fujiki, M., Brinton, B., Isaacson, T., & Summers, C. (2001). Social behaviors of children with language impairment on the playground: A pilot study. *Language, Speech, and Hearing Services in Schools, 32*, 101–113.

Fujiki, M., Brinton, B., Morgan, M., & Hart, C. (1999). Withdrawn and sociable behavior of children with language impairment. *Language, Speech, and Hearing Services in Schools, 30*, 183–195.

German, D. (2015). *Test of word finding—3*. Austin, TX: PRO-ED.

German, D. (2016). *Test of adolescent/adult word finding—2*. Austin, TX: PRO-ED.

Gillam, R., & Pearson, N. (2004). *Test of narrative language*. Austin, TX: PRO-ED.

Graham, S., & Harris, K. (1999). Assessment and intervention in overcoming writing difficulties: An illustration from the self-regulated strategy development model. *Language, Speech, and Hearing Services in Schools, 30*, 255–264.

Gray, D., Achilles, J., Keller, T., Tate, D., Haggard, L., Rolfs, R., ... McMahon, W. (2002). Utah youth suicide study. *Journal of the American Academy of Child and Adolescent Psychiatry, 41*, 427–434.

Hall, P., & Tomblin, J. B. (1978). A follow-up study of children with articulation and language disorders. *Journal of Speech and Hearing Disorders, 43*, 227–241.

Hammill, D. (1998). *Detroit tests of learning aptitude—4*. Austin, TX: PRO-ED.

Hammill, D., Brown, V., Larsen, S., & Wiederholt, J. (2007). *Test of adolescent and adult language—4* (4th ed.). Austin, TX: PRO-ED.

Hammill, D., & Bryant, B. (1991). *Detroit Tests of Learning Aptitude—Adult*. Austin, TX: PRO-ED.

Hammill, D., Mather, N., & Roberts, R. (2001). *Illinois test of psycholinguistic abilities—3*. Austin, TX: PRO-ED.

Hammill, D., & Newcomer, P. (2008). *Test of language development: Intermediate—4*. Austin, TX: PRO-ED.

Henry, F., Reed, V. A., & McAllister, L. (1995). Adolescents' perceptions of the relative importance of selected communication skills in their positive peer relationships. *Language, Speech, and Hearing Services in Schools, 26*, 263–272.

Hollo, A., Wehby, J., & Oliver, R. (2014). Unidentified language deficits in children with emotional and behavioral disorders: A meta-analysis. *Exceptional Children, 80*, 169–186.

Hopkins, T., Clegg, J., & Stackhouse, J. (2016). Young offenders' perspectives on their literacy and communication skills. *International Journal of Language and Communication Disorders, 51*, 95–109.

Huang, R., Hopkins, J., & Nippold, M. (1997). Satisfaction with standardized language testing: A survey of speech-language pathologists. *Language, Speech, and Hearing Services in Schools, 28*, 12–29.

Huber, M., Reed, V. A., Patchell, F., & Conrad, T. (2011, November). *SLI adolescents' verb morphology: Patterns from two narrative elicitation tasks*. Paper presented at the Annual Convention of the American Speech-Language-Hearing Association, San Diego.

Hughes, D., Turkstra, L., & Wulfeck, B. (2009). Parent and self-ratings of executive function in adolescents with specific language impairment. *International Journal of Language and Communication Disorders, 44*, 901–916.

Hummel, L., & Prizant, B. (1993). A socioemotional perspective for understanding social difficulties of school-age children with language disorders. *Language, Speech, and Hearing Services in Schools, 24*, 216–224.

Jerome, A., Fujiki, M., Brinton, B., & James, S. (2002). Self-esteem in children with specific language impairment. *Journal of Speech, Language, and Hearing Research, 45*, 700–714.

Joffe, V., & Black, E. (2012). Social, emotional, and behavioral functioning of secondary school students with low academic and language performance: Perspectives from students, teachers, and parents. *Language, Speech, and Hearing Services in Schools, 43*, 461–473.

Joffe, V., & Nippold, M. (2012). Progress in understanding adolescent language disorders. *Language, Speech, and Hearing Services in Schools, 43*, 438–444.

Johnson, C., Beitchman, J., & Brownlie, E. (2010). Twenty-year follow-up of children with and without speech-language impairments: Family, educational, occupational, and quality of life outcomes. *American Journal of Speech-Language Pathology, 19*, 51–65.

Johnson, C., Beitchman, J., Young, A., Escobar, M., Atkinson, L., Wilson, B., ... Wang, M. (1999). Fourteen-year follow up of children with and without speech/language impairments: Speech/language stability and outcomes. *Journal of Speech, Language, and Hearing Research, 42*, 744–760.

Kamhi, A. (2014). Improving clinical practices for children with language and learning disorders. *Language, Speech, and Hearing Services in Schools, 45*, 92–103.

Kamhi, A. (2009). The case for the narrow view of reading. *Language, Speech, and Hearing Services in Schools, 40*, 174–177.

Kaplan, J., & Kies, D. (1994). Strategies to increase critical thinking in the undergraduate classroom. *College Student Journal, 28*, 24–31.

Kauffman, J. (2001). *Characteristics of emotional and behavioral disorders of children and youth.* (7th ed.). Columbus, OH: Merrill.

Keith, R. (2009a). *SCAN—3: A Tests for auditory processing disorders in adolescents and adults (SCAN-3:A)* (3rd ed.). San Antonio, TX: Pearson.

Keith, R. (2009b). *SCAN—3: C Tests for auditory processing disorders for children (SCAN-3:C)*. San Antonio, TX: Pearson.

Kirk, J., & Reid, G. (2001). An examination of the relationship between dyslexia and offending in young people and the implications for the training system. *Dyslexia, 7*, 77–84.

Larson, V., & McKinley, N. (1985). General intervention principles with language impaired adolescents. *Topics in Language Disorders, 5*, 70–77.

Larson, V., & McKinley, N. (1987). *Communication assessment and intervention strategies for adolescents.* Eau Claire, WI: Thinking Publications.

Larson, V., & McKinley, N. (1995). *Language disorders in older students: Preadolescents and adolescents.* Eau Claire, WI: Thinking Publications.

Larson, V., & McKinley, N. (2003). *Communication solutions for older students.* Eau Claire, WI: Thinking Publications.

Law, J., Rush, R., Schoon, I., & Parsons, S. (2009). Modeling developmental language difficulties from school entry into early adulthood: Literacy, mental health, and employment outcomes. *Journal of Speech, Language, and Hearing Research, 52*, 1401–1416.

Lenz, B. K., Bulgren, J., & Kissam, B. (1995). *Pedagogies for academic diversity in secondary schools: Smarter planning.* Lawrence, KS: University of Kansas Center for Research on Learning.

Leonard, L., Miller, C., & Finneran, D. (2009). Grammatical morpheme effects on sentence processing by school-aged adolescents with specific language impairment. *Language and Cognitive Processes, 24*, 678–689.

Lindamood, P. C., & Lindamood, P. (2004). *Lindamood auditory conceptualization test (LAC-3)* (3rd ed.). San Antonio, TX: Pearson.

Lindsay, G., & Dockrell, J. (2004). Whose job is it? Parents' concerns about the needs of their children with language problems. *The Journal of Special Education, 37*, 225–235.

Lindsay, G., & Dockrell, J. (2012). Longitudinal patterns of behavioral, emotional, and social difficulties and self-concepts in adolescents with a history of specific language impairment. *Language, Speech, and Hearing Services in Schools, 43*, 445–460.

Lindsay, G., Dockrell, J., & Mackie, C. (2008). Vulnerability to bullying in children with a history of specific speech and language difficulties. *European Journal of Special Needs Education, 23*, 1–16.

Lindsay, G., Dockrell, J., & Strand, S. (2007). Longitudinal patterns of behaviour problems in children with specific speech and language difficulties: Child and contextual factors. *British Journal of Educational Psychology in the Schools, 77*, 811–828.

Loban, W. (1976). *Language development: Kindergarten through grade twelve.* Urbana, IL: National Council of Teachers of English.

Lunday, A. (1996). A collaborative communication skills program for Job Corps centers. *Topics in Language Disorders, 16*, 23–36.

Marcon, R. (1998, March). *Impact of language deficits on maladaptive behavior of inner-city early adolescents: A longitudinal analysis.* Paper presented at the Biennial Conference on Human Development, Mobile, AL.

Martin, N., & Brownell, R. (2005). *Test of auditory processing skills—3 (TAPS-3).* East Moline, IL: LinguiSystems.

Martin, N., & Brownell, R. (2010). *Receptive one-word picture vocabulary test—4.* Novato, CA: Academic Therapy Publications.

Martin, N., & Brownell, R. (2011). *Expressive one-word picture vocabulary test—4.* Novato, CA: Academic Therapy Publications.

Massa, J., & Eggert, L. (2001). Activity involvement among suicidal and nonsuicidal high-risk and typical adolescents. *Suicide and Life-Threatening Behavior, 31*, 265–281.

McCormick, L. (2003). Ecological assessment and planning. In L. McCormick, D. Loeb, & R. Schiefelbusch (Eds.), *Supporting children with communication difficulties in inclusive settings* (pp. 235–258). Boston: Allyn & Bacon.

McKinley, N., & Larson, V. (1989). Students who can't communicate: Speech-language services at the secondary level. *Curriculum Report, 19*, 1–8.

Miller, J., Andriacchi, K., & Nockerts, A. (2015). *Assessing language production using SALT software: A clinician's guide to language sample analysis* (2nd ed.). Middleton, WI: SALT Software LLC.

Mok, P., Pickles, A., Durkin, K., & Conti-Ramsden, G. (2014). Longitudinal trajectories of peer relations in children with specific language impairment. *Journal of Child Psychology and Psychiatry, 55*, 516–527.

National Governors Association Center for Best Practices and Council of Chief State School Officers. (2010). *Common Core State Standards Initiative.* Retrieved August 29, 2016, from http://www.corestandards.org/read-the-standards/

Nelson, N. (1998). *Childhood language disorders in context: Infancy through adolescence* (2nd ed.). Boston: Allyn & Bacon.

Nelson, N., Plante, E., Helm-Estabrooks, N., & Hotz, G. (2016). *Test of integrated language and literacy skills.* Baltimore: Paul H. Brookes.

Nippold, M. (1995). School-age children and adolescents: Norms for word definition. *Language, Speech, and Hearing Services in Schools, 26*, 320–325.

Nippold, M. (2007). *Later language development: School-age children, adolescents, and young adults.* Austin, TX: PRO-ED.

Nippold, M. (2010a). Explaining complex matters: How knowledge of a domain drives language. In M. Nippold & C. Scott (Eds.), *Expository discourse in children, adolescents, and adults: Development and disorders* (pp. 41–61). New York: Psychology Press.

Nippold, M. (2010b). It's NOT too late to help adolescents succeed in school. *Language, Speech, and Hearing Services in Schools, 41*, 137–138.

Nippold, M. (2011). Language intervention in the classroom: What it looks like. *Language, Speech, and Hearing Services in Schools, 42*, 393–394.

Nippold, M. (2012). Different service delivery models for different communication disorders. *Language, Speech, and Hearing Services in Schools, 43*, 117–120.

Nippold, M. (2014a). Language intervention at the middle school: Complex talk reflects complex thought. *Language, Speech, and Hearing Services in Schools, 45*, 153–156.

Nippold, M. (2014b). *Language sampling with adolescents: Implications for intervention* (2nd ed.). San Diego, CA: Plural Publishing.

Nippold, M., Hesketh, L., Duthie, J., & Mansfield, T. (2005). Conversational versus expository discourse: A study of syntactic development in children, adolescents, and adults. *Journal of Speech, Language, and Hearing Research, 48*, 1048–1064.

Nippold, M., Mansfield, T., & Billow, J. (2007). Peer conflict explanations in children, adolescents, and adults: Examining the development of complex syntax. *American Journal of Speech-Language Pathology, 16*, 179–188.

Nippold, M., Mansfield, T., Billow, J., & Tomblin, J. B. (2008). Expository discourse in adolescents with language impairments: Examining syntactic development. *American Journal of Speech-Language Pathology, 17*, 356–366.

Nippold, M., Mansfield, T., Billow, J., & Tomblin, J. B. (2009). Syntactic development in adolescents with a history of language impairments: A follow-up investigation. *American Journal of Speech-Language Pathology, 18*, 241–251.

Nys, J., Content, A., & Leybaerta, J. (2013). Impact of language abilities on exact and approximate number skills development: Evidence from children with specific language impairment. *Journal of Speech, Language, and Hearing Research, 56*, 956–970.

Pandolfe, J., Wittke, K., & Spaulding, T. (2016). Do adolescents with specific language impairment understand driving terminology? *Language, Speech, and Hearing Services in Schools, 47*, 324–333.

Phelps-Terasaki, D., & Phelps-Gunn, T. (2007). *Test of pragmatic language—2* (2nd ed.). Austin, TX: PRO-ED.

Poll, G., Betz, S., & Miller, C. (2010). Identification of clinical markers of specific language impairment in adults. *Journal of Speech, Language, and Hearing Research, 53*, 414–429.

Pratt, C., Botting, N., & Conti-Ramsden, G. (2006). The characteristics and concerns of mothers of adolescents with a history of SLI. *Child Language Teaching and Therapy, 22*, 177–196.

Prizant, B., Audet, L., Burke, G., Hummel, L., Maher, S., & Theadore, G. (1990). Communication disorders and emotional and behavioral disorders in children and adolescents. *Journal of Speech and Hearing Disorders, 55*, 179–192.

Raffaelli, M., & Duckett, E. (1989). "We were just talking . . .": Conversations in early adolescence. *Journal of Youth and Adolescence, 18*, 567–582.

Redmond, S. (2011). Peer victimization among students with specific language impairment, attention-deficit/hyperactivity disorder, and typical development. *Language, Speech, and Hearing Services in Schools, 42*, 520–535.

Reed, V. A., Bradfield, M., & McAllister, L. (1998). The relative importance of selected communication skills for successful adolescent peer interactions: Speech pathologists' opinions. *Clinical Linguistics and Phonetics, 12*, 205–220.

Reed, V. A., & Brammall, H. (2006). Methodological adaptations for investigating the perceptions of language-impaired adolescents regarding the relative importance of selected communication skills. *Clinical Linguistics and Phonetics, 20*, 573–582.

Reed, V. A., & Brammall, H. (2008). Importance of selected communication skills to adolescents: Effects of data collection methods. *Asia Pacific Journal of Speech, Language and Hearing, 11*, 63–71.

Reed, V. A., Conrad, T., & Patchell, F. (2006, June). *Verb morphological patterns of 16-year-old adolescents with and without specific language impairment.* Paper presented at the 11th Symposium of the International Clinical Phonetics and Linguistics Association, Dubrovnik, Croatia.

Reed, V. A., & Evernden, A. (2001, November). *Verb morphology of older children with reading difficulties.* Paper presented at the Annual Convention of the American Speech-Language-Hearing Association, New Orleans, LA.

Reed, V. A., Griffith, F., & Rasmussen, A. (1998). Morphosyntactic structures in the spoken language of older children and adolescents. *Clinical Linguistics and Phonetics, 12*, 163–181.

Reed, V. A., McLeod, K., & McAllister, L. (1999). Importance of selected communication skills for talking with peers and teachers: Adolescents' opinions. *Language, Speech and Hearing Services in Schools, 30*, 32–49.

Reed, V. A., & Miles, M. (1989). *Adolescent language disorders: A video inservice for educators.* Eau Claire, WI: Thinking Publications.

Reed, V. A., & Patchell, F. (2004, March). *Verb morphological patterns of adolescents with specific language impairment.* Paper presented at the 46th Annual Conference of the Speech-Language-Hearing Association of Virginia, Fredericksburg, VA.

Reed, V. A., & Patchell, F. (2010, April). *Discerning differences in the verb morphology of adolescents with specific language impairment.* Paper presented at the Annual Conference of the New Zealand Speech-Language Therapy Association, Wellington, New Zealand.

Reed, V. A., Patchell, F., & Conrad, T. (2006, November). *Verb morphology of younger and older adolescents with SLI.* Paper presented at the Annual Convention of the American Speech-Language-Hearing Association, Miami.

Reed, V. A., & Spicer, L. (2003). The relative importance of selected communication skills for adolescents' interactions with their teachers: High school teachers' opinions. *Language, Speech and Hearing Services in Schools, 34*, 343–357.

Rescorla, L. (2009). Age 17 language and reading outcomes in later-talking toddlers: Support for a dimensional perspective of language delay. *Journal of Speech, Language, and Hearing Research, 52*, 16–30.

Rice, M. (2000). Grammatical symptoms of specific language impairment. In D. V. M. Bishop & L. Leonard (Eds.), *Speech and language impairment in children: Causes, characteristics, intervention and outcome* (pp. 17–34). East Sussex, UK: Psychology Press.

Rice, M. (2013). Language growth and genetics of specific language impairment. *International Journal of Speech-Language Pathology, 15*, 223–233.

Rice, M., & Hoffman, L. (2015). Predicting vocabulary growth in children with and without specific language impairment: A longitudinal study from 2;6 to 21 years of age. *Journal of Speech, Language, and Hearing Research, 58*, 345–359.

Rice, M., Hoffman, L., & Wexler, K. (2009). Judgments of omitted BE and DO in questions as extended finiteness clinical markers of specific language impairment (SLI) to 15 years: A study of growth and asymptote. *Journal of Speech, Language, and Hearing Research, 52*, 1417–1433.

Rice, M., Wexler, K., & Hershberger, S. (1998). Tense over time: The longitudinal course of tense acquisition in children with specific language impairment. *Journal of Speech, Language, and Hearing Research, 41*, 1412–1431.

Rosta, G., & McGregor, K. (2012). Miranda rights comprehension in young adults with specific language impairment. *American Journal of Speech-Language Pathology, 21*, 101–108.

Sanger, D. (1999). The communication skills of female juvenile delinquents: A selected review. *Journal of Correctional Education, 50*, 90–94.

Sanger, D., Creswell, J., Dworak, J., & Schultz, L. (2000). Cultural analysis of communication behaviors among juveniles in a correctional facility. *Journal of Communication Disorders, 33*, 31–57.

Sanger, D., Hux, K., & Belau, D. (1997). Language skills of female juvenile delinquents. *American Journal of Speech-Language Pathology, 6*, 70–76.

Sanger, D., Hux, K., & Ritzman, M. (1999). Female juvenile delinquents' pragmatic awareness of conversational interactions. *Journal of Communication Disorders, 32*, 281–295.

Sanger, D., Moore-Brown, B., Magnuson, G., & Svoboda, N. (2001). Prevalence of language problems among adolescent delinquents: A closer look. *Communication Disorders Quarterly, 23*, 17–26.

Schleppegrell, M. (2001). Linguistic features of the language of schooling. *Linguistics and Education, 12*, 431–459.

Schmidt, J., Deshler, D., Schumaker, J., & Alley, G. (1989). Effects of generalization instruction on the written language performance of adolescents with learning disabilities in the mainstream classroom. *Journal of Reading, Writing and Learning Disabilities, 4*, 291–311.

Scott, C. (2014). One size does not fit all: Improving clinical practice in older children and adolescents with language and learning disorders. *Language, Speech, and Hearing Services in Schools, 45*, 145–152.

Scott, C., & Balthazar, C. (2010). The grammar of information: Challenges for older students with language impairments. *Topics in Language Disorders, 30*, 288–307.

Scott, C., & Windsor, J. (2000). General language performance measures in spoken and written narrative and expository discourse of school-age children with language learning disabilities. *Journal of Speech, Language, and Hearing Research, 43*, 324–339.

Semel, E., Wiig, E., & Secord, W. (1995). *Clinical Evaluation of Language Fundamentals—3.* San Antonio, TX: The Psychological Corporation.

Simon, C. (1987). *Classroom communication screening procedure for early adolescents.* Tempe, AZ: Communi-Cog Publications.

Simon, C. (1998). When big kids don't learn: Contextual modifications and intervention strategies for age 8–18 at-risk students. *Clinical Linguistics and Phonetics, 12*, 249–280.

Simon, C., & Holway, C. (1991). Presentation of communication evaluation information. In C. Simon (Ed.), *Communication skills and classroom success: Assessment and therapy methodologies for language and learning disabled students.* (pp. 151–197). Eau Claire, WI: Thinking Publications.

Singer, B., & Bashir, A. (1999). What are executive functions and self-regulation and what do they have to do with language-learning disorders? *Language, Speech and Hearing Services in Schools, 30*, 265–273.

Snow, P. (2000). Language disabilities: Comorbid developmental disorders and risk for drug abuse in adolescence. *Brain Impairment, 1*, 165–176.

Snow, P., & Powell, M. (2011). Oral language competence in incarcerated young offenders: Links with offending severity. *International Journal of Speech Language Pathology, 13*, 480–489.

Snow, P., Powell, M., & Sanger, D. (2012). Oral language competence, young speakers, and the law. *Language, Speech, and Hearing Services in Schools, 43*, 496–506.

Snowling, M., Adams, J., Bowyer-Crane, C., & Tobin, V. (2000). Levels of literacy among juvenile offenders: The incidence of specific reading difficulties. *Criminal Behaviour and Mental Health, 10*, 229–241.

Snowling, M., Bishop, D. V. M., Stothard, S., Chipchase, B., & Kaplan, C. (2006). Psychosocial outcomes at 15 years of children with a preschool history of speech-language impairment. *Journal of Child Psychology and Psychiatry, 47*, 759–765.

Snyder, L., & Caccamise, D. (2010). Comprehension processes for expository text: Building meaning and making sense. In M. Nippold & C. Scott (Eds.), *Expository discourse in children, adolescents, and adults: Development and disorders* (pp. 13–39). New York: Psychology Press.

St Clair, M., Pickles, A., Durkin, K., & Conti-Ramsden, G. (2011). A longitudinal study of behavioral, emotional and social difficulties in individuals with a history of specific language impairment (SLI). *Journal of Communication Disorders, 44*, 186–199.

Stanovich, K. (1986). Matthew effects in reading: Some consequences of individual differences in the acquisition of literacy. *Reading Research Quarterly, 21*, 360–364.

Stothard, S., Snowling, M., Bishop, D. V. M., Chipchase, B., & Kaplan, C. (1998). Language-impaired preschoolers: A follow-up into adolescence. *Journal of Speech, Language, and Hearing Research, 41*, 407–418.

Svensson, I., Lundberg, I., & Jacobson, C. (2001). The prevalence of reading and spelling difficulties among inmates of institutions for compulsory care of juvenile delinquents. *Dyslexia, 7*, 62–76.

Taliaferro, M., Reed, V. A., & Patchell, F. (2015, November). *Verb morphology of young adolescents with SLI: Patterns from two narrative elicitation tasks.* Paper presented at the Annual Convention of the American Speech-Language-Hearing Association, Denver.

Thorum, A. (1986). *Fullerton language test for adolescents* (2nd ed.). Austin, TX: PRO-ED.

Thurlow, C. (2005). Deconstructing adolescent communication. In A. Williams & C. Thurlow (Eds.), *Talking adolescence: Perspectives on communication in the teenage years* (pp. 1–20). New York: Peter Lang Publishing.

Tobin, K. (1986). Effects of teacher wait time on discourse characteristics in mathematics and language arts classes. *American Educational Research Journal, 23*, 191–200.

Tobin, K. (1987). The role of wait time in higher cognitive level learning. *Review of Educational Research, 57*, 69–95.

Tomblin, J. B., Freese, P., & Records, N. (1992). Diagnosing specific language impairment in adults for the purpose of pedigree analysis. *Journal of Speech and Hearing Research,* 35, 832–843.

Tomblin, J. B., Records, N., Buckwalter, P., Zhang, X., Smith, E., & O'Brien, M. (1997). Prevalence of specific language impairment in kindergarten children. *Journal of Speech and Hearing Research, 40*, 1245–1260.

U.S. Department of Education. (1999). *Twenty-first annual report to Congress on the implementation of the Individuals with Disabilities Education Act.* Washington: Author.

U.S. Department of Education. (2001). *Twenty-third annual report to Congress on the implementation of the Individuals with Disabilities Education Act.* Washington: Author.

U.S. Department of Education. (2006). *Twenty-eighth annual report to Congress on the implementation of the Individuals with Disabilities Education Act.* Washington: Author.

U.S. Department of Education. (2015). *37th Annual Report to Congress on the Implementation of the Individuals with Disabilities Education Act.* Washington: Author.

Vance, M., & Clegg, J. (2010). Editorial: Research and practice in the language and communication needs of adolescents in secondary education. *Child Language Teaching and Therapy, 26*, 101–103.

Wadman, R., Durkin, K., & Conti-Ramsden, G. (2008). Self-esteem, shyness, and sociability in adolescents with specific language impairment (SLI). *Journal of Speech, Language, and Hearing Research, 51*, 938–952.

Wagner, R., Torgesen, J., Rashotte, C., & Pearson, N. (2013). *Comprehensive test of phonological processing—2.* Austin, TX: PRO-ED.

Wallace, G., & Hammill, D. (2013). *Comprehensive receptive and expressive vocabulary test—3.* Austin, TX: PRO-ED.

Walsh, I., Scullion, M., Burns, S., MacEvilly, D., & Brosnan, G. (2014). Identifying demographic and language profiles of children with a primary diagnosis of attention deficit hyperactivity disorder. *Emotional and Behavioural Difficulties, 19*, 59–70.

Weiner, P. (1974). A language-delayed child at adolescence. *Journal of Speech and Hearing Disorders, 39*, 202–212.

Westby, C., & Atencio, D. (2002). Computers, culture, and learning. *Topics in Language Disorders, 22*, 70–90.

Wetherell, D., Botting, N., & Conti-Ramsden, G. (2007). Narrative in adolescent specific language impairment (SLI): A comparison with peers across two different narrative genres. *International Journal of Language and Communication Disorders, 42*, 583–605.

Whitehouse, A., Watt, H., Line, E., & Bishop, D. V. M. (2009). Adult psychosocial outcomes of children with specific language impairment, pragmatic language impairment and autism. *International Journal of Language and Communication Disorders, 44*, 511–528.

Whitmire, K., Rivers, K., Mele-McCarthy, J., & Staskowski, M. (2014). Building an evidence base for speech-language services in the schools: Challenges and recommendations. *Communication Disorders Quarterly, 35*, 84–92.

Wiig, E. (1990). Linguistic transitions and learning disabilities: A strategic learning perspective. *Learning Disability Quarterly, 13*, 128–140.

Wiig, E. (1995). Assessment of adolescent language. *Seminars in Speech and Language, 16*, 14–30.

Wiig, E., & Secord, W. (1989). *Test of language competence—Expanded edition.* San Antonio, TX: Pearson.

Wiig, E., & Secord, W. (1992). *Test of word knowledge.* San Antonio, TX: Pearson.

Wiig, E., & Secord, W. (2014). *Clinical Evaluation of Language Fundamentals—5 Metalinguistics.* San Antonio, TX: Pearson.

Wiig, E., Semel, E., & Secord, W. (2013). *Clinical Evaluation of Language Fundamentals—5.* San Antonio, TX: Pearson.

Williams, K. (2007). *Expressive vocabulary test—2.* San Antonio, TX: Pearson.

Woodcock, R., Muñoz-Sandoval, A., Ruef, M., Alvarado, C., Schrank, F., McGrew, K., . . . Dailey, D. (2017). *Woodcock-Muñoz Language Survey®-III.* Boston: Houghton Mifflin Harcourt.

Work, R., Cline, J., Ehren, B., Keiser, D., & Wujek, C. (1993). Adolescent language programs. *Language, Speech, and Hearing Services in Schools, 24*, 43–53.

Yew, S., & O'Kearney, R. (2013). Emotional and behavioural outcomes later in childhood and adolescence for children with specific language impairments: Meta-analyses of controlled prospective studies. *Journal of Child Psychology and Psychiatry 54*, 516–524.

Chapter 6

AAIDD. (2010). *Intellectual Disability: Definition, classification, and systems of supports* (11th ed.). Washington: American Association on Intellectual and Developmental Disabilities.

Abbeduto, L., Brady, N., & Kover, S. (2007). Language development and Fragile X syndrome: Profiles, syndrome specificity, and within-syndrome differences. *Mental Retardation and Developmental Disabilities Research Reviews, 13*, 36–46.

Abbeduto, L., & Murphy, M. (2004). Language, social cognition, maladaptive behavior, and communication in Down syndrome and Fragile X syndrome. In M. Rice & S. Warren (Eds.), *Developmental language disorders: From phenotypes to etiologies.* Mahwah, NJ: Lawrence Erlbaum Associates.

Abbeduto, L., Murphy, M., Richmond, E., Amman, A., Beth, P., Weissman, M., . . . Karadottir, S. (2006). Collaboration in referential communication: Comparison of youth with Down syndrome or fragile X syndrome. *American Journal on Mental Retardation, 111*, 170–183+227. doi: 10.1352/0895-8017(2006)111[170:CIRCCO]2.0.CO;2.

Abbeduto, L., Warren, S., & Conners, F. (2007). Language development in Down syndrome: From the prelinguistic period to the acquisition of literacy. *Mental Retardation and Developmental Disabilities Research Review, 13*, 247–261. doi: 10.1002/mrdd.20158.

Abel, E., & Sokol, R. (1987). Incidence of fetal alcohol syndrome and economic impact of FAS-related anomalies. *Drug and Alcohol Dependence, 19*, 51–70. doi: 10.1016/0376-8716(87)90087-1.

Adnams, C., Sorour, P., Kalberg, W., Kodituwakku, P., Perold, M., Kotze, A., . . . May, P. (2007). Language and literacy outcomes from a pilot intervention study for children with fetal alcohol spectrum disorders in South Africa. *Alcohol, 41*, 403–414. doi: 10.1016/j.alcohol.2007.07.005

Allor, J., Mathes, P., Roberts, J., Cheatham, J., & Otaiba, S. (2014). Is scientifically based reading instruction effective for students with below-average IQs? *Exceptional Children, 80*, 287–306. doi: 10.1177/0014402914522208.

Alvares, R., & Downing, S. (1998). A survey of expressive communication skills in children with Angelman Syndrome. *American Journal of Speech-Language Pathology, 7*, 14–24.

American Speech-Language-Hearing Association. (2001). Roles and responsibilities of speech-language pathologists with respect to reading and writing in children and adolescents [Guidelines]. Available from www.asha.org/policy.

American Speech-Language-Hearing Association. (2005). Roles and responsibilities of speech-language pathologists in service delivery for persons with mental retardation/developmental disabilities [Position statement]. From http://www.asha.org/policy/PS2005-00106.htm.

Andersen, W., Rasmussen, R., & Strømme, P. (2001). Levels of cognitive and linguistic development in Angelman syndrome: A study of 20 children. *Logopedics Phoniatrics Vocology, 26*, 2–9.

Aragón, A., Coriale, G., Fiorentino, D., Kalberg, W., Buckley, D., Phillip Gossage, J., . . . May, P. (2008). Neuropsychological characteristics of Italian children with fetal alcohol spectrum disorders. *Alcoholism: Clinical and Experimental Research, 32*(11), 1909–1919. doi: 10.1111/j.1530-0277.2008.00775.x

Barnes, E., Roberts, J., Long, S., Martin, G., Berni, M., Mandulak, K., & Sideris, J. (2009). Phonological accuracy and intelligibility in connected speech of boys with fragile X syndrome or down syndrome. *Journal of Speech, Language, and Hearing Research, 52*, 1048–1061. doi: 10.1044/1092-4388(2009/08-0001).

Bayley, N. (2006). *Bayley Scales of Infant and Toddler Development—Third Edition.* San Antonio: Harcourt Assessment.

Bertrand, J., Floyd, R., Weber, M., O'Connor, M., Riley, E., Johnson, K., & Cohen, D. (2004). *National task force on fetal alcohol syndrome and fetal alcohol effect. Fetal alcohol syndrome: Guidelines for referral and diagnosis.* Atlanta: Centers for Disease Control and Prevention.

Bhatara, V., Loudenberg, R., & Ellis, R. (2006). Association of attention deficit hyperactivity disorder and gestational alcohol exposure: An exploratory study. *Journal of Attention Disorders, 9*, 515–522. doi: 10.1177/1087054705283880

Bonati, M., Russo, S., Finelli, P., Valsecchi, M., Cogliati, F., Cavalleri, F., . . . Larizza, L. (2007). Evaluation of autism traits in Angelman syndrome: A resource to unfold autism genes. *Neurogenetics, 8*, 169–178. doi: 10.1007/s10048-007-0086-0

Boudreau, D., & Chapman, R. (2000). The relationship between event representation and linguistic skill in narratives of children and adolescents with Down syndrome. *Journal of Speech and Hearing Research, 43*, 1146–1159.

Brady, N., Bredin-Oja, S., & Warren, S. (2008). Prelinguistic and early language interventions for children with Down syndrome or fragile X syndrome. In J. Roberts, R. Chapman, & S. Warren (Eds.), *Speech and Language Development & Intervention in Down Syndrome & Fragile X Syndrome* (pp. 173–192). Baltimore: Paul H. Brookes.

Brady, N., Marquis, J., Fleming, K., & McLean, L. (2004). Prelinguistic predictors of language growth in children with developmental disabilities. *Journal of Speech, Language, and Hearing Research, 47*, 663–677. doi: 10.1044/1092-4388(2004/051).

Brady, N., Steeples, T., & Fleming, K. (2005). Effects of prelinguistic communication levels on initiation and repair of communication with children with disabilities. *Journal of Speech, Language, and Hearing Research, 48*, 1098–1113.

Brock, J. (2007). Language abilities in Williams syndrome: A critical review. *Development and Psychopathology, 19*, 97–127. doi: 10.1017/S095457940707006X.

Buckley, S., & Johnson-Glenberg, M. (2008). Increasing literacy learning for individuals with Down syndrome and Fragile X syndrome. In J. Roberts, R. Chapman, & S. Warren (Eds.), *Speech and Language Development & Intervention in Down Syndrome & Fragile X Syndrome* (pp. 233–254). Baltimore: Paul H. Brookes.

Burack, J. (1990). Differentiating mental retardation: The two-group approach and beyond. In R. Hodapp, J. A. Burack, & E. Zigler (Eds.), *Issues in the developmental approach to mental retardation* (pp. 27–48). New York: Cambridge University Press.

Bybee, J., & Zigler, E. (1999). Outerdirectedness in individuals with and without mental retardation: A review. In E. Zigler & D. Bennett-Gates (Eds.), *Personality development in individuals with mental retardation* (pp. 165–205). Cambridge: Cambridge University Press.

Calculator, S. (2002). Use of enhanced natural gestures to foster interactions between children with Angelman syndrome and their parents. *American Journal of Speech-Language Pathology, 11*, 340–355.

Carney, L., & Chermak, G. (1991). Performance of American Indian children with fetal alcohol syndrome on the test of language development. *Journal of Communication Disorders, 24*, 123–134. doi: 10.1016/0021-9924(91)90016-C.

Carter, J., Capone, G., Gray, R., Cox, C., & Kaufmann, W. (2007). Autistic-spectrum disorders in Down syndrome: Further delineation and distinction from other behavioral abnormalities. *American Journal of Medical Genetics, Part B: Neuropsychiatric Genetics, 144B*, 87–94. doi: 10.1002/ajmg.b.30407.

Centers for Disease Control and Prevention [CDC]. (2015). Birth Defects: Research and Tracking. Retrieved January 28, 2016, from http://www.cdc.gov/ncbddd/birthdefects/research.html.

Chamberlain, C., & Strode, R. (1999). *The source for Down syndrome.* East Moline, IL: LinguiSystems.

Chapman, R. (2003). Language and communication in individuals with Down syndrome. *International Review of Research in Mental Retardation* (Vol. 27, pp. 1–34).

Cirrin, F., Schooling, T., Nelson, N., Diehl, S., Flynn, P., Staskowski, M., . . . Adamczyk, D. (2010). Evidence-based systematic review: Effects of different service delivery models on communication outcomes for elementary school-age children. *Language, Speech, and Hearing Services in Schools, 41*, 233–264. doi: 10.1044/0161-1461(2009/08-0128).

Clifford, S., Dissanayake, C., Bui, Q., Huggins, R., Taylor, A., & Loesch, D. (2007). Autism spectrum phenotype in males and females with Fragile X full mutation and premutation. *Journal of Autism and Developmental Disorders, 37*, 738–747. doi: 10.1007/s10803-006-0205-z.

Coggins, T., Timler, G., & Olswang, L. (2007a). Identifying and treating social communication deficits in school-age children with fetal alcohol spectrum disorders. In K. O'Malley (Ed.), *ADHD and Fetal Alcohol Spectum Disorders (FASD)* (pp. 161–178). New York: Nova Science Publishers, Inc.

Coggins, T., Timler, G., & Olswang, L. (2007b). A state of double jeopardy: Impact of prenatal alcohol exposure and adverse environments on the social communicative abilites of school-age children with fetal alcohol spectrum disorder. *Language, Speech, and Hearing Services in Schools, 38*, 117–127.

Cone-Wesson, B. (2005). Prenatal alcohol and cocaine exposure: Influences on cognition, speech, language, and hearing. *Journal of Communication Disorders, 38*, 279–302. doi: 10.1016/j.jcomdis.2005.02.004.

Didden, R., Korzilius, H., Duker, P., & Curfs, L. M. G. (2004). Communicative functioning in individuals with Angelman syndrome: A comparative study. *Disability and Rehabilitation, 26*, 1263–1267. doi: 10.1080/09638280412331280271

Dimitropoulos, A., Ferranti, A., & Lemler, M. (2013). Expressive and receptive language in Prader-Willi syndrome: Report on genetic subtype differences. *Journal of Communication Disorders, 46*, 193–201. doi: 10.1016/j.jcomdis.2012.12.001.

Dulaney, C., & Ellis, N. (1997). Rigidity in the behavior of mentally retarded persons. In W. E. MacLean Jr. (Ed.), *Ellis' handbook of mental deficiency, psychological theory and research* (3rd ed., pp. 175—195). Mahwah, NJ: Lawrence Erlbaum.

Dykens, E., Hodapp, R., & Evans, D. (2006). Profiles and development of adaptive behavior in children with Down syndrome. *Down's Syndrome, Research and Practice: The Journal of the Sarah Duffen Centre/University of Portsmouth, 9*, 45–50. doi: 10.3104/reprints.293

Fey, M. (1986). *Language intervention with young children.* San Diego, CA: College-Hill Press.

Finestack, L., & Abbeduto, L. (2010). Expressive language profiles of verbally expressive adolescents and young adults with Down syndrome or fragile X syndrome. *Journal of Speech, Language, and Hearing Research, 53*, 1334–1348. doi: 10.1044/1092-4388(2010/09-0125).

Finestack, L., Palmer, M., & Abbeduto, L. (2012). Macrostructural narrative language of adolescents and young adults with Down syndrome or fragile X syndrome. *American Journal of Speech-Language Pathology, 21*, 29–46. doi: 10.1044/1058-0360(2011/10-0095).

Finestack, L., Sterling, A., & Abbeduto, L. (2013). Discriminating Down syndrome and fragile X syndrome based on language ability. *Journal of Child Language, 40*, 244–265. doi: 10.1017/S0305000912000207.

Frankenberger, W., & Harper, J. (1988). States' definitions and procedures for identifying children with mental retardation: Comparison of 1981–1982 and 1985–1986 guidelines. *Mental Retardation, 26*, 133–136.

Fryer, S., McGee, C., Matt, G., Riley, E., & Mattson, S. (2007). Evaluation of psychopathological conditions in children with heavy prenatal alcohol exposure. *Pediatrics, 119*, e733–e741. doi: 10.1542/peds.2006-1606.

Garbarino, J., & de Lara, E. (2002). *And words can hurt forever*. New York: Free Press.

Gathercole, S., & Alloway, T. (2006). Practitioner review: Short-term and working memory impairments in neurodevelopmental disorders: Diagnosis and remedial support. *Journal of Child Psychology and Psychiatry and Allied Disciplines, 47*, 4–15. doi: 10.1111/j.1469-7610.2005.01446.x.

Gathercole, S., Alloway, T., Willis, C., & Adams, A. (2006). Working memory in children with reading disabilities. *Journal of Experimental Child Psychology, 93*, 265–281. doi: 10.1016/j.jecp.2005.08.003.

Gierut, J. (2001). Complexity in phonological treatment: Clinical factors. *Language, Speech, and Hearing Services in Schools, 32*, 229–241.

Gierut, J. (2005). Phonological intervention: The how or the what? In A. Kamhi & K. Pollock (Eds.), *Phonological disorders in children: Clinical decision making in assessment and intervention* (pp. 201–210). Baltimore: Paul H. Brookes.

Grieco, J., Pulsifer, M., Seligsohn, K., Skotko, B., & Schwartz, A. (2015). Down syndrome: Cognitive and behavioral functioning across the lifespan. *American Journal of Medical Genetics, Part C: Seminars in Medical Genetics, 169*, 135–149. doi: 10.1002/ajmg.c.31439.

Grossman, H. J. (1983). *Classification in mental retardation*. Washington: American Association on Mental Deficiency.

Hagerman, R. (2002). Physical and behavioral phenotype. In R. Hagerman & P. Hagerman (Eds.), *Fragile X syndrome: Diagnosis, treatment and research* (3rd ed.). Baltimore: The John Hopkins University Press.

Hagerman, R. (2006). Lessons from fragile X regarding neurobiology, autism, and neurodegeneration. *Developmental and Behavioral Pediatrics, 27*, 63–74.

Hagerman, R. (2008). Etiology, diagnosis, anddevelopment in fragile X syndrome. In J. Roberts, R. Chapman, & S. Warren (Eds.), *Speech & Language Development & Intervention in Down Syndrome & Fragile X Syndrome* (pp. 27–49). Baltimore: Paul H. Brookes.

Hall, S., Burns, D., Lightbody, A., & Reiss, A. (2008). Longitudinal changes in intellectual development in children with fragile X syndrome. *Journal of Abnormal Child Psychology, 36*, 927–939. doi: 10.1007/s10802-008-9223-y.

Hansen, B., Wadsworth, J., Roberts, M., & Poole, T. (2014). Effects of naturalistic instruction on phonological awareness skills of children with intellectual and developmental disabilities. *Research in Developmental Disabilities, 35*, 2790–2801. doi: 10.1016/j.ridd.2014.07.011.

Harrison, P., & Oakland, T. (2015). *Adaptive Behavior Assessment System—Third Edition ABAS-3*. New York: Pearson.

Hickson, L., & Khemka, I. (2014). The psychology of decision making. *International Review of Research in Developmental Disabilities, 47*, 185–229.

Hodson, B. (2006). Identifying phonological patterns and projecting remediation cycles: Expediting intelligibility gains of a 7 year old Australian child. *Advances in Speech Language Pathology, 8*, 257–264. doi: 10.1080/14417040600824936.

Hoffmann, A., Martens, M., Fox, R., Rabidoux, P., & Andridge, R. (2013). Pragmatic language assessment in Williams syndrome: A comparison of the Test of Pragmatic Language—2 and the Children's Communication Checklist-2. *American Journal of Speech-Language Pathology, 22*, 198–204. doi: 10.1044/1058-0360(2012/11-0131).

Janzen, L., Nanson, J., & Block, G. (1995). Neuropsychological evaluation of preschoolers with fetal alcohol syndrome. *Neurotoxicology and Teratology, 17*, 273–279. doi: 10.1016/0892-0362(94)00063-J.

Jarrold, C., Cowan, B., Hewes, A., & Riby, D. (2004). Speech timing and verbal short-term memory: Evidence for contrasting deficits in Down syndrome and Williams syndrome. *Journal of Memory and Language, 51*, 365–380.

Jenkinson, J. (1999). Factors affecting decision-making by young adults with intellectual disabilities. *American Journal on Mental Retardation, 104*, 320–329.

John, A., Dobson, L., Thomas, L., & Mervis, C. (2012). Pragmatic abilities of children with Williams syndrome: A longitudinal examination. *Frontiers in Psychology, 3*(JUN). doi: 10.3389/fpsyg.2012.00199.

Jolleff, N., & Ryan, M. (1993). Communication development in Angelman's syndrome. *Archives of Disease in Childhood, 69*, 148–150.

Kaiser, A., & Roberts, M. (2013). Parent-implemented enhanced milieu teaching with preschool children who have intellectual disabilities. *Journal of Speech, Language, and Hearing Research, 56*, 295–309. doi: 10.1044/1092-4388(2012/11-0231).

Kaufmann, W., Cortell, R., Kau, A., Bukelis, I., Tierney, E., Gray, R., . . . Stanard, P. (2004). Autism spectrum disorder in fragile X syndrome: Communication, social interaction, and specific behaviors. *American Journal of Medical Genetics, 129 A*, 225–234. doi: 10.1002/ajmg.a.30229.

Keil, V., Paley, B., Frankel, F., & O'Connor, M. J. (2010). Impact of a social skills intervention on the hostile attributions of children with prenatal alcohol exposure. *Alcoholism: Clinical and Experimental Research, 34*, 231–241. doi: 10.1111/j.1530-0277.2009.01086.x.

Kent, R., & Vorperian, H. (2013). Speech impairment in down syndrome: A review. *Journal of Speech, Language, and Hearing Research, 56*, 178–210. doi: 10.1044/1092-4388(2012/12-0148).

Khemka, I., & Hickson, L. (2006). The role of motivation in the decision making of adolescents with mental retardation. *International Review of Research in Mental Retardation* (Vol. 31, pp. 73–115).

Kleppe, S., Katayama, K., Shipley, K., & Foushee, D. (1990). The speech and language characteristics of children with Prader-Willi syndrome. *Journal of Speech and Hearing Disorders, 55*, 300–308.

Kumin, L. (2008a). *Helping children with Down syndrome communicate better: Speech and language skills for ages 6–14*. Bethesda, MD: Woodbine House.

Kumin, L. (2008b). Language intervention to encourage complex language use. In J. Roberts, R. Chapman, & S. Warren (Eds.), *Speech and Language Development and Intervention in Down Syndrome and Fragile X Syndrome* (pp. 193–218). Baltimore: Paul H. Brookes.

Laws, G., & Bishop, D. V. M. (2004a). Pragmatic language impairment and social deficits in Williams syndrome. A comparison with Down syndrome and specific language impairment. *International Journal of Language and Communication Disorders, 39*, 45–64.

Laws, G., & Bishop, D. V. M. (2004b). Verbal deficits in Down syndrome and specific language impairment: A comparison. *International Journal of Language and Communication Disorders, 39*, 423–451.

Lesniak-Karpiak, K., Mazzocco, M., & Ross, J. (2003). Behavioral assessment of social anxiety in females with Turner or fragile X syndrome. *Journal of Autism and Developmental Disorders, 33*, 55–67. doi: 10.1023/A:1022230504787.

Lewis, B., Freebairn, L., Heeger, S., & Cassidy, S. (2002). Speech and language skills of individuals with Prader-Willi syndrome. *American Journal of Speech-Language Pathology, 11*, 285–294.

MacMillan, D., & Siperstein, G. (2001). *Learning disabilities as operationally defined by schools.* Paper presented at the Learning Disabilities Summit: Building a Foundation for the Future, Washington.

Marler, J., Elfenbein, J., Ryals, B., Urban, Z., & Netzloff, M. (2005). Sensorineural hearing loss in children and adults with Williams syndrome. *American Journal of Medical Genetics, 138A*, 318–327.

Martin, G., Losh, M., Estigarribia, B., Sideris, J., & Roberts, J. (2013). Longitudinal profiles of expressive vocabulary, syntax and pragmatic language in boys with fragile X syndrome or Down syndrome. *International Journal of Language and Communication Disorders, 48*, 432–443. doi: 10.1111/1460-6984.12019.

Mattson, S., Crocker, N., & Nguyen, T. (2011). Fetal alcohol spectrum disorders: Neuropsychological and behavioral features. *Neuropsychology Review, 21*, 81–101. doi: 10.1007/s11065-011-9167-9.

May, P., Gossage, J., Kalberg, W., Robinson, L., Buckley, D., Manning, M., & Hoyme, H. (2009). Prevalence and epidemiologic characteristics of FASD from various research methods with an emphasis on recent in-school studies. *Developmental Disabilities Research Reviews, 15*, 176–192. doi: 10.1002/ddrr.68.

McGee, C., Bjorkquist, O., Riley, E., & Mattson, S. (2009). Impaired language performance in young children with heavy prenatal alcohol exposure. *Neurotoxicology and Teratology, 31*, 71–75. doi: 10.1016/j.ntt.2008.09.004.

Mervis, C. (2009). Language and literacy development of children with Williams syndrome. *Topics in Language Disorders, 29*, 149–169. doi: 10.1097/TLD.0b013e3181a72044.

Mervis, C., & John, A. (2010). Cognitive and behavioral characteristics of children with Williams syndrome: Implications for intervention approaches. *American Journal of Medical Genetics, Part C: Seminars in Medical Genetics, 154*, 229–248. doi: 10.1002/ajmg.c.30263.

Miles, S., & Chapman, R. (2002). Narrative content as described by individuals with Down syndrome and typically developing children. *Journal of Speech, Language, and Hearing Research, 45*, 175–189.

Miller, J. (1995). Individual differences in vocabulary acquisition in children with Down syndrome. *Progress in Clinical and Biological Research, 393*, 93–103.

Miolo, G., Chapman, R., & Sindberg, H. (2005). Sentence comprehension in adolescents with Down syndrome and typically developing children: Role of sentence voice, visual context, and auditory-verbal short-term memory. *Journal of Speech, Language, and Hearing Research, 48*, 172–188.

Moreau, M. (2006). *Story grammar marker*. Greenville, SC: Super Duper.

Moss, J., Howlin, P., Hastings, R., Beaumont, S., Griffith, G., Petty, J., . . . Oliver, C. (2013). Social behavior and characteristics of autism spectrum disorder in Angelman, Cornelia de Lange, and Cri du Chat syndromes. *American Journal on Intellectual and Developmental Disabilities, 118*, 262–283. doi: 10.1352/1944-7558-118.4.262.

NOFAS. (2014). FASD: What everyone should know. Retrieved January 28, 2016, from http://www.nofas.org/wp-content/uploads/2014/08/Fact-sheet-what-everyone-should-know_old_chart-new-chart1.pdf.

O'Connor, M., Frankel, F., Paley, B., Schonfeld, A., Carpenter, E., Laugeson, E., & Marquardt, R. (2006). A controlled social skills training for children with fetal alcohol spectrum disorders. *Journal of Consulting and Clinical Psychology, 74*, 639–648. doi: 10.1037/0022-006X.74.4.639.

O'Malley, K. (2007a). *ADHD and fetal alcohol spectrum disorders (FASD) [electronic resource]*. New York: Nova Science Publishers.

O'Malley, K. (2007b). Multi-modal management strategies in FASD through the lifespan. In K. O'Malley (Ed.), *ADHD and fetal alcohol spectrum disorders (FASD)* (pp. 217–236). New York: Nova Science Publishers.

Parker-McGowan, Q., Chen, M., Reichle, J., Pandit, S., Johnson, L., & Kreibich, S. (2014). Describing treatment intensity in milieu teaching interventions for children with developmental disabilities: A review. *Language, Speech, and Hearing Services in Schools, 45*, 351–364. doi: 10.1044/2014_LSHSS-13-0087.

Patterson, D., & Lott, I. (2008). Etiology, diagnosis, and development in Down syndrome. In J. Roberts, R. Chapman, & S. Warren (Eds.), *Speech and language development and intervention in Down syndrome and fragile X syndrome* (pp. 1–25). Baltimore: Paul H. Brookes.

Peadon, E., & Elliott, E. (2010). Alcohol consumption in pregnancy. *Medicine Today, 11*, 70–72.

Polloway, E., Smith, J., Patton, J., Lubin, A., & Antoine, K. (2009). State guidelines for mental retardation and intellectual disabilities: A re-visitation of previous analyses in light of changes in the field. *Education and Training in Developmental Disabilities, 44*, 14–24.

Price, J., Roberts, J., Hennon, E., Berni, M., Anderson, K., & Sideris, J. (2008). Syntactic complexity during conversation of boys with fragile X syndrome and Down syndrome. *Journal of Speech, Language, and Hearing Research, 51*, 3–15.

Quattlebaum, J., & O'Connor, M. (2013). Higher functioning children with prenatal alcohol exposure: Is there a specific neurocognitive profile? *Child Neuropsychology, 19*, 561–578. doi: 10.1080/09297049.2012.713466.

Rakap, S., & Rakap, S. (2014). Parent-implemented naturalistic language interventions for young children with disabilities: A systematic review of single-subject experimental research studies. *Educational Research Review, 13*, 35–51. doi: 10.1016/j.edurev.2014.09.001.

Richard, G., & Hoge, D. (1999). *The source for syndromes*. East Moline, IL: LinguiSystems.

Roberts, J., Chapman, R., Martin, G., & Moskowitz, L. (2008). Language of preschool and school-age children with Down syndrome and fragile X syndrome. In J. Roberts, R. Chapman, & S. Warren (Eds.), *Speech and language development and intervention in Down syndrome and fragile X syndrome* (pp. 77–115). Baltimore: Paul H. Brookes.

Roberts, J., Mirrett, P., & Burchinal, M. (2001). Receptive and expressive communication development of young males with fragile X syndrome. *American Journal on Mental Retardation, 106*, 216–230. doi: 10.1352/0895-8017(2001)106<0216:RAECDO>2.0.CO;2.

Roberts, M., & Kaiser, A. (2011). The effectiveness of parent-implemented language interventions: A meta-analysis. *American Journal of Speech-Language Pathology, 20*, 180–199. doi: 10.1044/1058-0360(2011/10-0055).

Roberts, M., Kaiser, A., Wolfe, C., Bryant, J., & Spidalieri, A. (2014). Effects of the teach-model-coach-review instructional approach on caregiver use of language support strategies and children's expressive language skills. *Journal of Speech, Language, and Hearing Research, 57*, 1851–1869. doi: 10.1044/2014_JSLHR-L-13-0113.

Roid, G. (2003). *Stanford-Binet intelligence scales* (5th ed.). Scarborough, ON, Canada: Thomson-Nelson.

Roid, G., Miller, L., Pomplun, M., & Koch, C. (2013). *Leiter International Performance Scale-3*. Los Angeles: Western Psychological Services.

Roizen, N., & Patterson, D. (2003). Down's syndrome. *Lancet, 361*, 1281–1289. doi: 10.1016/S0140-6736(03)12987-X.

Schalock, R., Luckasson, R., Shogren, K., Borthwick-Duffy, S., Bradley, V., Buntinx, W., & Yeager, M. (2007). The renaming of mental retardation: Understanding the change to the term intellectual disability. *Intellectual and Developmental Disabilities, 45*, 116–124.

Scharfenaker, S., O'Connor, R., Stackhouse, T., Braden, M., & Gray, K. (2002). An integrated approach to intervention. In R. J. Hagerman & P. J. Hagerman (Eds.), *Fragile X syndrome: diagnosis, treatment, and research* (3 ed., pp. 363–427). Baltimore: The Johns Hopkins University Press.

Schreibman, L., Dawson, G., Stahmer, A., Landa, R., Rogers, S., McGee, G., . . . Halladay, A. (2015). Naturalistic developmental behavioral interventions: Empirically validated treatments for autism spectrum disorder. *Journal of Autism and Developmental Disorders, 45*, 2411–2428. doi: 10.1007/s10803-015-2407-8.

Seltzer, M., Baker, M., Hong, J., Maenner, M., Greenberg, J., & Mandel, D. (2012). Prevalence of CGG expansions of the *FMR1* gene in a US population-based sample. *American Journal of Medical Genetics, Part B: Neuropsychiatric Genetics, 159 B*, 589–597. doi: 10.1002/ajmg.b.32065.

Shott, S., Amin, R., Chini, B., Heubi, C., Hotze, S., & Akers, R. (2006). Obstructive sleep apnea: Should all children with Down syndrome be tested? *Archives of Otolaryngology and Head and Neck Surgery, 132*, 432–436.

Shprintzen, R. (1997). *Genetics, syndromes, and communication disorders*. San Diego, CA: Singular.

Shprintzen, R. (2000). *Syndrome identification for speech-language pathology: An illustrated pocket guide*. San Diego, CA: Singular Publishing Group.

Sparrow, S., Cicchetti, D., & Balla, D. (2005). *Vineland-II: Vineland adaptive behavior scales, Second Edition*. Boston: Pearson.

Sterling, A., & Warren, S. (2008). Communication and language development in infants and toddlers with Down syndrome or fragile X syndrome. In J. Roberts, R. Chapman, & S. Warren (Eds.), *Speech and language development and intervention in down syndrome & fragile X syndrome* (pp. 53–76). Baltimore: Paul H. Brookes.

Stevens, S., Dudek, J., Nash, K., Koren, G., & Rovet, J. (2015). Social perspective taking and empathy in children with fetal alcohol spectrum disorders. *Journal of the International Neuropsychological Society, 21*, 74–84. doi: 10.1017/S1355617714001088.

Stores, R. (1993). Sleep problems in children with Down syndrome: A summary report. *Down Syndrome Research and Practice, 1*, 72–74.

Tassé, M., & Havercamp, S. (2006). The role of motivation and psychopathology in understanding the IQ–adaptive behavior discrepancy. *International Review of Research in Mental Retardation 31*, 231–259.

Taylor, R., & Kaufmann, S. (1991). Trends in classification usage in the mental retardation literature. *Mental Retardation, 29*, 367–371.

Thorne, J., & Coggins, T. (2008). A diagnostically promising technique for tallying nominal reference errors in the narratives of school-aged children with foetal alcohol spectrum disorders (FASD). *International Journal of*

Language and Communication Disorders, 43, 570–594. doi: 10.1080/13682820701698960.

Thorne, J., Coggins, T., Olson, H., & Astley, S. (2007). Exploring the utility of narrative analysis in diagnostic decision making: Picture-bound reference, elaboration, and fetal alcohol spectrum disorders. *Journal of Speech, Language, and Hearing Research, 50*, 459–474.

Timler, G., Olswang, L., & Coggins, T. (2005a). "Do I know what I need to do?" A social communication intervention for children with complex clinical profiles. *Language, Speech, and Hearing Services in Schools, 36*, 73–85.

Timler, G., Olswang, L., & Coggins, T. (2005b). Social communication interventions for preschoolers: Targeting peer interactions during peer group entry and cooperative play. *Seminars in Speech and Language, 26*, 170–180. doi: 10.1055/s-2005-917122.

Van Borsel, J., Defloor, T., & Curfs, L. (2007). Expressive language in persons with Prader-Willi syndrome. *Genetic Counseling, 18*, 17–28.

Van Borsel, J., Dor, O., & Rondal, J. (2008). Speech fluency in fragile X syndrome. *Clinical Linguistics and Phonetics, 22*, 1–11. doi: 10.1080/02699200701601997.

van der Schuit, M., Segers, E., van Balkom, H., Stoep, J., & Verhoeven, L. (2010). Immersive communication intervention for speaking and non-speaking children with intellectual disabilities. *AAC: Augmentative and Alternative Communication, 26*, 203–218. doi: 10.3109/07434618.2010.505609.

Voss, K. (2006). *Teaching by design*. Bethesda, MD: Woodbine House.

Wechsler, D. (2014). *Wechsler Intelligence Scale for Children—Fifth Edition*. San Antonio, TX: Pearson.

Williams, C. (2005). Neurological aspects of the Angelman syndrome. *Brain and Development, 27*, 88–94. doi: 10.1016/j.braindev.2003.09.014.

Williams, C., Peters, S., & Calculator, S. (2009). Facts About Angelman Syndrome. Retrieved December 3, 2015, from http://www.angelman.org/wp-content/uploads/2015/11/facts_about_as_2009_3-19-10.pdf.

Wyper, K., & Rasmussen, C. (2011). Language impairments in children with fetal alcohol spectrum disorder. *Journal of Population Therapeutics and Clinical Pharmacology, 18*, e364–e376.

Yoder, P., Woynaroski, T., Fey, M., & Warren, S. (2014). Effects of dose frequency of early communication intervention in young children with and without Down syndrome. *American Journal on Intellectual and Developmental Disabilities, 119*, 17–32. doi: 10.1352/1944-7558-119.1.17.

Zigler, E., & Balla, D. (1982). Introduction: The developmental approach to mental retardation. In E. Zigler & D. Balla (Eds.), *Mental retardation: The developmental–difference controversy* (pp. 3–8). Hillsdale, NJ: Erlbaum.

Zigler, E., & Hodapp, R. (1986). *Understanding mental retardation*. New York: Cambridge University Press.

Zigler, E., & Hodapp, R. (1991). Behavioral functioning in individuals with mental retardation. *Annual Review of Psychology, 42*, 29–50.

Zurawski, L. (2014). Speech-language pathologists and inclusive service delivery: What are the first steps? *SIG 16 Perspectives on School-Based Issues, 15*, 5–14. doi: 10.1044/sbi15.1.5.

Chapter 7

American Psychiatric Association (APA). (2013). *Diagnostic and statistical manual of mental disorder* (5th ed.). Arlington, VA: Author.

Autism Speaks. (2016). DSM-5 Diagnostic Criteria. From https://www.autismspeaks.org/what-autism/diagnosis/dsm-5-diagnostic-criteria.

Bailey, H. (2006). Rapid word learning in preverbal children with autism. *Dissertation Abstracts International, DAI-B 66/08*, 157. (UMI No. 3187386).

Baldwin, D. (1991). Infant's contribution to the achievement of joint reference. *Child Development, 62*, 875–890.

Baldwin, D., & Moses, L. (2001). Links between social understanding and early word learning: Challenges to current account. *Social Development, 10*, 309–329.

Ballaban-Gil, K., & Tuchman, R. (2000). Epilepsy and epileptiform EEG: Association with autism and language disorders. *Mental Retardation and Developmental Disabilities Research Reviews, 6*, 300–308.

Baranek, G. (1999). Autism during infancy: A retrospective video analysis of sensory-motor and social behaviors at 9-12 months of age. *Journal of Autism and Developmental Disorders, 29*, 213–224.

Baranek, G. (2002). Efficacy of sensory and motor interventions for children with autism. *Journal of Autism and Developmental Disorders, 32*, 397–422. doi: 10.1023/A:1020541906063.

Baron-Cohen, S., Allen, J., & Gilberg, C. (1992). Can autism be detected at 18 months? The needle, the haystack, and the CHAT. *British Journal of Psychiatry, 161*, 839–843.

Baron-Cohen, S., Leslie, A., & Frith, U. (2007). Does the autistic child have a 'theory of mind'? In B. Gertler & L. Shapiro (Eds.), *Arguing about the mind* (pp. 310–318). New York: Routledge.

Baron-Cohen, S., Wheelwright, S., Cox, A., Baird, G., Charman, T., Swettenham, J., . . . Doehring, P. (2000). Early identification of autism: The CHecklist for Autism in Toddlers (CHAT). *Journal of the Royal Society of Medicine, 93*, 521–525.

Bass, J. D., & Mulick, J. (2007). Social play skills enhancement of children with autism usign peers and siblings as therapists. *Psychology in the Schools, 44*, 727–735.

Beukelman, D., & Mirenda, P. (2005). *Augmentative and alternative communication: Supporting children and adults with complex communication needs* (3rd ed.). Baltimore: Paul H. Brookes.

Bonneh, Y. S., Levanon, Y., Dean-Pardo, O., Lossos, L., & Adini, Y. (2011). Abnormal speech spectrum and increased pitch variability in young autistic children. *Frontiers in Human Neuroscience, 4*, 237. doi: 10.3389/fnhum.2010.00237.

Boutot, E., & Myles, B. (2011). *Autism spectrum disorders: Foundations, characteristics, and effective strategies*. Upper Saddle River, NJ: Pearson Education.

Bryson, S. E., Bradley, E. A., Thompson, A., & Wainwright, A. (2008). Prevalence of autism among adolescents with intellectual disabilities. *Canadian Journal of Psychiatry. Revue Canadienne De Psychiatrie, 53*, 449–459.

Buffington, D., Krantz, P., McClannahan, L., & Poulson, C. (1998). Procedures for teaching appropriate gestural communication skills to children with autism. *Journal of Autism and Developmental Disorders, 28*, 535–545.

Bundy, A., Lane, S., & Murray, E. (2002). *Sensory integration: Theory and practice* (2nd ed.). Philadelpha, PA: F.A. Davis Company.

Buschbacher, P., & Fox, L. (2003). Understanding and intervening with the challenging behavior of young children with autism spectrum disorder. *Language, Speech, and Hearing Services in Schools, 34*, 217–227.

Calculator, S. (1999). Look who's pointing now: Cautions related to the clinical use of facilitated communication. *Language, Speech, and Hearing Services in Schools, 30*, 408–414.

CDC. (2014). Autism Spectrum Disorders (ASD): Data and Statistics. Retrieved February 12, 2016, from http://www.cdc.gov/ncbddd/autism/data.html.

Cleland, J., Gibbons, F., Peppé, S., O'Hare, A., & Rutherford, M. (2010). Phonetic and phonological errors in children with high functioning autism and Asperger syndrome. *International Journal of Speech-Language Pathology, 12*, 69–76.

Clifford, S., & Dissanayake, C. (2008). The early development of joint attention in infants with autistic disorder using home video observations and parental interview. *Journal of Autism and Developmental Disorders, 38*, 791–805.

Coggins, T., & Frederickson, R. (1988). The communicative role of a highly frequent repeated utterance in the conversations of an autistic boy. *Journal of Autism and Developmental Disorders, 18*, 687–694.

Courchesne, E., Karns, C. M., Davis, H. R., Ziccardi, R., Carper, R. A., Tigue, Z. D., . . . Courchesne, R. Y. (2001). Unusual brain growth patterns in early life in patients with autistic disorder: An MRI study. *Neurology, 57*, 245–254.

Cowan, R., & Allen, K. (2007). Using naturalistic procedures to enhance learning in individuals with autism: A focus on generalized teaching within the school setting. *Psychology in the Schools, 44*, 701–715.

Crais, E., Watson, L., Baranek, G., & Reznick, J. (2006). Early identification of autism: How early can we go? *Seminars in Speech and Language, 27*, 143–160.

Curcio, F., & Paccia, J. (1987). Conversations with autistic children: Contingent relationships between features of adult input and children's response adequacy. *Journal of Autism and Developmental Disorders, 17*, 81–93.

Dahl, E., Cohen, D., & Provence, S. (1986). Clinical and multivariate approaches to the nosology of pervasive developmental disorders. *Journal of the American Academy of Child Psychiatry, 25*, 170–180.

Dawson, G., Hill, D., Spencer, A., Galpert, L., & Watson, L. (1990). Affective exchanges between young autistic children and their mothers. *Journal of Abnormal Child Psychology, 18*, 335–345.

Dewey, D., Dentell, M., & Crawford, S. (2007). Motor and gestural performance in children with autistic spectrum disorders, developmental coordination disorder, and/or attention deficit hyperactive disorder. *Journal of the International Neuropsychological Society, 13*, 246–256.

Dobbinson, S., Perkins, M., & Boucher, J. (2003). The interactional significance of formulas in autistic language. *Clinical Linguistics and Phonetics, 17*, 299–307.

Dyer, K., Williams, L., & Luce, S. (1991). Training teachers to use naturalistic communication strategies in classrooms for students with autism and other severe handicaps. *Language, Speech, and Hearing Services in Schools, 22*, 313–321.

Edelson, M. G. (2006). Are the majority of children with autism mentally retarded: A systematic evaluation of the data. *Focus on Autism and Other Developmental Disabilities, 21*, 66–83.

Eikeseth, S., Smith, T., Jahr, E., & Eldevik, S. (2002). Intensive behavioral treatment at school for 4- to 7-year-old children with autism: A 1-year comparison controlled study. *Behavior Modification, 26*, 49–68.

El Achkar, C., & Spence, S. (2015). Clinical characteristics of children and young adults with co-occurring autism spectrum disorder and epilepsy. *Epilepsy and Behavior, 47*, 183–190.

Erba, H. (2000). Early intervention programs for children with autism: Conceptual frameworks for implementation. *American Journal of Orhopsychiatry, 70*, 82–94.

Gallaudet Research Institute. (2011). Regional and national summary report of data from the 2009-2010 annual survey of deaf and hard of hearing children and youth. Washington, DC: GRI, Gallaudet University.

Gerrans, P. (2009). Imitation and theory of mind. *Handbook of neuroscience for the behavioral sciences* (vol. VI, pp. 905– 922). New York: Wiley.

Gilliam, J. (2014). *Gilliam autism rating scale* (3rd ed.). Austin, TX: PRO-ED.

Gonzalez-Lopez, A., & Kamps, D. (1997). Social skills training to increase social interactions between children with autism and their typical peers. *Focus on Autism and Other Developmental Disabilities, 12*, 2–14.

Gordon, R., & Barker, J. (2007). Autism and the 'theory of mind' debate. In B. Gertler & L. Shapiro (Eds.), *Arguing about the mind* (pp. 319–332). New York: Routledge.

Grecucci, A., Brambilla, P., Siugzdaite, R., Londero, D., Fabbro, F., & Rumiati, R. (2013). Emotional resonance deficits in autistic children. *Journal of Autism and Developmental Disorders, 43*, 616–628.

Greenspan, S. (1992). *Infancy and early childhood: The practice of clinical assessment and intervention with emotional and developmental challenges*. Madison, CT: International Universities Press.

Greenspan, S., & Wieder, S. (2006). *Engaging autism: Using the floortime approach to help children relate, communicate, and think*. Philadelphia: Da Capo Press.

Ha, S., Sohn, I., Kim, N., Hyeon, J., & Cheon, K. (2015). Characteristics of brains in autism spectrum disorder: Structure, function and connectivity across the lifespan. *Experimental Neurobiology, 24*, 273—284.

Hobson, R., Lee, A., & Hobson, J. (2010). Personal pronouns and communicative engagement in autism. *Journal of Autism and Developmental Disorders, 40*, 653–664.

Hughes, J. (2008). A review of recent reports on autism: 1000 studies published in 2007. *Epilepsy and Behavior, 13*, 425–437.

Hurwitz, S., & Yirmiiya, N. (2014). Autism diagnostic observation schedule (ADOS) and its uses in research and practice. In V. B. Patel, V. R. Preedy & C. R. Martin (Eds.), *Comprehensive guide to autism* (pp. 345–353). New York: Springer.

Jawaid, A., Riby, D. M., Owens, J., White, S., Tarar, T., & Schulz, P. (2012). 'Too withdrawn' or 'too friendly': Considering social vulnerability in two neuro-developmental disorders. *Journal of Intellectual Disability Research, 56*, 335–350.

Johnson, C., Myers, S., & Councils on Children with Disabilities. (2007). Idenfication and evaluation of children with autistic spectrum disorders. *Pediatrics, 120*, 1183–1215.

Jones, C. D., & Schwartz, I. S. (2004). Siblings, peers and adults: Differential effects of models for children with autism. *Topics in Early Childhood Special Education, 24*, 187–198.

Kanner, L. (1943). Autistic disturbances of affective contact. *Nervous Child, 2*, 217–250.

Kasari, C., Freeman, S., & Paparella, T. (2006). Joint attention and symbolic play in young children with autism: A randomized controlled intervention study. *Journal of Child Psychology and Psychiatry, 47*, 611–620.

Kazdin, A. (1993). Replication and extension of behavioral treatment of autistic disorder. *American Journal of Mental Retardation, 97*, 377–379.

Key, A., Ibanex, L., Henderson, H., Warren, Z., Messinger, D., & Stone, W. L. (2015). Positive affect processing and joing attention in infants at high risk for autism: An exploratory study. *Journal of Autism and Developmental Disorders, 45*, 4051–4062. doi: 10.1007/s10803-014-2191-x.

Kiln, A. (1991). Young autistic children's listening preferences in regard to speech: A possible characterization of the symptom of social withdrawal. *Journal of Autism and Developmental Disorders, 21*, 29–42.

Koegel, L., Koegel, R., Frea, W., & Green-Hopkins, I. (2003). Priming as a method of coordinating educational services for students with autism. *Language, Speech, and Hearing Services in Schools, 34*, 228–235.

Kuo, H., Orsmond, B., Coster, W., & Cohn, E. (2014). Media use among adolscents with autism spectrum disorder. *Autism, 18*, 914–923.

Landa, R., & Holman, K. C. (2005). The effects of targeting interpersonal synchrony on social and communication development in toddlers with autism. Paper presented at the Annual Collaborative Programs Excellence in Autism/Studies to Advance Autism Research and Treatment Meeting, Washington, DC.

Lang, R., O'Reilly, M., Sigafoos, J., Lancioni, G., Machalicek, W., Rispoli, M., & White, P. (2009). Enhancing the effectiveness of a play intervention by abolishing the reinforcing value of stereotypy: A pilot study. *Journal of Applied Behavior Analysis, 42*, 889–894.

Lathe, R. (2006). *Autism, brain, and environment*. Philadelphia: Jessica Kingsley Publishers.

Levy, S. E., Giarelli, E., Lee, L. C., Schieve, L. A., Kirby, R. S., Cunniff, C., . . . Rice, C. E. (2010). Autism spectrum disorder and co-occuring developmental, psychiatric, and medical conditions among children in multiple populations of the United States. *Journal of Developmental and Behavioral Pediatrics, 31*, 267–275.

Lewis, M. (2004). Environmental complexity and central nervous system development and function. *Mental Retardation and Developmental Disabilities Research Reviews, 10*, 91–5.

Lord, C., Rutter, M., DiLavore, P. C., Risi, S., Gotham, K., & Bishop, S. (2012). *Autism Dianostice Observation Schedule, (ADOS-2)* (2nd ed.). Torrance, CA: Western Psychological Services.

Lord, C., & Volkmar, F. (2002). Genetics of childhood disorders: XLII. Autism, Part 1: Diagnosis and assessment in autistic spectrum disorders. *Journal of the American Academy of Child and Adolescent Psychiatry, 41*, 1134–1136.

Lovaas, O. (1987). Behavioral treatment and normal educational and intellectural functioning in young autistic children. *Journal of Consulting and Clinical Psychology, 55*, 3–9.

Lovaas, O., Schaeffer, B., & Simmons, J. (1965). Building social behavior in autistic children by use of electric shock. *Journal of Experimental Research in Personality, 1*, 99–109.

Matson, J., & LoVullo, S. (2008). A review of behavioral treatments for self-injurious behaviors of persons with autism spectrum disorders. *Behavior Modification, 32*, 61–76.

Matson, J., & Nebel-Schwalm, M. (2007). Assessing challenging behaviors in children with autism spectrum disorders: A review. *Research in Developmental Disabilities, 28*, 567–579.

Matson, J., & Shoemaker, M. (2009). Intellectual disability and its relationship to autism spectrum disorders. *Research in Developmental Disabilities, 30*, 1107–1114.

McEachin, J., Smith, T., & Lovaas, O. (1993). Long-term outcome for children with autism who received early intensive treatment. *American Journal of Mental Retardation, 97*, 359–372.

McLean, J. (1992). Facilitated communication: Some thoughts of Biklen's and Caclulator's interaction. *American Journal of Speech-Language Pathology, 1*, 25–27.

Metz, B., Mulick, J., & Butter, E. (2005). Autism: A late 20th-Century fad magnet. In J. W. Jacobson, R. M. Foxx & J. A. Mulick (Eds.), *Controversial therapies for developmental disabilities: Fad, fashion, and science in professional practice* (pp. 237–263). Mahwah, NJ: Lawrence Erlbaum Associates.

Minshew, N. J., & Keller, T. A. (2010). The nature of brian dysfunction in autism: Functional brain imaging studies. *Current Opinion in Neurology, 23*, 124–130.

Mullegama, S., Alaimo, J., Chen, L., & Elsea, S. (2015). Phenotypic and molecular convergence of 2q23.1 deletion syndrome with other neurodevelopmental syndromes associated with autism spectrum disorder. *International Journal of Molecular Sciences, 16*, 7627-7643.

Myers, S., Johnson, C., & Councils on Children with Disabilities. (2007). Management of children with autism spectrum disorders. *Pediatrics, 120*, 1162–1182.

Myles, B. S., Trautman, M., & Schelvan, R. L. (2004). *The hidden curriculum: Practical solutions for understanding unstated rules in social situations*. Shawnee Mission, KS: Autism Asperger Publishing Company.

O'Reilly, M., Rispoli, M., Davis, T., Machalicek, W., Lang, R., Sigafoos, J., . . . Didden, R. (2010). Functional analysis of challenging behavior in children with autism spectrum disorders: A summary of 10 cases. *Research in Autism Spectrum Disorders, 4*, 1–10.

Oberman, L., Hubbard, E., McCleery, J., Altschuler, E., Ramachandran, V., & Pineda, J. (2005). EEG evidence for mirror neuron dysfunction in autism. *Cognitive Brain Research, 24*, 190–198.

Odom, S., Boyd, B., Hall, L., & Hume, K. (2010). Evaluationof comprehensive treatment models for individuals with autism spectrum disorders. *Journal of Autism and Developmental Disorders, 40*, 425–436.

Odom, S., & Watts, E. (1991). Reducing teacher prompts in peer-mediated interventions for young children with autism. *Journal of Special Education, 25*, 26–43.

Ogletree, B., Oren, T., & Fischer, M. (2007). Examining effective intervention practices for communication impairment in autism spectrum disorder. *Exceptionality, 15*, 233–247.

Oller, J., & Oller, S. (2010). *Autism: The diagnosis, treatment, and etiology of the undeniable epidemic*. Burlington, MA: Jones and Bartlett Learning.

Paul, R., Augustyn, A., Klin, A., & Volkmar, F. (2005). Perception and production of prosody by speakers with autism spectrum disorders. *Journal of Autism and Developmental Disorders, 35*, 205–220.

Prelock, P. (2006). *Autism spectrum disorders: Issues in assessment and intervention*. Austin, TX: PRO-ED.

Prelock, P., & Contompasis, S. (2006). Autism and related disorders: Trends in diagnosis and neurobiologic considerations. In P. A. Prelock (Ed.), *Autism spectrum disorders: Issues in assessment and intervention* (pp. 3–63). Austin, TX: PRO-ED.

Prizant, B., Schuler, A., Wetherby, A., & Rydell, P. (1997). Enhancing language and communication development: Language approaches. In D. Cohen & F. Volkmar (Eds.), *Handbook of autism and pervasive developmental disorders* (2nd ed., pp. 572–605). New York: Wiley.

Reed, F., & Reed, D. (2015). Autism service delivery: Bridging the gap between science and practice. In F. Reed & D. Reed (Eds.), *Autism and child psychopathology series*. New York: Springer.

Reichow, B. (2012). Overview of meta-analyses on early intensive behavioral intervention for young children with autism spectrum disorders. *Journal of Autism and Developmental Disorders, 42*, 512–520.

Robins, D., Fein, D., Barton, M., & Green, J. (2001). The modified checklist for autism in toddlers: An initial study investigating the early detection of autism and pervasive developmental disorders. *Journal of Autism and Developmental Disorders, 31*, 131–144.

Rogers, S. (2000). Interventions that facilitate socialization in children with autism. *Journal of Autism and Developmental Disorders, 30*, 399–409.

Rosenberg, R., Mandell, D., Farmer, J., Law, J., Marvin, A., & Law, P. (2010). Psychotropic medication use among children with autism spectrum disorders enrolled in a national registry, 2007-2008. *Journal of Autism and Developmental Disorders, 40*, 342–351.

Rutherford, M., Baron-Cohen, S., & Wheelwright, S. (2002). Reading the mind in the voice: A study with normal adults and adults with Aspergers syndrome and high functioning autism. *Journal of Autism and Developmental Disorders, 32*, 189–194.

Schopler, E., Short, A., & Mesibov, G. (1989). Relation of behavioral treatment to "normal functioning:" Comment on Lovaas. *Journal of Consulting and Clinical Psychology, 57*, 162–164.

Schopler, E., Van Bourgondien, M., Wellman, G., & Love, S. (2010). *Childhood Autism Rating Scale* (2nd ed.). Austin, TX: PRO-ED.

Shavelle, R., Strauss, D., & Pickett, J. (2001). Causes of death in autism. *Journal of Autism and Developmental Disorders, 31*, 569–576.

Shriberg, L., Paul, R., McSweeny, J., Klin, A., Cohen, D., & Volkmar, F. (2001). Speech and prosody characteristics of adolescents and adults with high-functioning autism and Aspergers syndrome. *Journal of Speech, Language, and Hearing Research, 44*, 1097–1115.

Siegel, B., Vukicevic, J., Elliot, G., & Kraemer, H. (1989). The use of signal detection theory to assess DSM-III-R criteria for autistic disorder. *Journal of the American Academy of Child and Adolescent Psychiatry, 28*, 542–548.

Sillman, E., Diehl, S., Bahr, R., Hnath-Chisolm, T., Zenko, C., & Friedman, S. (2003). A new look at performance on theory-of-mind tasks by adolescents with autism spectrum disorder. *Language, Speech, and Hearing Services in Schools, 34*, 236–252.

Simon, N. (1975). Echolalic speech in childhood autism. *Archives of General Psychiatry, 32*, 1439–1446.

Simpson, R. L. (2001). ABA and students with autism spectrum disorders: Issues and consideration for effective practice. *Focus on Autism and Other Developmental Disabilities, 1*, 68–71.

Smith, T. (2013). What is evidence-based behavior analysis? *The Behavior Analyst, 36*, 7–33.

Smith, T., Klorman, R., & Mruzek, D. (2015). Predicting outcome of community-based early intensive behavioral intervention for children with autism. *Journal of Abnormal Child Psychology, 43*, 1271–1282.

Spengler, S., Bird, G., & Brass, M. (2010). Hyperimitation of actions is related to reduced understanding of others' minds in autism spectrum conditions *Biological Psychiatry, 68*, 1148–1155.

Stahmer, A. (1999). Using pivotal response training to faciliate appropriate play in children with austistic spectrum disorders. *Child Language Teaching and Therapy, 15*, 29–40.

Sterponi, L., & Shankey, J. (2014). Rethinking echolalia: Repetition as interactional resource in the communication of a child with autism. *Journal of Child Language, 42*, 275–304.

Stiegler, L. (2015). Examining the echolalia literature: Where do speech-language pathoologists stand? *American Journal of Speech-Language Pathology, 24*, 750–762.

Stockbridge, M. D., Happe, F. G., & White, S. (2014). Impaired comprehension of alternating syntactic construction in autism. *Autism Research, 7*, 314–321.

Stothers, M. E., & Cardy, J. O. (2012). Oral language impairments in developmental disorders characterized by language strengths: A comparison of Asperger syndrome and nonverbal learning disabilities. *Research in Autism Spectrum Disorders, 6*, 519–534.

Surén, P., Roth, C., Bresnahan, M., Haugen, M., Hornig, M., Hirtz, D., . . . Stoltenberg, C. (2013). Association between maternal use of folic acid supplements and risk of autism spectrum disorders in children *Journal of the American Medical Association, 309*, 570–577.

Tager-Flusberg, H., Paul, R., & Lord, C. (2005). Language and communication in autism. In F. Volkmar, R. Paul, A. Kiln & D. Cohen (Eds.), *Handbook of autism and pervasive developmental disorder* (3rd ed., vol. 1, pp. 335–364). New York: Wiley.

Tonge, B. (2002). Autism, autistic spectrum and teh need for better definition. *Medical Journal of Australia, 176*, 412–413.

Trevarthen, C., & Daniel, S. (2005). Disorganized rhythm and synchrony: Early signs of autism and Rett syndrome. *Brain Development, 27*, S25–S34.

Van der Paelt, S., Warreyn, P., & Roeyers, H. (2014). Social-communicative abilities and language in preschoolers with autism spectrum disorders: Associations differ depending on language age. *Research in Autism Spectrum Disorders, 8*, 518–528.

Volden, J., Magill-Evans, J., Goulden, K., & Clarke, M. (2007). Varying language register according to listener needs in speakers with autism spectrum disorders. *Journal of Autism and Developmental Disorders, 37*, 1139–1154.

Volden, J., & Sorenson, A. (2009). Bossy and nice requests: Varying language register in speakers with autism spectrum disorder (ASD). *Journal of Communication Disorders, 42*, 58–73.

Volkmar, F., & Wiesner, L. (2004). *Health care for children on the autism spectrum: A guide to medical, nuritional, and behavioral issues*. Bethesda, MD: Woodbine House.

Williams, G., Donley, C., & Keller, J. (2000). Teaching children with autism to ask questions about hidden objects. *Journal of Applied Behavior Analysis, 33*, 627–630.

Wong, C., Odom, S., Hume, K., Cox, A. W., Fettig, A., Kucharczyk, S., . . . Schultz, T. (2015). Evidence-based practices for children, youth, and young adults with autism spectrum disorder: A comprehensive review. *Journal of Autism and Developmental Disorders, 45*, 1951–1966.

Woods, J., & Wetherby, A. (2003). Early identification of and intervention for infants and toddlers who are at risk for autism spectrum disorder. *Language, Speech, and Hearing Services in Schools, 34*, 180–193.

Wray, A., & Perkins, M. (2000). The functions of formulaic language: An integrated model. *Language and Communication, 20*, 1–28.

Yuen, R. K., Thiruvahindrapuram, B., Merico, D., Walker, S., Tammimies, K., Hoang, N., . . . Scherer, S. W. (2015). Whole-genome sequencing of quartet families with autism spectrum disorder. *Nature Medicine, 21*, 185–191.

Zane, T., Carlson, M., Estep, D., & Quinn, M. (2014). Using functional assessment to treat behavior problems of deaf and hard of hearing children diagnosed with autism spectrum disorder. *American Annals of the Deaf, 158*, 555–566.

Zane, T., Davis, C., & Rosswurm, M. (2008). The cost of fad treatments in autism. *Journal of Early and Intensive Behavior Intervention, 5*, 44–51.

Chapter 8

Akdogan, O., Selcuk, A., Ozcan, I., & Dere, H. (2008). Vestibular nerve functions in children with auditory neuropathy. *International Journal of Pediatric Otorhinolaryngology, 72*, 415–419.

American Academy of Audiology. (2003). Pediatric amplification protocol. Retrieved September 21, 2009, from http://www.audiology.org/resources/documentlibrary/Documents/pedamp.pdf

American Academy of Audiology. (2004). Pediatric amplification guidelines. *Audiology Today, 16*, 46–53.

American Speech-Language-Hearing Association (ASHA). (1996). Taskforce on Central Auditory Processing Consensus Development: Central auditory processing: Current status of research and implications for clinical practice. *American Journal of Audiology, 5*, 41–54.

American Speech-Language-Hearing Association (ASHA). (2005). (Central) auditory processing disorders [Technical report]. Rockville, MD: Author.

Anderson, K. L. (2004). The problem of classroom acoustics: The typical classroom soundscape barrier to learning. *Seminars in Hearing, 25*, 117–129.

Anita, S. D., Reed, S., & Kreimeyer, K. H. (2005). Written language of deaf and hard-of-hearing students in public schools. *Journal of Deaf Studies and Deaf Education, 10*, 244–255.

Archbold, S. M., Nikolopoulous, T. P., & O'Donoghue, G. M. (2006, March). *Reading ability after cochlear implantation: The effect of age of implantation*. Paper presented at the European Society for Pediatric Cochlear Implantation, Venice, Italy.

Beauchaine, K. L., Barlow, N. L., & Stelmachowicz, P. G. (1990). Special considerations in amplification for young children. *ASHA, 32*, 44–46.

Bellis, T. J. (2003). *Assessment and management of central auditory processing disorders in the educational setting: From science to practice* (2nd ed.). New York: Thomson Delmar Learning.

Bellis, T. J. (2006). Interpretation of APD test results. In T. K. Parthasarathy (Ed.), *An introduction to auditory processing disorders in children* (pp. 145–160). Mahwah, NJ: Lawrence Erlbaum Associates.

Bellis, T. J. (2014). The nature of central auditory processing disorders. In F. E. Musiek & G. D. Chermak (Eds.), *Handbook of central auditory processing disorders: Auditory neuroscience and diagnosis* (2nd ed., Vol. 1). San Diego, CA: Plural Publishing.

Belzner, K., & Seal, B. (2009). Children with cochlear implants: A review of demographics and communication outcomes. *American Annals of the Deaf, 154*, 311–333.

Berg, A. L., Spitzer, J. B., Towers, H. M., Bartosiewicz, C., & Diamond, B. E. (2005). Newborn hearing screening in the NICU: Profile of failed auditory brainstem response/passed otoacoustic emission. *Pediatrics, 116*, 933–938.

Berg, F. S. (1987). *Facilitating classroom listening: A handbook for teachers of normal and hard-of-hearing students*. Boston, MA: College-Hill Press/Little Brown.

Berlin, C. (2000). Managing patients with auditory neuropathy/auditory dyssynchrony. Retrieved July 17, 2003, from www.medschool.lsumc.edu/otor/dys.htm

Berlin, C., Bordelon, J., St. John, P., Wilensky, D., Hurley, A., Kluka, E., & Hood, L. (1998). Reversing click polarity may uncover neuropathy in infants. *Ear and Hearing, 19*, 37–47.

Berlin, C., Hood, L., Morlet, T., Rose, K., & Brashears, S. (2002). Auditory neuropathy/dyssynchrony: After diagnosis, then what? *Seminars in Hearing, 23*, 209–214.

Berlin, C., Hood, L., & Rose, K. (2001). On renaming auditory neuropathy as auditory dys-synchrony. *Audiology Today, 13*, 15–17.

Berlin, C., Morlet, T., & Hood, L. (2003). Auditory neuropathy/dyssynchrony: Its diagnosis and management. *Pediatric Clinical of North America, 50*, 331–340.

Bess, F. H., Klee, T., & Culbertson, J. L. (1986). Identification, assessment and management of children with unilateral sensorineural hearing loss. *Ear and Hearing, 7*, 43–51.

Bess, F. H., & Tharpe, A. M. (1988). Performance and management of children with unilateral sensorineural hearing loss. *Scandinavian Audiology Supplement, 30*, 75–79.

Blamey, P., Sarant, J., Paatsch, L. E., Barry, J. G., Bow, C. P., Wales, R. J., . . . Tooher, R. (2001). Relationships among speech perception, production, language, hearing loss, and age in children with impaired hearing. *Journal of Speech, Language, and Hearing Research, 44*, 246–285.

Boothroyd, A. (1982). *Hearing impairments in young children*. Englewood Cliffs, NJ: Prentice Hall.

Boothroyd, A. (1984). Auditory perception of speech contrasts by subjects with sensorineural hearing loss. *Journal of Speech and Hearing Research, 27*, 134–144.

Brannon, J. (1968). Linguistic word classes in the spoken language of normal, hard-of-hearing, and deaf children. *Journal of Speech and Hearing Research, 11*, 279–287.

Breier, J., Fletcher, J., Foorman, B., Klaas, P., & Gray, L. (2003). Auditory temporal processing in children with specific reading disability with and without attention deficit/hyperactivity disorder. *Journal of Speech, Language, and Hearing Research, 46*, 31–42.

Brenta, B., Kricos, P., & Lasky, E. (1981). Comprehension and production of basic semantic concepts by older hearing impaired children. *Journal of Speech and Hearing Research, 24*, 414–419.

Brill, R. G., MacNeil, B., & Newman, L. R. (1986). Framework for appropriate programs for deaf children: Conference of educational administrators serving the deaf. *American Annals of the Deaf, 131*, 65–77.

Brown, J. (1984). Examination of grammatical morphemes in the language of hard-of-hearing children. *Volta Review, 86*, 229–238.

Cacace, A. T., & McFarland, D. J. (1998). Central auditory processing disorder in school–aged children: A critical review. *Journal of Speech, Language, and Hearing Research, 41*, 355–373.

Cacace, A. T., & McFarland, D. J. (2005). The importance of modality specificity in diagnosing central auditory processing disorder. *American Journal of Audiology, 14*, 112–123.

Cacace, A. T., & McFarland, D. J. (2006). Delineating auditory processing disorder (APD) and attention deficit hyperactivity disorder (ADHD): A conceptual, theoretical, and practical framework. In T. K. Parthasarathy (Ed.), *An introduction to auditory processing disorders in children* (pp. 39–61). Mahwah, NJ: Lawrence Erlbaum Associates.

Carrow-Woolfolk, E. (1999). *Comprehensive assessment of spoken language (CASL)*. Circle Pines, MN: American Guidance Services.

Centers for Disease Control and Prevention. (2010). Identifying infants with hearing loss—United States, 1999–2007. *Morbidity and Mortality Weekly Report, 59*, 220–223.

Chermak, G., & Musiek, F. (1997). *Central auditory processing disorders: New perspectives*. San Diego, CA: Singular.

Clarkson, R., Eimas, P., & Marean, G. (1989). Speech perception in children with histories of recurrent otitis media. *Journal of the Acoustical Society of America, 85*, 926–933.

Cognitive Concepts Inc. (1998). *Earobics auditory development and phonics program step 2*. Evanston, IL: Author.

Cognitive Concepts Inc. (2000a). *Earobics step 1*. Evanston, IL: Hougton Mifflin.

Cognitive Concepts Inc. (2000b). *Earobics step 2*. Evanston, IL: Houghton Mifflin.

Cohen, W., Hodson, A., O'Hare, A., Boyle, J., Durrani, T., McCartney, E., . . . Watson, J. (2005). Effects of computer-based intervention through acoustically modified speech (Fast ForWord) in severe mixed receptive-expressive language impairment: Outcomes from a randomized controlled trial. *Journal of Speech, Language, and Hearing Research, 48*, 715–729.

Cole, E., & Paterson, M. (1984). Assessment and treatment of phonologic disorders in the hearing impaired. In J. Costello (Ed.), *Speech disorders in children: Recent advances*. San Diego, CA: College-Hill Press.

Cone-Wesson, B., Rance, G., & Sininger, Y. S. (2001). Amplification and rehabilitation strategies for patients with auditory neuropathy. In Y. S. Sininger & A. Starr (Eds.), *Auditory neuropathy* (pp. 233–250). San Diego, CA: Singular

Connor, C. M., Craig, H., Raudenbush, S. W., Heavner, K., & Zwolan, T. A. (2006). The age at which young deaf children receive their cochlear implants and their vocabulary and speech-production growth. Is there an added value for early implantation? *Ear and Hearing, 27*, 628–644.

Connor, C. M., & Zwolan, T. A. (2004). Examining multiple sources of influence on the reading comprehension skills of children who use cochlear implants. *Journal of Speech, Language, and Hearing Research, 47*, 509–526.

Cornett, R. (1985). Diagnostic factors bearing on the use of cued speech with hearing impaired children. *Ear and Hearing, 6*, 33–35.

Cross, T., Johnson-Morris, J., & Nienhuys, T. (1980). Linguistic feedback and maternal speech: Comparison of mothers addressing hearing and hearing-impaired children. *First Language, 1*, 163–189.

Cunningham, M., Cox, E. O., & The Committee on Practice and Ambulatory Medicine: The Section on Otolaryngology and Brochoesophagology (2003). Hearing assessment in infant and children: Recommendations beyond neonatal screening. *Pediatrics, 111*, 436–440.

Curtiss, S., Prutting, C., & Lowell, E. (1979). Pragmatic and semantic development in young children with impaired hearing. *Journal of Speech and Hearing Research, 22*, 534–552.

Davis, J. (1974). Performance of young hearing impaired children on a test of basic concepts. *Journal of Speech and Hearing Research, 17*, 342–351.

Davis, J. (1990). *Our forgotten children: Hard-of-hearing pupils in the schools* (2nd ed.). Washington, DC: Self-Help for the Hard-of-Hearing.

Davis, J., & Blasdell, R. (1975). Perceptual strategies employed by normal hearing and hearing-impaired children in the comprehension of sentences containing relative clauses. *Journal of Speech and Hearing Research, 18*, 281–295.

Davis, J., Elfenbein, J., Schum, R., & Bentler, R. (1986). Effects of mild and moderate hearing impairments on language, educational and psychosocial behaviour of children. *Journal of Speech and Hearing Disorders, 51*, 53–62.

Davis, J., & Hardick, E. (1981). *Rehabilitative audiology for children and adults*. New York: Wiley.

Dawes, P., & Bishop, D. V. M. (2009). Auditory processing disorder in relation to developmental disorders of language, communication and attention: A review and critique. *International Journal of Communication Disorders, 44*, 440–465.

Dawes, P., Bishop, D. V. M., Sirimanna, T., & Bamiou, D. E. (2008). Profile and aetiology of children diagnosed with auditory processing disorder (APD). *International Journal of Pediatric Otorhinolaryngology, 72*, 483–489.

Dawson, P. W., Blamey, P., Dettman, S. J., Barker, E., & Clark, G. M. (1995). A clinical report on receptive vocabulary skills in cochlear implant users. *Ear and Hearing, 16*, 287–294.

De Raeve, L., & Lichert, G. (2012). Changing trends within the population of children who are deaf or hard of hearing in Flanders (Belgium): Effects of 12 years of universal newborn hearing screening, early intervention, and early cochlear implantation. *Volta Review, 112*, 131–148.

DeBonis, D. A., & Donohue, C. L. (2008). *Survey of audiology: Fundamentals for audiologists and health professionals* (2nd ed.). Boston: Allyn & Bacon.

DeBonis, D. A., & Moncrieff, D. (2008). Auditory processing disorders: An update for speech–language pathologists. *American Journal of Speech-Language Pathology, 17*, 4–18.

Declau, F., Boudewyns, A., Van den Ende, J., Peeters, A., & van den Heyning, P. (2008). Etiologic and audiologic evaluations after universal neonatal hearing screening: Analysis of 170 referred neonates. *Pediatrics, 121*, 1119–1126.

Dermody, P., Katsch, R., & Mackie, K. (1983). Auditory processing limitations in low verbal children. *Ear and Hearing, 4*, 272–277.

Dermody, P., Mackie, K., & Katsch, R. (1983). Dichotic listening in good and poor readers. *Journal of Speech and Hearing Research, 26*, 341–348.

DiSimoni, F. (1978). *The token test for children*. Rolling Meadows, IL: Riverside.

Dodd, B., Hua, Z., Crosbie, S., Holm, A., & Ozanne, A. (2002). *Diagnostic evaluation of articulation and phonology (DEAP)*. London: The Psychological Corporation.

Duchan, J. (1988). Assessing communication of hearing-impaired children: Influences from pragmatics. *Journal of the Academy of Rehabilitative Audiology, 21*(Suppl.), 19–40.

Dunkley, C., Farnsworth, A., Mason, S., Dodd, M., & Gibbin, K. (2003). Screening and follow up assessment in three cases of auditory neuropathy. *Archives of Disease in Childhood, 88*, 25–26.

Dunn, L., & Dunn, L. (1997). *Peabody picture vocabulary test-III*. Circle Pines, MN: American Guidance Service.

Eilers, R. E., Cobo-Lewis, A. B., Vergara, K. C., & Oller, D. K. (1997). Longitudinal speech perception performance of young children with cochlear implants and tactile aids plus hearing aids. *Scandinavian Audiology Supplement, 26*(Suppl 47), 50–54.

Eisenson, J. (1972). *Aphasia in children*. New York: Harper & Row.

Elfenbein, J. L., Hardin-Jones, M. A., & Davis, J. M. (1994). Oral communication skills of children who are hard-of-hearing. *Journal of Speech and Hearing Research, 37*, 216–225.

Elliot, C. D. (1996). *The British ability scales (BAS)* (2nd ed.). Windsor, UK: NFER-Nelson.

Engen, E., & Engen, T. (1983). *Rhode Island test of language structure (RITLS)*. Baltimore: University Park Press.

English, K. (2007a). Audiological rehabilitation services in the school setting. In R. L. Schow & M. A. Nerbonne (Eds.), *Introduction to audiological rehabilitation* (5th ed., pp. 269–300). Boston, MA: Allyn & Bacon.

English, K. (2007b). Psychological aspects of hearing impairment and counseling basics. In R. L. Schow & M. A. Nerbonne (Eds.), *Introduction to audiological rehabilitation* (5th ed., pp. 245–268). Boston, MA: Allyn & Bacon.

Erber, N., & Alencewicz, C. (1976). Audiologic evaluation of deaf children. *Journal of Speech and Hearing Disorders, 41*, 256–267.

Estabrooks, W. (1994). *Auditory verbal therapy for parents and professionals*. Washington, DC: A.G. Bell Association for the Deaf.

Farrell, J. M. (2009). Developing a strong early hearing detection and intervention program. *The ASHA Leader, 14*, 8–11.

Ferre, J. M. (2006). Management strategies for APD. In T. K. Parthasarathy (Ed.), *An introduction to auditory processing disorders in children* (pp. 161–185). Mahwah, NJ: Lawrence Erlbaum Associates.

Fey, M., Richard, G. J., Geffner, D., Kamhi, A., Medwetsky, L., Paul, D., . . . Schooling, T. (2011). Auditory processing disorder and auditory/language interventions: An evidence-based systematic review. *Language, Speech, and Hearing Services in Schools, 42*, 246–264.

Flexer, C. (1990). Audiological rehabilitation in the schools. *ASHA, 32*, 44–45.

Flowers, A., Costello, M., & Small, V. (1970). *Manual for the Flowers-Costello test of central auditory abilities*. Dearborn, MI: Perceptual Learning Systems.

Franck, K. H., Rainey, D. M., Montoya, L. A., & Gerdes, M. (2002). Developing a multidisciplinary clinical protocol to manage pediatric patients with auditory neuropathy. *Seminars in Hearing, 23*, 225–237.

Frederickson, N., Firth, U., & Reason, R. (1997). *Phonological assessment battery (PhAB)*. Windsor: NFER-Nelson.

Friel-Patti, S. (1999). Clinical decision-making in the assessment and intervention of central auditory processing disorders. *Language, Speech, and Hearing Services in the Schools, 30*, 345–352.

Friel-Patti, S., Desbarres, K., & Thibodeau, L. (2001). Case studies of children using Fast ForWard. *American Journal of Speech-Language Pathology, 10*, 203–215.

Friel-Patti, S., & Finitzo, T. (1990). Language learning in a prospective study of otitis media with effusion in the first 2 years of life. *Journal of Speech and Hearing Research, 33*, 188–194.

Gallaudet Research Institute. (2005). Regional and national summary report of data from the 2003–2004 annual survey of deaf and hard-of-hearing children and youth. Washington, DC: Gallaudet Research Institute, Gallaudet University.

Geers, A. (2002). Factors affecting the development of speech, language, and literacy in children with early cochlear implantation. *Language, Speech, and Hearing Services in the Schools, 33*, 172–183.

Geers, A. (2003). Predictors of reading skill development in children with early cochlear implantation. *Ear and Hearing, 24*(Suppl. 1), 59S–68S.

Geers, A. (2004). Speech, language, and reading skills after early cochlear implantation. *Archives of Otolaryngology – Head and Neck Surgery, 130*, 634–638.

Geers, A. (2005). *Factors associated with academic achievement by children who received a cochlear implant by 5 years of age.* Paper presented at the annual meeting of the Society for Research in Child Development, Atlanta, GA.

Geers, A., & Brenner, C. (2003). Background and educational characteristics of prelingually deaf children implanted by five years of age. *Ear and Hearing, 24*(Suppl. 1), 2S–14S.

Geers, A., & Moog, J. (1994a). The effectiveness of cochlear implants and tactile aids for deaf children: A report of the CID sensory aids study. *Volta Review, 96*, 1–232.

Geers, A., & Moog, J. (1994b). Spoken language results: Vocabulary, syntax, and communication. *Volta Review, 96*, 131–148.

Geers, A., Nicholas, J., & Sedey, A. (2002). Language skills of children with early cochlear implantation. *Ear and Hearing, 24*(Suppl. 1), 46S–58S.

Geffner, D. (2013). Central auditory processing disorders: Definition, description, and behaviors. In D. Geffner & D. Ross-Swain (Eds.), *Auditory processing disorders: Assessment, management, and treatment* (2nd ed., pp. 59–89). San Diego, CA: Plural Publishing.

Geffner, D., & Freeman, L. R. (1980). Assessment of language comprehension of six-year-old deaf children. *Journal of Communication Disorders, 13*, 455–470.

Gérard, J. M., Deggoui, N., Hupin, C., Buisson, A. L., Monteyne, V., Lavis, C., . . . Gersdorff, M. (2010). Evolution of communication abilities after cochlear implantation in prelingually deaf children. *International Journal of Pediatric Otorhinolaryngology, 74*, 642–648.

Gibson, W., & Graham, J. (2008). Editorial: "Auditory neuropathy" and cochlear implantation—Myths and facts. *Cochlear Implants International, 9*, 1–7.

Gillam, R. (1999). Computer-assisted language intervention using Fast ForWord: Theoretical and empirical considerations for clinical decision-making. *Language, Speech, and Hearing Services in the Schools, 30*, 363–370.

Gillam, R., Loeb, D., Hoffman, L., Bohman, T., Champlin, C. A., Thibodeau, L., . . . Friel-Patti, S. (2008). The efficacy of Fast ForWord Language intervention in school-age children with language impairment: A randomized controlled trial. *Journal of Speech, Language, and Hearing Research, 51*, 97–119.

Gillam, R., & Ukrainetz, T. M. (2006). Language intervention through literacy-based units. In T. M. Ukrainetz (Ed.), *Literate language intervention: Scaffolding PreK–12 literacy achievement* (pp. 59–94). Eau Claire, WI: Thinking Publications.

Gold, T., & Levitt, H. (1975). *Comparison of articulatory errors in hard-of-hearing and deaf children*. New York: Communication Science Laboratory Graduate School and University Center-City University of New York.

Gravel, J., & Wallace, I. (1992). Listening and language at 4 years of age. *Journal of Speech and Hearing Research, 35*, 588–595.

Greenberg, M. (1980). Mode use in deaf children: The effects of communication method and communication competence. *Applied Psycholinguistics, 1*, 65–79.

Haggard, M., Birkin, J., & Pringle, D. (1994). Consequences of otitis media for speech and language. In B. McCormick (Ed.), *Pediatric audiology*. London: Whurr.

Hammill, D., & Larsen, S. (1974). The effectiveness of psycholinguistic training. *Exceptional Children, 41*, 5–14.

Hay-McCutcheon, M. J., Kirk, K. I., Henning, S. C., Gao, S., & Qi, R. (2008). Using early language outcomes to predict later language ability in children with cochlear implants. *Audiology and Neurotology, 13*, 370–380.

Hind, S. E., Haines-Bazrafshan, R., Benton, C. L., Brassington, W., Towle, B., & Moore, D. R. (2011). Prevalence of clinical referrals having hearing thresholds within normal limits. *International Journal of Audiology, 50*, 708–716.

Holden-Pitt, L., & Diaz, J. A. (1998). Thirty years of the annual survey of deaf and hard-of-hearing children & youth: A glance over the decades. *American Annals of the Deaf, 142*, 72–76.

Holm, V., & Kunze, L. (1969). Effects of chronic otitis media on language and speech development. *Paediatrics, 43*, 833–839.

Holmes, A. E., & Rodriguez, G. P. (2007). Cochlear implants and vestibular/tinnitus rehabilitation. In *Introduction to audiologic rehabilitation* (5th ed., pp. 77–112). Boston: Allyn & Bacon.

Hood, L. J. (1998). Auditory neuropathy: What is it and what can we do about it. *The Hearing Journal, 51*, 10–18.

Howie, V. (1975). Natural history of otitis media. *Annals of Otolaryngology, Rhinology, and Laryngology, 84*(Part 2, Suppl. 19), 67–72.

Israelite, N., Ower, J., & Goldstein, G. (2002). Hard-of-hearing adolescents and identity construction: Influences of school experiences, peers, and teachers. *Journal of Deaf Studies and Deaf Education, 7*, 134–148.

JCIH. (1995). Joint Committee on Infant Hearing 1994 position statement. *Paediatrics, 85*, 152–156.

JCIH. (2000). Joint Committee on Infant Hearing: Year 2000 position statement. Principles and guidelines for early hearing detection and intervention programs. *Audiology Today, Special Issue* (August), 6–27.

JCIH. (2007). Year 2007 position statement: Principles and guidelines for early hearing detection and intervention programs. *Pediatrics, 120*, 898–921.

Jensema, C., & Trybus, R. (1978). Communication patterns and educational achievement of hearing impaired students. Washington, DC: Office of Demographic Studies, Gallaudet College.

Jerger, J. (1998). Controversial issues in central auditory processing disorders. *Seminars in Hearing, 19*, 393–397.

Jerger, J., & Musiek, F. (2000). Report on the consensus conference on the diagnosis of auditory processing disorders in school-aged children. *Journal of the Academy of Audiology, 11*, 467–474.

Jerger, J., & Musiek, F. (2002). On the diagnosis of auditory processing disorder: A reply to "Clinical and research concerns regarding Jerger & Musiek (2000) APD recommendation." *Audiology Today, 16*, 100–106.

Jerger, S., & Jerger, J. (1983). Evaluation of diagnostic audiometric tests. *Audiology, 22*, 144–161.

Johnson, C. A., & Goswami, U. C. (2005, July). *Phonological skills, vocabulary development and reading development in children with cochlear implants*. Paper presented at the International Congress of the Education of the Deaf, Maastricht, Netherlands.

Johnson, D. L., McCormick, D. P., & Baldwin, C. D. (2008). Early middle ear effusion and language at age seven. *Journal of Communication Disorders, 41*, 20–32.

Joint Committee on Infant Hearing [JCIH], American Academy of Audiology, American Academy of Pediatrics, & ASHA Directors of Speech and Hearing Programs in State Health and Welfare Agencies. (2000). Year 2000 position statement: Principles and guidelines for early hearing detection and intervention programs. *Pediatrics, 106*, 798–817.

Jutras, B., Loubert, M., Dupuis, J. L., Maroux, C., Dumont, V., & Baril, M. (2007). Applicability of central auditory processing disorder models. *American Journal of Audiology, 16*, 100–106.

Katz, J., Johnson, C. D., Brander, S., Delagange, T., Ferre, J. M., King, J., . . . Stecker, N. A. (2002). Clinical and research concerns regarding the 2000 APD consensus report and recommendations. *Audiology Today, 14*, 14–17.

Katz, W., Curtiss, S., & Tallal, P. (1992). Rapid automatized naming and gesture by normal and language-impaired children. *Brain and Language, 43*, 623–641.

Keith, R. (1986). *SCAN: A screening test for auditory processing disorders*. San Diego, CA: The Psychological Corporation.

Keith, R. (1999). Clinical issues in central auditory processing disorders. *Language, Speech, and Hearing Services in the Schools, 30*, 339–344.

Kent, R. D., Osberger, M. J., Netsell, R., & Hustedde, C. G. (1987). Phonetic development in identical twins differing in auditory function. *Journal of Speech and Hearing Disorders, 52*, 64–75.

Kenworthy, O. T. (1986). Caregiver-child interaction and language acquisition of hearing-impaired children. *Topics in Language Disorders, 6*, 1–11.

Kiese-Himmel, C. (2002). Unilateral sensorineural hearing impairment in childhood: Analysis of 31 consecutive cases. *International Journal of Audiology, 41*, 57–63.

Kirk, K. I., Miyamoto, R. T., Lento, C. L., Ying, E., O'Neill, T., & Fears, B. (2002). Effects of age at implantation in young children. *Annals of Otololaryngology, Rhinology, and Laryngology, 111*(189), 69–73.

Knowledge Adventure Inc. (1999). Dinosaur adventure 3-D (Version 4.0.1). Torrance, CA: Author.

Kraus, N., Bradlow, A. R., Cheatham, J., Cunningham, C. D., King, D. B., Koch, T. G., . . . Wright, B. A. (2000). Consequences of neural asynchrony: A case of auditory neuropathy. *Journal of the Association for Research in Otolaryngology, 1*, 33–45.

Kretschmer, R., & Kretschmer, L. (1980). Pragmatics: Development in normal-hearing and hearing-impaired children. In J. Subtenly (Ed.), *Speech assessment and speech improvement for the hearing impaired*. Washington, DC: A.G. Bell Association for the Deaf.

Lee, J. S., McPherson, B., Yuen, K. C. P., & Wong, L. L. N. (2001). Screening for auditory neuropathy in a school for hearing impaired children. *International Journal of Pediatric Otorhinolaryngology, 61*, 39–46.

Leigh, J., Dettman, S., Dowell, R., & Briggs, R. (2013). Communication development in children who receive a cochlear implant by 12 months of age. *Otology and Neurotolgy, 34*, 443–450.

Leonard, L. (1979). Language impairment in children. *Merrill-Palmer Quarterly, 25*, 205–232.

Levitt, H. (1987). Interrelationships among the speech and language levels. In H. Levitt, N. McGarr, & D. Geffner (Eds.), *Development of language and communication skills in hearing-impaired children: ASHA monographs* (Vol. 26, pp. 123–139). Rockville, MD: ASHA.

Levitt, H., McGarr, N., & Geffner, D. (1987). Concluding commentary. In H. Levitt, N. McGarr, & D. Geffner (Eds.), *Development of language and communication skills in hearing-impaired children: ASHA monographs* (Vol. 26, pp. 140–144). Rockville, MD: ASHA.

Lindamood, C. H., & Lindamood, P. C. (1998). *Lindamood phoneme sequencing program (LIPS)*. Austin, TX: PRO-ED.

Loeb, D., Stoke, C., & Fey, M. (2001). Language changes associated with Fast ForWord Language: Evidence from case studies. *American Journal of Speech-Language Pathology, 10*, 216–230.

Lucker, J. R. (2013). The history of auditory processing disorders in children. In D. Geffner & D. Ross-Swain (Eds.), *Auditory processing disorders: Assessment, management, and treatment* (2nd ed., pp. 33–57). San Diego, CA: Plural Publishing.

Mackie, K., & Dermody, P. (1986). Use of monosyllabic adaptive speech test (MAST) with young children. *Journal of Speech and Hearing Research, 29*, 275–281.

Madden, C., Rutter, M., Hilbert, L., Greinwald, J. Jr., & Choo, D. (2002a). Clinical and audiological features in auditory neuropathy. *Archives of Otoloaryngology – Head and Neck Surgery, 128*, 1026–1030.

Madden, C., Rutter, M., Hilbert, L., Greinwald, J. Jr., & Choo, D. (2002b). Pediatric cochlear implantation in auditory neuropathy. *Otology and Neurotology, 23*, 163–168.

Markides, A. (1970). The speech of deaf and partially hearing children with special reference to factors affecting intelligibility. *British Journal of Disorders of Communication, 5*, 126–140.

Markides, A. (1983). *The speech of hearing-impaired children*. Manchester: Manchester University Press.

Marler, J., Champlin, C. A., & Gillam, R. B. (2001). Backward and simultaneous masking measured in language-learning impaired children who received intervention with Fast ForWord or Laureate learning systems software. *American Journal of Speech-Language Pathology, 10*, 258–268.

Marschark, M., Mouradian, V., & Halas, M. (1994). Discourse rules in the language production of deaf and hearing children. *Journal of Experimental Child Psychology, 57*, 89–107.

Marschark, M., Rhoten, C., & Fabich, M. (2007). Effects of cochlear implants on children's reading and academic achievement. *Journal of Deaf Studies and Deaf Education, 12*, 269–282.

Martin, F. N., & Clark, J. G. (2006). *Introduction to audiology* (9th ed.). Boston: Allyn & Bacon.

Mauk, G., White, K. R., & Mortensen, L. B. (1991). The effectiveness of hearing screening programs based on high risk characteristics in early identification of hearing impairment. *Ear and Hearing, 12*, 312–319.

Maxwell, M. M., & Falick, T. G. (1992). Cohesion and quality in deaf and hearing children's written English. *Sign Language Studies, 77*, 345–371.

Mayberry, R. I., & Eichen, E. B. (1991). The long lasting advantage of learning sign language in childhood: Another look at the critical period of language acquisition. *Journal of Memory and Language, 30*, 486–512.

McAnally, K. I., Castles, A., & Bannister, S. (2004). Auditory temporal pattern discrimination and reading ability. *Journal of Speech, Language, and Hearing Research, 47*, 1237–1243.

McCaffrey, H. (1999). Multichannel cochlear implantation and the organization of the early speech. *Volta Review, 101*, 5–29.

McClure, W. (1966). Current problems and trends in the education of the deaf. *The Deaf American, 18*, 8–14.

McFarland, D. J., & Cacace, A. T. (1997). Modality specificity of auditory and visual pattern recognition: Implication for assessment of central auditory processing disorders. *Audiology, 36*, 249–260.

McFarland, D. J., & Cacace, A. T. (2006). Current controversies in CAPD: From Procrustes' bed to Pandora's box. In T. K. Parthasarathy (Ed.), *An introduction to auditory processing disorders in children* (pp. 247–263). Mahwah, NJ: Lawrence Erlbaum Associates.

McFarland, D. J., & Cacace, A. T. (2009). Modality specificity and auditory processing disorders. In A. T. Cacace & D. J. McFarland (Eds.), *Controversies in central auditory processing disorder* (pp. 199–216). San Diego, CA: Plural Publishing.

McKay, S., Gravel, J., & Tharpe, A. M. (2008). Amplification considerations for children with minimal or mild bilateral hearing loss and unilateral hearing loss. *Trends in Amplification, 12*, 43–54.

McKirdy, L., & Blank, M. (1982). Dialogue in deaf and hearing preschoolers. *Journal of Speech and Hearing Research, 25*, 487–499.

Mehl, A. L., & Thomson, V. (1998). Newborn hearing screening: The great omission. *Paediatrics, 101*, 1–6.

Meinzen-Derr, J., Wiley, S., Grether, S., & Choo, D. I. (2011). Children with cochlear implants and developmental disabilities: A language skills study with developmentally matched hearing peers. *Research in Developmental Disabilties, 32*, 757–767.

Merzenich, M., Jenkins, W., Johnson, P., Schreiner, C., Miller, S., & Tallal, P. (1996). Temporal processing deficits of language-learning impaired children ameliorated by training. *Science, 271*, 77–81.

Michalewski, H. J., Starr, A., Nguyen, T. T., Kong, Y. Y., & Zeng, F. G. (2005). Auditory temporal processes in normal-hearing individuals and in patients with auditory neuropathy. *Clinical Neurophysiology, 116*, 669–680.

MindWeavers Inc. (1996). MindWeavers history. Retrieved from www.mindweavers.co.uk

Mody, M., Studdert-Kennedy, M., & Brady, S. (1997). Speech perception deficits in poor readers: Auditory processing or phonological coding? *Journal of Experimental Child Psychology, 64*, 199–231.

Moeller, M. P., & Lukete-Stahlman, B. (1990). Parents' use of SEE-II: A descriptive analysis. *Journal of Speech and Hearing Disorders, 55*, 327–338.

Moeller, M. P., McConkey, A. J., & Osberger, M. J. (1983). Evaluation of the communicative skills of hearing-impaired children. *Audiology, 8*, 113–128.

Moncrieff, D. (2006). Identification of binaural integration deficits in children with competing words subtest: Standard score versus interaural asymmetry. *International Journal of Audiology, 45*, 545–558.

Montgomery, G. (1966). The relationship of oral skills to manual communication in profoundly deaf adolescents. *American Annals of the Deaf, 111*, 557-565.

Moog, J. S., Geers, A. E., Gustus, C., & Brenner, C. (2011). Psychosocial adjustment in adolescents who have used cochlear implants since preschool. *Ear and Hearing, 32*(Suppl. 1), 75S–83S.

Moore, D. R. (2006). Auditory processing disorder (APD): Definition, diagnosis, neural basis, and intervention. *Audiological Medicine, 4*, 4–11.

Moore, D. R. (2011). The diagnosis and management of auditory processing disorder. *Language, Speech, and Hearing Services in Schools, 42*, 303–308.

Moore, D. R., Cowan, J. C., Riley, A., Edmondson-Jones, A. M., & Ferguson, M. A. (2011). Development of auditory processing in 6–11 year old children. *Ear and Hearing, 32*, 269–285.

Moore, D. R., Ferguson, M. A., Edmondson-Jones, A. M., & Ratib, S. (2010). The nature of auditory processing disorder in children. *Pediatrics, 126*, e382–e390.

Moores, D. (1987). *Educating the deaf: Psychology, principles, and practices* (3rd ed.). Boston: Houghton Mifflin.

Moores, D., Weiss, K., & Goodwin, M. (1978). Early education programs for hearing-impaired children: Major findings. *American Annals of the Deaf, 123*, 925–936.

Mueller, H., Johnson, E. E., & Carter, A. (2007). Hearing aids and assistive devices. In R. L. Schow & M. A. Nerbonne (Eds.), *Introduction to audiological rehabilitation* (5th ed., pp. 31–76). Boston: Allyn & Bacon.

Musiek, F. (1999). Central auditory tests. *Scandinavian Audiology, 28*(Suppl. 51), 33–46.

Musiek, F., Bellis, T. J., & Chermak, G. (2005). Non-modularity of the central auditory nervous system: Implications for (central) auditory processing disorder. *American Journal of Audiology, 14*, 128–138.

Musselman, C., & Szanto, G. (1998). The written language of deaf adolescents: Patterns of performance. *Journal of Deaf Studies and Deaf Education, 3*, 245–257.

Myklebust, H. (1954). *Auditory disorders in children: A manual for different diagnosis*. New York: Grune & Stratton.

National Institutes of Health. (2006). Fact sheet: Newborn hearing screening. Washington, DC: U.S. Department of Health and Human Services.

Needleman, H. (1977). Effects of hearing loss from early recurrent otitis media on speech and language development. In B. Jaffe (Ed.), *Hearing loss in children*. Baltimore: University Park Press.

Nevins, H., & Chute, P. (1996). *Children with cochlear implants in educational setting*. London: Singular.

Newcomer, P. L., & Hammill, D. D. (1997). *Test of language development–Primary, (TOLD-P:3)* (3rd ed.). Austin, TX: PRO-ED.

Nicholas, J., & Geers, A. (2003a). Hearing status, language modality, and young children's communicative and linguistic behavior. *Journal of Deaf Studies and Deaf Education, 8*, 422–437.

Nicholas, J., & Geers, A. (2003b). Personal, social and family adjustment in school-aged children with cochlear implant. *Ear and Hearing, 24*(Suppl. 1), 69S–81S.

Nicholas, J., & Geers, A. (2007). Will they catch up? The role of age at cochlear implantation in the spoken language development of children with severe to profound hearing loss. *Journal of Speech, Language, and Hearing Research, 50*, 1048–1062.

Nordic Software Inc. (1999). Coin critters (Version 2.1.4A). Lincoln, NE: Author.

Norris, J. (1989). Providing language remediation in the classroom: An integrated language-to-reading intervention method. *Language, Speech, and Hearing Services in the Schools, 20*, 205–218.

Northern, J., & Downs, M. (1991). *Hearing in children* (4th ed.). Baltimore: Williams & Wilkins.

Northern, J., & Downs, M. (2002). *Hearing in children* (5th ed.). Baltimore: Lippincott Williams & Wilkins.

Oller, D. K., & Eilers, R. E. (1988). The role of audition in infant babbling. *Child Development, 59*, 441–449.

Osberger, M. J. (1986). Summary and implications for research and educational management. In M. J. Osberger (Ed.), *Language and learning skills of hearing-impaired students. ASHA Monograph* (Vol. 23, pp. 92–98). Rockville, MD: ASHA.

Osberger, M. J. (1990). Audiological rehabilitation with cochlear implants and tactile aids. *ASHA, 32*, 38–43.

Osberger, M. J., & Hesketh, L. (1988). Speech and language disorders related to hearing impairment. In N. Lass, L. McReynolds, J. Northern, & D. Yoder (Eds.), *Handbook of speech-language pathology and audiology* (pp. 858–886). Toronto: B.C. Decker.

Osberger, M. J., & McGarr, N. (1982). Speech production characteristics of the hearing impaired. In N. Lass (Ed.), *Speech and language: Advances in basic science and research*. New York: Academic Press.

Osberger, M. J., Robbins, A. M., Berry, S., Todd, S., Hesketh, L., & Sedey, A. (1991). Analysis of the spontaneous speech samples of children with cochlear implants or tactile aids. *American Journal of Otology, 12*, 151–164.

Osberger, M. J., Robbins, A. M., Miyamoto, R. T., Berry, S., Myres, W., Kessler, K., & Pope, M. (1991). Speech perception abilities of children with cochlear implants, tactile aids or hearing aids. *American Journal of Otology, 12*, 80–88.

Osberger, M. J., Robbins, M., Todd, S., & Riley, A. (1996). Cochlear implants and tactile aids for children with profound hearing impairment. In F. Bess, J. Gravel, & A. Tharpe (Eds.), *Amplification for children with auditory deficits* (pp. 283–308). Nashville, TN: Bill Wilkerson Press.

Oyler, R., Oyler, A., & Matkin, N. (1987). Warning: A unilateral hearing loss may be detrimental to a child's academic career. *Hearing Journal, 40*, 18–22.

Oyler, R., Oyler, A., & Matkin, N. (1988). Unilateral hearing loss: Demographics and educational impact. *Language, Speech, and Hearing Services in the Schools, 19*, 201–210.

Parving, A., Hauch, A., & Christensen, B. (2003). Hearing loss in children: Epidemiology, age at identification and causes through 30 years [in Danish]. *Ugeskr Laeger, 165*, 574–579.

Peterson, N. R., Pisoni, D. B., & Miyamoto, R. T. (2010). Cochlear implants and spoken language processing abilities: Review and assessment of the literature. *Restorative Neurology and Neuroscience, 28*, 237–250. doi: 10.3233/RNN-2010-0535

Pipp-Siegel, S., & Biringen, Z. (2000). Assessing the quality of relationships between parents and children: The Emotional Availability Scales. *Volta Review, 100*, 237–249.

Pokorini, J., Worthington, C., & Jamison, P. (2004). Phonological awareness intervention comparison of Fast ForWord, Earobics, and LiPS. *Journal of Educational Research, 97*, 147–157.

Presnell, L. (1973). Hearing-impaired children's comprehension and production of syntax in oral language. *Journal of Speech and Hearing Research, 16*, 12–21.

Quigley, S. (1969). *The influence of fingerspelling on the development of language, communication and educational achievement in deaf children*. Champaign: Department of Special Education, University of Illinois.

Rance, G. (2005). Auditory neuropathy/dys-synchrony and its perceptual consequences. *Trends in Amplification, 9*, 1–43.

Rance, G. (2013). Auditory processing in individuals with auditory neuropathy spectrum disorder. In D. Geffner & D. Ross-Swain (Eds.), *Auditory processing disorders: Assessment, management, and treatment* (2nd ed., pp. 185–209). San Diego, CA: Plural Publishing.

Rance, G. (Ed.). (2007). *Auditory processing in individuals with auditory neuropathy/dyssynchrony*. San Diego, CA: Plural Publishing.

Rance, G., & Barker, E. (2008). Speech perception in children with auditory neuropathy/dyssynchrony managed with either hearing aids or cochlear implants. *Otology and Neurotology, 29*, 179–182.

Rance, G., Barker, E., Sarant, J., & Ching, T. Y. C. (2007). Receptive language and speech production in children with auditory neuropathy/dyssynchrony type hearing loss. *Ear and Hearing, 28*, 694–702.

Rance, G., Beer, D., Cone-Wesson, B., Sheperd, R., Dowell, R., King, A., . . . Clark, G. (1999). Clinical findings for a group of infants and young children with auditory neuropathy. *Ear and Hearing, 20*, 238–252.

Rance, G., Cone-Wesson, B., Wunderlich, J., & Dowell, R. (2002). Speech perception and cortical event related potentials in children with auditory neuropathy. *Ear and Hearing, 23*, 239–253.

Rance, G., McKay, C., & Grayden, D. (2004). Perceptual characterization of children with auditory neuropathy. *Ear and Hearing, 25*, 34–46.

Raphael, L., Borden, G., & Harris, K. (2007). *Speech science primer* (5th ed.). Baltimore: Lippincott Williams & Wilkins.

Rapin, I., & Gravel, J. (2003). "Auditory neuropathy": Physiologic and pathologic evidence calls for more diagnostic specificity. *International Journal of Pediatric Otorhinolaryngology, 67*, 707–728.

Rattigan, K., Reed, V. A., & Lee, K. (2002). *An investigation into the phonological processing and literacy skills of children using cochlear implants*. Paper presented at the annual meeting of the A.G. Bell Association for the Deaf and Hard-of-Hearing, St. Louis, MO.

Raveh, E., Buller, N., Badrana, O., & Attias, J. (2007). Auditory neuropathy: Clinical characteristics and therapeutic approach. *American Journal of Otolaryngology – Head and Neck Medicine and Surgery, 28*, 302–308.

Rees, N. (1973). Auditory processing factors in language disorders: The view from Procrustes' bed. *Journal of Speech and Hearing Disorders, 38*, 304–315.

Rees, N. (1981). Saying more than we know: Is it a meaningful concept? In R. Keith (Ed.), *Central auditory and language disorders in children*. San Diego, CA: College-Hill Press.

Reichman, J., & Healey, W. (1989). Amplification monitoring and maintenance in schools. *ASHA, 31*, 43–45.

Renfrew, C. (1997). *Bus story test* (4th ed.). Bicester, UK: Winslow Press.

Roberts, J., Burchinal, M., Davis, B., Collier, A., & Henderson, F. (1991). Otitis media in early childhood and later language. *Journal of Speech and Hearing Research, 34*, 1158–1168.

Roberts, J., Burchinal, M., & Zeisel, A. (2002). Otitis media in early childhood in relation to children's school-age language and academic skills. *Paediatrics, 110*, 696–706.

Roberts, J., Hunter, L., Gravel, J., Rosenfeld, R., Berman, S., Haggard, M., . . . Wallace, I. (2002). Otitis media, hearing loss, and language learning: Controversies and current research. *Journal of Developmental and Behavioral Pediatrics, 25*, 110–122.

Robertson, C., & Salter, W. (1997). *The phonological awareness test*. East Moline, IL: LinguiSystems.

Rosen, S. (2003). Auditory processing in dyslexia and specific language impairment: Is there a deficit? What is its nature? Does it explain anything? *Journal of Phonetics, 31*(3–4), 509–527.

Ross, M. (1982). *Hard-of-hearing children in regular schools*. Englewood Cliffs, NJ: Prentice Hall.

Ross, M., Brackett, D., & Maxon, A. (1991). *Assessment and management of mainstream hearing-impaired children: Assessment and principles*. Austin, TX: PRO-ED.

Roush, J. (2001). Screening for hearing loss and otitis media: Basic principles. In J. Roush (Ed.), *Screening for hearing loss and otitis media in children* (pp. 3–32). San Diego, CA: Singular.

Rubinstein, J. (2002). Pediatric cochlear implantation: Prosthetic hearing and language development. *Lancet, 360*(9331), 483–487.

Russell, W., Power, D., & Quigley, S. (1976). *Linguistics and deaf children*. Washington, DC: A.G. Bell Association for the Deaf.

Sainsbury, S. (1986). *Deaf worlds: A study of integration, segregation, and disability*. London: Hutchinson.

Sarant, J. (2012). Cochlear implants in children: A review. In S. Naz (Ed.), *Hearing loss* (pp. 331–382). Rijeka, Croatia: InTech.

Schildroth, A. (1986). Hearing-impaired children under age 6: 1977 and 1984. *American Annals of the Deaf, 131*, 85–89.

Scholastic Inc. (2001). *The magic school bus discovers flight*. New York: Author.

Schorr, E., Roth, F., & Fox, N. (2008). A comparison of speech and language skills of children with cochlear implants and children with normal hearing. *Communication Disorders Quarterly, 29*, 195–210.

Scientific Learning Corporation. (1999). *Fast ForWord companion: A comprehensive guide to the training exercises*. Berkeley, CA: Authors.

Scientific Learning Corporation. (2000). *Guide to implementation for training programs Fast ForWard, 4wd, Step 4word*. Berkeley, CA: Author.

Scientific Learning Corporation. (1997). *Fast ForWord training program for children: Procedure manual for professionals*. Berkeley, CA: Author.

Scientific Learning Corporation. (1998). Fast ForWord Language. Berkeley, CA: Author.

Scientific Learning Corporation. (2001). Fast ForWord Language (Version 2.01). Oakland, CA: Author.

Seewald, R., Ross, M., Giolas, T., & Yonovitz, A. (1985). Primary modality for speech perception in children with normal and impaired hearing. *Journal of Speech and Hearing Research, 28*, 38–46.

Semel, E. (2000). *Following directions*. Winooski, VT: Laureate Learning Systems.

Semel, E., Wiig, E., & Secord, W. (1995). *Clinical evaluation of language fundamentals–3*. San Antonio, TX: The Psychological Corporation.

Semel, E., Wiig, E., & Secord, W. (2000). *Clinical evaluation of language fundamentals*. London: The Psychological Corporation.

Seyfried, D., & Kricos, P. (1996). Language and speech of the deaf and hard-of-hearing. In R. L. Schow & M. A. Nerbonne (Eds.), *Introduction to audiological rehabilitation* (3rd ed., pp. 168–228). Boston: Allyn & Bacon.

Sharma, A., & Nash, A. (2009). Brain maturation in children with cochlear implants. *The ASHA Leader*, 14–17.

Siebein, G., Gold, M., Siebein, G., & Ermann, M. (2000). Ten ways to provide a high-quality acoustical environment in schools. *Language, Speech, and Hearing Services in the Schools, 31*, 376–384.

Simmons, J., & Beauchaine, K. L. (2000). Auditory neuropathy: Case study with hyperbilirubinemia. *Journal of American Academy of Audiology, 11*, 337–347.

Sininger, Y. S., & Oba, S. (2001). Patients with auditory neuropathy: Who are they and what can they hear? In Y. S. Sininger & A. Starr (Eds.), *Auditory neuropathy*. San Diego, CA: Singular.

Spencer, L., & Oleson, J. (2008). Early listening and speaking skills predict later reading proficiency in pediatric cochlear implant users. *Ear and Hearing, 29*, 270–280.

Starr, A., McPherson, D., Patterson, J., Don, M., Luxford, W., Shannon, R., . . . Waring, M. (1991). Absence of both auditory evoked potentials and auditory percepts dependent on timing cues. *Brain, 114*, 1157–1180.

Starr, A., Picton, T., Sininger, Y., Hood, L., & Berlin, C. (1996). Auditory neuropathy. *Brain, 119*, 741–753.

Starr, A., Sininger, Y., & Pratt, H. (2000). The varieties of auditory neuropathy. *Journal of Basic Clinical Physiology and Pharmacology, 11*, 215–230.

Stephens, J. (2006). Longer-term aspects of the language development of children with cochlear implants. *Audiological Medicine, 4*, 151–163.

Stoel-Gammon, C. (1988). Prelinguistic vocalizations of hearing-impaired and normally hearing subjects: A comparison of consonantal inventories. *Journal of Speech and Hearing Disorders, 53*, 302–315.

Stoel-Gammon, C., & Kehoe, M. (1994). Hearing impairment in infants and toddlers. In J. Bernthal & N. Bankson (Eds.), *Child phonology: Characteristics, assessment and intervention in special populations* (pp. 163–181). New York: Thieme.

Strong, C., & Hoggan, K. (1996). *The magic of stories: Literature-based language intervention.* Eau Claire, WI: Thinking Publications.

Svirsky, M., Chin, S., Miyamoto, R. T., Sloan, R., & Cadwell, M. (2002). Speech intelligibility of profoundly deaf pediatric hearing aid users. *Volta Review, 102*, 175–198.

Svirsky, M., Teoh, S., & Neuburger, H. (2004). Development of language and speech perception in congenitally, profoundly deaf children as a function of age at cochlear implantation. *Audiology and Neuro-Otology, 9*, 224–233.

Tallal, P. (1975). Perceptual and linguistic factors in the language impairment of developmental dysphasics: An experimental investigation with the Token Test. *Cortex, 11*, 196–205.

Tallal, P. (1976). Rapid auditory processing in normal and disordered language development. *Journal of Speech and Hearing Research, 19*, 561–571.

Tallal, P. (1980). Language and reading: Some perceptual prerequisites. *Bulletin of the Orton Society, 30*, 170–178.

Tallal, P., Miller, S., Bedi, G., Byma, G., Wang, X., Nagarajan, S., . . . Merzenich, M. (1996). Language comprehension in language-learning impaired children improved with acoustically modified speech. *Science, 271*(5245), 81–84.

Tallal, P., & Piercy, M. (1973a). Defects of nonverbal auditory perception in children with development dysphagia. *Nature, 241*, 468–499.

Tallal, P., & Piercy, M. (1973b). Developmental aphasia: Impaired rate of non-verbal processing as a function of sensory modality. *Neuropsychologia, 11*, 389–398.

Tallal, P., & Piercy, M. (1974). Developmental aphasia: Rate of auditory processing and selective impairment of consonant perception. *Neuropsychologia, 12*, 83–93.

Tallal, P., & Piercy, M. (1975). Developmental aphasia: The perception of brief vowels and extended stop consonants. *Neuropsychologia, 13*, 69–74.

Tallal, P., Stark, R., & Curtiss, B. (1976). The relation between speech perception impairment and speech production impairment in children with developmental dysphagia. *Brain and Language, 3*, 305–317.

Tang, T., McPherson, D., Yuen, K. C. P., Wong, L. L. N., & Lee, J. S. (2004). Auditory neuropathy/auditory dyssynchrony in school children with hearing loss: Frequency of occurrence. *International Journal of Pediatric Otorhinolaryngology, 68*, 175–183.

Taylor, L. (1969). *A language analysis of the writing of deaf children*, Unpublished doctoral dissertation. Florida State University, Tallahassee.

Teasdale, T., & Sorenson, M. (2007). Hearing loss in relation to educational attainment and cognitive abilities: A population study. *International Journal of Audiology, 46*, 172–175.

Templin, M. (1966). Vocabulary problems of the deaf child. *International Journal of Audiology, 5*, 349–354.

Tharpe, A. (2007). Assessment and management of minimal, mild, and unilateral hearing loss in children. Retrieved September 21, 2009, from http://www.audiologyonline.com/articles/pf_article_detail.asp?article.html

Thibodeau, L., Friel-Patti, S., & Britt, L. (2001). Psychoacoustic performance in children completing Fast ForWord training. *American Journal of Speech-Language Pathology, 10*, 248–257.

Tomblin, J. B., Barker, B., Spencer, L., Zhang, X., & Grantz, B. (2005). The effect of age at cochlear implant stimulation on expressive language growth in infants and toddlers. *Journal of Speech, Language, and Hearing Research, 48*, 853–867.

Tomblin, J. B., Spencer, L., Flock, S., Tyler, R., & Gantz, B. (1999). A comparison of language achievement in children with cochlear implants and children using hearing aids. *Journal of Speech, Language, and Hearing Research, 42*, 497–511.

Tooher, R. (2002). *Making their way in the world: An investigation into the outcomes of cochlear implantation for adolescents using biopsychosocial approach.* Sydney: University of Sydney.

Tooher, R., Hogan, A., & Reed, V. A. (2002a, September). *"The hearing's not enough, it's just enough to get by . . ." What is life like for young people who use cochlear implants to hear?* Paper presented at the International Cochlear Implant Conference, Manchester, United Kingdom.

Tooher, R., Hogan, A., & Reed, V. A. (2002b, March). *Quality of life and psychosocial outcomes of pediatric cochlear implantation in adolescents.* Paper presented at the International Congress of Audiology, Melbourne, Australia.

Troia, G. (2003). Auditory perceptual impairments and learning disabilities: Theoretical and empirical considerations. *Learning Disabilities: A Contemporary Journal, 1*, 27–37.

Trybus, R., & Karchmer, M. (1977). School achievement scores of hearing impaired children: National data on achievement patterns and growth patterns. *American Annals of the Deaf Directory of Programs and Service, 122*, 62–69.

Turner, R., Robinette, M., & Bauch, C. (1999). Clinical decisions. In F. Musiek & W. Rintelmann (Eds.), *Contemporary perspectives in hearing assessment* (pp. 437–464). Boston: Allyn & Bacon.

Tye-Murray, N. (1998). *Foundations of aural rehabilitation: Children, adults, and their family members.* San Diego, CA: Singular.

Tye-Murray, N. (2009). *Foundations of aural rehabilitation: Children, adults, and their family members* (3rd ed.). New York: Delmar Cengage Learning.

Tye-Murray, N., & Kirk, K. I. (1993). Vowel and diphthong production by young users of cochlear implants and the relationship between the phonetic level evaluation and spontaneous speech. *Journal of Speech and Hearing Research, 36*, 488–502.

U.S. Department of Education. (2004). *Individuals with Disabilities Education Act of 2004, PL 108-446.* Washington, DC: Author.

U.S. Preventive Services Task Force. (2008). Universal screening for hearing loss in newborns: U.S. Preventive Services Task Force recommendation statement. *Pediatrics, 122*, 143–148.

van Straaten, H., Tibosch, C., Dorrepaal, F., & Kok, J. (2001). Efficacy of automated auditory brainstem response hearing screening in very preterm newborns. *Journal of Pediatrics, 138*, 674–678.

Ventry, I. (1983). Research design issues in studies of the effects of middle ear effusion. *Pediatrics, 71*, 644.

Wagner, R., Torgesen, J., & Rashotte, C. (1999). *Comprehensive test of phonological processing (CTOPP).* Austin, TX: PRO-ED.

Wake, M., & Poulakis, Z. (2004). Slight and mild hearing loss in primary school children. *Journal of Paediatric Child Health, 40*(1–2), 11–13.

Wallach, G. (2011). Peeling the onion of auditory processing disorder: A language/curricular-based perspective. *Language, Speech, and Hearing Services in Schools, 42*, 273–285.

Waltzman, S., Cohen, N., Gomolin, R., Green, J., Shapiro, W., Brackett, D., & Zara, C. (1997). Perception and production results in children implanted between 2 and 5 years of age. *Advances in Otorhinolaryngology, 52*, 177–180.

Watson, C., Kidd, G., Horner, D., Connell, P., Lowther, A., Eddins, D., . . . Watson, B. (2003). Sensory, cognitive, and linguistic factors in the early academic performance of elementary school children: The Benton-IU Project. *Journal of Learning Disabilities, 36*, 165–197.

Watson, C. S., & Kidd, G. R. (2009). Assocations between auditory abilities reading and other language skills in children and adults. In A. T. Cacace & D. J. McFarland (Eds.), *Controversies in central auditory processing disorders* (pp. 217–242). San Diego, CA: Plural Publishing.

White, S., & White, R. (1987). The effects of hearing status of the family and age of intervention on receptive and expressive oral language skills in hearing-impaired infants. In H. Levitt, N. McGarr, & D. Geffner (Eds.), *Development of language and communication skills in hearing-impaired children* (Vol. 26, pp. 9–24). Washington, DC: ASHA.

Wilcox, J., & Tobin, H. (1974). Linguistic performance of hard-of-hearing and normal hearing children. *Journal of Speech and Hearing Research, 17*, 286–293.

Willeford, J. (1977). Assessing central auditory behaviour in children: A test battery approach. In R. W. Keith (Ed.), *Central auditory dysfunction* (pp. 43–72). New York: Grune and Stratton.

Wilson, M., & Fox, B. (1997). *Micro-LADS*. Winoski, VT: Laureate Learning Systems.

Winskel, H. (2006). The effects of an early history of otitis media on children's language and literacy skill development. *British Journal of Educational Psychology, 76*, 727–744.

Woodcock, R. (1991). *Woodcock language proficiency battery–Revised*. Itasca, IL: Riverside.

Wright, B. A., Lombardino, L., King, W., Puranik, C., Leonard, C., & Merzenich, M. (1997). Deficits in auditory temporal and spectral resolution in language impaired children. *Nature, 387*, 176–178.

Wright, M., Purcell, A., & Reed, V. A. (2001a, March). *Cochlear implants for babies: Expectations and outcomes*. Paper presented at the Symposium on Cochlear Implants in Children, Los Angeles, CA.

Wright, M., Purcell, A., & Reed, V. A. (2001b, June). *Communicative intents in infants pre- and post-cochlear implantation*. Paper presented at the Symposium on Research in Child Language Disorders, Madison, WI.

Wright, M., Purcell, A., & Reed, V. A. (2002). Cochlear implants and infants: Expectations and outcomes. *Annals of Otololaryngology, Rhinology, and Laryngology, 111*, 131–137.

Yoshinaga-Itano, C. (1998). Development of audition and speech: Implications for early intervention with infants who are deaf or hard-of-hearing. *Volta Review, 100*, 212–234.

Yoshinaga-Itano, C., Coulter, D., & Thomson, V. (2000). The Colorado newborn hearing screening project: Effects on speech and language development for children with hearing loss. *Journal of Perinatology, 20*(Part 2), 132–137.

Yoshinaga-Itano, C., & Gravel, J. (2001). The evidence for universal newborn hearing screening. *American Journal of Audiology, 10*, 62–64.

Yoshinaga-Itano, C., Snyder, L., & Mayberry, R. I. (1996a). Can lexical/semantic skills differentiate deaf or hard-of-hearing readers and non-readers. *Volta Review, 98*, 39–61.

Yoshinaga-Itano, C., Snyder, L., & Mayberry, R. I. (1996b). How deaf and normally hearing students convey meaning within and between written sentences. *Volta Review, 98*, 9–38.

Yoshinaga-Itano, C., & Stredler-Brown, A. (1992). Learning to communicate: Babies with hearing impairments make their needs known. *Volta Review, 94*, 107–129.

Yoshinaga-Itano, C., Stredler-Brown, A., & Jancosek, E. (1992). From phone to phoneme: What can we understand from babble. *Volta Review, 94*, 283–313.

Zeisel, S., & Roberts, J. (2003). Otitis media in young children with disabilities. *Infants and Young Children, 16*, 106–119.

Zeng, F. G., Kong, Y. Y., Michalewski, H. J., & Starr, A. (2005). Perceptual consequences of disrupted auditory nerve activity. *Journal of Neurophysiology, 93*, 3050–3063.

Zeng, F. G., & Liu, S. (2006). Speech perception in individuals with auditory neuropathy. *Journal of Speech, Language, and Hearing Research, 49*, 367–380.

Zeng, F. G., Oba, S., Garde, S., Sininger, Y., & Starr, A. (1999). Temporal and speech processing deficits in auditory neuropathy. *NeuroReport, 10*, 3429–3435.

Chapter 9

American Educational Research Association, American Psychological Association, & National Council on Measurement and Education. (1999). *Standards for educational and psychological testing*. Washington, DC: American Psychological Association.

Anderson, R. (1996). Assessing the grammar of Spanish-speaking children: A comparison of two procedures. *Language, Speech, and Hearing Services in Schools, 27*, 333–344.

Arnold, K., & Reed, L. (1976). The grammatic closure subtest of the ITPA: A comparative study of black and white children. *Journal of Speech and Hearing Disorders, 41*, 477–485.

ASHA. (2001). Roles and responsibilities of speech-language pathologists with respect to reading and writing in children and adolescents (Position statement). Rockville, MD: Author.

ASHA. (2016). Demographic profile of ASHA members providing bilingual services. Rockville, MD: Author.

ASHA. (n.d.). Collaborating with interpreters (Practice portal). Retrieved October 20, 2016, from www.asha.org/Practice-Portal/Professional-Issues/Collaborating-with-Interpreters

ASHA Committee on the Status of Racial Minorities. (1983). Social dialects position paper. *ASHA, 25*, 23–24.

Baker, C. (2000). *A parents' and teachers' guide to bilingualism*. Clevedon, UK: Multilingual Matters.

Barlow, J. (2005). Phonological change and the representation of consonant clusters in Spanish: A case study. *Clinical Linguistics and Phonetics, 19*, 659–679.

Beah, I. (2007). *A long way gone: Memoirs of a boy soldier*. New York: Farrar, Straus and Giroux.

Bedore, L., Peña, E., Gillam, R., & Hoa, T.-H. (2010). Language sample measures and language ability in Spanish English bilingual kindergartners. *Journal of Communication Disorders, 43*, 498–510.

Blank, M., Rose, S., & Berlin, L. (1978). *Preschool language assessment instrument (PLAI)*. San Antonio, TX: The Psychological Corporation.

Bleile, K., McGowan, J., & Bernthal, J. (1997). Professional judgements about the relationship between speech and intelligence in African American preschoolers. *Journal of Communication Disorders, 30*, 367–383.

Bleile, K., & Wallach, H. (1992). A sociolinguistic investigation of the speech of African-American preschoolers. *American Journal of Speech-Language Pathology, 1*, 44–52.

Bracken, B. (2006a). *Bracken basic concept scale—Third Edition: Expressive (BBCS-3:E)—Spanish Adaptation*. San Antonio. TX: Pearson.

Bracken, B. (2006b). *Bracken basic concept scale—Third Edition: Receptive (BBCS-3:R)—Spanish Adaptation*. San Antonio, TX: Pearson.

Brice, A. (2002). *The Hispanic child: Speech, language, culture, and education*. Boston: Allyn & Bacon.

Brice, A., & Anderson, R. (1999). Code mixing in a young bilingual child. *Communication Disorders Quarterly, 21*, 17–22.

Butt, J., & Benjamin, C. (2000). *A new reference grammar of modern Spanish* (3rd ed.). London: Edward Arnold.

Carrow, E. (1973). *Test for auditory comprehension of language*. Austin, TX: Learning Concepts.

Champion, T., Hyter, Y., McCabe, A., & Bland-Stewart, L. (2003). "A matter of vocabulary": Performances of low-income African American Head Start children on the Peabody Picture Vocabulary Test—III. *Communication Disorders Quarterly, 24*, 121–127.

Charity, A., Scarborough, H., & Griffin, D. (2004). Familiarity with school English in African American children and its relation to early reading achievement. *Child Development, 75*, 1340–1356.

Cheng, L. (1987a). *Assessment and remediation of Asian language populations*. Rockville, MD: Aspen.

Cheng, L. (1987b). Cross-cultural and linguistic considerations in working with Asian populations. *ASHA, 29*, 33–38.

Cheng, L. (1998). Enhancing the communication skills of newly-arrived Asian American students. Retrieved December 2, 2002, from http://www.eric.ed.gov

Cheng, L. (2006, September). Lessons from the Da Vinci Code. *The ASHA Leader, 11*, 14–15.

Cheng, L. (2007a). Cultural intelligence (CQ): A quest for cultural competence. *Communication Disorders Quarterly, 29*, 36–42.

Cheng, L. (2007b). From the guest editor: Introduction to the special series on culture and SLPs. *Communication Disorders Quarterly, 29*, 5–6.

Cheng, L. (2009). *Working with multilingual/multicultural families: Implications for speech language pathologists*. Paper presented at the Third International Symposium on Communication Disorders in Multilingual Populations, Agros, Cyprus.

Cheng, L. (2010). Immigration, cultural-linguistic diversity, and topics in language disorders. *Topics in Language Disorders, 30*, 79–83.

Connor, C., & Craig, H. (2006). African American preschoolers' language, emergent literacy skills, and use of African American English: A complex relation. *Journal of Speech, Language, and Hearing Research, 49*, 771–792.

Craig, H., Thompson, C., Washington, J., & Potter, S. (2003). Phonological features of child African American English. *Journal of Speech and Hearing Research, 46*, 623–635.

Craig, H., & Washington, J. (2000). An assessment battery for identifying language impairments in African American children. *Journal of Speech, Language, and Hearing Research, 43*, 366–379.

Craig, H., & Washington, J. (2002). Oral language expectations for African American preschoolers and kindergartners. *American Journal of Speech-Language Pathology, 11*, 59–70.

Craig, H., & Washington, J. (2004). Grade-related changes in the production of African American English. *Journal of Speech, Language, and Hearing Research, 47*, 450–463.

Craig, H., Zhang, L., Hensel, S., & Quinn, E. (2009). African American English–speaking students: An examination of the relationship between dialect shifting and reading outcomes. *Journal of Speech, Language, and Hearing Research, 52*, 839–855.

Crystal, D. (1997). *The Cambridge encyclopedia of language* (2nd ed.). New York: Cambridge University Press.

Cummins, J. (2000). *Language, power and pedagogy: Bilingual children in the crossfire*. Clevedon, UK: Multilingual Matters.

Day-Vines, N., Barto, H., Booker, B., Smith, K., Barna, J., Maiden, B., . . . Felder, M. (2009). African American English: Implications for school counseling professionals. *Journal of Negro Education, 78*, 70–82.

De Houwer, A. (1995). Bilingual language acquisition. In P. Fletcher & B. MacWhinney (Eds.), *Handbook of child language* (pp. 219–250). London: Blackwell.

De Houwer, A. (1999). Two or more languages in early childhood: Some general points and practical recommendations. Retrieved December 2, 2002, from http://www.cal.org/ericcll/digest/earlychild.html

Deal-Williams, V. (2002). Celebrating our differences. Retrieved December 2, 2012, from http://professional.asha.org/news/020402a.cfm

Dogruoz, A. (2008). Dutch influence on Turkish constructions in Turkish-Dutch contact. Tilburg: Tilburg University.

Dunn, L. (1965). *Peabody picture vocabulary test*. Circle Pines, MN: American Guidance Service.

Dunn, L., & Dunn, L. (1981). *Peabody picture vocabulary test—Revised*. Circle Pines, MN: American Guidance Service.

Dunn, L., & Dunn, L. (1997). *Peabody picture vocabulary test—III*. Circle Pines, MN: American Guidance Services.

Fagundes, D., Haynes, W., Haak, N., & Moran, M. (1998). Task variability effects on the language test performance of southern lower socioeconomic class African American and Caucasian five-year-olds. *Language, Speech, and Hearing Services in Schools, 29*, 148–157.

Fleischman, H., & Hopstock, P. (1993). Descriptive study of services to limited English proficient students: Vol. 1 Summary of findings and conclusions. Retrieved July 21, 2002, from www.ncbe.gwu.edu/miscpubs/siac/descript/part2.htm

Freire, P. (2004). *Pedagogy of the heart*. New York: Continuum.

Freire, P. (2006). *Pedagogy of the oppressed*. New York: Continuum.

Gardner, M. (1979). *Expressive one-word picture vocabulary test*. Novato, CA: Academic Therapy.

Gardner, M. (1983). *Expressive one-word picture vocabulary test—Upper extension*. Novato, CA: Academic Therapy.

Genesse, F., Nicoladis, E., & Paradis, J. (1995). Language differentiation in early bilingual development. *Journal of Child Language, 22*, 611–631.

Goldstein, B. (2001). Transcription of Spanish and Spanish-influenced English. *Communication Disorders Quarterly, 23*, 54–60.

Global Slavery Index. (2016). Retrieved October 22, 2016, from http://www.globalslaveryindex.org/findings/

Goldstein, B., & Iglesias, A. (2001). The effect of dialect on phonological analysis: Evidence from Spanish-speaking children. *American Journal of Speech-Language Pathology, 10*, 394–406.

Gottardo, A. (2002). The relationship between language and reading skills in bilingual Spanish-English speakers. *Topics in Language Disorders, 22*, 46–70.

Grosjean, F. (1982). *Life with two languages: An introduction to bilingualism*. Cambridge, MA: Harvard University Press.

Gutiérrez-Clellen, V. (1999). Language choice in intervention with bilingual children. *American Journal of Speech-Language Pathology, 8*, 291–302.

Gutiérrez-Clellen, V., Restrepo, M., Bedore, L., Peña, E., & Anderson, R. (2000). Language sample analysis in Spanish-speaking children: Methodological considerations. *Language, Speech, and Hearing Services in Schools, 31*, 88–98.

Hall, E. (1990). *The silent language*. New York: Anchor Books.

Hammer, C., Pennock-Roman, M., Rzasa, S., & Tomblin, J. B. (2002). An analysis of the Test of Language Development—Primary for item bias. *American Journal of Speech-Language Pathology, 11*, 274–284.

Harris, G. (1985). Considerations in assessing English language performance of Native American children. *Topics in Language Disorders, 5*, 42–52.

Hart, B., & Risley, T. (1995). *Meaningful differences in the everyday experience of young American children*. Baltimore: Paul H. Brookes.

Haynes, W., Haak, N., Moran, M., Rice, R., & Johnson, V. (1995, December). *The preschool language assessment instrument (PLAI): Performance differences in rural southern African American and white Head Start children*. Paper presented at the Annual

Convention of the American Speech-Language-Hearing Association, Orlando, FL.

Hemsley, G., Holm, A., & Dodd, B. (2014). Identifying language difference versus disorder in bilingual children. *Speech, Language and Hearing, 17*, 101–115.

Hirata, Y., Whitehurst, E., & Cullings, E. (2007). Training native English speakers to identify Japanese vowel length contrast with sentences at varied speaking rates. *Journal of the Acoustical Society of America, 121*, 3837–3845.

Hirshoren, A., & Ambrose, W. (1976). The Wepman Auditory Discrimination Test and southern Piedmont children. *Language, Speech, and Hearing Services in Schools, 7*, 86–90.

Horton-Ikard, R., & Ellis Weismer, S. (2007). A preliminary examination of vocabulary and word learning in African American toddlers from middle and low socioeconomic status homes. *American Journal of Speech-Language Pathology, 16*, 381–392.

Hwa-Froelich, D., Hodson, B., & Edwards, H. (2002). Characteristics of Vietnamese phonology. *American Journal of Speech-Language Pathology, 11*, 264–273.

Hyter, Y. (1998). Ties that bind: The sounds of African American English. Retrieved December 2, 2002, from http://www.asha.ucf.edu/hyter.html

Iglesias, A., & Anderson, N. (1993). Dialectal variations. In J. Bernthal & N. Bankson (Eds.), *Articulation and phonological disorders* (3rd ed.). Englewood Cliffs, NJ: Prentice Hall.

Jackson-Maldonado, D., Thal, D., Marchman, V., Newton, T., Fenson, L., & Conboy, B. (2003). *MacArthur inventarios del desarrollo de habilidades comunicativas: User's guide and technical manual*. Baltimore: Paul H. Brookes.

Jia, G., & Fuse, A. (2007). Acquisition of English grammatical morphology by native Mandarin-speaking children and adolescents: Age-related differences. *Journal of Speech, Language, and Hearing Research, 50*, 1280–1299.

John-Steiner, V., & Panofsky, C. (1992). Narrative competence: Cross-cultural comparisons. *Journal of Narrative and Life History, 2*, 219–233.

Juan-Garau, M., & Perez-Vidal, C. (2001). Mixing and pragmatic parental strategies in early bilingual acquisition. *Journal of Child Language, 28*, 59–86.

Kaplan, R. (1966). Cultural thought patterns in intercultural education. *Language Learning, 16*, 1–20.

Kay-Raining Bird, E., & Vetter, D. (1994). Storytelling in Chippewa-Cree children. *Journal of Speech and Hearing Research, 37*, 1354–1368.

Kirk, S., McCarthy, J., & Kirk, W. (1968). *The Illinois test of psycholinguistic abilities* (Rev. ed.). Urbana: University of Illinois Press.

Koeppe, R. (1996). Language differentiation in bilingual children: The development of grammatical and pragmatic competence. *Linguistics, 34*, 927–954.

Kohnert, K., Bates, E., & Hernandez, A. (1999). Balancing bilinguals: Lexical-semantic production and cognitive processing in children learning Spanish and English. *Journal of Speech, Language, and Hearing Research, 42*, 1400–1413.

Kohnert, K., Kennedy, M., Glaze, L., Kan, P., & Carney, E. (2003). World view, breadth and depth of diversity in Minnesota: Challenges to clinical competency. *American Journal of Speech-Language Pathology, 12*, 259–272.

Kohnert, K., Windsor, J., & Ebert, K. (2009). Primary or "specific" language impairment and children learning a second language. *Brain and Language, 109*, 101–103.

Kreschek, J., & Nicolosi, L. (1973). A comparison of black and white children's scores on the Peabody Picture Vocabulary Test. *Language, Speech, and Hearing Services in Schools, 4*, 37–40.

Langdon, H. (2012). *Spanish structured photographic expressive language test—3 (SPELT-3)*. DeKalb, IL: Janelle Publications.

Langdon, H., & Cheng, L. (2009). *Infusing cultural and linguistic diversity within CSD curriculum*. Paper presented at the Council of Academic Programs in Communication Sciences and Disorders, Newport, CA.

Leap, W. (1993). *American Indian English*. Salt Lake City, UT: University of Utah Press.

Lee, L. L. (1974). *Developmental sentence analysis: A grammatical assessment procedure for speech and language clinicians*. Evanston, IL: Northwestern University Press.

Levey, S. (2004). Discrimination and production of English vowels by bilingual speakers of Spanish and English. *Perceptual and Motor Skills, 99*, 445–462.

Linares-Orama, N., & Sanders, L. (1977). Evaluation of syntax in three-year-old Spanish-speaking Puerto Rican children. *Journal of Speech and Hearing Research, 20*, 350–357.

Long, E. (1998). Native American children's performance on the Preschool Language Scale—3. *Journal of Children's Communication Development, 19*, 43–47.

Long, E., & Christensen, J. (1998). Indirect language assessment tool for English-speaking Cherokee Indian children. *Journal of American Indian Education, 38*, 1–14.

Martin Luther King Jr. Elementary School children v. Ann Arbor School District Board. (1997). 473 Federal Supplement 1371c ED. Michigan.

Martin, N. (2012a). *Expressive one-word picture vocabulary test—4: Spanish-Bilingual Edition (EOWPVT-4:SBE)*. Novato, CA: Academic Therapy Publications.

Martin, N. (2012b). *Receptive one-word picture vocabulary test—4: Spanish-Bilingual Edition (ROWPVT-4:SBE)*. Novato, CA: Academic Therapy Publications.

Mattock, K., & Burnham, D. (2006). Chinese and English infants' tone perception: Evidence for perceptual reorganization. *Infancy, 10*, 241–265.

McGregor, K., Williams, D., Hearst, S., & Johnson, A. (1997). The use of contrastive analysis in distinguishing difference from disorder: A tutorial. *American Journal of Speech-Language Pathology, 6*, 45–56.

Miller, J., Andriacchi, K., & Nockerts, A. (2015). *Assessing language production using SALT software: A clinician's guide to language sample analysis* (2nd ed.). Middleton, WI: SALT Software LLC.

Mugitani, R., Fais, L., Dietrich, C., Werker, J., Pons, F., & Amano, S. (2009). Perception of vowel length by Japanese- and English-learning infants. *Developmental Psychology, 45*, 236–247.

Mujica, M. (2009). Fact sheet: States with official English. Retrieved February 7, 2010, from http://www.us-english.org/view/302/

National Center for Children in Poverty. (2016). Basic facts about low-income children: Children under 18 years, 2014. Retrieved September 30, 2016, from http://www.nccp.org/publications/pub_1145.html

Nelson, N., & Hyter, Y. (1990). *Black English sentence scoring: Development and use as a tool for non-biased assessment*. Paper presented at the Annual Convention of the American Speech-Language-Hearing Association, Seattle, WA.

Newcomer, P., & Hammill, D. (1977). *Test of language development*. Austin, TX: PRO-ED.

Newcomer, P., & Hammill, D. (1991). *Test of language development—Primary: 2*. Austin, TX: PRO-ED.

Nicoladis, E., & Secco, G. (2000). The role of a child's productive vocabulary in the language choice of a bilingual family. *First Language, 20*, 3–28.

Pajewski, A., & Enriquez, L. (1996). Teaching from a Hispanic perspective: A handbook for non-Hispanic adult educators. Retrieved December 2, 2012, from http://literacynet.org/lp/hperspectives/

Peacock, T., & Day, D. (1999). Teaching American Indian and Alaska Native languages in the schools: What has been learned. Retrieved July 6, 2002, from www.ed.gov/databases/ERIC_Digests/ed438155.html

Pearson, B., Fernandez, S., & Oller, D. (1995). Lexical development in bilingual infants and toddlers: Comparison to monolingual norms. *Language Learning, 43*, 93–120.

Peña, E., & Bedore, L. (2011, November 1). It takes two: Improving assessment accuracy in bilingual children. *The ASHA Leader, 16*, 20–22.

Peña, E., Bedore, L., Iglesias, A., Gutiérrez-Clellen, V., & Goldstein, B. (2008). *Bilingual English Spanish Oral Screener—Experimental Version (BESOS)*. Unpublished instrument.

Peña, E., Bedore, L., & Rappazzo, C. (2003). Comparison of Spanish, English, and bilingual children's performance across semantic tasks. *Language, Speech, and Hearing Services in Schools, 34*, 5–16.

Peña, E., Bedore, L., & Zlatic-Giunta, R. (2002). Category-generation performance of bilingual children: The influence of condition, category, and language. *Journal of Speech, Language, and Hearing Research, 45*, 938–947.

Peña, E., Gutiérrez-Clellen, V., Iglesias, A., Goldstein, B., & Bedore, L. (2014). *Bilingual English Spanish Assessment (BESA)*. San Rafael, CA: AR Clinical Publications.

Peña, E., Iglesias, A., & Lidz, C. (2001). Reducing test bias through dynamic assessment of children's word learning ability. *American Journal of Speech-Language Pathology, 10*, 138–154.

Philips, S. (1983). *The invisible culture: Communication in classroom and community on the Warm Springs Indian Reservation*. New York: Longman.

Pollock, K. (2001). Phonological features of African American Vernacular English. Retrieved December 2, 2002, from http://www.ausp.memphis.edu/phonology/features.htm

Qi, C., Kaiser, A., Milan, S., Yzquierdo, Z., & Hancock, T. (2003). The performance of low-income, African American children on the Preschool Language Scale—3. *Journal of Speech, Language, and Hearing Research, 43*, 576–590.

Qi, C., Kaiser, A., Milan, S., Yzquierdo, Z., & Hancock, T. (2006). Language performance of low-income African-American and European American preschool children on the PPVT-III. *Language, Speech, and Hearing Services in Schools, 37*, 5–16.

Quiroga, T., Lemos-Britton, Z., Mostafapour, E., Abbott, R., & Berninger, V. (2002). Phonological awareness and beginning reading in Spanish-speaking ESL first graders: Research into practice. *Journal of School Psychology, 40*, 85–111.

Ramos, M., Ramos, J., Hresko, W., Reid, D., & Hammill, D. (2007). *Test of early language development—3: Spanish (TELD-3: S)*. Austin, TX: PRO-ED.

Restrepo, M. (1998). Identifiers of Spanish-speaking children with specific language impairment. *Journal of Speech, Language, and Hearing Research, 41*, 1398–1411.

Restrepo, M., Schwanenflugel, P., Blake, J., Neuharth-Pritchett, S., Cramer, S., & Ruston, H. (2006). Performance on the PPVT-III and the EVT: Applicability of the measure with African American and European American preschool children. *Language, Speech, and Hearing Services in Schools, 37*, 17–27.

Restrepo, M., & Silverman, S. (2001). Validity of the Spanish Preschool Language Scale—3 for use with bilingual children. *American Journal of Speech-Language Pathology, 10*, 382–393.

Rethfeldt, W. (2009). *The bilingual patient's profile as an approach to logopedic intervention*. Paper presented at the Seventh European CPLOL Congress, Ljubljana, Slovenia.

Rickford, J. (1998). The creole origins of African American Vernacular English: Evidence from copula absence. In S. Mufwene, J. Rickford, G. Bailey, & J. Baugh (Eds.), *African-American English: Structure, history, and usage*. London: Routledge.

Robinson-Zañartu, C. (1996). Serving Native American children and families: Considering cultural variables. *Language, Speech, and Hearing Services in Schools, 27*, 373–384.

Rossetti, L. (2006). *The Rossetti infant-toddler scale* (Spanish translation). East Moline, IL: LinguiSystems.

Rueda, R., & Perozzi, J. (1977). A comparison of two Spanish tests of receptive language. *Journal of Speech and Hearing Disorders, 42*, 210–215.

Saad, C., & Polovoy, C. (2009, May). Differences or disorder? In the 1980s, research focused on culturally and linguistically diverse populations. *The ASHA Leader, 14*, 24–25.

Salas-Provance, M., Erickson, J., & Reed, J. (2002). Disabilities as viewed by four generations of one Hispanic family. *American Journal of Speech-Language Pathology, 11*, 151–162.

Sattler, J. (2001). *Assessment of children: Cognitive applications* (4th ed.). San Diego, CA: Jerome M. Sattler.

Semel, E., Wiig, E., & Secord, W. (2005). *Clinical evaluation of language fundamentals (CELF-4) (Spanish)*. San Antonio, TX: Pearson.

Seymour, H., Bland-Stewart, L., & Green, L. (1998). Difference versus deficit in child African American English. *Language, Speech, and Hearing Services in Schools, 29*, 96–108.

Seymour, H., Roeper, T., deVilliers, J., & deVilliers, P. (2003). *Diagnostic evaluation of language variance—Screening text (DELV-Screening)*. San Antonio, TX: The Psychological Corporation.

Seymour, H., Roeper, T., deVilliers, J., & deVilliers, P. (2005). *Diagnostic evaluation of language variation—Norm-referenced (DELV-Norm-referenced)*. San Antonio, TX: Pearson.

Smitherman, G. (2000). *Words and phrases from the Hood to the Amen Corner* (Rev. ed.). Boston: Houghton Mifflin.

Snow, C., Burns, M., & Griffin, P. (Eds.). (1998). *Preventing reading difficulties in young children*. Washington, DC: National Academies Press.

St. Charles, J., & Costantino, M. (2000). *Reading and the Native American learner* (Research Report). Olympia, WA: Office of Superintendent of Public Instruction, Office of Indian Education.

Stephens, M. (1976). Elicited imitation of selected features of two American English dialects in Head Start children. *Journal of Speech and Hearing Research, 19*, 493–508.

Stockman, I. (1996a). Phonological development and disorders in African American children. In A. Kamhi, K. Pollock, & J. Harris (Eds.), *Communication development and disorders in African American children: Research, assessment and intervention* (pp. 117–153). Baltimore: Paul H. Brookes.

Stockman, I. (1996b). The promises and pitfalls of language sample analysis as an assessment tool for linguistic minority children. *Language, Speech, and Hearing Services in Schools, 27*, 355–366.

Taylor, O. (1987). Clinical practice as a social occasion. In V. Deal (Ed.), *Communication disorders in multicultural populations*. Rockville, MD: American Speech-Language-Hearing Association.

Tempest, P. (1998). Local Navajo norms for the Wechsler Intelligence Scale for Children—Third Edition. *Journal of American Indian Education, 37*, 18–30.

Terrell, S., Arensberg, K., & Rosa, M. (1992). Parent-child comparative analysis: A criterion-referenced method for the nondiscriminatory assessment a child who spoke a relatively uncommon dialect of English. *Language, Speech, and Hearing Services in Schools, 23*, 34–42.

Teuber, J., & Furlong, M. (1985). The concurrent validity of the Expressive One-Word Picture Vocabulary Test for Mexican-American children. *Psychology in the Schools, 22*, 269–273.

Thal, D., Jackson-Maldonado, D., & Acosta, D. (2000). Validity of a parent report measure of vocabulary and grammar for Spanish-speaking toddlers. *Journal of Speech, Language, and Hearing Research, 43*, 1087–1100.

Thurston, K. (1998). Mitigating barriers to Navajo students' success in English courses. *Teaching English in the Two-Year College, 26*, 29–38.

Toppelberg, C., Medrano, L., Pena Morgens, L., & Nieto-Castanon, A. (2002). Bilingual children referred for psychiatric services:

Associations of language disorders, language skills, and psychopathology. *Journal of the American Academy of Child and Adolescent Psychiatry, 41*, 712–722.

Toppelberg, C., Snow, C., & Tager-Flusberg, H. (1999). Severe developmental disorders and bilingualism. *Journal of the American Academy of Child and Adolescent Psychiatry, 38*, 1197–1199.

Toronto, A. (1976). Developmental assessment of Spanish grammar. *Journal of Speech and Hearing Disorders, 41*, 150–171.

Trueba, H., Cheng, L., & Ima, K. (1993). *Myth or reality: Adaptive strategies of Asian Americans in California*. Washington, DC: Falmer Press.

Ukrainetz, T., Harpell, S., Walsh, C., & Coyle, C. (2000). A preliminary investigation of dynamic assessment with Native American kindergartners. *Language, Speech, and Hearing Services in Schools, 31*, 142–154.

UN High Commissioner for Refugees. (2012). The State of the World's Refugees: In Search of Solidarity. Retrieved October 22, 2016, from http://www.refworld.org/docid/5100fec32.html

U.S. Bureau of the Census. (2010). Statistical abstract of the United States (129th ed.). Washington, DC: U.S. Department of Commerce.

U.S. Department of Education. (2001). *Twenty-third annual report to Congress on the implementation of the Individuals with Disabilities Education Act*. Washington, DC: Author.

Volterra, V., & Taeschner, R. (1978). The acquisition and development of language by bilingual children. *Journal of Child Language, 5*, 311–326.

Walk Free Foundation. (2016). Global Slavery Index 2016. Retrieved October 22, 2016, from http://www.globalslaveryindex.org/45-8-million-people-enslaved-across-world/

Washington, J. (2015). The dialect features of AAE and their importance in LSA. In J. Miller, K. Andriacchi, & A. Nockerts (Eds.), *Assessing language production using SALT software: A clinician's guide to language sample analysis* (2nd ed.). Middleton, WI: SALT Software LLC.

Wepman, J. (1958). *Wepman auditory discrimination test*. Chicago: Language Research Association.

Westby, C. (2009). *Communicating across cultures: Serving diverse populations*. Paper presented at the Third International Symposium on Communication Disorder in Multilingual Populations, Argos, Cyprus.

Westby, C., & Roman, R. (1995). Finding the balance: Learning to live in two worlds. *Topics in Language Disorders, 15*, 68–88.

Wiener, F., Lewnau, L., & Erway, E. (1983). Measuring language competency in speakers of Black American English. *Journal of Speech and Hearing Disorders, 48*, 76–84.

Wiig, E., & Langdon, H. (2006). *W-ABC Spanish version*. Greenville, SC: Super-Duper Publications.

Wiig, E., Secord, W., & Semel, E. (2009). *Clinical evaluation of language fundamentals (Preschool-2) (Spanish edition)*. San Antonio, TX: Pearson.

Wilcox, K., & Aasby, S. (1988). The performance of monolingual and bilingual Mexican children on the TACL. *Language, Speech, and Hearing Services in Schools, 19*, 34–40.

Wolfram, W., & Schilling-Estes, N. (1998). *American English: Dialects and variation*. Oxford: Blackwell.

Work, R. (1991). Children of poverty: What is their future? *ASHA, 33*, 61.

Zimmerman, I., Steiner, V., & Pond, R. (1992). *Preschool language scales—3*. San Antonio, TX: The Psychological Corporation.

Zimmerman, I., Steiner, V., & Pond, R. (1993). *Preschool language scales—3: Spanish edition*. San Antonio, TX: The Psychological Corporation.

Zimmerman, I., Steiner, V., & Pond, R. (2002). *Preschool language scales—4: Spanish edition*. San Antonio, TX: Pearson.

Zimmerman, I., Steiner, V., & Pond, R. (2012a). *Preschool language scales—Fifth Edition Spanish (PLS-5 Spanish)*. Bloomington, MN: NCS Pearson.

Zimmerman, I., Steiner, V., & Pond, R. (2012b). *Preschool language scales: Spanish screening test—Fifth Edition*. Bloomington, MN: NCS Pearson.

Chapter 10

Almli, C. R., & Finger, S. (1992). Brain injury and recovery of function: Theories and mechanisms of functional reorganization. *Journal of Head Trauma Rehabilitation, 7*, 70–77.

Anderson, V., Catroppa, C., Morse, S., Haritou, F., & Rosenfeld, J. (2005). Functional plasticity or vulnerability after early traumatic brain injury. *Pediatrics, 116*, 1374–1382.

Anderson, V., Morse, S. A., Catroppa, C., Haritou, F., & Rosenfeld, J. V. (2004). Thirty month outcome from early childhood head injury: A prospective analysis of neurobehavioural recovery. *Brain, 127*, 2608–2620.

Anderson, V., Morse, S. A., Klug, G., Catroppa, C., Haritou, F., & Rosenfeld, J. V. (1997). Predicting recovery from head injury in young children: A prospective analysis. *Journal of the International Neuropsychological Society, 3*, 568–580.

Aram, D. (1988). Language sequelae of unilateral brain lesions in children. In F. Plum (Ed.), *Language, communication, and the brain* (pp. 171–198). New York: Raven Press.

Aram, D., Ekelman, B. L., & Whitaker, H. (1986). Spoken syntax in children with acquired left and right hemisphere lesions. *Brain and Language, 27*, 75–100.

Aram, D., Ekelman, B. L., & Whitaker, H. (1987). Lexical retrieval in left and right lesioned children. *Brain and Language, 31*, 75–100.

Bagnato, S. J., Mayes, S. D., Nichter, C., Domoto, V., Hamann, L., Keener, S., . . . Telenko, A. (1988). An interdisciplinary neurodevelopmental assessment model for brain-injured infants and preschool children. *Journal of Head Trauma Rehabilitation, 3*, 75–86.

Ballantyne, A. O., Spilkin, J. H., Hesselink, J., & Trauner, D. A. (2008). Plasticity in the developing brain: Intellectual, language and academic functions in children with ischaemic perinatal stroke. *Brain, 131*, 2975–2985.

Barnes, M. A., & Dennis, M. (2001). Knowledge-based inferencing after childhood head injury. *Brain and Language, 76*, 253–265.

Bates, E., & Roe, K. (2001). Language development in children with unilateral brain injury. In C. A. Nelson & M. Luciana (Eds.), *Handbook of developmental cognitive neuroscience* (pp. 281–307). Cambridge, MA: MIT Press.

Bey, T., & Ostick, B. (2009). Second impact syndrome. *West Journal of Emergency Medicine, 10*, 6–10.

Blosser, J., & DePompei, R. (1994). *Pediatric traumatic brain injury*. San Diego, CA: Singular.

Braga, L., Da Paz Júnior, A., & Ylvisaker, M. (2005). Direct clinician-delivered versus indirect family-supported rehabilitation of children with traumatic brain injury: A randomized controlled trial. *Brain Injury, 19*, 819–831.

Brain Injury Association of Virginia (BIAV). (2013). Brain Injury in the Schools: A Guide for Educators. Retrieved March 1, 2017 from http://biav.net/brain-injury-children.htm

Brookshire, B. L., Chapman, S. B., Song, J., & Levin, H. S. (2000). Cognitive and linguistic correlates of children's discourse after closed head injury: A three-year follow-up. *Journal of the International Neuropsychological Society, 6*, 741–751.

Burd, L., Gascon, G., Swenson, R., & Hankey, R. (1990). Crossed aphasia in early childhood. *Developmental Medicine and Child Neurology, 32*, 539–546.

Campbell, T., & Dollaghan, C. (1990). Expressive language recovery in severely brain-injured children and adolescents. *Journal of Speech and Hearing Disorders, 55*, 564–581.

Campbell, T., & Dollaghan, C. (1995). Speaking rate, articulatory speed, and linguistic processing in children and adolescents with severe traumatic brain injury. *Journal of Speech and Hearing Research, 38*, 864–875.

Carroll, L. J., Cassidy, D., Peloso, P. M., Borg, J., Von Holst, H., Holm, L., . . . Pepin, M. (2004). Prognosis for mild traumatic brain injury: Results of the WHO Collaborating Centre Task Force on Mild Traumatic Brain Injury. *Journal of Rehabilitation Medicine, 43*, 84–105.

Catroppa, C., & Anderson, V. (1999). Recovery of educational skills following pediatric head-injury. *Pediatric Rehabilitation, 3*, 167–175.

Catroppa, C., & Anderson, V. (2003). Children's attentional skills 2 years posttraumatic brain injury. *Developmental Neuropsychology, 23, 359–373.*

Catroppa, C., & Anderson, V. (2004). Recovery and predictors of language skills two years following pediatric traumatic brain injury. *Brain and Language, 88*, 68–78.

Catroppa, C., Anderson, V., Morse, S., Haritou, F., & Rosenfeld, J. (2008). Outcome and predictors of functional recovery 5 years following pediatric traumatic brain injury (TBI). *Journal of Pediatric Psychology, 33*, 707–718.

CDC. (2011). *Nonfatal traumatic brain injuries related to sports and recreation activities among persons aged <19 years—United States, 2001–2009*. Bethesda, MD: CDC.

Chapman, S. B., Levin, H. S., Wanek, A., Weyrauch, J., & Kufera, J. (1998). Discourse after closed head injury in young children. *Brain and Language, 61*, 420–449.

Chapman, S. B., McKinnon, L., Levin, H. S., Song, J., Meier, M. C., & Chiu, S. (2001). Longitudinal outcome of verbal discourse in children with traumatic brain injury: Three-year follow-up. *Journal of Head Trauma Rehabilitation, 16*, 441–455.

Chilosi, A. M., Cipriani, P., Pecini, C., Brizzolara, D., Biagi, L., Montanaro, D., . . . Cioni, G. (2008). Acquired focal brain lesions in childhood: Effects on development and reorganization of language. *Brain and Language, 106*, 211–225.

Cohen, S. B., Joyce, C. M., Rhoades, K. W., & Welks, D. M. (1985). Educational programming for head injured students. In M. Ylvisaker (Ed.), *Head injury rehabilitation: Children and adolescents* (pp. 395–427). Austin, TX: PRO-ED.

Cooper, J. A., & Flowers, C. R. (1987). Children with a history of acquired aphasia: Residual language and academic impairments. *Journal of Speech and Hearing Disorders, 52*, 251–262.

Cornwell, P. L., Murdoch, B., Ward, E. C., & Kellie, S. (2003). Perceptual evaluation of motor speech following treatment for childhood cerebellar tumour. *Clinical Linguistics and Phonetics, 17*, 597–615.

Dapretto, M., Woods, R. P., & Bookheimer, S. Y. (2000). *Enhanced cortical plasticity early in development: Insights from an FMRI study of language processing in children and adults*. Paper presented at the Annual Meeting of the Neuroscience Society, Los Angeles.

de Bode, S., & Curtiss, S. (2001). *Exploring neuronal plasticity: Language development in pediatric hemispherectomies*. Paper presented at the 23rd Annual Conference of the Cognitive Science Society, Edinburgh, Scotland.

Dennis, M. (1980). Strokes in childhood: Communicative intent, expression, and comprehension after left hemisphere arteriopathy in a right-handed nine-year-old. In R. W. Rieber (Ed.), *Language development and aphasia in children* (pp. 45–67). New York: Academic Press.

Dennis, M. (1992). Word finding in children and adolescents with a history of brain injury. *Topics in Language Disorders, 13*, 66–82.

Dennis, M. (2000). Developmental plasticity in children: The role of biological risk, development, time, and reserve. *Journal of Communication Disorders, 33*, 321–332.

Dennis, M., & Barnes, M. A. (2001). Comparison of literal, inferential, and intentional text comprehension in children with mild or severe closed head injury. *Journal of Head Trauma Rehabilitation, 16*, 456–468.

Dennis, M., Barnes, M. A., Wilkinson, M., & Humphreys, R. P. (1998). How children with head injury represent real and deceptive emotion in short narratives. *Brain and Language, 61*, 450–483.

Dennis, M., Purvis, K., Barnes, M. A., Wilkinson, M., & Winner, E. (2001). Understanding of literal truth, ironic criticism, and deceptive praise following childhood head injury. *Brain and Language, 78*, 1–16.

DePompei, R., & Blosser, J. (1987). Strategies for helping head-injured children successfully return to school. *Language, Speech, and Hearing Services in Schools, 18*, 292–300.

DePompei, R., Gillette, Y., Goetz, E., Xenopoulos-Oddsson, A., Bryen, D., & Dowds, M. (2008). Practical applications for use of PDAs and smartphones with children and adolescents who have traumatic brain injury. *NeuroRehabilitation, 23*, 487–499.

Dollaghan, C., & Campbell, T. (1992). A procedure for classifying disruptions in spontaneous language samples. *Topics in Language Disorders, 12*, 56–68.

Duff, M. C., Proctor, A., & Haley, K. (2002). Mild traumatic brain injury (MTBI): Assessment and treatment procedures used by speech-language pathologists (SLPs). *Brain Injury, 16*, 773–787.

Duhaime, A. C., Christian, C. W., Rorke, L. B., & Zimmerman, R. A. (1998). Nonaccidental head injury in infants—The "shaken-baby syndrome." *New England Journal of Medicine, 338*, 1822–1829.

Durham, S. R., Clancy, R. R., Leuthardt, E., Sun, P., Kamerling, S., Dominguez, T., & Duhaime, A. C. (2000). Chop infant coma scale ("infant face scale"): A novel coma scale for children less than two years of age. *Journal of Neurotrauma, 17*, 729–737.

Eisele, J., & Aram, D. (1995). Lexical and grammatical development in children with early hemisphere damage: A cross-sectional view from birth to adolescence. In P. Fletcher & B. MacWhinney (Eds.), *The handbook of child language* (pp. 664–689). Oxford: Basil Blackwell.

Ewing-Cobbs, L., & Barnes, M. (2002). Linguistic outcomes following traumatic brain injury in children. *Seminars in Pediatric Neurology: Diagnosis and Management of Language Disabilities, 9*, 209–217.

Ewing-Cobbs, L., Barnes, M., Fletcher, J. M., Levin, H. S., Swank, P. R., & Song, J. (2004). Modeling of longitudinal academic achievement scores after pediatric traumatic brain injury. *Developmental Neuropsychology, 25*, 107–133.

Ewing-Cobbs, L., Brookshire, B., Scott, M. A., & Fletcher, J. M. (1998). Children's narratives following traumatic brain injury: Linguistic structure, cohesion, and thematic recall. *Brain and Language, 61*, 395–419.

Ewing-Cobbs, L., Fletcher, J. M., Landry, S. H., & Levin, H. S. (1985). Language disorders after pediatric head injury. In J. K. Darby (Ed.), *Speech and language evaluation in neurology: Childhood disorders* (pp. 97–111). Orlando, FL: Grune and Stratton.

Ewing-Cobbs, L., Levin, H. S., & Fletcher, J. M. (1998). Neuropsychological sequelae after pediatric traumatic brain injury: Advances since 1985. In M. Ylvisaker (Ed.), *Traumatic brain injury rehabilitation: Children and adolescents* (2nd ed., pp. 11–26). Woburn, MA: Butterworth-Heinemann.

Ewing-Cobbs, L., Prasad, M. R., Kramer, L., Cox, C. S., Jr., Baumgartner, J., Fletcher, S., . . . Swank, P. (2006). Late intellectual and academic outcomes following traumatic brain injury sustained during early childhood. *Journal of Neurosurgery, 105*, 287–296.

Faul, M., Xu, L., Wald, M. M., & Coronado, V. G. (2010). *Traumatic brain injury in the United States: Emergency department visits, hospitalizations, and deaths 2002–2006*. Atlanta, GA: Centers for Disease Control and Prevention, National Center for Injury Prevention and Control.

Felberg, R. A., Burgin, W. S., & Grotta, J. C. (2000). Neuroprotection and the ischemic cascade. *CNS Spectrums, 5*, 52–58.

Foreman, B. P., Caesar, R. R., Parks, J., Madden, C., Gentilello, L. M., Shafi, S., . . . Diaz-Arrastia, R. R. (2007). Usefulness of the abbreviated injury score and the injury severity score in comparison to the Glasgow Coma Scale in predicting outcome after traumatic brain injury. *The Journal of Trauma Injury, Infection, and Critical Care, 62*, 946–950.

Fullerton, H. J., Wu, Y. W., Zhao, S., & Johnston, C. S. (2003). Risk of stroke in children: Ethnic and gender disparities. *Neurology, 61*, 189–194.

Gaddes, W. H., & Crockett, D. J. (1975). The Spreen-Benton aphasia tests, normative data as a measure of normal language development. *Brain and Language, 2*, 257–280.

Ghosh, A., Wilde, E. A., Hunter, J. V., Bigler, E. D., Chu, Z., Li, X., . . . Levin, H. S. (2009). The relation between Glasgow Coma Scale score and later cerebral atrophy in paediatric traumatic brain injury. *Brain Injury, 23*, 228–233.

Giza, C. C., Kutcher, J. S., Barth, J., Getchius, T. S. D., Giaoia, G. A., Guskiewicz, K., . . . Zafonte, R. (2013). Summary of evidence-based guidelines update: Evaluation and management of concussion in sports. *Neurology, 80*, 2250–2257.

Haley, S. M., Cioffi, M. I., Lewin, J. E., & Barqza, M. J. (1990). Motor dysfunction in children and adolescents after traumatic brain injury. *Journal of Head Trauma Rehabilitation, 5*, 77–90.

Hawley, C. A., Ward, A. B., Magnay, A. R., & Long, J. (2003). Parental stress and burden following traumatic brain injury amongst children and adolescents. *Brain Injury, 17*, 1–23.

Hawley, C. A., Ward, A. B., Magnay, A. R., & Mychalkiw, W. (2004). Return to school after brain injury. *Archives of Disease in Childhood, 89*, 136–142.

Heather, N. L., Derraik, J. G., Beca, J., Hofman, P. L., Dansey, R., Hamill, J., & Cutfield, W. S. (2013). Glasgow Coma Scale and outcomes after structural traumatic head injury in early childhood. *PLoS One, 8*, e82245. doi: 10.1371/journal.pone.0082245

Hécaen, H. (1976). Acquired aphasia in children and the ontogenesis of hemispheric functional specialization. *Brain and Language, 3*, 114–134.

Helm-Estabrooks, N., & Albert, M. (2004). *Manual of aphasia and aphasia therapy* (2nd ed.). Austin, TX: PRO-ED.

Hotz, G., Helm-Estabrooks, N., & Nelson, N. W. (2001). Development of the pediatric test of traumatic brain injury. *Journal of Head Trauma Rehabilitation, 16*, 426–440.

Hux, K. (2011). *Assisting survivors of traumatic brain injury: The role of the speech-language pathologist* (2nd ed.). Austin, TX: PRO-ED.

Hux, K., Walker, M., & Sanger, D. (1996). Traumatic brain injury: Knowledge and self-perceptions of school speech-language pathologists. *Language, Speech, and Hearing Services in Schools, 27*, 171–184.

Jantz, P. B., & Coulter, G. A. (2007). Child and adolescent traumatic brain injury: Academic, behavioural, and social consequences in the classroom. *Support for Learning, 22*, 84–89.

Janusz, J. A., Kirkwood, M. W., Yeates, K. O., & Taylor, H. G. (2002). Social problem-solving skills in children with traumatic brain injury: Long-term outcomes and prediction of social competence. *Child Neuropsychology, 8*, 179–194.

Johansson, B. (2004). Brain plasticity in health and disease. *The Keio Journal of Medicine, 53*, 231–246.

Jordan, F., & Ashton, R. (1996). Language performance of severely closed head injured children. *Brain Injury, 10*, 91–97.

Jordan, F., Cremona-Meteyard, S., & King, A. (1996). High-level linguistic disturbances subsequent to childhood closed head injury. *Brain Injury, 10*, 729–738.

Jordan, F., & Murdoch, B. (1994). Severe closed-head injury in childhood: Linguistic outcomes into adulthood. *Brain Injury, 8*, 501–508.

Jordan, F., Murdoch, B., Hudson-Tennent, L., & Boon, D. (1996). Naming performance of brain-injured children. *Aphasiology, 10*, 755–766.

Kirkwood, M., Yeates, K., Taylor, G., Randolph, C., McCrea, M., & Anderson, V. (2008). Management of pediatric mild traumatic brain injury: A neuropsychological review from injury through recovery. *Clinical Neuropsychology*, 22, 769–800.

Koch, M. A., Narayan, R. K., & Timmons, S. D. (2007). Traumatic brain injury. Retrieved March 24, 2009, from http://www.merck.com/mmpe/sec21/ch310/ch310a.html?qt=Traumatic%20Brain%20Injury&alt=sh

Kochanek, P. M., Berger, R., Bayr, H., Wagner, A. K., Jenkins, L. W., & Clark, R. (2008). Biomarkers of primary and evolving damage in traumatic and ischemic brain injury: Diagnosis, prognosis, probing mechanisms, and therapeutic decision making. *Neuroscience, 14*, 135–141.

Laatsch, L., Harrington, D., Hotz, G., Marcantuono, J., Mozzoni, M., Walsh, V., & Hersey, K. (2007). An evidence-based review of cognitive and behavioural rehabilitation treatment studies in children with acquired brain injury. *Journal of Head Trauma Rehabilitation, 22*, 248–256.

Lenneberg, E. (1967). *Biological foundations of language*. New York: Wiley.

Levin, H. S., Hanten, G., Zhang, L., Swank, P. R., Ewing-Cobbs, L., Dennis, M., . . . Hunter, J. V. (2004). Changes in working memory after traumatic brain injury in children. *Neuropsychology, 18*, 240–247.

Mandalis, A., Kinsella, G., Ong, B., & Anderson, V. (2007). Working memory and new learning following pediatric traumatic brain injury. *Developmental Neuropsychology, 32*, 683–701.

Martins, I. P., & Ferro, J. M. (1992). Recovery of acquired aphasia in children. *Aphasiology, 6*, 431–438.

Mason, C. N. (2013). Mild traumatic brain injury in children. *Continuing Nursing Education, 39*, 267–272.

McDonald, S. (1993). Pragmatic language skills after closed head injury: Ability to meet the informational needs of the listener. *Brain and Language, 44*, 28–46.

McDonald, S., & Turkstra, L. (1998). Adolescents with traumatic brain injury: Assessing pragmatic language function. *Clinical Linguistics and Phonetics, 12*, 237–248.

Mills, D. L., Coffey-Corina, S. A., & Neville, H. J. (1993). Language acquisition and cerebral specialization in 20-month-old infants. *Journal of Cognitive Neuroscience, 5*, 317–334.

Minino, A. M., & Smith, B. L. (2001). Deaths: Preliminary data for 2000. *National Vital Statistics Reports, 49*, 1–40.

Msall, M. E., DiGaudio, K., Rogers, B. T., LaForest, S., Catanzaro, N. L., Campbell, J., . . . Duffy, L. C. (1994). The Functional Independence Measure for Children (WeeFIM): Conceptual basis and pilot use in children with developmental disabilities *Clinical Pediatrics, 33*, 421–430.

National Center for Injury Prevention and Control (NCIPC). (2003). *Report to Congress on mild traumatic brain injury in the United States: Stets to prevent a serious public health problem*. Atlanta, GA: Centers for Disease Control and Prevention, National Center for Injury Prevention and Control.

National Head Injury Foundation. (1985). *An educator's manual: What educators need to know about students with traumatic brain injury*. Framingham, MA: Author.

New Zealand Guidelines Group. (1998). Traumatic brain injury rehabilitation guidelines. Retrieved December 2, 2002, from http://www.nzgg.org.nz/library/gl_complete/tbiTBI_guideline.pdf

Ottenbacher, K. J., Taylor, E. L., Msall, M. E., Braun, S., Lane, S. J., Granger, C. V., . . . Duffy, L. C. (2008). The stability and equivalence reliability of the Functional Independence Measure for Children (WeeFIM). *Developmental Medicine and Child Neurology, 38*, 907–916.

Porch, B. (1979). *Porch index of communicative ability in children*. Palo Alto, CA: Consulting Psychologists Press.

Raybarman, C. (2002). Landau-Kleffner syndrome: A case report. *Neurology India, 50*, 212–213.

Reilly, P., Simpson, D., Sprod, R., & Thomas, L. (1988). Assessing the conscious level in infants and young children: A pediatric version of the Glasgow Coma Scale. *Child's Nervous System, 4*, 30–33.

Roger, V. L., Go, A. S., Lloyd-Jones, D. M., Adams, R. J., Berry, J. D., Brown, T. M., . . . Wylie-Rosett, J. (2011). Heart disease and stroke statistics—2011 update: A report from the American Heart Association. *Circulation, 123*, e18–e209.

Ross, K., Dorris, L., & McMillan, T. (2011). A systematic review of psychological interventions to alleviate cognitive and psychosocial problems in children with acquired brain injury. *Developmental Medicine and Child Neurology, 53*, 692–701.

Sander, A. (2002). The Center for Outcome Measurement in Brain Injury. Retrieved April 23, 2009, from www.tbims.org/combi/lcfs

Sarno, M. T. (1998). Recovery and rehabilitation in aphasia. In M. T. Sarno (Ed.), *Acquired aphasia* (3rd ed., pp. 595–631). San Diego, CA: Academic Press.

Satz, P., & Bullard-Bates, C. (1981). Acquired aphasia in children. In M. T. Sarno (Ed.), *Acquired aphasia* (2nd ed.). New York: Academic Press.

Savage, R. C. (1991). Identification, classification, and placement issues for students with traumatic brain injuries. *Journal of Head Trauma Rehabilitation, 6*, 1–9.

Savage, R. C., DePompei, R., Tyler, J., & Lash, M. (2005). Paediatric traumatic brain injury: A review of pertinent issues. *Pediatric Rehabilitation, 8*, 92–103.

Savage, R. C., & Wolcott, G. (1994). *Educational dimensions of acquired brain injury*. Austin, TX: PRO-ED.

Semel, E., Wiig, E., & Secord, W. (2013). *Clinical evaluation of language fundamentals—5*. San Antonio, TX: The Psychological Corporation.

Simpson, D. A., Cockington, R. A., Hanieh, A., Raftos, J., & Reilly, P. L. (1991). Head injuries in infants and young children: The value of Pediatric Coma Scale: Review of literature and report on a study. *Child's Nervous System, 7*, 183–190.

Statler, K. D., Swank, S., Abildskov, T., Bigler, E. D., & White, H. S. (2008). Traumatic brain injury during development reduces minimal clonic seizure thresholds at maturity. *Epilepsy Research, 80*, 163–170.

Sullivan, J., & Riccio, C. (2010). Language functioning and deficits following pediatric traumatic brain injury. *Applied Neuropsychology, 17*, 93–98.

Swisher, L. (1985). Language disorders in children. In J. K. Darby (Ed.), *Speech and language evaluation in neurology: Childhood disorders*. Orlando, FL: Grune and Stratton.

Tate, R., & Douglas, J. (2002). Editorial: Evidence-based clinical practice in rehabilitation. *Brain Impairment, 3*, ii–iv.

Taylor, H. G., Yeates, K. O., Wade, S. L., Drotar, D., Stancin, T., & Minich, N. (2002). A prospective study of short- and long-term outcomes after traumatic brain injury in children: Behavior and achievement. *Neuropsychology, 16*, 15–27.

Teasdale, G., & Jennett, B. (1974). Assessment of coma and impaired consciousness: A practical scale. *Lancet, 2*, 81–84.

Tucker, B. F., & Colson, S. E. (1992). Traumatic brain injury: An overview of school re-entry. *Intervention in School and Clinic, 27*, 198–206.

Turkstra, L. (1999). Language testing in adolescents with brain injury: A consideration of the CELF-3. *Language, Speech, and Hearing Services in Schools, 30*, 132–140.

Turkstra, L., & Holland, A. (1998). Assessment of syntax after adolescent brain injury: Effects of memory on test performance. *Journal of Speech, Language, and Hearing Research, 41*, 137–149.

Turkstra, L., Politis, A. M., & Forsyth, R. (2015). Cognitive-communication disorders in children with traumatic brain injury. *Developmental Medicine and Child Neurology, 57*, 217–222.

van Dongen, H. R., Paquier, P. F., Creten, W. L., van Borsel, J., & Catsman-Berrevoets, C. E. (2001). Clinical evaluation of conversational speech fluency in the acute phase of acquired childhood aphasia: Does a fluency/nonfluency dichotomy exist? *Journal of Child Neurology, 16*, 345–351.

van Mourik, M., Catsman-Berrevoets, C. E., Yousef-Bak, E., Paquier, P. F., & van Dongen, H. R. (1998). Dysarthria in children with cerebellar or brainstem tumors. *Pediatric Neurology, 18*, 411–414.

Watamori, T. S., Sasanuma, S., & Ueda, S. (1990). Recovery and plasticity in child-onset aphasics: Ultimate outcome at adulthood. *Aphasiology, 4*, 9–30.

Wright, J. (2000). The FIM™. Retrieved April 23, 2009, from www.tbims.org/combi/FIM

Yeates, K. O., & Taylor, H. G. (2006). Behavior problems in school and their educational correlates among children with traumatic brain injury. *Exceptionality, 14*, 141–154.

Ylvisaker, M. (1989). Cognitive and psychosocial outcome following head injury in children. In J. T. Hoff, T. Anderson, & T. Cole (Eds.), *Mild to moderate head injury* (Vol. 3 of Contemporary Issues in Neurological Surgery). Boston: Blackwell Scientific Publications, Inc.

Ylvisaker, M., & Feeney, T. (2007). Pediatric brain injury: Social, behavioral, and communication disability. *Physical Medicine and Rehabilitation Clinics of North America*, 18, 133–144.

Ylvisaker, M., & Gioia, G. A. (1998). Cognitive assessment. In M. Ylvisaker (Ed.), *Traumatic brain injury rehabilitation: Children and adolescents* (2nd ed., pp. 159–179). Boston: Butterworth-Heinemann.

Ylvisaker, M., Hartwick, P., & Stevens, M. (1991). School reentry following head injury: Managing the transition from hospital to school. *Journal of Head Trauma Rehabilitation, 6*, 10–22.

Ylvisaker, M., & Holland, A. (1984). Head injury. In W. H. Perkins (Ed.), *Language handicaps in children*. New York: Thieme-Stratton.

Ylvisaker, M., & Szekeres, S. F. (1989). Metacognitive and executive impairments in head-injured children and adults. *Topics in Language Disorders, 9*, 34–49.

Ylvisaker, M., Turkstra, L., & Coelho, C. (2005). Behavioral and social interventions for individuals with traumatic brain injury: A summary of the research with clinical implications. *Seminars in Speech and Language, 26*, 256–267.

Yorkston, K. M., Jaffe, K. M., Liao, S., & Polissar, N. L. (1999). Recovery of written language production in children with traumatic brain injury: Outcomes at one year. *Aphasiology, 13*, 691–700.

Ziviani, J., Ottenbacher, K. J., Shepard, K., Foreman, S., Astbury, W., & Ireland, P. (2001). Concurrent validity of the Functional Independence Measure for Children (WeeFIM) and the Pediatric Evaluation of Disabilities Inventory in children with developmental disabilities and acquired brain injury. *Physical and Occupational Therapy in Pediatrics, 21*, 91–101.

Chapter 11

Alexander, P., & Muia, J. (1982). *Gifted education: A comprehensive roadmap*. Rockville, MD: Aspen.

Andersen, E. S., Dunlea, A., & Kekelis, L. (1984). Blind children's language: Resolving some differences. *Journal of Child Language, 11*, 645–664.

Arndt, J., & Healey, E. (2001). Concomitant disorders in school-age children who stutter. *Language, Speech, and Hearing Services in Schools, 32*, 68–78.

Assouline, S., Nicpon, M., & Huber, D. (2006). The impact of vulnerabilities and strengths on the academic experiences of twice-exceptional students: A message to school counselors. *Professional School Counseling, 10*, 14–24.

Bajaj, A. (2007). Analysis of oral narratives of children who stutter and their fluent peers: Kindergarten through second grade. *Clinical Linguistics and Phonetics, 21*, 227–245.

Barlow-Brown, F., & Connelly, V. (2002). The role of letter knowledge and phonological awareness in young Braille readers. *Journal of Research in Reading, 25*, 259–270.

Bernstein Ratner, N. (1995). Language complexity and stuttering in children. *Topics in Language Disorders, 15*, 32–47.

Blood, G., & Seider, R. (1981). The concomitant problems of young stutterers. *Journal of Speech and Hearing Research, 46*, 31–33.

Bottcher, L., Flachs, E. M., & Uldall, P. (2010). Attentional and executive impairments in children with spastic cerebral palsy. *Developmental Medicine and Child Neurology, 52*, 42–47.

Broder, H., Richman, L., & Matheson, P. (1998). Learning disability, school achievement, and grade retention among children with cleft: A two-center study. *Cleft Palate-Craniofacial Journal, 35*, 127–131.

Brody, L., & Mills, C. (1997). Gifted children with learning disabilities: A review of the issues. *Journal of Learning Disabilities, 30*, 282–286.

Broen, P., Doyle, S., Moller, K., & Prouty, J. (1991). *Early language development in children with cleft palate.* Paper presented at the Annual Convention of the American Speech-Language-Hearing Association, Atlanta, GA.

Butcher, C., McFadden, D., Quinn, B., & Ryan, B. (2003). The effects of language training on stuttering in young children, without and with contingency management. *Journal of Developmental and Physical Disabilities, 15*, 255–280.

Byrd, K., & Cooper, E. (1989). Expressive and receptive language skills in stuttering children. *Journal of Fluency Disorders, 14*, 121–126.

Byrne, K., Abbeduto, L., & Brooks, P. (1990). The language of children with spina bifida and hydrocephalus: Meeting task demands and mastering syntax. *Journal of Speech and Hearing Disorders, 55*, 118–123.

California Birth Defects Monitoring Program. (2002). Oral clefts: Racial/ethnic variation. Retrieved December 2, 2002, from www.cbdmp.org/bd_clefts_racial.htm

Carneol, S., Marks, S., & Weik, L. (1999). The speech-language pathologist: Key role in the diagnosis of velocardiofacial syndrome. *American Journal of Speech-Language Pathology, 8*, 23–32.

Ceponiene, R., Hukki, J., Cheour, M., Haapanen, M., Koskinen, M., Alho, K., & Naatanen, R. (2000). Dysfunction of the auditory cortex persists in infants with certain cleft types. *Developmental Medicine and Child Neurology, 42*, 258–265.

Ceponiene, R., Hukki, J., Cheour, M., Haapanen, M., Ranta, R., & Naatanen, R. (1999). Cortical auditory dysfunction in children with oral clefts: Relation with cleft types. *Clinical Neurophysiology, 110*, 1921–1926.

Chapman, K. (2004). Is presurgery and early postsurgery performance related to speech and language outcomes at 3 years of age for children with cleft palate? *Clinical Linguistics and Phonetics, 18*, 235–257.

Chapman, K., Hardin-Jones, M., & Halter, K. (2003). The relationship between early speech and later speech and language performance for children with cleft lip and palate. *Clinical Linguistics and Phonetics, 17*, 173–197.

Chapman, K., Hardin-Jones, M., Goldstein, J. A., Halter, K. A., Haylik, R. J., & Schulte, J. (2008). Timing of palatal surgery and speech outcome. *Cleft Palate-Craniofacial Journal, 45*, 297–308.

Chen, D. (1996). Parent-infant communication: Early intervention for very young children with visual impairment or hearing loss. *Infants and Young Children, 9*, 1–13.

Chen, L., & Whittington, D. (2006). Organizing language intervention relative to the client's personal experience: A clinical case study. *Clinical Linguistics and Phonetics, 20*, 563–571.

Cline, S., & Hegeman, K. (2005). Gifted children with disabilities. In S. Johnsen & J. Kendrick (Eds.), *Teaching gifted students with disabilities* (pp. 37–54). Waco, TX: Prufrock Press.

Cline, S., & Schwartz, D. (1999). *Diverse populations of gifted children.* Columbus, OH: Prentice Hall.

Cohen, L. (1990). Meeting the needs of gifted and talented minority language students. Retrieved July 23, 2002, from www.ed.gov/databases/ERIC_Digests/ed321485.html

Colburn, N., & Mysak, E. (1982a). Developmental disfluency and emerging grammar I. Disfluency in early syntactic utterances. *Journal of Speech and Hearing Research, 25*, 414–420.

Colburn, N., & Mysak, E. (1982b). Developmental disfluency and emerging grammar II. Cooccurrence of disfluency with specified semantic-syntactic structures. *Journal of Speech and Hearing Research, 25*, 421–427.

Conti-Ramsden, G., & Perez-Pereira, M. (1999). Conversational interactions between mothers and their infants who are congenitally blind, have low vision, or are sighted. *Journal of Visual Impairment and Blindness, 93*, 691–703.

Cotton, S., Voudouris, N., & Greenwood, K. (2001). Intelligence and Duchenne muscular dystrophy: Full-scale, verbal, and performance intelligence quotients. *Developmental Medicine and Child Neurology, 43*, 497–501.

Cramer, R. (1991). The education of gifted children in the United States: A Delphi study. *Gifted Child Quarterly, 35*, 84–91.

Cramond, B. (2004). Reading instruction for the gifted. *Illinois Reading Council Journal, 32*, 31–36.

Crawford, S., & Snart, F. (1994). Process-based remediation of decoding in gifted LD students: Three case studies. *Roeper Review, 16*, 247–253.

Croen, L., Shaw, G., Wasserman, C., & Tolarova, M. (1998). Racial and ethnic variations in the prevalence of orofacial clefts in California, 1983–1992. *American Journal of Medicine Genetics, 79*, 42–47.

Culp, D. (1984). The preschool fluency development program: Assessment and treatment. In M. Peins (Ed.), *Contemporary approaches to stuttering treatment* (pp. 39–71). Boston: Little, Brown.

Cutler, R. (1992). Neurology. In E. Rubenstein & D. Federman (Eds.), *Scientific American medicine.* New York: Scientific American.

Cyrulnik, S., Fee, R., Batchelder, A., Kiefel, J., Goldstein, E., & Hinton, V. (2008). Cognitive and adaptive deficits in young children with Duchenne muscular dystrophy (DMD). *Journal of the International Neuropsychological Society, 14*, 853–861.

Devers, M., & Broen, P. (1991). *Prelinguistic vocalizations of infants with and without cleft palate.* Paper presented at the Annual Convention of the American Speech-Language-Hearing Association, Atlanta, GA.

Fehrenbach, C. (1991). Gifted/average readers: Do they use the same reading strategies? *Gifted Child Quarterly, 35*, 125–127.

Fehrenbach, C. (1994). Cognitive style of gifted and average readers. *Roeper Review, 16*, 290–292.

Fenstermacher, G. (1982). To be or not to be gifted: That is the question. *Elementary School Journal, 82*, 299–303.

Fletcher, J., Barnes, M., & Dennis, M. (2002). Language development in children with spina bifida. *Seminars in Pediatric Neurology, 9*, 201–208.

Ford, D. (1996). *Reversing underachievement among gifted black students: Promising practices and programs.* New York: Teachers College Press.

Ford, D. (1997). Underachievement among gifted minority students: Problems and promises. Reston, VA: ERIC Clearinghouse on Disabilities and Gifted Education.

Frasier, M., Hunsaker, S., Lee, J., Mitchell, S., Cramond, B., Krisel, S., . . . Finley, V. S. (1995). Core attributes of giftedness: A foundation for recognizing the gifted potential of economically disadvantaged students. Storrs, CT: National Research Center on the Gifted and Talented, University of Connecticut.

Frederickson, M., Chapman, K., & Hardin-Jones, M. (2006). Conversational skills of children with cleft lip and palate: A replication and extension. *Cleft Palate-Craniofacial Journal, 43*, 179–188.

Freeman, J. (1979). *Gifted children: Their identification and development in a social context*. Baltimore: University Park Press.

Freeman, R., & Blockberger, S. (1987). Language development and sensory disorder: Visual and hearing impairments. In W. Yule & M. Rutter (Eds.), *Language development and disorders*. Philadelphia: Lippincott.

Gagne, F. (1998). The prevalence of gifted, talented, and multitalented individuals: Estimates from peer and teacher nominations. In R. Friedman & K. Rogers (Eds.), *Table in context: Historical and social perspectives on giftedness* (pp. 101–126). Washington, DC: American Psychological Association.

Galati, D. (1997). Voluntary facial expression of emotion: Comparing congenitally blind with normally sighted encoders. *Journal of Personality and Social Psychology, 73*, 1363–1379.

Geake, J., & Gross, M. (2008). Teachers' negative affect toward academically gifted students: An evolutionary psychological study. *Gifted Child Quarterly, 52*, 217–231.

Gentry, M. (2009). Myth 11: A comprehensive continuum of gifted education and talent development services: Discovering, developing, and enhancing young people's gifts and talents. *Gifted Child Quarterly, 53*, 262–265.

Gerdes, M., Solot, C., Wang, P., Moss, E., LaRossa, D., & Randall, P. (1999). Cognitive and behavior profile of preschool children with chromosome 22q11.2 deletion. *American Journal of Medical Genetics, 85*, 127–133.

Gillon, G., & Young, A. (2002). The phonological awareness skills of children who are blind. *Journal of Visual Impairment and Blindness, 96*, 38–49.

Gisel, E., Birnbaum, R., & Schwartz, S. (1998). Feeding impairments in children: Diagnosis and effective interventions. *International Journal of Orofacial Myology, 24*, 27–33.

Gothelf, D. (2007). Velocardiofacial syndrome. *Child Adolescent Psychiatric Clinics of North America, 16*, 677–693.

Gothelf, D., Schaer, M., & Eliez, S. (2008). Genes, brain development and psychiatric phenotypes in velo-cardio-facial syndrome. *Developmental Disabilities Research Review, 14*, 59–68.

Grunwell, P., & Russell, J. (1987). Vocalisations before and after cleft palate surgery: A pilot study. *British Journal of Disorders of Communication, 22*, 1–17.

Hall, N., Yamashita, T., & Aram, D. (1993). Relationship between language and fluency in children with developmental language disorders. *Journal of Speech and Hearing Research, 36*, 568–579.

Hardin-Jones, M. A., & Chapman, K. (2011). Cognitive and language issues associated with cleft lip and palate. *Seminars in Speech and Language, 32*, 127–140.

Hardin-Jones, M., Chapman, K., & Schulte, J. (2003). The impact of cleft type on early vocal development in babies with cleft palate. *Cleft Palate-Craniofacial Journal, 40*, 453–459.

Himpens, P., Van den Broeck, C., Oostra, A., Calders, P., & Vanhaesebrouck, P. (2008). Prevalence, type, distribution, and severity of cerebral palsy in relation to gestational age: A meta-analytic review. *Developmental Medicine and Child Neurology, 50*, 334–340.

Hinton, V., De Vivo, D., Fee, R., Goldstein, E., & Stern, Y. (2004). Investigation of poor academic achievement in children with Duchenne muscular dystrophy. *Learning Disabilities Research and Practice, 19*, 146–154.

Hinton, V., Fee, R., Goldstein, E., & De Vivo, D. (2007). Verbal and memory skills in males with Duchenne muscular dystrophy. *Developmental Medicine and Child Neurology, 49*, 123–128.

Hoh, P. (2005). The linguistic advantage of the intellectually gifted child: An empirical study of spontaneous speech. *Roeper Review, 27*, 178–185.

Howe, M. (1990). *The origins of exceptional abilities*. Cambridge, MA: Basil Blackwell.

Howell, P., Davis, S., & Au-Yeung, J. (2003). Syntactic development in fluent children, children who stutter, and children who have English as an additional language. *Child Language Teaching and Therapy, 19*, 311–337.

Hustad, K. C., Allison, K., McFadd, E., & Riehle, K. (2013). Speech and language development in 2-year-old children with cerebral palsy. *Developmental Neurorehabilitation, 17*, 167–175.

Iverson, J. (2000). The relation between gesture and speech in congenitally blind and sighted language-learners. *Journal of Nonverbal Behavior, 24*, 105–130.

Jackson, N. (1988). Precocious reading ability: What does it mean? *Gifted Child Quarterly, 32*, 200–204.

Jackson, N., Donaldson, G., & Cleland, L. (1988). The structure of precocious reading ability. *Journal of Educational Psychology, 80*, 234–243.

Jackson, N., & Kearney, J. (1995). Achievement of precocious readers in middle childhood and young adulthood. In N. Colangelo & S. Assouline (Eds.), *Talent development III* (pp. 203–218). Scottsdale, AZ: Gifted Psychology Press.

James, D. M., & Stojanovik, V. (2007). Communication skills in blind children: A preliminary investigation. *Child: Care, Health and Development, 33*, 4–10.

Jan, J., Groenveld, M., Sykanda, A., & Hoyt, C. (1987). Behavioral characteristics of children with permanent cortical visual impairment. *Developmental Medicine and Child Neurology, 29*, 571–576.

Kirby, R. S., Wingate, M. S., Van Naarden Braun, K., Doernberg, N. S., Arneson, C. L., Benedict, R. E., . . . Yeargin-Allsopp, M. (2011). Prevalence and functioning of children with cerebral palsy in four areas of the United States in 2006: A report from the Autism and Developmental Disabilities Monitoring Network. *Developmental Disabilities, 32*, 462–469.

Kitzinger, M. (1984). The role of repeated and echoed utterances in communication with a blind child. *British Journal of Disorders of Communication, 19*, 135–146.

Kummer, A. W. (2014). *Cleft palate and craniofacial anomalies: The effects on speech and resonance* (3rd ed.). New York: Delmar Cengage Learning.

Landau, B., & Gleitman, L. (1985). *Language and experience: Evidence from the blind child*. Cambridge, MA: Harvard University Press.

Lee, S., Olszewski-Kubilius, P., & Thomson, D. (2012). Academically gifted students' perceived interpersonal competence and peer relationships. *Gifted Child Quarterly, 56*, 90–104.

Lomax-Bream, L., Taylor, H., Landry, S., Barnes, M., Fletcher, J., & Swank, P. (2007). Role of early parenting and motor skills on development in children with spina bifida. *Journal of Applied Developmental Psychology, 28*, 250–263.

Loots, G., Devisé, I., & Sermijn, J. (2003). The interaction between mothers and their visually impaired infants: An intersubjective developmental perspective. *Journal of Visual Impairment and Blindness, 97*, 403–418.

Louis, B., & Lewis, M. (1992). Prenatal beliefs about giftedness in young children and their relation to actual ability level. *Gifted Child Quarterly, 36*, 27–31.

March of Dimes Birth Defects Foundation. (2002). March of Dimes: Health library: Infant health statistics. Retrieved July 8, 2002, from www.modimes.org/HealthLibrary/334_606.htm

Marchant, J. (1992). Deaf-blind handicapping conditions. In P. McLaughlin & P. Wehman (Eds.), *Developmental disabilities: A handbook for best practices*. Boston: Andover Medical.

McClain, M., & Pfeiffer, S. (2012). Identification of gifted students in the United States today: A look at state definitions, policies, and practices. *Journal of Applied School Psychology, 28*, 59–88.

McCluckey, K., & Walker, K. (1986). *The doubtful gift*. Kingston: Ronald P. Frye.

McWilliams, B., Morris, H., & Shelton, R. (1990). *Cleft palate speech*. Philadelphia: BC Decker.

Mendaglio, S. (1993). Counseling techniques. In L. Silverman (Ed.), *Counseling the gifted and talented* (pp. 131–149). Denver, CO: Love.

Mervis, C., Yeargin-Allsopp, M., Winter, S., & Boyle, C. (2000). Aetiology of childhood vision impairment, metropolitan Atlanta, 1991–93. *Paediatric and Perinatal Epidemiology, 14*, 70–77.

Mills, C., & Durden, W. (1992). Cooperative learning and ability grouping: An issue of choice. *Gifted Child Quarterly, 36*, 11–16.

Mindell, P., & Stracher, D. (1980). Assessing reading and writing of the gifted: The warp and woof of the language program. *Gifted Child Quarterly, 24*, 72–80.

Morris, S., & Klein, K. (1987). *Pre-feeding skills: A comprehensive resource for therapists*. Tucson, AZ: Therapy Skill Builders.

Muscular Dystrophy Campaign. (2002). Duchenne MD. Retrieved December 2, 2002, from http://www.muscular-dystrophy.org/information/KeyFacts/duchenne.html

National Joint Committee on Learning Disabilities. (1998). Operationalizing the NJCLD definition of learning disabilities for ongoing assessment in schools. *Learning Disabilities Quarterly, 21*, 186–193.

Nippold, M. (2004). Phonological and language disorders in children who stutter: Impact on treatment recommendations. *Clinical Linguistics and Phonetics, 18*, 145–159.

Nopoulos, P., Berg, S., Canady, J., Van Demark, D., Richman, L., & Andreasen, N. C. (2000). Abnormal brain morphology in patients with isolated cleft lip, cleft palate, or both: A preliminary analysis. *Cleft Palate-Craniofacial Journal, 37*, 441–446.

Nordberg, A., Miniscalco, C., Lohmander, A., & Himmelmann, K. (2013). Speech problems affect more than one in two children with cerebral palsy: Swedish population-based study. *Acta Paediatrica, 102*, 161–166.

Ntourou, K., Conture, E. G., & Lipsey, M. W. (2011). Language abilities of children who stutter: A meta-analytical review. *American Journal of Speech-Language Pathology, 20*, 163–179.

O'Connor, J. (2012). Is it good to be gifted? The social construction of the gifted child. *Children and Society, 26*, 293–303.

O'Gara, M., & Logemann, J. (1988). Phonetic analyses of the speech development of babies with cleft palate. *Cleft Palate Journal, 25*, 122–134.

Olenchak, F. (1994). Talent development. *Journal of Secondary Gifted Education, 5*, 40–52.

Olson, L., Evans, J., & Keckler, W. (2006). Precocious readers: Past, present, and future. *Journal for the Education of the Gifted, 30*, 205–235.

Paradise, J., Elster, B., & Lingshi, T. (1994). Evidence in infants with cleft lip and palate that breast milk protects against otitis media. *Pediatrics, 94*, 853–860.

Parette, H., Hourcade, J., & Ginny, S. (2000). The importance of structured computer experiences for young children with and without disabilities. *Early Childhood Education Journal, 27*, 243–250.

Parke, K., Shallcross, R., & Anderson, R. (1980). Differences in coverbal behavior between blind and sighted persons during dyadic communication. *Journal of Visual Impairment and Blindness, 74*, 142–146.

Perez-Pereira, M., & Conti-Ramsden, G. (1999). *Language development and social interaction in blind children*. Hove: Psychology Press.

Perez-Pereira, M., & Conti-Ramsden, G. (2001). The use of directives in verbal interactions between blind children and their mothers. *Journal of Visual Impairments and Blindness, 95*, 133–149.

Pfeiffer, S. (2012). Current perspectives on the identification and assessment of gifted students. *Journal of Psychoeducational Assessment, 30*, 3–9.

Pharoah, P., Cooke, T., Johnson, M., King, R., & Mutch, L. (1998). Epidemiology of cerebral palsy in England and Scotland, 1984–9. *Archives of Disease in Childhood: Fetal and Neonatal Edition, 79*, F21–F25.

Pirila, S., van der Meer, J., Pentikainen, T., Ruusu-Niem, P., & Korpela, R. (2007). Language and motor speech skills in children with cerebral palsy. *Journal of Communication Disorders, 40*, 116–128.

Powls, A., Botting, N., Cooke, R., Stephenson, G., & Marlow, N. (1997). Visual impairment in very low birth-weight children. *Archives of Disease in Childhood, 76*, F82–F87.

Price, E. (1976). How 37 gifted children learned to read. *The Reading Teacher, 30*, 44–48.

Rettig, M. (1994). The play of young children with visual impairment: Characteristics and interventions. *Journal of Visual Impairments and Blindness, 88*, 410–420.

Richman, L., & Eliason, M. (1993). Disorders of communication, developmental language disorders and cleft palate. In C. Walker & M. Roberts (Eds.), *Handbook of child clinical psychology—Revised* (pp. 537–552). New York: Wiley.

Richman, L., Eliason, M., & Lindgren, S. (1988). Reading disability in children with clefts. *Cleft Palate Journal, 25*, 21–25.

Richman, L., & Ryan, S. (2003). Do the reading disabilities of children with cleft fit into current models of developmental dyslexia? *Cleft Palate-Craniofacial Journal, 40*, 154–157.

Riley, G., & Riley, J. (1984). A component model of treating stuttering in children. In M. Peins (Ed.), *Contemporary approaches to stuttering treatment* (pp. 123–172). Boston: Little, Brown.

Robert, E., Kallen, B., & Harris, J. (1996). The epidemiological characteristics. *Journal of Craniofacial Genetics and Developmental Biology, 16*, 234–241.

Rogers, K., & Silverman, L. (1997). A study of 241 profoundly gifted children. Retrieved July 2002, from www.gifteddevelopment.com/Articles/Astudyof241ExtraordGC.htm

Ross, P. (1993). National excellence: A case for developing America's talent. Washington, DC: Office of Educational Research and Improvement, U.S. Department of Education.

Runco, M. (1997). Is every child gifted? *Roeper Review, 19*, 220–224.

Sankar, C., & Mundkur, N. (2005). Cerebral palsy—Definition, classification, etiology and early diagnosis. *Indian Journal of Pediatrics, 72*, 865–868.

Sardegna, J., & Otis, T. (1991). *The encyclopedia of blindness and vision impairment*. New York: Facts on File.

Scherer, N., & D'Antonio, L. (1997). Language and play development in toddlers with cleft lip and/or palate. *American Journal of Speech-Language Pathology, 6*, 48–54.

Scherer, N., D'Antonio, L., & Kalbfleisch, J. (1999). Early speech and language development in children with velo-cardiofacial syndrome. *American Journal of Medical Genetics, 88*, 714–723.

Scherer, N., Williams, A., & Proctor-Williams, K. (2008). Early and later vocalization skills in children with and without cleft palate. *International Journal of Pediatric Otorhynolaryngology, 72*, 827–840.

Schiff, M., Kaufman, A., & Kaufman, N. (1981). Scatter analysis of WISC-R profiles for learning disabled children with superior intelligence. *Journal of Learning Disabilities, 14*, 400–404.

Sigurdardottir, S., & Vik, T. (2011). Speech, expressive language, and verbal cognition of preschool children with cerebral palsy in Iceland. *Developmental Medicine and Child Neurology, 53*, 74–80.

Silverman, S., & Bernstein Ratner, N. (2002). Measuring lexical diversity in children who stutter: Applications of VOCD. *Journal of Fluency Disorders, 27*, 289–304.

Skidmore, M., Rivers, A., & Hack, M. (1990). Increased risk of cerebral palsy among very low-birthweight infants with chronic lung disease. *Developmental Medicine and Child Neurology, 32*, 325–332.

Snyder, L., & Scherer, N. (2004). The development of symbolic play and language in toddlers with cleft palate. *American Journal of Speech-Language Pathology, 13*, 66–80.

Solow, R. (1995). Parents' reasoning about the social and emotional development of their intellectually gifted children. *Roeper Review, 18*, 142–146.

Speltz, M., Endriga, M., Hill, S., Maris, C., Jones, K., & Omnell, M. (2000). Brief report: Cognitive and psychomotor development of infants with orofacial clefts. *Journal of Pediatric Psychology, 25*, 185–190.

Tadic, V., Pring, L., & Dale, N. (2010). Are language and social communication intact in children with congenital visual impairment at school age? *Journal of Child Psychology and Psychiatry, 51*, 696–705.

Tew, B. (1991). The effects of spina bifida upon learning and behaviour. In C. M. Bannister & B. Tew (Eds.), *Current concepts in spina bifida and hydrocephalus*. London: MacKeith Press.

United Cerebral Palsy. (2002). Cerebral palsy facts and figures. Retrieved December 2, 2002, from www.ucpa.org/ucp_generaldoc.cfm/1/9/37/37-37/447

Uresti, R., Goertz, J., & Bernal, E. (2002). Maximizing achievement for potentially gifted and talented and regular minority students in a primary classroom. *Roeper Review, 25*, 27–32.

U.S. Department of Education. (1993). Office of Educational Research and Improvement. Retrieved March 12, 2010, from https://www2.ed.gov/pubs/TeachersGuide/oeri.html

U.S. Department of Education. (2007). *Twenty-ninth annual report to Congress on the implementation of the Individuals with Disabilities Education Act (IDEA)*. Washington, DC: Author.

van Kleeck, A., & Richardson, A. (1988). Language delay in the child. In N. Lass, L. McReynolds, J. Northern, & D. Yoder (Eds.), *Handbook of speech-language pathology and audiology*. Philadelphia: BC Decker.

Vanderslice, R. (1998). Hispanic children and giftedness: Why the difficulty in identification? *The Delta Kappa Gamma Bulletin, 64*, 18–23.

VanTassel-Baska, J. (1992). Educational decision making on acceleration and grouping. *Gifted Child Quarterly, 36*, 68–72.

Waldron, K., & Saphire, D. (1990). An analysis of WISC-R factors for gifted students with learning disabilities. *Journal of Learning Disabilities, 23*, 491–498.

Watkins, R., & Yairi, E. (1997). Language production abilities of children whose stuttering persisted or recovered. *Journal of Speech, Language, and Hearing Research, 40*, 385–399.

Watkins, R., Yairi, E., & Ambrose, N. (1999). Early childhood stuttering III: Initial status of expressive language abilities. *Journal of Speech, Language, and Hearing Research, 42*, 1125–1135.

Webb, J. (1993). Nuturing social-emotional development of gifted children. In K. Heller, F. Monks, & A. Passow (Eds.), *International handbook for research on giftedness and talent* (pp. 525–538). Oxford: Pergamon Press.

Weinfeld, R., Barnes-Robinson, L., Jeweler, S., & Shevitz, B. (2002). Academic programs for gifted and talented/learning disabled students. *Roeper Review, 24*, 226–234.

Wiegner, S., & Donders, J. (2000). Predictors of parental distress after congenital disabilities. *Journal of Developmental and Behavioral Pediatrics, 21*, 271–277.

Wilcox, M. J. (1989). Delivering communication-based services to infants, toddlers, and their families: Approaches and models. *Topics in Language Disorders, 10*, 68–79.

Willadsen, E., & Enemark, H. (2000). A comparative study of prespeech vocalizations in two groups of toddlers with cleft palate and noncleft group. *Cleft Palate-Craniofacial Journal, 37*, 172–178.

Williams, P., Williams, A., Graff, J., Hanson, S., Stanton, A., & Hafeman, C. (2002). Interrelationships among variables affecting well siblings and mothers families of children with a chronic illness or disability. *Journal of Behavioral Medicine, 25*, 411–424.

Winebrenner, S. (2003). Teaching strategies for twice-exceptional students. *Intervention in School and Clinic, 38*, 131–137.

World Health Organization. (2014). Visual impairment and blindness. Retrieved December 22, 2014, from http://222.who.int/mediacentre/factsheets/fs282/en/

Yates, C., Berninger, V., & Abbott, R. (1995). Specific writing difficulties in intellectually gifted children. *Journal for the Education of the Gifted, 18*, 131–155.

Chapter 12

American Speech-Language-Hearing Association (ASHA). (2002). Augmentative and alternative communication: Knowledge and skills for service delivery [Knowledge and Skills]. Retrieved December 30, 2008, from www.asha.org/policy

American Speech-Language-Hearing Association (ASHA). (2005). Roles and responsibilities of speech-language pathologists with respect to augmentative and alternative communication: Position statement. Retrieved December, 30, 2008, from http://www.asha.org/docs/html/PS2005-00113.html

Bailey, R. L., Angell, M. E., & Stoner, J. B. (2011). Improving literacy skills in students with complex communication needs who use augmentative/alternative communication systems. *Education and Training in Autism and Developmental Disabilities, 46*, 352–368.

Bailey, R. L., Paretter, H. P., Stoner, J. B., Angell, M. E., & Carroll, K. (2006). Family members' perceptions of augmentative and alternative communication device use. *Language, Speech, and Hearing Services in Schools, 37*, 50–60.

Baker, B. (1982). Minspeak: A semantic compaction system that makes self-expression easier for communicatively disabled individuals. *Byte, 7*, 186–202.

Balandin, S. (1994). Symbol board vocabularies. *Sixth Biennial Conference of the International Society for Augmentative and Alternative Communication* (pp. 548–550). Maastricht: IRV.

Balandin, S., & Iacono, T. (1993). Symbol vocabularies: A study of vocabulary found on communication boards used by adults with cerebral palsy. In The Crippled Children's Association of SA Inc. (Ed.), *Australian Conference on Technology for People with Disabilities* (pp. 85–87). Adelaide: The Crippled Children's Association of SA Inc.

Barker, R. M., Akaba, S., Brady, N. C., & Thiemann-Bourque, K. (2013). Support for AAC use in preschool, and growth in language skills, for young children with developmental disabilities. *AAC: Augmentative and Alternative Communication, 29*, 334–346. doi: 10.3109/07434618.2013.848933

Bax, M., Cockerill, H., & Carroll-Few, L. (2001). Who needs augmentative and alternative communication and when? In L. Carroll-Few & H. Cockerill (Eds.), *Communication without speech: Practical augmentative and alternative communication for children* (pp. 65–72). Cambridge, MA: Mac Keith Press.

Baxter, S., Enderby, P., Evans, P., & Judge, S. (2012). Barriers and facilitators to the use of high-technology augmentative and alternative communication devices: A systematic review and qualitative synthesis. *International Journal of Language and Communication Disorders, 47*, 115–129. doi: 10.1111/j.1460-6984.2011.00090.x

Baynes, K., Kegl, J., Brentari, D., Kussmaul, C., & Poizner, H. (1998). Chronic auditory agnosia following Landau-Kleffner syndrome: A 23 year outcome study. *Brain and Language, 63*, 381–425.

Beck, A. R., Stoner, J. B., Bock, S. J., & Parton, T. (2008). Comparison of PECS and the use of a VOCA: A replication. *Education and Training in Developmental Disabilities, 43*, 198–216.

Beukelman, D., McGinnis, J., & Morrow, D. (1991). Vocabulary selection in augmentative and alternative communication. *AAC: Augmentative and Alternative Communication, 7*, 171–185.

Beukelman, D., & Mirenda, P. (2014). *Augmentative and alternative communication: Supporting children and adults with complex communication needs* (4th ed.). Baltimore: Paul H. Brookes.

Bialik, P., & Seligman-Wine, J. (2002). I see, I hear, I speak: So what's the problem? In K. Erickson, D. Koppenhaver, & D. Yoder (Eds.), *Waves of words: Augmented communicators read and write* (pp. 133–141). Toronto: ISAAC Press.

Biklen, D. (1990). Communication unbound: Autism and praxis. *Harvard Educational Review, 60*, 291–314.

Binger, C., Berens, J., Kent-Walsh, J., & Taylor, S. (2008). The effects of aided AAC interventions on AAC use, speech, and symbolic gestures. *Seminars in Speech and Language, 29*, 101–111.

Binger, C., & Light, J. (2006). Demographics of preschoolers who require AAC. *Language, Speech, and Hearing Services in Schools, 37*, 200–208.

Blischak, D. M., & Lloyd, L. L. (1996). Multimodal augmentative and alternative communication: Case study. *AAC: Augmentative and Alternative Communication, 12*, 37–46.

Blischak, D. M., Lombardino, L. J., & Dyson, A. T. (2003). Use of speech-generating devices: In support of natural speech. *AAC: Augmentative and Alternative Communication, 19*, 29–35.

Bliss, C. K. (1965). *Semantography—Blissymobolics*. Sydney, Australia: Semantography Publications.

Boesch, M. C., Wendt, O., Subramanian, A., & Hsu, N. (2013). Comparative efficacy of the Picture Exchange Communication System (PECS) versus a speech-generating device: Effects on social-communicative skills and speech development. *AAC: Augmentative and Alternative Communication, 29*, 197–209. doi: 10.3109/07434618.2013.818059

Boisvert, M., Lang, R., Andrianopoulos, M., & Boscardin, M. L. (2010). Telepractice in the assessment and treatment of individuals with autism spectrum disorders: A systematic review. *Developmental Neurorehabilitation, 13*, 423–432.

Bondy, A., & Frost, L. (1994). The Picture Exchange Communication System. *Topics in Language Disorders, 19*, 373–390.

Brady, N., Skinner, D., Roberts, J., & Hennon, E. (2006). Communication in young children with fragile X syndrome: A qualitative study of mothers' perspectives. *American Journal of Speech-Language Pathology, 15*, 353–364. doi: 10.1044/1058-0360(2006/033)

Brady, N. C., Thiemann-Bourque, K., Fleming, K., & Matthews, K. (2013). Predicting language outcomes for children learning augmentative and alternative communication: Child and environmental factors. *Journal of Speech Language and Hearing Research, 56*, 1595–1612. doi: 10.1044/1092-4388(2013/12-0102)

Branson, D., & Demchak, M. (2009). The use of augmentative and alternative communication methods with infants and toddlers with disabilities: A research review. *AAC: Augmentative and Alternative Communication, 25*, 274–286. doi: 10.3109/07434610903384529

Browder, D. M., Mims, P. J., Spooner, F., Ahlgrim-Delzell, L., & Lee, A. (2008). Teaching elementary students with multiple disabilities to participate in shared stories. *Research and Practice for Persons with Severe Disabilities, 33*, 3–12.

Brown, B. B., & Edwards, M. (1989). *Developmental disorders of language*. London: Whurr.

Cafiero, J. M., Acheson, M., & Zins, J. E. (2007). Autism spectrum disorders and augmentative and alternative communication: From research to practice. *Perspectives on Augmentative and Alternative Communication, 16*, 3–8.

Cafiero, J. M., & Delsack, B. S. (2007). AAC and autism: Compelling issues, promising practices and future directions. *Perspectives on Augmentative and Alternative Communication, 16*, 23–26.

Calculator, S. (1999). Look who's pointing now: Cautions related to the clinical use of facilitated communication. *Language, Speech, and Hearing Services in Schools, 30*, 408–414.

Calculator, S. (2002). Use of enhanced natural gestures to foster interactions between children with Angelman syndrome and their parents. *American Journal of Speech-Language Pathology, 11*, 340–355.

Calculator, S., & Dollaghan, C. (1982). The use of communication boards in a residential setting: An evaluation. *Journal of Speech and Hearing Disorders, 47*, 281–287.

Calculator, S. (2013). Parents' reports of patterns of use and exposure to practices associated with AAC acceptance by individuals with Angelman syndrome. *AAC: Augmentative and Alternative Communication, 29*, 146–158. doi: 10.3109/07434618.2013.784804

Campbell, P. H., Milbourne, S., Dugan, L. M., & Wilcox, M. J. (2006). A review of evidence on practices for teaching young children to use assistive technology devices. *Topics in Early Childhood Special Education, 26*, 3–13. doi: 10.1177/02711214060260010101

Carr, E., & Durand, V. M. (1985). Reducing behavior problems through functional communication training. *Journal of Applied Behavior Analysis, 18*, 111–126.

Chan, J., & Iacono, T. (2001). Gesture and word production in children with Down syndrome. *AAC: Augmentative and Alternative Communication, 17*, 73–87.

Cockerill, H., Elbourne, D., Allen, E., Scrutton, D., Will, E., McNee, A., . . . Baird, G. (2014). Speech, communication and use of augmentative communication in young people with cerebral palsy: The SH&PE population study. *Child: Care, Health and Development, 40*, 149–157. doi: 10.1111/cch.12066

Cockerill, H., & Fuller, P. (2001). Assessing children for augmentative and alternative communication. In L. Carroll-Few & H. Cockerill (Eds.), *Communicating without speech: Practical augmentative and alternative communication for children* (pp. 73–87). New York: Cambridge University Press.

Costello, J. M. (2000). AAC intervention in the intensive care unit: The Children's Hospital Boston model. *AAC: Augmentative and Alternative Communication, 16*, 137–153.

Costello, J. M., Patak, L., & Pritchard, J. (2010). Communication vulnerable patients in the pediatric ICU: Enhancing care through augmentative and alternative communication. *Journal of Pediatric Rehabilitation Medicine, 3*, 289–301. doi: 10.3233/prm-2010-0140

Crossley, R. (1994). *Facilitated communication training*. New York: Teachers College Press.

Culp, D. M. (1987). Outcome measurement: The impact of communication augmentation. *Seminars in Speech and Language, 8*, 169–185.

DeVeney, S. L., Hoffman, L., & Cress, C. J. (2012). Communication-based assessment of developmental age for young children with developmental disabilities. *Journal of Speech Language and Hearing Research, 55*, 695–709. doi: 10.1044/1092-4388(2011/10-0148)

Donnellan, A. M., Mirenda, P., Mesaros, R. A., & Fassbender, L. L. (1984). Analysing the communicative functions of aberrant behavior. *Journal of the Association for Persons with Severe Handicaps, 9*, 201–212.

Drager, K., & Light, J. (2006). Designing dynamic display AAC systems for young children with complex communication needs. *Perspectives on Augmentative and Alternative Communication, 15*, 3–7.

Drager, K., Light, J., Speltz, J. C., Fallon, K., & Jeffries, L. (2003). The performance of typically developing 2 1/2-year-olds on dynamic display AAC technologies with different system layouts and language organizations. *Journal of Speech, Language, and Hearing Research, 46*, 298–312.

Drager, K., Light, J. , & McNaughton, D. (2010). Effects of AAC interventions on communication and language for young children with complex communication needs. *Journal of Pediatric Rehabilitation Medicine, 3*, 303–310. doi: 10.3233/prm-2010-0141

Erickson, K. A., & Clendon, S. A. (2005). Responding to individual needs: Promoting the literacy development of students who use AAC. *Perspectives on School-Based Issues, 6*, 12–17.

Fager, S., & Spellman, C. (2010). Augmentative and alternative communication intervention in children with traumatic brain injury and spinal cord injury. *Journal of Pediatric Rehabilitation Medicine, 3*, 269–277. doi: 10.3233/prm-2010-0142

Flores, M., Musgrove, K., Renner, S., Hinton, V., Strozier, S., Franklin, S., & Hil, D. (2012). A comparison of communication using the Apple iPad and a picture-based system. *AAC: Augmentative and Alternative Communication, 28*, 74–84. doi: 10.3109/07434618.2011.644579

Fristoe, M., & Lloyd, L. (1980). Planning an initial expressive sign lexicon for persons with severe communication impairment. *Journal of Speech and Hearing Disorders, 45*, 170–180.

Gandell, T., & Filippelli, F. (2002). Face-to-face, computer-to-computer: Telecommunications in adult literacy. In K. Erickson, D. Koppenhaver, & D. Yoder (Eds.), *Waves of words: Augmented communicators read and write* (pp. 105–114). Toronto: ISAAC.

Ganz, J. B., Davis, J. L., Lund, E. M., Goodwyn, F. D., & Simpson, R. L. (2012). Meta-analysis of PECS with individuals with ASD: Investigation of targeted versus non-targeted outcomes, participant characteristics, and implementation phase. *Research in Developmental Disabilities, 33*, 406–418. doi: 10.1016/j.ridd.2011.09.023

Ganz, J. B., Earles-Vollrath, T. L., Mason, R. A., Rispoli, M. J., Heath, A. K., & Parker, R. I. (2011). An aggregate study of single-case research involving aided AAC: Participant characteristics of individuals with autism spectrum disorders. *Research in Autism Spectrum Disorders, 5*, 1500–1509. doi: 10.1016/j.rasd.2011.02.011

Geytenbeek, J., Harlaar, L., Stam, M., Ket, H., Becher, J. G., Oostrom, K., & Vermeulen, J. (2010). Utility of language comprehension tests for unintelligible or non-speaking children with cerebral palsy: A systematic review. *Developmental Medicine and Child Neurology, 52*, E267–E277. doi: 10.1111/j.1469-8749.2010.03807.x

Goossens, C., & Crain, S. (1986). *Guidelines for selecting an initial core vocabulary for early intervention.* Wauconda, IL: Don Johnston, Inc.

Goossens, C., Crain, S., & Elder, P. S. (1992). *Engineering the preschool environment for interactive, symbolic communication.* Birmingham, AL: Southeast Augmentative Communication Conference Publications.

Grandin, T. (1995). *Thinking in pictures and other reports from my life with autism.* New York: Doubleday.

Hart, P., Scherz, J., Apel, K., & Hodson, B. (2007). Analysis of spelling error patterns of individuals with complex communication needs and physical impairments. *AAC: Augmentative and Alternative Communication, 23*, 16–29. doi: 10.1080/07434610600802737

Hemsley, B., & Balandin, S. (2014). A metasynthesis of patient-provider communication in hospital for patients with severe communication disabilities: Informing new translational research. *AAC: Augmentative and Alternative Communication, 30*, 329–343.

Horner, R. H., & Budd, C. M. (1985). Acquisition of manual sign use: Collateral reduction of maladaptive behavior, and factors limiting generalization. *Education and Training of the Mentally Retarded, 20*, 39–47.

Hunt, P., Soto, G., Maier, E., Muller, E., & Goetz, L. (2002). Collaborative teaming to support students with augmentative and alternative communication needs in general classrooms. *AAC: Augmentative and Alternative Communication, 18*, 20–35.

Iacono, T., Chan, J. B., & Waring, R. E. (1998). Efficacy of a parent implemented early language intervention based on collaborative consultation. *International Journal of Language and Communication Disorders, 33*, 281–303.

Iacono, T., & Duncum, J. E. (1995). Comparison of sign alone and in combination with an electronic communication device in early language intervention: Case study. *AAC: Augmentative and Alternative Communication, 11*, 249–254.

Iacono, T., Mirenda, P., & Beukelman, D. (1993). Comparison of unimodal and multimodal AAC techniques for children with intellectual disabilities. *AAC: Augmentative and Alternative Communication, 9*, 83–94.

Jackson, C. W., Wahlquist, J., & Marquis, C. (2011). Visual supports for shared reading with young children: The effect of static overlay design. *AAC: Augmentative and Alternative Communication, 27*, 91–102. doi: 10.3109/07434618.2011.576700

Johnston, S. S., Reichle, J., & Evans, J. (2004). Supporting augmentative and alternative communication use by beginning communicators with severe disabilities. *American Journal of Speech-Language Pathology, 13*, 20–30.

Jurgens, A., Anderson, A., & Moore, D. W. (2009). The effect of teaching PECS to a child with autism on verbal behaviour, play, and social functioning. *Behavior Change, 26*, 66–81.

Kagohara, D. M., van der Meer, L., Achmadi, D., Green, V. A., O'Reilly, M. F., Lancioni, G. E., . . . Sigafoos, J. (2012). Teaching picture naming to two adolescents with autism spectrum disorders using systematic instruction and speech-generating devices. *Research in Autism Spectrum Disorders, 6*, 1224–1233. doi: 10.1016/j.rasd.2012.04.001

Kangas, K. A., & Lloyd, L. L. (1988). Early cognitive skills as prerequisites to augmentative and alternative communication use: What are we waiting for? *AAC: Augmentative and Alternative Communication, 4*, 211–221.

Keen, D., Woodyatt, G., & Sigafoos, J. (2002). Verifying teacher perceptions of the potential communicative acts of children with autism. *Communication Disorders Quarterly, 23*, 133–142.

King, A. M., Hengst, J. A., & DeThorne, L. S. (2013). Severe speech sound disorders: An integrated multimodal intervention. *Language Speech and Hearing Services in Schools, 44*, 195–210. doi: 10.1044/0161-1461(2012/12-0023)

Larsson, M., & Sandberg, A. D. (2008). Memory ability of children with complex communication needs. *AAC: Augmentative and Alternative Communication, 24*, 139–148. doi: 10.1080/07434610801897239

Launonen, K. (2003). Manual sign as a tool of communicative interaction and language: The development of children with Down syndrome and their parents. In S. von Tetzchner & N. Grove (Eds.), *Developmental issues in augmentative and alternative communication* (pp. 83–122). London: Whurr.

Leech, E. R., & Cress, C. J. (2011). Indirect facilitation of speech in a late talking child by prompted production of picture symbols or signs. *AAC: Augmentative and Alternative Communication, 27*, 40–52. doi: 10.3109/07434618.2010.550062

Lerna, A., Esposito, D., Russo, L., & Massagli, A. (2009). *The efficacy of the PECS for improving the communicative, relational and social skills in children with autistic disorder: Preliminary results.* Paper presented at the 17th European Congress of Psychiatry, Lisbon, Portugal.

Light, J. (1997). "Let's go star fishing": Reflections on the contexts of language learning for children who use aided AAC. *AAC: Augmentative and Alternative Communication, 13*, 158–171.

Light, J., Collier, B., & Parnes, P. (1985a). Communicative interaction between young nonspeaking physically disabled children and their primary caregivers: Part 1—Discourse patterns. *AAC: Augmentative and Alternative Communication, 1*, 74–83.

Light, J., Collier, B., & Parnes, P. (1985b). Communicative interaction between young nonspeaking physically disabled children and their primary caregivers: Part II—Communicative function. *AAC: Augmentative and Alternative Communication, 1*, 98–107.

Light, J., Collier, B., & Parnes, P. (1985c). Communicative interaction between young nonspeaking physically disabled children and their primary caregivers: Part III—Modes of communication. *AAC: Augmentative and Alternative Communication, 1*, 125–133.

Light, J., & McNaughton, D. (2013). Putting people first: Rethinking the role of technology in augmentative and alternative communication intervention. *AAC: Augmentative and Alternative Communication, 29*, 299–309. doi: 10.3109/07434618.2013.848935

Light, J., Page, R., Curran, J., & Pitkin, L. (2007). Children's ideas for the design of AAC assistive technologies for young children with complex communication needs. *AAC: Augmentative and Alternative Communication, 23*, 274–287. doi: 10.1080/07434610701390475

Light, J., Roberts, B., Dimarco, R., & Greiner, N. (1998). Augmentative and alternative communication to support receptive and expressive communication for people with autism. *Journal of Communication Disorders, 31*, 153–180.

Lorah, E. R., Tincani, M., Dodge, J., Gilroy, S., Hickey, A., & Hantula, D. (2013). Evaluating Picture Exchange and the iPad™ as a speech generating device to teach communication to young children with autism. *Journal of Developmental and Physical Disabilities, 25*, 637–649. doi: 10.1007/s10882-013-9337-1

MacDuff, G., Krantz, P., & McClannahan, I. (1993). Teaching children with autism to use photographic activity schedules: Maintenance and generalization of complex response chains. *Journal of Applied Behavior Analysis, 26*, 89–98.

Marvin, C. (1994). Cartalk! Conversational topics of preschool children en route home from preschool. *Language, Speech, and Hearing Services in Schools, 25*, 146–155.

Marvin, C., Beukelman, D. R., & Bilyeu, D. (1994). Vocabulary-use patterns in preschool children: Effects of context and time sampling. *AAC: Augmentative and Alternative Communication, 10*, 224–136.

McNaughton, D. (1991). Augmentative and alternative communication intervention for a child with acquired aphasia with convulsive disorder: A case study. *Journal of Speech-Language Pathology and Audiology, 15*, 35–41.

McNaughton, D. (2002). What to look for on the literacy voyage. In K. Erickson, D. Koppenhaver, & D. Yoder (Eds.), *Waves of words: Augmented communicators read and write* (pp. 63–73). Toronto: ISAAC Press.

McNaughton, D., & Light, J. (2013). The iPad and mobile technology revolution: Benefits and challenges for individuals who require augmentative and alternative communication. *AAC: Augmentative and Alternative Communication, 29*, 107–116. doi: 10.3109/07434618.2013.784930

Merchen, M. A. (1984). Technology and people. *Communication Outlook, 6*, 12–13.

Merchen, M. A. (1990). Some reasons for being passive from a personal perspective. *Communication Outlook, 12*, 10–11.

Millar, D. C., Light, J. , & Schlosser, R. W. (2006). The impact of augmentative and alternative communication intervention on the speech production of individuals with developmental disabilities: A research review. *Journal of Speech, Language, and Hearing Research, 49*, 248–264.

Mirenda, P. (1997). Supporting individuals with challenging behavior through functional communication training and AAC: Research review. *AAC: Augmentative and Alternative Communication, 13*, 207–225.

Mirenda, P. (2001). Autism, augmentative communication and assistive technology: What do we really know? *Focus on Autism and Other Developmental Disabilities, 16*, 141–151.

Mirenda, P., & Brown, K. (2007). Supporting individuals with autism and problem behavior using AAC. *Perspectives on Augmentative and Alternative Communication, 16*, 26–31.

Mirenda, P., & Locke, P. A. (1989). A comparison of symbol transparency in nonspeaking persons with intellectual disabilities. *Journal of Speech and Hearing Disorders, 54*, 131–140.

Morrow, D. R., Mirenda, P., Beukelman, D. R., & Yorkston, K. M. S. (1993). Vocabulary selection for augmentative communication systems: A comparison of three techniques. *American Journal of Speech-Language Pathology, 2*, 19–30.

Morse, J. L. (1988). Assessment procedures for people with mental retardation: The dilemma and suggested adaptive procedures. In S. Calculator & J. L. Bedrosian (Eds.), *Communication assessment and intervention for adults with mental retardation* (pp. 109–138). London: Taylor & Francis.

Murray, J., & Goldbart, J. (2009). Cognitive and language acquisition in typical and aided language learning: A review of recent evidence from an aided communication perspective. *Child Language Teaching and Therapy, 25*, 31–58. doi: 10.1177/0265659008098660

National Joint Committee for the Communication Needs for Persons with Severe Disabilities. (2002). Supporting documentation for the position statement of access to communication services and supports: Concerns regarding the application of restrictive "eligibility" policies. *Communication Disorders Quarterly, 23*, 145–153.

Norwell, S. H. (2007). Literacy learning: An intervention for children with autism. *Perspectives on Augmentative and Alternative Communication, 16*, 8–18.

Nunes da Ponte, M. M. (2002). When I grow up, I want to help my mother at the shop. In K. Erickson, D. Koppenhaver, & D. Yoder (Eds.), *Waves of words: Augmented communicators read and write*. Toronto: ISAAC Press.

O'Reilly, M. F., Edrisinha, C., Sigafoos, J., Lancioni, G., & Andrews, A. (2006). Isolating the evocative and abative effects of an establishing operation on challenging behavior. *Behavioral Interventions, 21*, 195–204.

Ogletree, B., & Pierce, H. (2010). AAC for individuals with severe intellectual disabilities: Ideas for nonsymbolic communicators. *Journal of Developmental and Physical Disabilities, 22*, 273–287. doi: 10.1007/s10882-009-9177-1

Paul, R. (1997). Introduction: Special section on language development in children who use AAC. *AAC: Augmentative and Alternative Communication, 13*, 139–140.

Pearce, P. S., & Darwish, H. (1984). Correlation between EEG and auditory perceptual measures in auditory agnosia. *Brain and Language, 22*, 41–48.

Pless, M., & Granlund, M. (2012). Implementation of the International Classification of Functioning, Disability and Health (ICF) and the ICF Children and Youth Version (ICF-CY) within the context of augmentative and alternative communication. *AAC: Augmentative and Alternative Communication, 28*, 11–20. doi: 10.3109/07434618.2011.654263

Pousada Garcia, T., Pereira Loureiro, J., Groba Gonzalez, B., Nieto Riveiro, L., & Pazos Sierra, A. (2011). The use of computers and augmentative and alternative communication devices by children and young with cerebral palsy. *Assistive Technology, 23*, 135–149. doi: 10.1080/10400435.2011.588988

Proctor, L. A., & Oswalt, J. (2008). Augmentative and alternative communication: Assessment in the schools. *Perspectives on Augmentative and Alternative Communication, 17*, 13–19.

Romski, M. A., & Sevcik, R. A. (1996). *Breaking the speech barrier: Language development through augmented means*. Baltimore: Paul H. Brookes.

Romski, M. A., & Sevcik, R. A. (2005). Augmentative communication and early intervention: Myths and realities. *Infants and Young Children, 18*, 174–185.

Romski, M. A., Sevcik, R. A., & Adamson, L. B. (1997). Framework for studying how children with developmental disabilties develop language through augmented means. *AAC: Augmentative and Alternative Communication, 13,* 172–178.

Romski, M. A., Sevcik, R. A., Adamson, L. B., Cheslock, M., Smith, A., Barker, R. M., & Bakeman, R. (2010). Randomized comparison of augmented and nonaugmented language Interventions for toddlers with developmental delays and their parents. *Journal of Speech Language and Hearing Research, 53,* 350–364. doi: 10.1044/1092-4388(2009/08-0156)

Romski, M. A., Sevcik, R. A., & Forrest, S. (2000). Assistive technology and augmentative and alternative communication in early childhood programs. In M. J. Guralnick (Ed.), *Early childhood inclusion* (pp. 465–479). Baltimore: Paul H. Brookes.

Romski, M. A., Sevicik, M., Cheslock, M., & Barton, A. (2006). The system for augmenting language: AAC and emerging language intervention. In R. J. McCauley & M. E. Fey (Eds.), *Treatment of language disorders in children* (pp. 123–147). Baltimore: Paul H. Brookes.

Rowe, M. L., & Goldin-Meadow, S. (2009). Early gesture selectively predicts later language learning. *Developmental Science, 12,* 182–187.

Rowland, C., Fried-Oken, M., Steiner, S. A. M., Lollar, D., Phelps, R., Simeonson, R. J., & Granlund, M. (2012). Developing the ICF-CY for AAC profile and code set for children who rely on AAC. *AAC: Augmentative and Alternative Communication, 28,* 21–32. doi: 10.3109/07434618.2012.654510

Rowland, C., & Schweigert, P. (1990). *Tangible symbols: Symbolic communication for individuals with multisensory impairments.* Tucson, AZ: Communication Skill Builders.

Sandberg, A. D., & Liliedahl, M. (2008). Patterns in early interaction between young preschool children with severe speech and physical impairments and their parents. *Child Language Teaching and Therapy, 24,* 9–30. doi: 10.1177/0265659007084566

Sandberg, A. D., Smith, M., & Larsson, M. (2010). An analysis of reading and spelling abilities of children using AAC: Understanding a continuum of competence. *AAC: Augmentative and Alternative Communication, 26,* 191–202. doi: 10.3109/07434618.2010.505607

Schepis, M. M. (2007). Evidence-based practice and research support for the use of speech generating devices as a functional communication mode for individuals with autism. *Perspectives on Augmentative and Alternative Communication, 16,* 18–21.

Schlosser, R. W., Balandin, S., Hemsley, B., Iacono, T., Probst, P., & von Tetzchner, S. (2014). Facilitated communication and authorship: A systematic review. *AAC: Augmentative and Alternative Communication, 30,* 359–368. doi: 10.3109/07434618.2014.971490

Schlosser, R. W., Sigafoos, J., Luiselli, J. K., Angermeier, K., Harasymowyz, U., Schooley, K., & Belfiore, P. J. (2007). Effects of synthetic speech output on requesting and natural speech production in children with autism: A preliminary study. *Research in Autism Spectrum Disorders, 1,* 139–163. doi: 10.1016/j.rasd.2006.10.001

Schlosser, R. W., & Wendt, O. (2008). Effects of augmentative and alternative communication intervention on speech production in children with autism: A systematic review. *American Journal of Speech-Language Pathology, 17,* 212–230. doi: 10.1044/1058-0360(2008/021)

Sevcik, R. A., Barton-Hullsey, A., & Romski, M. A. (2008). Early intervention, AAC, and transition to school for young children with significant spoken communication disorders and their families. *Seminars in Speech and Language, 29,* 92–100. doi: 10.1055/s-2008-1079123

Siegel, E. B., & Cress, C. (2002). Overview of the emergence of early AAC behaviors: Progression from communicative to symbolic skills. In J. Reichle, D. Beukelman, & J. Light (Eds.), *Exemplary practices for beginning AAC users and their partners* (pp. 25–58). Baltimore: Paul H. Brookes.

Sieratzki, J. S., Calvert, G. A., Brammer, M., David, A., & Woll, B. (2001). Accessibility of spoken, written, and sign language in Landau-Kleffner syndrome: A linguistic and functional MRI study. *Epileptic Disorders, 3,* 79–89.

Sigafoos, J., Arthur-Kelly, M., & Butterfield, N. (2006). *Enhancing everyday communication.* Baltimore: Paul H. Brookes.

Sigafoos, J., & Iacono, T. (1993). Selecting augmentative communication devices for persons with severe disabilities: Some factors for educational teams to consider. *Australia and New Zealand Journal of Developmental Disabilities, 18,* 133–146.

Sigafoos, J., Kerr, M., Roberts, D., & Couzens, D. (1994). Increasing opportunities for requesting in classrooms serving children with developmental disabilities. *Journal of Autism and Developmental Disabilities, 24,* 631–645.

Sigafoos, J., & Tucker, M. (2000). Brief assessment and treatment of multiple challenging behaviors. *Behavioral Intervention, 15,* 53–70.

Smith, M. (2006). Literacy instruction and AAC: A mysterious mosaic? *Perspectives on Augmentative and Alternative Communication, 15,* 2–7.

Snodgrass, M. R., Stoner, J. B., & Angell, M. E. (2013). Teaching conceptually referenced core vocabulary for initial augmentative and alternative communication. *AAC: Augmentative and Alternative Communication, 29,* 322–333. doi: 10.3109/07434618.2013.848932

Spragale, D., & Micucci, D. (1990). Signs of the week: A functional approach to manual sign training. *AAC: Augmentative and Alternative Communication, 6,* 29–37.

Stefanini, S., Caselli, M. C., & Volterra, V. (2007). Spoken and gestural production in a naming task by young children with Down syndrome. *Brain and language, 101,* 208–221.

Stefanini, S., Recchia, M., & Caselli, M. C. (2008). The relationship between spontaneous gesture production and spoken lexical ability in children with Down syndrome in a naming task. *Gesture, 8,* 197–218.

Stephenson, J. (2010). Book reading as an intervention context for children beginning to use graphic symbols for communication. *Journal of Developmental and Physical Disabilities, 22,* 257–271. doi: 10.1007/s10882-009-9164-6

Sturm, J., & Clendon, S. A. (2004). AAC, language, and literacy: Fostering the relationship. *Topics in Language Disorders, 24,* 76–91.

Sulzer-Azaroff, B., Hoffman, A., Horton, C., Bondy, A., & Frost, L. (2009). The Picture Exchange Communication System (PECS): What do the data say? *Focus on Autism and Other Developmental Disabilities, 24,* 89–103.

Sundqvist, A., Plejert, C., & Ronnberg, J. (2010). The role of active participation in interaction for children who use augmentative and alternative communication. *Communication and Medicine, 7,* 165–175.

Sutton, A., Trudeau, N., Morford, J., Rios, M., & Poirier, M. (2010). Preschool-aged children have difficulty constructing and interpreting simple utterances composed of graphic symbols. *Journal of Child Language, 37,* 1–26. doi: 10.1017/s0305000909009477

Tan, X. Y., Trembath, D., Bloomberg, K., Iacono, T., & Caithness, T. (2014). Acquisition and generalization of key word signing by three children with autism. *Developmental Neurorehabilitation, 17,* 125–136.

Taylor, R., & Iacono, T. (2003). AAC and scripting activities to facilitate communication and play. *Advances in Speech-Language Pathology, 5,* 79–93.

Thal, D., & Tobias, S. (1992). Communicative gestures in children with delayed onset of oral expressive vocabulary. *Journal of Speech and Hearing Research, 35,* 1281–1289.

Thal, D., & Tobias, S. (1994). Relationships between language and gesture in normally developing and late-talking toddlers. *Journal of Speech and Hearing Research, 37*, 157–170.

Thunberg, G., Sandberg, A. D., & Ahlsen, E. (2009). Speech-generating devices used at home by children with autism spectrum disorders: A preliminary assessment. *Focus on Autism and Other Developmental Disabilities, 24*, 104–114. doi: 10.1177/1088357608329228

Trembath, D., Balandin, S., Togher, L., & Stancliffe, R. (2009). Peer-mediated teaching and augmentative and alternative communication for preschool-aged children with autism. *Journal of Intellectual and Developmental Disability, 34*, 173–186.

Truxler, J. E., & O'Keefe, B. M. (2007). The effects of phonological awareness instruction on beginning word recognition and spelling. *AAC: Augmentative and Alternative Communication, 23*, 164–176.

United Nations. (2006). Convention on the Rights of Persons with Disabilities. New York: United Nations.

van der Meer, L., Didden, R., Sutherland, D., O'Reilly, M. F., Lancioni, G. E., & Sigafoos, J. (2012). Comparing three augmentative and alternative communication modes for children with developmental disabilities. *Journal of Developmental and Physical Disabilities, 24*, 451–468. doi: 10.1007/s10882-012-9283-3

van der Meer, L., Kagohara, D., Achmadi, D., O'Reilly, M. F., Lancioni, G. E., Sutherland, D., & Sigafoos, J. (2012). Speech-generating devices versus manual signing for children with developmental disabilities. *Research in Developmental Disabilities, 33*, 1658–1669. doi: 10.1016/j.ridd.2012.04.004

van der Meer, L., Kagohara, D., Roche, L., Sutherland, D., Balandin, S., Green, V. A., . . . Sigafoos, J. (2013). Teaching multi-step requesting and social communication to two children with autism spectrum disorders with three AAC options. *AAC: Augmentative and Alternative Communication, 29*, 222–234. doi: 10.3109/07434618.2013.815801

van der Meer, L., Sigafoos, J., O'Reilly, M. F., & Lancioni, G. E. (2011). Assessing preferences for AAC options in communication interventions for individuals with developmental disabilities: A review of the literature. *Research in Developmental Disabilities, 32*, 1422–1431. doi: 10.1016/j.ridd.2011.02.003

van der Schuit, M., Segers, E., van Balkom, H., Stoep, J., & Verhoeven, L. (2010). Immersive communication intervention for speaking and non-speaking children with intellectual disabilities. *AAC: Augmentative and Alternative Communication, 26*, 203–220. doi: 10.3109/07434618.2010.505609

Vicker, B. (1996). *Using tangible symbols for communication purposes: An optional step in building the two-way communication process*. Bloomington: Indiana Resource Center for Autism, Indiana University.

von Tetzchner, S., & Martinsen, H. (2000). *Introduction to augmentative and alternative communication* (2nd ed.). London: Whurr.

Walker, M. (1976). *Language programmes for use with the Revised Makaton Vocabulary*. Surry, UK: Author.

Walker, V. L., & Snell, M. E. (2013). Effects of augmentative and alternative communication on challenging behavior: A meta-analysis. *AAC: Augmentative and Alternative Communication, 29*, 117–131. doi: 10.3109/07434618.2013.785020

Wershing, A., & Hughes, C. (2002). Just give me words. In K. Erickson, D. Koppenhaver, & D. Yoder (Eds.), *Waves of words: Augmented communicators read and write* (pp. 45–56). Toronto: ISAAC Press.

Wilkinson, K. M., & Rosenquist, C. (2006). Demonstration of a method for assessing semantic organization and category membership in individuals with autism spectrum disorders and receptive vocabulary limitations. *AAC: Augmentative and Alternative Communication, 22*, 242–257. doi: 10.1080/07434610600650375

Williams, M. B. (2000). Just an independent guy who leads a busy life. In M. Fried-Oken & H. Bersani (Eds.), *Speaking up and spelling it out* (pp. 231–235). Baltimore: Paul H. Brookes.

Yoder, P., & Lieberman, R. (2010). Brief report: Randomized test of the efficacy of Picture Exchange Communication System on highly generalized picture exchanges in children with ASD. *Journal of Autism and Developmental Disabilities, 40*, 629–632.

Yoder, P., & Stone, W. (2006a). A randomized comparison of the effect of two prelinguistic communication interventions on the acquistion of spoken communication in preschoolers with ASD. *Journal of Speech, Language, and Hearing Research, 49*, 698–711.

Yoder, P., & Stone, W. (2006b). Randomized comparison of two communication interventions for preschoolers with autism spectrum disorders. *Journal of Consulting and Clinical Psychology, 74*, 426–435.

Zampini, L., & D'Odorico, L. (2011). Gesture production and language development: A longitudinal study of children with Down syndrome. *Gesture, 11*, 174–193.

Chapter 13

Apel, K. (1999). Checks and balances: Keeping the science in our profession. *Language, Speech, and Hearing Services in Schools, 30*, 98–107.

Applebee, A. (1978). *The child's concept of story: Ages two to seventeen*. Chicago: University of Chicago Press.

Balason, D., & Dollaghan, C. (2002). Grammatical morpheme production in 4-year-old children. *Journal of Speech, Language, and Hearing Research, 45*, 961–969.

Barrow, I., Holbert, D., & Rastatter, M. (2000). Effect of color on developmental picture-vocabulary naming of 4-, 6-, and 8-year-old children. *American Journal of Speech-Language Pathology, 9*, 310–318.

Betz, S., Eickhoff, J., & Sullivan, S. (2013). Factors influencing the selection of standardized tests for the diagnosis of specific language impairment. *Language, Speech, and Hearing Services in Schools, 44*, 133–146.

Botting, N., Faragher, B., Simkin, Z., Knox, E., & Conti-Ramsden, G. (2001). Predicting pathways of specific language impairment: What differentiates good and poor outcomes? *Journal of Child Psychology and Psychiatry, 42*, 1013–1020.

Bracken, B., & McCallum, R. (2016). *Universal Nonverbal Intelligence Test—2 (UNIT—2)*. Boston: Houghton Mifflin Harcourt.

Braden, J. (1994). *Deafness, deprivation and IQ*. London: Plenum Press.

Brown, L., Sherbenou, R., & Johnsen, S. (2010). *Test of nonverbal intelligence—4* (4th ed.). Austin, TX: Pearson.

Brown, R. (1973). *A first language: The early stages*. Cambridge, MA: Harvard University Press.

Burgemeister, B., Blum, L., & Lorge, I. (1971). *Columbia mental maturity scale* (3rd ed.). San Antonio, TX: The Psychological Corporation.

Channell, R. (1998). GramCats (Version 1.0) [MS-DOS computer software]. Provo, UT: Department of Audiology and Speech-Language Pathology, Brigham Young University.

Channell, R., & Johnson, B. (1999). Automated grammatical tagging of child language samples. *Journal of Speech, Language, and Hearing Research, 42*, 727–734.

Chapman, R. (1981). Exploring children's communicative intents. In J. Miller (Ed.), *Assessing language production in children: Experimental procedures* (pp. 111–138). Boston: Allyn & Bacon.

Chiat, S., & Roy, P. (2007). The Preschool Repetition Test: An evaluation of performance in typically developing and clinically referred children. *Journal of Speech, Language, and Hearing Research, 50*, 429–443.

Conti-Ramsden, G., Botting, N., Simkin, Z., & Knox, E. (2001). Follow-up of children attending infant language units:

Outcomes at 11 years of age. *International Journal of Language and Communication Disorders, 36*, 207–219.

Crystal, D. (1982). *Profiling linguistic disability*. London: Edward Arnold.

Crystal, D., Fletcher, P., & Garman, M. (1989). *The grammatical analysis of language disability: A procedure for assessment and remediation* (2nd ed.). London: Cole & Whurr.

de Villiers, J., & de Villiers, P. (1973). A cross-sectional study of the acquisition of grammatical morphemes in child speech. *Journal of Psycholinguistic Research, 2*, 267–278.

DeThorne, L., & Schaefer, B. (2004). A guide to child nonverbal IQ measures. *American Journal of Speech-Language Pathology, 13*, 275–290

Dollaghan, C., & Campbell, T. (1992). A procedure for classifying disruptions in spontaneous language samples. *Topics in Language Disorders, 12*, 56–68.

Dollaghan, C., & Campbell, T. (1998). Nonword repetition and child language impairment. *Journal of Speech, Language, and Hearing Research, 41*, 1136–1146.

Dollaghan, C., Campbell, T., Paradise, J., Feldman, H., Janosky, J., Pitcairn, D., & Kurs-Lasky, M. (1999). Maternal education and measures of early speech and language. *Journal of Speech, Language, and Hearing Research, 42*, 1432–1443.

Dore, J. (1979). Conversational acts and the acquisition of language. In E. Ochs & B. Schieffelin (Eds.), *Developmental pragmatics*. New York: Academic Press.

Dunn, L. (1965). *Peabody picture vocabulary test*. Circle Pines, MN: American Guidance Service.

Dunn, L., & Dunn, D. (2007). *Peabody picture vocabulary test—IV*. San Antonio, TX: Pearson.

Ebert, K., & Scott, C. (2014). Relationships between narrative language samples and norm-referenced test scores in language assessments of school-age children. *Language, Speech, and Hearing Services in Schools, 45*, 337–350.

Eickhoff, J., Betz, S., & Ristow, J. (2010, June). *Clinical procedures used by speech-language pathologists to diagnose SLI*. Paper presented at the Symposium on Research in Child Language Disorders, Madison, WI.

Eisenberg, S., Fersko, T., & Lundgren, C. (2001). The use of MLU for identifying language impairment in preschool children: A review. *American Journal of Speech-Language Pathology, 10*, 323–342.

Eisenberg, S., & Guo, L.-Y. (2015). Sample size for measuring grammaticality in preschool children from picture-elicited language samples. *Language, Speech, and Hearing Services in Schools, 46*, 81–93.

Evans, J., & Craig, H. (1992). Language sample collection and analysis: Interview compared to freeplay assessment contexts. *Journal of Speech and Hearing Research, 35*, 343–353.

Fey, M. (1986). *Language intervention with young children*. San Diego, CA: College-Hill Press.

Friberg, J. (2010). Considerations for test selection: How do validity and reliability impact diagnostic decisions? *Child Language Teaching and Therapy, 26*, 77–92.

Gathercole, S., Willis, C., Baddeley, A., & Emslie, H. (1994). The Children's Test of Nonword Repetition: A test of phonological working memory. *Memory, 2*, 103–127.

Gavin, W., & Giles, L. (1996). Temporal reliability of language sample measures. *Journal of Speech and Hearing Research, 39*, 1258–1262.

Gillam, R., & Pearson, N. (2004). *Test of narrative language (TNL)*. Austin, TX: PRO-ED.

Gillam, R., Peña, E., & Miller, L. (1999). Dynamic assessment of narrative and expository discourse. *Topics in Language Disorders, 20*, 33–47.

Glenn, C., & Stein, N. (1980). *Syntactic structures and real world themes in stories generated by children*. Urbana, IL: University of Illinois Center for the Study of Reading.

Gray, S. (2003). Diagnostic accuracy and test-retest reliability of nonword repetition and digit span tasks administered to preschool children with specific language impairment. *Journal of Communication Disorders, 36*, 129–151.

Gray, S., Plante, E., Vance, R., & Henrichsen, M. (1999). The diagnostic accuracy of four vocabulary tests administered to preschool-age children. *Language, Speech, and Hearing Services in Schools, 30*, 196–206.

Greenslade, K., Plante, E., & Vance, R. (2009). The diagnostic accuracy and construct validity of the Structured Photographic Expressive Language Test—Preschool 2. *Language, Speech, and Hearing Services in Schools, 40*, 150–160.

Gummersall, D., & Strong, C. (1999). Assessment of complex sentence production in a narrative context. *Language, Speech, and Hearing Services in Schools, 30*, 152–164.

Guo, L.-Y., & Eisenberg, S. (2015). Sample length affects the reliability of language sample measures in 3-year-olds: Evidence from parent-elicited conversational samples. *Language, Speech, and Hearing Services in Schools, 46*, 141–153.

Guo, L.-Y., Tomblin, J. B., & Samelson, V. (2008). Speech disruptions in the narratives of English-speaking children with specific language impairment. *Journal of Speech, Language, and Hearing Research, 51*, 722–738.

Gutiérrez-Clellen, V., & Peña, E. (2001). Dynamic assessment of diverse children: A tutorial. *Language, Speech, and Hearing Services in Schools, 32*, 212–224.

Hadley, P. (1998). Language sampling protocols for eliciting text-level discourse. *Language, Speech, and Hearing Services in Schools, 29*, 132–147.

Hadley, P., & Short, H. (2005). The onset of tense marking in children at risk for specific language impairment. *Journal of Speech, Language, and Hearing Research, 48*, 1344–1362.

Hammill, D. (1998). *Detroit test of learning aptitude—4*. Austin, TX: PRO-ED.

Hammill, D., Pearson, N., & Wiederholt, J. (2009). *Comprehensive test of nonverbal intelligence—2* (2nd ed.). San Antonio, TX: Pearson.

Hannah, E. (1977). *Applied linguistic analysis II*. Pacific Palisades, CA: SenCom Associates.

Heilmann, J., Miller, J., Nockerts, A., & Dunaway, C. (2010). Properties of the Narrative Scoring Scheme using narrative retells in young school-age children. *American Journal of Speech-Language Pathology, 19*, 154–166.

Heilmann, J., Nockerts, A., & Miller, J. (2010). Language sampling: Does the length of the transcript matter? *Language, Speech, and Hearing Services in Schools*. Published online on July 2, 2010. doi:10.1044/0161-1461(2009/09-0023).

Hoffman, L., Loeb, D., Brandel, J., & Gillam, R. (2011). Concurrent and construct validity of oral language measures with school-age children with specific language impairment. *Journal of Speech, Language, and Hearing Research, 54*, 1597–1608.

Huang, R., Hopkins, J., & Nippold, M. (1997). Satisfaction with standardized language testing: A survery of speech-language pathologists. *Language, Speech, and Hearing Services in Schools, 28*, 12–29.

Huber, M., Reed, V. A., Patchell, F., & Conrad, T. (2011). *SLI adolescents' verb morphology: Patterns from two narrative elicitation tasks*. Paper presented at the Annual Convention of the American Speech-Language-Hearing Association, San Diego, CA.

Hughes, D. (1998). Effects of preparation time for two quantitative measures of narrative production. *Perceptual and Motor Skills, 87*, 343–352.

Hughes, D., McGillivray, L., & Schmidek, M. (1997). *Guide to narrative language*. Eau Claire, WI: Thinking Publications.

Hunt, K. (1965). *Grammatical structures written at three grade levels*. Urbana, IL: National Council of Teachers of English.

Hutson-Nechkash, P. (1990). *Storybuilding: A guide to structuring oral narratives*. Eau Claire, WI: Thinking Publications.

Hux, K., Morris-Friehe, M., & Sanger, D. (1993). Language sampling practices: A survey of nine states. *Language, Speech, and Hearing Services in Schools, 24*, 84–91.

Johnston, J. (2001). An alternate MLU calculation: Magnitude and variability. *Journal of Speech, Language, and Hearing Research, 44*, 156–164.

Kaufman, A., & Kaufman, N. (2004a). *Kaufman assessment battery for children—2 (KABC-2)*. San Antonio, TX: Pearson.

Kaufman, A., & Kaufman, N. (2004b). *Kaufman brief intelligence test—II (KBIT-2)*. San Antonio, TX: Pearson.

Kemp, K., & Klee, T. (1997). Clinical language sampling practices: Results of a survey of speech-language pathologists in the United States. *Child Language Teaching and Therapy, 13*, 161–176.

Klee, T., Pearce, K., & Carson, D. (2000). Improving the positive predictive value of screening for developmental language disorder. *Journal of Speech, Language, and Hearing Research, 43*, 821–833.

Lahey, M. (1988). *Language disorders and language development*. Columbus, OH: Macmillan.

Lahey, M. (1994). Grammatical morpheme acquisition: Do norms exist? [Letter to the editor]. *Journal of Speech and Hearing Research, 37*, 1192–1194.

Lee, L. L. (1974). *Developmental sentence analysis: A grammatical assessment procedure for speech and language clinicians*. Evanston, IL: Northwestern University Press.

Leonard, L. (2014). *Children with specific language impairment* (2nd ed.). Cambridge, MA: MIT Press.

Leonard, L., Prutting, C., Perozzi, J., & Berkley, R. (1978). Nonstandard approaches to the assessment of language behaviors. *ASHA, 20*, 371–379.

Lieberman, R., & Michael, A. (1986). Content relevance and content coverage in tests of grammatical ability. *Journal of Speech and Language Disorders, 51*, 71–81.

Liles, B. (1985). Cohesion in the narratives of normal and language-disordered children. *Journal of Speech and Hearing Disorders, 28*, 123–133.

Loban, W. (1976). *Language development: Kindergarten through grade twelve*. Urbana, IL: National Council of Teachers of English.

Loeb, D., Kinsler, K., & Bookbinder, L. (2000, November). *Current language sampling practices in preschools*. Paper presented at the American Speech-Language-Hearing Association, Washington, DC.

Long, S. (1999a). About time: A comparison of computerized and manual procedures for grammatical and phonological analysis. *Clinical Linguistics and Phonetics, 15*, 399–426.

Long, S. (1999b). Technology applications in the assessment of children's language. *Seminars in Speech and Hearing, 20*, 117–132.

Long, S. (2010). Computerized Profiling (Version 9.7.0) [MS-DOS computer software]. Milwaukee, WI: Author.

Long, S., & Channell, R. (2001). Accuracy of four language analysis procedures performed automatically. *American Journal of Speech-Language Pathology, 10*, 180–188.

Long, S., Fey, M., & Channell, R. (2000). Computerized Profiling (CP) (Version 9.2.7) [MS-DOS computer software]. Cleveland, OH: Department of Communication Sciences, Case Western Reserve University.

MacWhinney, B. (1996). The CHILDES system. *American Journal of Speech-Language Pathology, 5*, 5–14.

MacWhinney, B. (2000). *The CHILDES project: Tools for analyzing talk* (3rd ed.). Mahwah, NJ: Lawrence Erlbaum.

Marchman, V., Wulfeck, B., & Ellis Weismer, S. (1999). Morphological productivity in children with normal language and SLI: A study of the English past tense. *Journal of Speech, Language, and Hearing Research, 42*, 206–219.

Masterson, J., & Kamhi, A. (1992). Linguistic trade-offs in school-age children with and without language disorders. *Journal of Speech and Hearing Research, 35*, 1064–1075.

McCauley, R. (1996). Familiar strangers: Criterion-referenced measures in communication disorders. *Language, Speech, and Hearing Services in Schools, 27*, 122–131.

McFadden, T., & Gillam, R. (1996). An examination of the qualitiy of narratives produced by children with language disorders. *Language, Speech, and Hearing Services in Schools, 27*, 48–56.

Merrell, A., & Plante, E. (1997). Norm-referenced test interpretation in the diagnostic process. *Language, Speech, and Hearing Services in Schools, 28*, 50–58.

Miller, J. (1981). *Assessing language production in children: Experimental procedures*. Boston: Allyn & Bacon.

Miller, J. (1996). Progress in assessing, describing, and defining child language disorder. In K. Cole, P. Dale, & D. Thal (Eds.), *Assessment of communication and language* (pp. 309–324). Baltimore, MD: Paul H. Brookes.

Miller, J., Andriacchi, K., & Nockerts, A. (2015). *Assessing language production using SALT software: A clinician's guide to language sample analysis* (2nd ed.). Middleton, WI: SALT Software LLC.

Mordecai, D., & Palin, M. (1982). Lingquest 1 & 2 [Computer software]. Napa, CA: Lingquest Software Inc.

Nelson, N. (1998). *Childhood language disorders in context: Infancy through adolescence* (2nd ed.). Boston: Allyn & Bacon.

Nettelbaldt, U., & Hansson, K. (1999). Mazes in Swedish preschool children with specific language impairment. *Clinical Linguistics and Phonetics, 13*, 483–497.

Nippold, M. (2014). *Language sampling with adolescents: Implications for intervention* (2nd ed.). San Diego, CA: Plural Publishing.

Nippold, M., Hesketh, L., Duthie, J., & Mansfield, T. (2005). Conversational versus expository discourse: A study of syntactic development in children, adolescents, and adults. *Journal of Speech, Language, and Hearing Research, 48*, 1048–1064.

Nippold, M., Mansfield, T., Billow, J., & Tomblin, J. B. (2008). Expository discourse in adolescents with language impairments: Examining syntactic development. *American Journal of Speech-Language Pathology, 17*, 356–366.

Nippold, M., Ward-Lonergan, J., & Fanning, J. (2005). Persuasive writing in children, adolescents, and adults: A study of syntactic, semantic, and pragmatic development. *Language, Speech, and Hearing Services in Schools, 36*, 125–138.

O'Neill, D. (2007). The language use inventory for young children: A parent-report measure of pragmatic language development for 18- to 47-month-old children. *Journal of Speech, Language, and Hearing Research, 50*, 214–228.

Olswang, L., & Bain, B. (1991). Intervention issues for toddlers with specific language impairments. *Topics in Language Disorders, 11*, 69–86.

Owen, A., & Leonard, L. (2002). Lexical diversity in the spontaneous speech of children with specific langauge impairment: Application of D. *Journal of Speech, Language, and Hearing Research, 45*, 927–937.

Pankratz, M. E., Plante, E., Vance, R., & Insalaco, D. M. (2007). The diagnostic and predictive validity of The Renfrew Bus Story. *Language, Speech, and Hearing Services in Schools, 38*, 390–399.

Paul, R., Hernandez, R., Taylor, L., & Johnson, K. (1996). Narrative development in late talkers: Early school age. *Journal of Speech and Hearing Research, 39*, 1295–1303.

Pavelko, S., Owens, R., Ireland, M., & Hahs-Vaughn, D. (2016). Use of language sample analysis by school-based SLPs: Results of a nationwide survey. *Language, Speech, and Hearing Services in Schools, 47*, 246–258.

Peña, E. (1996). Dynamic assessment: The model and its language applications. In K. Cole, P. Dale, & D. Thal (Eds.), *Assessment of communicaiton and language* (pp. 281–307). Baltimore, MD: Paul H. Brookes.

Perona, K., Plante, E., & Vance, R. (2005). Diagnostic accuracy of the Structured Photographic Expressive Language Test: Third Edition (SPELT-3). *Language, Speech, and Hearing Services in Schools, 36*, 103–115.

Petersen, D., Gillam, S., & Gillam, R. (2008). Emerging procedures in narrative assessment: The Index of Narrative Complexity. *Topics in Language Disorders, 28*, 115–130.

Plante, E., & Vance, R. (1994). Selection of preschool language tests: A data-based approach. *Language, Speech, and Hearing Services in Schools, 25*, 15–24.

Plante, E., & Vance, R. (1995). Diagnostic accuracy of two tests of preschool language. *American Journal of Speech-Language Pathology, 4*, 70–76.

Price, J., & Jackson, S. (2015). Procedures for obtaining and analyzing writing samples of school-age children and adolescents. *Language, Speech, and Hearing Services in Schools, 46*, 277–293.

Pye, C. (1987). Pye Analysis of Language (PAL) [DOS computer software]. Lawrence, KS: University of Kansas.

Ram, G., Marinellie, S., Benigno, J., & McCarthy, J. (2013). Morphological analysis in context versus isolation: Use of a dynamic assessment task with school-age children. *Language, Speech, and Hearing Services in Schools, 44*, 32–47.

Raven, C. (2003). *Raven's Coloured Progressive Matrices (CPM)—* 1998 edition, 2003 updates. San Antonio, TX: Pearson.

Reed, V. A. (1992). Associations between phonology and other language components in children's communicative performance. *Australian Journal of Human Communication Disorders, 20*, 75–87.

Reed, V. A., & Evernden, A. (2001, November). *Verb morphology of older children with reading difficulties.* Paper presented at the Annual Convention of the American Speech-Language-Hearing Association, New Orleans, LA.

Reed, V. A., MacMillan, V., & McLeod, S. (2001). Elucidating the effects of different definitions of "utterance" on selected syntactic measures of older children's language samples. *Asia Pacific Journal of Speech, Language, and Hearing, 6*, 39–45.

Rescorla, L., & Achenbach, T. (2002). Use of the Language Development Survery (LDS) in a national probability sample of children 18 to 35 months old. *Journal of Speech, Language, and Hearing Research, 45*, 733–743.

Retherford, K. (2000). *Guide to analysis of language transcripts* (3rd ed.). Eau Claire, WI: Thinking Publications.

Reynolds, C., & Bigler, E. (1994). *Test of memory and learning.* Austin, TX: PRO-ED.

Rice, M., Sell, M., & Hadley, P. (1990). The social interactive coding system (SICS): An online, clinically relevant descriptive tool. *Language, Speech, and Hearing Services in Schools, 21*, 2–14.

Rice, M., & Wexler, K. (2001). *Rice/Wexler test of early grammatical impairment.* San Antonio, TX: The Psychological Corporation.

Rice, M., Wexler, K., & Cleave, P. (1995). Specific language impairment as a period of extended optional infinitive. *Journal of Speech and Hearing Research, 38*, 850–863.

Rice, M., Wexler, K., & Hershberger, S. (1998). Tense over time: The longitudinal course of tense acquitision in children with specific language impairment. *Journal of Speech, Language, and Hearing Research, 41*, 1412–1431.

Roy, P., & Chiat, S. (2004). A prosodically controlled word and nonword repetition task for 2- to 4-year-olds: Evidence from typically developing children. *Journal of Speech, Language, and Hearing Research, 47*, 223–234.

Sabers, D. (1996). By their tests we will know them. *Language, Speech, and Hearing Services in Schools, 27*, 102–108.

Scarborough, H. (1990). Index of Productive Syntax (IPSyn). *Applied Psycholinguistics, 11*, 1–22.

Schwartz, R., Leonard, L., Folger, M., & Wilcox, M. (1980). Early phonological behavior in normal-speaking and language disordered children: Evidence for a synergistic view of linguistic disorders. *Journal of Speech and Hearing Disorders, 45*, 357–377.

Shipley, K., & McAfee, J. (2009). *Assessment in speech-language pathology: A resource manual* (4th ed.). Clifton Park, NY: Delmar Cengage Learning.

Simkin, Z., & Conti-Ramsden, G. (2001). Non-word repetition and grammatical morphology: Normative data for children in their final year of primary school. *International Journal of Language and Communication Disorders, 36*, 395–404.

Stein, N., & Glenn, C. (1979). An analysis of story comprehension in elementary school children. In R. Freedle (Ed.), *New directions in discourse processing* (Vol. 2, pp. 53–120). Norwood, NJ: Ablex.

Stokes, S., & Klee, T. (2009). The diagnostic accuracy of a new Test of Early Nonword Repetition for differentiating late talking and typically developing children. *Journal of Speech, Language, and Hearing Research, 52*, 872–882.

Strong, C. (1998). *Strong narrative assessment procedure.* Eau Claire, WI: Thinking Publications.

Sullivan, P. (1978). *A comparison of administration modifications on the WISC-R perfomance scale with different categories of deaf children.* (Doctoral dissertation). University of Iowa, Iowa City.

Taliaferro, M., Reed, V. A., & Patchell, F. (2015). *Verb morphology of young adolescents with SLI: Patterns from two narrative elicitation tasks.* Paper presented at the Annual Convention of the American Speech-Language-Hearing Association, Denver, CO.

Terman, L., & Merrill, M. (1973). *Stanford-Binet intelligence scale.* Boston: Houghton Mifflin.

Thal, D., Miller, S., Carlson, J., & Vega, M. (2005). Nonword repetition and language development in 4-year-old children with and without a history of early language delay. *Journal of Speech, Language, and Hearing Research, 48*, 1481–1495.

Thordardottir, E., & Ellis Weismer, S. (2002). Content mazes and filled pauses in narrative language samples of children with specific language impairment. *Brain and Cognition, 48*, 587–592.

Tomblin, J. B., Hardy, J., & Hein, H. (1991). Predicting poor-communication status in preschool children using risk factors present at birth. *Journal of Speech and Hearing Research, 34*, 1096–1105.

Tommerdahl, J. (2010, June). *Reliability of spontaneous language samples.* Paper presented at the 13th Symposium of the International Clinical Phonetics and Linguistics Association, Oslo, Norway.

Tyack, D., & Venable, G. (1999). *Language sampling, analysis and training: A handbook* (3rd ed.). Austin, TX: PRO-ED.

Ukrainetz, T., & Gillam, R. (2009). The expressive elaboration of imaginative narratives by children with specific language impairment. *Journal of Speech, Language, and Hearing Research, 52*, 883–898.

Vygotsky, L. (1978). *Mind in society: The development of higher psychological processes.* Cambridge, MA: Harvard University Press.

Wagner, R., Torgesen, J., Rashotte, C., & Pearson, N. (2013). *Comprehensive test of phonological processing—2.* Austin, TX: PRO-ED.

Wechsler, D. (2012). *Wechsler preschool and primary scale of intelligence—IV.* San Antonio, TX: Pearson.

Wechsler, D. (2014). *Wechsler intelligence scale for children—V* (5th ed.). San Antonio, TX: Pearson.

Westby, C. (1998). Communicative refinement in school age and adolescence. In W. Hayes & B. Shulman (Eds.), *Communication development: Foundations, processes, and clinical applications* (pp. 311–360). Baltimore, MD: Williams & Wilkins.

Wetherell, D., Botting, N., & Conti-Ramsden, G. (2007). Narrative in adolescent specific language impairment (SLI): A comparison with peers across two different narrative genres. *International Journal of Language and Communication Disorders, 42*, 583–605.

Yont, K. (1998). *The source of conversational breakdowns in typically developing preschoolers.* Unpublished manuscript, Pennsylvania State University, University Park.

Yont, K., & Hewitt, L. (1999, November). *Nature of conversational breakdowns in children with specific language impairment.* Paper presented at the Annual Convention of the American Speech-Language-Hearing Association, San Francisco.

Yont, K., Hewitt, L., & Miccio, A. (2000). A coding system for describing conversational breakdowns in preschool children. *American Journal of Speech-Language Pathology, 9,* 300–309.

Young, E., & Perachio, J. (1993). *The patterned elictiation syntax test with morphological analysis.* Tuscon, AZ: Communication Skill Builders.

Chapter 14

American Speech-Language-Hearing Association. (2008). 2008 Schools survey: Caseload characteristics. Rockville, MD.

Bandura, A. (1971). *Psychological modeling.* Chicago: Aldine-Atherton.

Bandura, A. (1977). *Social learning theory.* Englewood Cliffs, NJ: Prentice Hall.

Bedore, L., & Leonard, L. (1995). Prosodic and syntactic bootstrapping and their applications: A tutorial. *American Journal of Speech-Language Pathology, 4,* 66–72.

Bjork, E. (2004). *Research on learning as a foundation for curricular reform and pedagogy.* Paper presented at the the Reinvention Center's Second National Conference: Integrating Research into Undergraduate Education: The Value Added, Washington, DC.

Bjork, R. (2011). On the symbiosis of remembering, forgetting, and learning. In A. S. Benjamin (Ed.), *Successful remembering and successful forgetting: A festschrift in honor of Robert A. Bjork* (pp. 1–22). London: Psychology Press.

Bock, J., & Loebell, H. (1990). Framing sentences. *Cognition, 35,* 1–39.

Bock, J., Loebell, H., & Morey, R. (1992). From conceptual roles to structural relations: Bridging the syntactic cleft. *Psychological Review, 99,* 150–171.

Boyle, J., McCartney, E., O'Hare, A., & Forbes, J. (2009). Direct versus indirect and individual versus group modes of language therapy for children with primary language impairment: Principal outcomes from a randomized controlled trial and economic evaluation. *International Journal of Language and Communication Disorders, 44,* 826–846.

Bunce, B. (1995). *Building a language-focused curriculum for the preschool classroom: A planning guide* (Vol. II). Baltimore, MD: Paul H. Brookes.

Buschmann, A., Jooss, B., Rupp, A., Feldhusen, F., Pietz, J., & Philippi, H. (2009). Parent based language intervention for 2-year-old children with specific expressive language delay: A randomized controlled trial. *Archives of Disease in Childhood, 94,* 110–116.

Camarata, S., & Nelson, K. (1992). Treatment efficiency as a function of target selection in the remediation of child language disorders. *Clinical Linguistics and Phonetics, 6,* 167–178.

Camarata, S., Nelson, K., & Camarata, M. (1994). Comparison of conversational recasting and imitative procedures for training grammatical structures in children with specific language impairment. *Journal of Speech and Hearing Research, 37,* 1414–1423.

Childers, J., & Tomasello, M. (2002). Two-year-olds learn novel nouns, verbs and conventional actions from massed or distributed exposures. *Developmental Psychology, 38,* 967–978.

Cirran, F., & Gillam, R. (2008). Language intervention practices for school-age children with spoken language disorders: A systematic review. *Language, Speech, and Hearing Services in Schools, 39,* S110–S137.

Cirrin, F., Schooling, T., Nelson, N., Diehl, S., Flynn, P., Staskowski, M., . . . Adamczyk, D. (2010). Evidence-based systematic review: Effects of different service delivery models on communication outcomes for elementary school-age children. *Language, Speech, and Hearing Services in Schools, 41,* 233–264.

Cleave, P., & Fey, M. (1997). Two approaches to the facilitation of grammar in children with language impairments: Rationale and description. *American Journal of Speech-Language Pathology, 6,* 22–32.

Connell, P. (1989). Facilitating generalization through induction teaching. In L. McReynolds & J. Spradlin (Eds.), *Generalization strategies in the treatment of communication disorders.* Philadelphia: BC Decker.

Connell, P., & Stone, C. (1992). Morpheme learning of children with specific language impairment under controlled instructional conditions. *Journal of Speech and Hearing Research, 35,* 844–852.

Conti-Ramsden, G. (1990). Maternal recasts and other contingent replies to language-impaired children. *Journal of Speech and Hearing Disorders, 55,* 262–274.

Conti-Ramsden, G., Botting, N., Simkin, Z., & Knox, E. (2001). Follow-up of children attending infant language units: Outcomes at 11 years of age. *International Journal of Language and Communication Disorders, 36,* 207–219.

Conti-Ramsden, G., Hutcheson, G., & Grove, J. (1995). Contingency and breakdown: Children with SLI and their conversations with mothers and fathers. *Journal of Speech and Hearing Research, 38,* 1290–1302.

Courtright, J., & Courtright, I. (1976). Imitative modeling as an instructional base for instructing language-disordered children. *Journal of Speech and Hearing Research, 19,* 655–663.

Dickson, K., Marshal, M., Boyle, J., McCartney, E., O'Hare, A., & Forbes, J. (2009). Cost analysis of direct versus direct and individual versus group modes of manual-based speech-langauge therapy for primary school-age children with primay language impairment. *International Journal of Language and Communication Disorders, 44,* 369–381.

Dollaghan, C. (1987). Fast mapping in normal and language-impaired children. *Journal of Speech and Hearing Disorders, 52,* 218–222.

Dore, J. (1975). Holophrase, speech acts, and language universals. *Journal of Child Language, 2,* 21–40.

Ellis Weismer, S. (1997). The role of stress in language processing and intervention. *Topics in Language Disorders, 18,* 41–52.

Ellis Weismer, S. (2000). Intervention for children with developmental language delay. In D. V. M. Bishop & L. Leonard (Eds.), *Speech and language impairment in children: Causes, characteristics, intervention and outcome* (pp. 157–176). East Sussex, UK: Psychology Press.

Ellis Weismer, S., & Hesketh, L. (1993). The influence of prosodic and gestural cues on novel word acquisition by children with specific language impairment. *Journal of Speech and Hearing Research, 36,* 1013–1025.

Ellis Weismer, S., & Hesketh, L. (1996). Lexical learning by children with specific language impairment: Effects of linguistic input presented at varying speaking rates. *Journal of Speech and Hearing Research, 39,* 177–190.

Ellis Weismer, S., & Hesketh, L. (1998). The impact of emphatic stress on novel word learning by children with specific language impairment. *Journal of Speech, Language, and Hearing Research, 41,* 1444–1458.

Ellis Weismer, S., & Schraeder, T. (1993). Discourse characteristics and verbal reasoning: Wait time effects on the performance of children with language-learning disabilities. *Exceptionality Education Canada, 3,* 71–92.

Evans, J., Viele, K., & Kass, R. (1997). Response latency and verbal complexity: Stochastic models of individual differences in children with specific language impairments. *Journal of Speech, Language, and Hearing Research, 40,* 754–764.

Farrar, M. (1990). Discourse and the acquisition of grammatical morphemes. *Journal of Child Language, 17,* 607–624.

Fey, M. (1986). *Language intervention with young children.* San Diego, CA: College-Hill Press.

Fey, M., Cleave, P., & Long, S. (1997). Two models of grammar facilitation in children with language impairments: Phase 2. *Journal of Speech, Language, and Hearing Research, 40*, 5–19.

Fey, M., Cleave, P., Long, S., & Hughes, D. (1993). Two approaches to the facilitation of grammar in language-impaired children: An experimental evaluation. *Journal of Speech and Hearing Research, 36*, 141–157.

Fey, M., Krulik, T., Loeb, D., & Proctor-Williams, K. (1999). Sentence recast use by parents of children with typical language and specific language impairment. *American Journal of Speech-Language Pathology, 8*, 273–286.

Fey, M., Long, S., & Finestack, L. (2003). Ten principles of grammar facilitation for children with specific language impairments. *American Journal of Speech Language Pathology, 12*, 3–15.

Fey, M., & Proctor-Williams, K. (2000). Recasting, elicited imitation and modelling in grammar intervention for children with specific language impairments. In D. V. M. Bishop & L. Leonard (Eds.), *Speech and language impairment in children: Causes, characteristics, intervention and outcome* (pp. 177–194). East Sussex, UK: Psychology Press.

Fokes, J. (1976). *Fokes sentence builder*. Hingham, MA: Teaching Resources.

Fokes, J. (1977). *Fokes sentence builder expansion*. Hingham, MA: Teaching Resources.

Gerken, L. (1994). Young children's representaions of prosodic phonology: Evidence from English-speakers' weak syllable productions. *Journal of Memory and Language, 33*, 19–38.

Gerken, L., & McGregor, K. (1998). An overview of prosody and its role in normal and disordered child language. *American Journal of Speech-Language Pathology, 7*, 38–48.

Gertner, B., Rice, M., & Hadley, P. (1994). Influence of communicative competence on peer preferences in a preschool classroom. *Journal of Speech and Hearing Research, 37*, 913–923.

Girolametto, L., Greenberg, J., & Manolson, H. (1986). *Developing dialogue skills: The Hanen early language parent program*. New York: Thieme Medical Publishers.

Girolametto, L., Pearce, P., & Weitzman, E. (1996). Interactive focused stimulation for toddlers with expressive vocabulary delays. *Journal of Speech and Hearing Research, 39*, 1274–1283.

Gray, S. (2003). Word-learning by preschoolers with specific language impairment: What predicts success? *Journal of Speech, Language, and Hearing Research, 46*, 56–67.

Halliday, M. (1975). *Learning how to mean: Explorations in the development of language*. London: Edward Arnold.

Hirst, E., & Britton, L. (1998). Specialised service to children with specific language impairment in mainstream schools. *International Journal of Language and Communication Disorders, 33*(Suppl.), 593–598.

Hoffman, L., Ireland, M., Hall-Mills, S., & Flynn, P. (2013). Evidence-based speech-language pathology practices in schools: Findings from a national survey. *Language, Speech, and Hearing Services in Schools, 44*, 266–280.

Holland, A. (1975). Language therapy for children: Some thoughts on context. *Journal of Speech and Hearing Disorders, 40*, 514–523.

Hughes, D. (1998). Effects of preparation time for two quantitative measures of narrative production. *Perceptual and Motor Skills, 87*, 343–352.

Jacoby, G., Levin, L., Lee, L., Creaghead, N., & Kummer, A. (2002). The number of individual treatment units necessary to facilitate functional communication improvements in the speech and language of young children. *American Journal of Speech-Language Pathology, 11*, 370–380.

Kamhi, A. (2014). Improving clinical practices for children with language and learning disorders. *Language, Speech, and Hearing Services in Schools, 45*, 92–103.

Law, J., Garrett, Z., & Nye, C. (2004). The efficacy of treatment children with developmental speech and language delay/disorder: A meta-analysis. *Journal of Speech, Language, and Hearing Research, 47*, 924–943.

Lee, L. L., Koenigsknecht, R., & Mulhern, S. (1975). *Interactive language development teaching: The clinical presentation of grammatical structure*. Evanston, IL: Northwestern University Press.

Leonard, L. (1998). *Children with specific language impairment*. Cambridge, MA: MIT Press.

Leonard, L. (2009). Is expressive language disorder an accurate diagnostic category? *American Journal of Speech-Language Pathology, 18*, 115–123.

Leonard, L., Miller, C., Deevy, P., Rauf, L., Gerber, E., & Charest, M. (2002). Production operations and the use of nonfinite verbs by children with specific language impairment. *Journal of Speech, Language, and Hearing Research, 45*, 744–758.

Leonard, L., Miller, C., Grela, B., Holland, A., Gerber, E., & Petucci, M. (2000). Production operations contribute to the grammatical morpheme limitations of children with specific language impairment. *Journal of Memory and Language, 43*, 362–378.

McGregor, K. (1997). Prosodic influences on children's grammatical morphology. *Topics in Language Disorders, 17*, 63–75.

Miller, C., & Deevy, P. (2006). Structural priming in children with and without specific language impairment. *Clinical Linguistics and Phonetics, 20*, 387–399.

Nelson, K., Camarata, S., Welsh, J., Butovsky, L., & Camarata, M. (1996). Effects of imitative and conversational recasting treatment on the acquisition of grammar in children with specific language impairment and younger language-normal children. *Journal of Speech and Hearing Research, 39*, 850–859.

Olswang, L., & Bain, B. (1991a). Intervention issues for toddlers with specific language impairments. *Topics in Language Disorders, 11*, 69–86.

Olswang, L., & Bain, B. (1991b). When to recommend intervention. *Language, Speech, and Hearing Services in Schools, 22*, 255–263.

Paul, R., & Norbury, C. (2012). *Language disorders from infancy through adolescence: Listening, speaking, reading, writing, and communicating* (4th ed.). St. Louis, MO: Elsevier.

Proctor-Williams, K., Fey, M., & Loeb, D. (2001). Parental recasts and production of copulas and articles by children with specific language impairment and typical language. *American Journal of Speech-Language Pathology, 10*, 155–168.

Rice, M., & Wilcox, K. (Eds.). (1995). *Building a language-focused curriculum for the preschool classroom: A foundation for lifelong communication* (Vol. I). Baltimore, MD: Paul H. Brookes.

Riches, N., Tomasello, M., & Conti-Ramsden, G. (2005). Verb learning in children with SLI: Frequency and spacing effects. *Journal of Speech, Language, and Hearing Research, 48*, 1397–1411.

Schwartz, R., & Terrell, B. (1983). The role of input frequency in lexical acquisition. *Journal of Child Language, 10*, 57–64.

Smith-Lock, K., Leitão, S., Prior, P., & Nickels, L. (2015). The effectiveness of two grammar treatment procedures for children with SLI: A randomized clinical trial. *Language, Speech, and Hearing Services in Schools, 46*, 312–324.

Starling, J., Munro, N., Togher, L., & Arciuli, J. (2012). Training secondary school teachers in instructional language modification techniques to support adolescents with language impairment: A randomized controlled trial. *Language, Speech, and Hearing Services in Schools, 43*, 474–495.

Swanson, L., & Leonard, L. (1994). Duration of function-word vowels in mothers' speech to young children. *Journal of Speech and Hearing Research, 37*, 1394–1405.

Swenson, N. (2000). Comparing traditional and collaborative settings for language intervention. *Communication Disorders Quarterly, 22*, 12–18.

Throneburg, R., Calvert, L., Sturm, J., Paramboukas, A., & Paul, P. (2000). A comparison of service delivery models: Effects on curricular vocabulary skills in the school setting. *American Journal of Speech-Language Pathology, 9*, 10–20.

Tomblin, J. B., & Zhang, X. (2006). The dimensionality of language ability in school-age children. *Journal of Speech, Language, and Hearing Research, 49*, 1193–1208.

Turkstra, L., Norman, R., Whyt, J., Dijkers, M., & Hart, T. (2016). Knowing what we're doing: Why specification of treatment methods is critical for evidence-based practice in speech-language pathology. *American Journal of Speech-Language Pathology, 25*, 164–171.

Vygotsky, L. (1978). *Mind in society: The development of higher psychological processes*. Cambridge, MA: Harvard University Press.

Yoder, P., Fey, M., & Warren, S. (2012). Studying the impact of intensity is important but complicated. *International Journal of Language and Communication Disorders, 14*, 410–413.

Zhang, X., & Tomblin, J. B. (2000). The association of intervention receipt with speech-language profiles and social-demographic variables. *American Journal of Speech-Language Pathology, 9*, 345–357.

Author Index

Subject Index